Hepatology

A Practical Approach

Hepatology

A Practical Approach

Editors

Bandar Al Knawy
Section of Gastroenterology / Hepatology
King Abdulaziz Medical City
Riyadh, Saudi Arabia

Mitchell L. Shiffman
Hepatology Section
Liver Transplant Program
Virginia Commonwealth University Health System
Richmond, VA, USA

Russell H. Wiesner
Mayo Clinic Transplant Center
Liver Transplantation
Rochester, MN, USA

2004

ELSEVIER
ACADEMIC
PRESS

Amsterdam – Boston – Heidelberg – London – New York – Oxford
Paris – San Diego – San Francisco – Singapore – Sydney – Tokyo

ELSEVIER B.V.
Radarweg 29
P.O. Box 211, 1000 AE Amsterdam
The Netherlands

ELSEVIER Inc.
525 B Street, Suite 1900
San Diego, CA 92101-4495
USA

ELSEVIER Ltd
The Boulevard, Langford Lane
Kidlington, Oxford OX5 1GB
UK

ELSEVIER Ltd
84 Theobalds Road
London WC1X 8RR
UK

First edition 2004

Library of Congress Cataloging in Publication Data
A catalog record is available from the Library of Congress.

British Library Cataloguing in Publication Data

Hepatology : a practical approach
1. Liver - Diseases
I. Al Knawy, Bandar II. Shiftman, Mitchell L. III. Wiesner, Russell H.
616.3′62

ISBN: 0-444-51344-2

The paper used in this publication meets the requirements of ANSI/NISO Z39.48-1992 (Permanence of Paper). Printed in The Netherlands.

Preface

Liver disease may be caused by a host of genetic or congenital abnormalities, immunologic disorders and following exposure to either infectious agents, pharmaceuticals or toxins. Worldwide, viral hepatitis B and C accounts for over half of all causes of chronic liver disease; although non-alcoholic fatty liver disease (NAFLD) may be more common in those populations where obesity has become a significant health issue. Regardless of etiology, acute and chronic liver disease contributes to morbidity and is a major cause of mortality throughout the world.

Liver disease and many of its complications have been recognized for centuries. However, it has been just within the past two decades that advances in technologies to image the liver, serologic and molecular genetic and virologic assays have revolutionized our understanding of many liver disorders and fueled the emergence of medical and surgical therapies for many liver diseases. Vaccines to prevent viral hepatitis A and B infection are now widely available. Antiviral agents and pharmaceuticals, which modulate the immune system have for the first time provided effective therapy for hundreds of millions of persons worldwide infected with viral hepatitis B or C. The refinement of liver transplant surgery has revolutionized our approach to patients with advanced cirrhosis. Such advances have enabled Hepatology to become recognized as an independent medical discipline.

Given the many advances which have occurred in our understanding and ability to effectively treat many forms of liver disease it has become increasingly important for the non-hepatologist to both recognize, evaluate and treat liver disease and its complications. *Hepatology: A Practical Approach* was conceived with this need in mind. Our goal was to produce a concise yet comprehensive reference textbook for the physician caring for patients with liver disease. Gastroenterology and Hepatology sub-specialists, internists, family physicians, general practioners, fellows and residents will find this text both informative and useful. Our international list of contributors represents a geographically diverse group of renowned Hepatologists from 4 continents and 8 different countries. The chapters they have produced are well written, appropriately referenced and contain easy to interpret illustrations and figures.

We would like to thank you for adding *Hepatology: A Practical Approach* to your reference collection and welcome your comments.

Bandar Al Knawy, Mitchell Shiffman, Russell Wiesner

List of Contributors

Dr. Hisham O. Akbar
King Abdulaziz University Hospital
P.O. Box 80215, Jeddah 21589
Saudi Arabia

Dr. Abdulmajeed Alabdulkareem
Department of Hepatobiliary Sciences
and Liver Transplantation
Liver Center, King Abdulaziz Medical City
National Guard, P.O. Box 22490
Riyadh 11246, Saudi Arabia

Dr. Joshua Aron
Center for Liver Disease and Transplantation
New York-Presbyterian Hospital
Columbia University College of
Physicians and Surgeons
622 West 168 St, PH 14
New York, NY 10032, USA

Dr. Hamad Al Ashgar
Section of Gastroenterology (MBC 46)
Department of Medicine
King Faisal Specialist Hospital and Research Centre
Post Box 3354, Riyadh 11211
Saudi Arabia

Dr. Bandar Al Knawy
Section of Gastroenterology/Hepatology
King Abdulaziz Medical City
P.O. Box 22490
Riyadh 11425, Saudi Arabia

Dr. Vicente Arroyo
Liver Unit, Institut de Malalties Digestives
Hospital Clinic, IDIBAPS
University of Barcelona
Barcelona, Spain

Dr. Bruce R. Bacon
Saint Louis University School of Medicine
3635 Vista Avenue at Grand Blvd.
St. Louis, MO 63110-0250, USA

Dr. L. Balart
Center for Digestive Diseases
2820 Napolean Avenue Suite 700
New Orleans, LA 70115, USA

Dr. Annika Bergquist
Department of Gastroenterology and Hepatology
Huddinge University Hospital
Karolinska Institute
Huddinge, Sweden

Dr. Ulrika Broomé
Department of Gastroenterology and Hepatology
Huddinge University Hospital
Karolinska Institute
Huddinge, Sweden

Dr. Robert S. Brown Jr.
Center for Liver Disease and Transplantation
New York-Presbyterian Hospital
Columbia University College of
Physicians and Surgeons
622 West 168 St, PH 14
New York, NY 10032, USA

Dr. Andrés Cárdenas
Division of Gastroenterology and Hepatology
Beth Israel Deaconess Medical Center
Harvard Medical School
Boston, MA, USA

Dr. William Carey
The Cleveland Clinic Foundation
9500 Euclid Avenue
Cleveland, OH 44195, USA

Dr. Michael R. Charlton
Division of Gastroenterology/Hepatology
Mayo Medical School
Mayo Clinic and Foundation
Rochester, MN, USA

Dr. Sanjiv Chopra
Harvard Medical School
Boston, MA, USA

Dr. R.T. Chung
Gastrointestinal Unit GRJ724
Massachusetts General Hospital, Fruit Street
Boston, MA 02114, USA

Dr. J. Craig
Department of Pathology
St Jude Medical Center
101 E Valencia mesa Drive
Fullerton, CA 92835, USA

Dr. Michael P. Curry
Harvard Medical School
Boston, MA, USA

Dr. Albert J. Czaja
Division of Gastroenterology and Hepatology
Mayo Clinic, 200 First Street SW
Rochester, MN 55905, USA

Dr. Valeria I. Descalzi
Hepatology and Liver Transplantation Unit
Fundación Favaloro
Avenida Belgrano 1782
Piso 5, 1093 Capital Federal
Buenos Aires, Argentina

Dr. Hashem B. El-Serag
Gastroenterology and Health Services
Research Sections, Baylor College of Medicine
The Houston VA Medical Center
Houston, TX, USA

Dr. Michael W. Fried
Division of Gastroenterology and Hepatology
University of North Carolina at Chapel Hill
Chapel Hill, NC, USA

Dr. Paul J. Gaglio
Center for Liver Disease and Transplantation
New York-Presbyterian Hospital
Columbia University College of
Physicians and Surgeons
622 West 168 St, PH 14
New York, NY 10032, USA

Dr. Todd W.B. Gehr
Divisions of Gastroenterology and Nephrology
Virginia Commonwealth University School of Medicine
Medical College of Virginia Hospitals
Richmond, VA, USA

Dr. Pere Ginès
Liver Unit, Institut de Malalties Digestives
Hospital Clinic, IDIBAPS
University of Barcelona, Villaroel 170
Barcelona 08036, Spain

Andrea Gossard, CNP
Division of Gastroenterology/Hepatology
Department of Internal Medicine
Mayo Clinic Rochester
200 First Street SW
Rochester, MN 55905, USA

Prof. Stephanos J. Hadziyannis
Department of Medicine and Hepatology
The Henry Dunant Hospital
107 Messogion Avenue
115 26 Athens, Greece

Dr. Robert A. Halvorsen
Radiology Department, Medical College
of Virginia Hospitals & Physicians

Virginia Commonwealth University Health System
Main Building, 3rd Floor
Room 3-407B, 1250 East Marshall Street
P.O. Box 980615, Richmond
VA 23298-0615, USA

Dr. Jenny Heathcote
Toronto Western Hospital
University of Toronto
399 Bathurst St., Toronto
Ont., Canada M5T 2S8

Suzanne Herten-Wittig
Center for Liver Diseases
Inova Fairfax Hospital
Falls Church, VA, USA

Dr. Saleem Kamili
Division of Viral Hepatitis
Centers for Disease Control and Prevention
Atlanta, GA, USA

Dr. Emmet B. Keeffe
Division of Gastroenterology and Hepatology
Department of Medicine
Stanford University School of Medicine
Stanford, CA, USA

Prof. Mohammad Sultan Khuroo
Consultant Transplant Hepatology (MBC 72)
Department of Liver Transplantation
Hepato-biliary and Pancreatic Surgery
King Faisal Specialist Hospital and Research Centre
Post Box 3354, Riyadh 11211
Saudi Arabia

Dr. Mehnaaz Sultan Khuroo
Department of Pathology
Shri-Ramachandra Medical College
and Research Institute
Porur, Chennai, India

Dr. Raymond S. Koff
University of Massachusetts Medical School
55 Lake Avenue North
Worcester, MA 01655, USA

Kris V. Kowdley
University of Washington
P.O. Box 356174
Seattle, WA 98195, USA

Dr. Michael J. Krowka
Division of Pulmonary and Critical Care
Mayo Clinic College of Medicine
Mayo Clinic, 200 First Street SW
Rochester, MN 55905, USA

Dr. Keith Lindor
Division of Gastroenterology/Hepatology
Department of Internal Medicine
Mayo Clinic Rochester
200 First Street SW
Rochester, MN 55905, USA

Dr. Arthur J. McCullough
MetroHealth Medical Center
Case Western Reserve University
2500, MetroHealth Drive
Cleveland, OH 44109, USA

Dr. K.V. Naraynan Menon
Division of Gastroenterology
Hepatology and Internal Medicine
Mayo Clinic, Mayo Medical School
Mayo Clinic College of Medicine
Rochester, MN, USA

Dr. Philippe Merle
Service d'Hépato-Gastroentérologie
Hôpital de l'Hôtel-Dieu
1 Place de l'Hôpital
69288 Lyon Cedex 02, France

Dr. Qurrat-Ul-Ain Nawab
Gastroenterology Division
University of Tennessee, Memphis
951 Court Ave., Room 555 D
Memphis, TN 38163, USA

Dr. Mindie H. Nguyen
Division of Gastroenterology and Hepatology
Department of Medicine
Stanford University School of Medicine
Stanford, CA, USA

Dr. Julia R. Nunley
Virginia Commonwealth University School of Medicine
P.O. Box 980164, Richmond, VA 23221, USA

Dr. George V. Papatheodoridis
2nd Academic Department of Medicine
Athens University School of Medicine
Hippokration General Hospital
114 Vas Sofias Ave.
115 21 Athens, Greece

Dr. Javier Parra
Albert Einstein Medical Center
Philadelphia, PA, USA

Dr. K. Rajender Reddy
University of Pennsylvania
3 Ravdin, 3400 Spruce Street
Philadelphia, PA 19104, USA

Dr. Caroline A. Riely
Gastroenterology Division
University of Tennessee, Memphis
951 Court Ave., Room 555 D
Memphis, TN 38163, USA

Dr. Mark W. Russo
Division of Gastroenterology and Hepatology
University of North Carolina at Chapel Hill
Chapel Hill, NC USA

Dr. Arun J. Sanyal
Division of Gastroenterology
Department of Internal Medicine
Medical College of Virginia Campus
of the Virginia Commonwealth University
Richmond, VA, USA

J.C. Servoss
Gastrointestinal Unit GRJ724
Massachusetts General Hospital
Fruit Street, Boston
MA 02114, USA

K.E. Sherman
Gastrointestinal Unit GRJ724
Massachusetts General Hospital
Fruit Street, Boston
MA 02114, USA

Dr. Mitchell L. Shiffman
Hepatology Section
Liver Transplant Program
Virginia Commonwealth University Health System
Richmond, VA, USA

Dr. Sonia M. Soria
Hepatology and Liver Transplantation Unit
Fundación Favaloro, Avenida Belgrano 1782
Piso 5, 1093 Capital Federal
Buenos Aires, Argentina

Dr. Richard K. Sterling
Divisions of Gastroenterology and Nephrology
Virginia Commonwealth University
School of Medicine
Medical College of Virginia Hospitals
Richmond, VA, USA

Dr. James K. Stoller
Department of Pulmonary/Critical Care Medicine
The Cleveland Clinic Foundation
Cleveland, OH, USA

Dr. Stephanie Straley
University of California, San Francisco
San Francisco, CA, USA

Dr. R. Todd Stravitz
Section of Hepatology
Virginia Commonwealth University
Richmond, VA 23298-0341, USA

Dr. Karen L. Swanson
Division of Pulmonary and Critical Care
Mayo Clinic College of Medicine
Mayo Clinic, 200 First Street SW
Rochester, MN 55905, USA

Dr. Jayant A. Talwalkar
Division of Gastroenterology/Hepatology
Mayo Medical School, Mayo Clinic and Foundation
Rochester, MN, USA

Dr. Norah Terrault
University of California, San Francisco
San Francisco, CA, USA

Prof. Christian Trépo
Service d'Hépato-Gastroentérologie
Hôpital de l'Hôtel-Dieu
1 Place de l'Hôpital
69288 Lyon Cedex 02, France

Dr. James Trotter
Division of Gastroenterology/Hepatology
University of Colorado Health Sciences Center
4200 E. 9th Avenue, B-154
Denver, CO 80262, USA

Dr. Dimitrios Vassilopoulos
2nd Academic Department of Medicine
Athens University School of Medicine
Hippokration General Hospital
114 Vas Sofias Ave.
115 21 Athens, Greece

Dr. Federico G. Villamil
Hepatology and Liver Transplantation Unit
Fundación Favaloro
Avenida Belgrano 1782
Piso 5, 1093 Capital Federal
Buenos Aires, Argentina

Dr. Shiobhan R. Weston
University of California
San Francisco, CA, USA

Dr. Zobair M. Younossi
Center for Liver Diseases
Inova Fairfax Hospital
Falls Church, VA, USA

Dr. Wael I. Youssef
MetroHealth Medical Center
Case Western Reserve University
2500, MetroHealth Drive
Cleveland, OH 44109, USA

Dr. Steven L. Zacks
Division of Gastroenterology and Hepatology
University of North Carolina at Chapel Hill
Chapel Hill, NC USA

Dr. Fabien Zoulim
Service d'Hépato-Gastroentérologie
Hôpital de l'Hôtel-Dieu
1 Place de l'Hôpital
69288 Lyon Cedex 02
France

Table of Contents

Preface v

List of Contributors vii

Section I: **Diagnostic Methodology**
Section Editor – R. Wiesner 1

Chapter
1. Recognition of Liver Disease in the Asymptomatic Patient
   K.V. Narayanan Menon 3
2. Interpretation and Evaluation of Liver Chemistries
   Andrea Gossard and Keith Lindor 11
3. Imaging the Liver
   Robert A. Halvorsen 21
4. Diagnostic Laparoscopy
   Javier Parra and K. Rajender Reddy 33
5. Liver Biopsy – A Pathologist's Perspective
   J. Craig 45

Section II: **Acute and Chronic Liver Disease**
Section Editor – M. Shiffman 55

Chapter
1. Hepatitis A
   Raymond S. Koff 57
2. Hepatitis B Virus Infection
   Philippe Merle, Fabien Zoulim and Christian Trepo 67
3. Hepatitis C
   Steven L. Zacks, Mark W. Russo and Michael W. Fried 87
4. Hepatitis D
   Stephanos J. Hadziyannis, Dimitrios Vassilopoulos and George V. Papatheodoridis 101
5. Hepatitis E
   Mohammad Sultan Khuroo, Saleem Kamili, Mehnaaz Sultan Khuroo and Hamad Al Ashgar 111
6. Other Hepatitis Viruses
   Federico G. Villamil, Sonia M. Soria, Valeria I. Descalzi 123
7. Liver Diseases in AIDS
   J.C. Servoss, K.E. Sherman and R.T. Chung 139
8. Non-Viral Infections of the Liver
   Mohammad Sultan Khuroo 155
9. Nonalcoholic Fatty Liver Disease
   Shiobhan R. Weston and Kris V. Kowdley 175
10. Alcohol-Induced Liver Disease
    W. Carey 191
11. Alpha 1-Antitrypsin Deficiency
    Suzanne Herten-Wittig, James K. Stoller and Zobair M. Younossi 201

12. Hereditary Hemochromatosis
Bruce R. Bacon . . . 211
13. Wilson's Disease
Hisham O. Akbar . . . 223
14. Autoimmune Hepatitis and Overlap Syndromes
Albert J. Czaja . . . 233
15. Primary Biliary Cirrhosis
Jenny Heathcote . . . 249
16. Primary Sclerosing Cholangitis
Annika Bergquist and Ulrika Broomé . . . 259
17. Hepatic Vascular Disorders
Michael P. Curry and Sanjiv Chopra . . . 273
18. Liver Disorders of Pregnancy
Qurrat-Ul-Ain Nawab and Caroline A. Riely . . . 289
19. Drug-Induced Liver Disease
Mitchell L. Shiffman . . . 299
20. Fulminant Hepatic Failure
Paul J. Gaglio, Joshua Aron and Robert S. Brown Jr. . . . 315
21. Benign Tumors and Evaluation of Liver Masses
Mindie H. Nguyen and Emmet B. Keeffe . . . 331

Section III: Complications of End-Stage Liver Disease
Section Editor – B. Al Knawy . . . 345

Chapter
1. Ascites
Andrés Cárdenas and Vicente Arroyo . . . 347
2. Management of Variceal Hemorrhage
Arun J. Sanyal . . . 361
3. Hepatic Encephalopathy
Bandar Al Knawy . . . 381
4. Hepatorenal Syndrome
Andrés Cárdenas and Pere Ginès . . . 389
5. Hepatopulmonary Syndrome
Karen L. Swanson and Michael J. Krowka . . . 399
6. Hepatocellular Carcinoma
Hashem B. El-Serag . . . 409

Section IV: Systemic Effect of Liver Diseases
Section Editor – B. Al Knawy . . . 421

Chapter
1. Nutrition in Liver Disease
Wael I. Youssef and Arthur J. McCullough . . . 423
2. Renal Involvement in Liver Disease
Richard K. Sterling and Todd W.B. Gehr . . . 443
3. Dermatologic Manifestations of Liver Disease
Julia R. Nunley . . . 455
4. Immune-Mediated Manifestations of Chronic Liver Diseases
Stephanie Straley and Norah Terrault . . . 465

5. The Liver in Systemic Diseases
L. Balart 491
6. Use and Misuse of Medications in Patients with Liver Disease
R. Todd Stravitz 501

Section V: Liver Transplantation
Section Editor – R. Wiesner 515

Chapter
1. Assessment and Timing of Liver Transplantation
Abdulmajeed Alabdulkareem 517
2. Surgical Issues in Cadaveric and Living Donor Liver Transplantation Recipients
James F. Trotter 531
3. Long-Term Management of the Liver Transplant Recipient
Jayant A. Talwalkar and Michael R. Charlton 545

Color Plates 561

Subject Index 591

Section I

Diagnostic Methodology

Section Editor – R. Wiesner

Hepatology: A Practical Approach
B. Al Knawy, M.L. Shiffman, R.H. Wiesner (editors)

Chapter 1

Recognition of Liver Disease in the Asymptomatic Patient

K.V. Narayanan Menon

Division of Gastroenterology, Hepatology and Internal Medicine, Mayo Clinic, Mayo Medical School, Mayo Clinic College of Medicine, Rochester, MN, USA

1. History 3
2. Symptoms 5
   2.1 Anorexia, nausea, and vomiting 5
   2.2 Fatigue 5
   2.3 Weight loss or gain 6
   2.4 Abdominal pain 6
   2.5 Pruritus 6
3. Physical Examination 6
   3.1 Skin 6
   3.2 Face and eyes 7
   3.3 Extremities 7
   3.4 Abdomen 8
   3.5 Cardiovascular and respiratory systems 8
   3.6 Nervous system 9
4. Conclusion 10
References 10

What the mind does not know, the eye cannot see.

Advanced, compensated liver disease is frequently present in patients with minimal signs and symptoms of liver disease. In addition, patients with liver disease may have symptoms and signs relating to other organ systems, with little clinical evidence of liver dysfunction. Recognition of liver disease in these situations requires an awareness by the clinician of the various manifestations of both acute and chronic liver diseases.

Liver disease may be detected at various stages during the physician–patient interaction. Abnormal results from routine laboratory testing may indicate the presence of liver disease in asymptomatic patients when blood screening panels include tests such as those for concentrations of bilirubin, aspartate aminotransferase, alanine aminotransferase, γ-glutamyl transpeptidase, and alkaline phosphatase. Frequently, though, initial clues come from the history and physical examination. The physician must be aware of the subtle nature of the presentation of patients with liver disease and know when to order appropriate investigations to determine whether significant liver disease is present. This chapter focuses on the history and physical examination of the patient, with particular reference to the recognition of liver disease in the asymptomatic patient.

1. HISTORY

Obtaining a complete history of the present illness is an important step in the recognition of liver disease in any patient. Liver disease is an obvious consideration when a patient has a history of jaundice, dark urine, hematemesis, or melena. However, patients may not always present with such specific symptoms. Nonspecific symptoms that may indicate the presence of liver disease include fatigue, pruritus, anorexia, weight loss, abdominal pain, and diarrhea. Patients may also present with signs and symptoms related to thrombocytopenia as a result of hypersplenism from liver disease; these include easy bruising, purpura, and prolonged bleeding after a minor surgical procedure.

In addition to presenting with these more common symptoms of liver disease, patients with unrecognized liver disease may present with symptoms referable to other organ systems in the absence of symptoms related to liver disease. For example, patients with pulmonary hypertension complicating cirrhosis (also known as portopulmonary hypertension) may present with dyspnea on exertion. Erectile dysfunction, commonly seen in male patients with end-stage liver disease, may be a presenting manifestation of previously unrecognized liver disease. Other examples include glomerulonephritis in patients with hepatitis B or C, joint pain, heart failure or diabetes in patients with hemochromatosis, and pruritus in patients with cholestatic liver disease. Therefore, a review of systems is necessary to recognize these aberrant manifestations of liver disease.

Drugs are a frequent cause of liver dysfunction, and a current or past drug history is extremely important because it may provide clues to the presence of drug-induced liver disease. Examples of drugs causing liver disease are shown in Table 1.

In addition to a thorough history of the present illness, a detailed past, social, and family history must be obtained for all patients. A past history of jaundice should alert the clinician to the possibility of chronic hepatitis, either viral or autoimmune. A history of blood transfusions, administration of blood products, or recreational drug use may have exposed the patient to the risk of viral hepatitis, such as hepatitis B or C, which can be detected easily by serologic testing. Travel to parts of the world where viral hepatitis is endemic may place the patient at risk for acquiring a disease such as hepatitis A. Incubation periods may be prolonged, and travelers may exhibit signs and symptoms after returning to their home countries. Therefore, to recognize these illnesses, the clinician should be aware of various possibilities.

Table 1. Histologic classification of liver disease induced by drugs and other agents.

Category	Examples of agents
Zonal necrosis	Acetaminophen, carbon tetrachloride
Nonspecific hepatitis	Aspirin, oxacillin
Viral hepatitis-like reactions	Halothane, isoniazid, phenytoin, diclofenac
Chronic hepatitis	
Autoimmune hepatitis-like	Methyldopa, dantrolene, diclofenac
Viral hepatitis-like	Isoniazid, halothane
Cholestasis	
Noninflammatory	Estrogens, 17α-substituted steroids
Inflammatory	Amoxicillin-clavulanate, piroxicam
Ductal	Flucloxacillin, thiabendazole
Sclerosing cholangitis	Floxuridine (FUDR)
Fatty liver	Ethanol, corticosteroids, tetracycline, valproic acid, didanosine, amiodarone, perhexiline maleate
Granulomas	Phenylbutazone, allopurinol
Fibrosis	Methotrexate, vitamin A
Vascular lesions	
Hepatic vein thrombosis	Estrogens
Veno-occlusive disease	Antineoplastic agents, azathioprine, pyrrolizidine alkaloids
Noncirrhotic portal hypertension	Vinyl chloride monomer, azathioprine, 6-thioguanine
Peliosis hepatis	Anabolic steroids, estrogens
Nodular regenerative hyperplasia	Azathioprine, 6-thioguanine
Tumors	
Adenoma	Estrogens
Hepatocellular carcinoma	Estrogens, anabolic steroids
Angiosarcoma	Vinyl chloride monomer

From Zakim, D. and Boyer, T.D. (eds.) (1996) Hepatology: A Textbook of Liver Disease, 3rd ed. (W.B. Saunders, Philadelphia), p. 966. By permission of the publisher.

A history of alcohol use is extremely important, especially if the patient presents with nonspecific signs and symptoms. A structured set of questions such as the CAGE questionnaire may help in detecting excessive alcohol use ("CAGE" is an acronym for "cut down," "annoyed by criticism," "guilty about drinking," and "eye-opener drinks"). Additionally, alcohol use markedly accelerates the progression of liver disease in patients with hepatitis C.

Obtaining a family history of liver disease is important in the process of recognition of liver disease in an asymptomatic patient. The presence of hereditary or metabolic conditions such as Wilson's disease, α_1-antitrypsin deficiency, or genetic hemochromatosis in family members should lead to testing for these conditions. Early recognition and management may help patients with Wilson's disease and hereditary hemochromatosis live a normal lifespan. With advances in molecular and genetic diagnostic techniques, the diagnosis of these disorders can be confirmed with the results of blood tests without the need for a more invasive procedure such as liver biopsy.

Several liver diseases are associated with disorders of other organ systems, such as primary biliary cirrhosis in patients with systemic sclerosis and CREST syndrome, primary sclerosing cholangitis in patients with ulcerative colitis, and Crohn's disease. The liver may also be involved in multisystem disorders such as systemic lupus erythematosus or sarcoidosis. Additionally, nonalcoholic steatohepatitis, which can progress silently to cirrhosis, may occur in obese patients. The physician must be aware of these associations to detect liver disease in these patients.

2. SYMPTOMS

2.1 Anorexia, nausea, and vomiting

Anorexia is a common symptom in patients with liver disease. Anorexia and influenza-like symptoms are commonly seen in the preicteric phase of acute viral hepatitis [1]. Elevated plasma levels of cholecystokinin and bombesin, hormones that regulate signals of feeding and satiety, may affect the occurrence of dyspepsia and anorexia in this condition [1]. Similar symptoms may also be present in patients with acute fatty liver of pregnancy, and the onset of nausea and vomiting in the second or third trimester of pregnancy should alert the clinician to this possibility. Anorexia occurs in patients with alcoholic hepatitis or cirrhosis of the liver and may contribute to the muscle wasting and malnutrition seen in these patients [2]. The mechanism is not entirely clear and may be partly related to alcohol use.

2.2 Fatigue

Fatigue is a common symptom in chronic liver disease, particularly in patients with hepatitis C and cholestatic conditions such as primary biliary cirrhosis [3–5]. Although fatigue is frequently seen in patients with chronic debilitating illnesses, the severity of fatigue in patients with cholestatic liver disease or hepatitis C is thought to be out of proportion to the severity of their liver disease.

Fatigue may be central or peripheral. Peripheral fatigue occurs in muscles after prolonged exercise and is thought to be unrelated to liver disease. Central fatigue, in contrast, is thought to be mediated through central mechanisms and may involve changes in the central nervous system. Patients with cholestasis are thought to have central fatigue rather than peripheral fatigue. Various theories have been offered to explain the pathogenesis of central fatigue in patients with cholestasis. In one theory, demonstrated in a rat model of cholestasis, an abnormally functioning hypothalamic–pituitary–adrenal axis may cause abnormal fatigue in patients with cholestasis [6]. Altered opioid-mediated neurotransmission has also been postulated to cause central fatigue. According to this theory, altered neurotransmission may affect the functional status of other neurotransmitter systems, such as the serotonin system, which may mediate central fatigue in patients with cholestasis [7].

In addition to being a prominent feature of cholestatic liver disease and hepatitis C, fatigue may also be a complaint of patients with cirrhosis due to other causes. Fatigue in these patients may be related partly to the loss of muscle mass seen in the later stages of cirrhosis, coupled with poor nutrition related to anorexia.

2.3 Weight loss or gain

Weight loss or gain is commonly seen in patients with end-stage liver disease. Weight loss occurs from loss of muscle mass in patients with cirrhosis. Although the exact mechanisms are unclear, poor nutrition related to anorexia may contribute to the loss of muscle bulk. These patients characteristically lose muscle bulk in their extremities and chest, a loss that becomes more pronounced as the liver disease progresses. Because liver disease may progress silently to cirrhosis, physicians must be aware of this symptom.

Weight gain in patients with liver disease usually results from retention of salt and water. Although this retention may appear as obvious ascites in patients with advanced liver disease, this symptom may sometimes be unrecognized in a patient with advancing liver disease who has no other manifestations, such as jaundice. Various mechanisms are thought to contribute to the fluid retention and ascites in patients with cirrhosis, including portal hypertension, increased splanchnic and hepatic lymph formation, retention of salt and water, and hypoalbuminemia. These mechanisms are discussed in greater detail in subsequent chapters.

2.4 Abdominal pain

Abdominal pain may be a symptom in patients with previously unrecognized liver disease. Although injury to the liver is painless, distention of the liver capsule causes pain that usually occurs as abdominal discomfort in the right upper quadrant. Common causes include alcoholic hepatitis and liver abscesses; patients with these conditions typically present with fever and discomfort in the right upper quadrant. Although painless when small, space-occupying lesions in the liver may grow large enough to distend the liver capsule and cause right upper quadrant discomfort. Other causes of abdominal pain related to the liver include thrombosis of the hepatic veins (resulting in Budd–Chiari syndrome), acute fatty liver of pregnancy, hemorrhage into or rupture of a hepatic adenoma, or, rarely, hepatic rupture from the HELLP syndrome (hemolysis, elevated liver enzymes, and low platelet count syndrome). Rarely, cholestatic disorders such as primary biliary cirrhosis may also result in right upper quadrant discomfort [8].

2.5 Pruritus

Pruritus is usually a sign of cholestasis and is seen in patients with intrahepatic or extrahepatic cholestasis. Although pruritus is usually seen in deeply jaundiced patients, in conditions such as primary biliary cirrhosis and benign intrahepatic cholestasis of pregnancy, it can sometimes be a presenting manifestation without overt evidence of advanced liver disease. The pathogenesis of pruritus in liver disease remains unknown, although evidence suggests that it may be centrally mediated through opioid receptors [9].

3. PHYSICAL EXAMINATION

The physical examination frequently provides many clues to the presence of liver disease, especially cirrhosis, in the asymptomatic patient. Therefore, a complete physical examination including all organ systems is necessary.

3.1 Skin

Various skin manifestations provide clues to the presence of underlying liver disease in the asymptomatic patient (Figure 1). For example, excessive bruising and sparse body hair have been described in patients with cirrhosis of the liver. Careful examination of the skin may reveal petechiae related to thrombocytopenia. Patients with cirrhosis may also exhibit palmar erythema, although this has been described in other conditions, such as pregnancy and rheumatoid arthritis.

In addition, a careful examination of the skin may reveal clues to the cause of liver disease. For example, deeply tanned skin may suggest the presence of hemochromatosis, and numerous spider nevi and Dupuytren's contractures of the palmar fascia may be seen in patients with alcoholism.

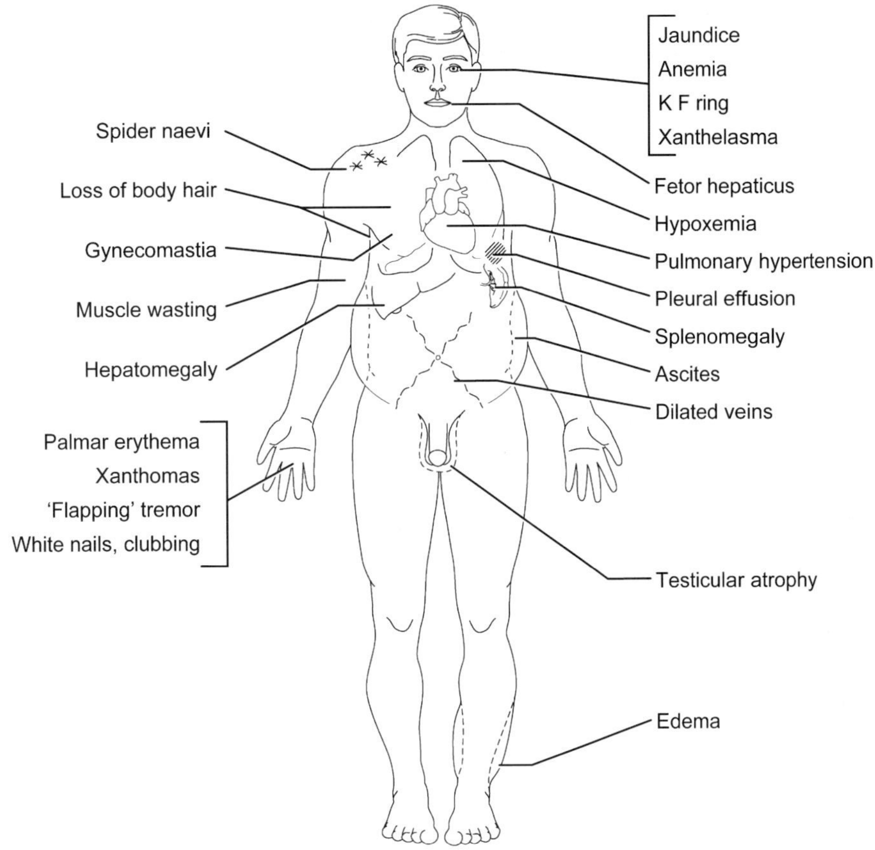

Figure 1. Clues to the presence of liver disease. K F, Kayser–Fleischer (Modified from Sherlock, S. and Dooley, J. (2002) Diseases of the Liver and Biliary System. 11th ed. (Blackwell Science, Oxford, UK) p. 209. By permission of the publisher.)

Cutaneous deposits of lipid in the skin are called xanthomas and are usually seen over the extensor surfaces of joints and eyelids (xanthelasmas) but can also occur over the face, hands, and buttocks. Xanthomas and xanthelasmas are commonly seen in patients with primary biliary cirrhosis. Cutaneous vasculitis, oral lichen planus, cryoglobulinemia, and porphyria cutanea tarda have been described in association with hepatitis C infection [10].

3.2 Face and eyes

Although the patient may not notice mild jaundice, the physician may observe it by carefully examining the sclera in natural light. Usually jaundice indicates the presence of liver disease, but occasionally it results from unconjugated hyperbilirubinemia due to either a hemolytic anemia or Gilbert's syndrome. Anemia may result from previously unrecognized portal hypertensive gastropathy. Bilateral parotid gland enlargement may be seen in patients with alcoholic liver disease. Rarely, an astute observer may note the Kayser–Fleischer ring, a green-brown ring at the periphery of the cornea in patients with Wilson's disease. However, detection usually requires a slit-lamp examination.

3.3 Extremities

Fluid retention, usually present as ascites or pedal edema, is common in patients with decompensated cirrhosis. Although minimal ascites is difficult to detect clinically, when patients have significant pedal edema, liver disease with portal hypertension must be considered in the differential diagnosis. Clubbing of the fingernails and toenails has been described in patients with cirrhosis of the liver. However, clubbing may also be seen in patients who have hypoxia associated with hepatopulmonary syndrome.

3.4 Abdomen

The presence of dilated veins on the anterior abdominal wall may indicate the presence of portal hypertension. In portal hypertension, blood flows from the left branch of the portal vein through the paraumbilical veins into the caval venous system. This results in a venous pattern called caput medusae, consisting of prominent veins radiating from the umbilicus. This finding is rare, however, and usually only one or two prominent veins are seen. Prominent veins may also be visible along the flank in patients with obstruction of the inferior vena cava. Determining the direction of blood flow is helpful. In portal hypertension, the direction of blood flow is away from the umbilicus, whereas in inferior vena caval obstruction, blood flows cranially to the superior vena caval system.

The finding of splenomegaly, ascites, or significant hepatomegaly in an otherwise asymptomatic patient must alert the clinician to the presence of liver disease. The presence of splenomegaly or ascites should always prompt a search for chronic liver disease and portal hypertension. Tender hepatomegaly usually occurs not only in patients with acute liver disease but also in patients with heart failure. Patients with cirrhosis may have a palpable, firm left lobe of the liver. The increased intra-abdominal pressure from ascites may cause abdominal wall hernias. Umbilical hernias, the most common, have a prevalence as high as 20% in patients with cirrhosis and ascites [11]. Groin and incisional hernias occur less frequently.

Investigations such as Doppler ultrasonography of the hepatic vasculature and diagnostic paracentesis with examination of the ascitic fluid provide further information about the presence or absence of liver disease. Doppler interrogation of the hepatic vasculature may show the presence of hepatic or portal vein thrombosis in patients with unexplained ascites or portal hypertension. A high serum-ascites albumin gradient (>1.1) is indicative of portal hypertension [12].

3.5 Cardiovascular and respiratory systems

Rarely, patients with cirrhosis of the liver present with pulmonary hypertension without overt symptoms of decompensated liver disease. This condition, called portopulmonary hypertension, is caused by elevated pulmonary artery pressures resulting from nonembolic pulmonary processes that are vasoconstrictive or obliterative (or both), and it may be seen in about 4% of patients with advanced cirrhosis of the liver and portal hypertension [13]. Clues to the presence of liver disease in these patients may be subtle, and patients with presumed primary pulmonary hypertension must be examined carefully for the presence of liver disease. The pathologic process is similar to that in patients with primary pulmonary hypertension. Diagnostic criteria for portopulmonary hypertension, derived from the National Institutes of Health criteria for primary pulmonary hypertension, are shown in Table 2. The use of intravenous prostacyclin analogues, which have pulmonary arterial vasodilatory effects, followed by liver transplantation, may be useful in a small group of patients.

A few patients with advanced liver disease may present with hypoxemia resulting from pulmonary vascular dilatations. This condition, called the hepatopulmonary syndrome, consists of a triad: liver disease, arterial hypoxemia, and intrapulmonary vascular dilatation. Diagnostic criteria are shown in Table 2. Although liver transplantation may be beneficial in these patients, mortality remains high (16–38% in the first year after transplantation) and is greatest in patients who have pretransplantation PaO_2 less than 50 mmHg and uptake in the brain greater than 30% during technetium-labeled macroaggregated lung scanning [14].

Table 2. Specific diagnostic criteria for hepatopulmonary syndrome and portopulmonary hypertension.

Criteria
Hepatopulmonary syndrome
Chronic liver disease[a]
$PaO_2 < 70$ mmHg or alveolar–arterial oxygen gradient > 20 mmHg[b]
Intrapulmonary vascular dilatations
Portopulmonary hypertension
Portal hypertension
MPAP > 25 mmHg
PCWP < 15 mmHg
PVR > 120 dynes.s.cm^{-5}[c]

CO, cardiac output; MPAP, mean pulmonary artery pressure; PCWP, capillary wedge pressure; PVR, pulmonary vascular resistance.
[a]Portal hypertension (cirrhotic or noncirrhotic) has been reported in most cases.
[b]Some investigators use an alveolar–arterial oxygen gradient > 15 mmHg.
[c]PVR = (MPAP − PCWP)/CO. This criterion helps to discern increased pulmonary artery pressures from high flow/hyperdynamic circulatory states (low PVR) caused by vasoconstriction (high PVR).
From Krowka, M.J. (2000) Hepatopulmonary syndromes. Gut **46**, 1–4. By permission of BMJ Publishing Group.

Pleural effusions, unilateral or bilateral, may be present in about 5% of patients with cirrhosis. This condition, called hepatic hydrothorax, results from the same physiologic process that results in ascites and is usually seen in patients with ascites. Rarely, these transudative effusions may be present without ascites [15,16]. It is important to recognize their association with liver disease because management of hepatic hydrothorax focuses on fluid management and aggressive diuretic therapy. Chest tube drainage for these effusions is usually not advised; in patients with refractory hepatic hydrothorax, liver transplantation may be an option.

In patients with α_1-antitrypsin deficiency, lung disease may result in severe panacinar emphysema and bullous emphysema, whereas liver disease may be evident as cirrhosis. Rarely, emphysema and cirrhosis occur in the same patient; therefore, patients with a predominance of respiratory manifestations must be examined carefully for hepatic manifestations of the disease. Additionally, with improved survival of patients with bullous lung disease, the increased risk of hepatocellular cancer in these patients must be borne in mind [17].

3.6 Nervous system

In the nervous system, manifestation of liver disease usually includes acute or chronic hepatic encephalopathy. Hepatic encephalopathy must be considered in all patients presenting with neuropsychiatric or neurologic manifestations. Although jaundice may be present in the majority of patients with fulminant hepatic failure, occasionally encephalopathy may precede the appearance of jaundice in these patients. They may present with agitation, delusional ideas, or hyperkinesis that may be mistaken for drug overdose or septicemia [18]. Cerebral edema, found in 75–80% of the patients whose condition progresses to coma, is the major cause of death in these patients [19]. Because progression to coma and death occurs quickly, early recognition of liver disease is essential for appropriate management. Patients with chronic hepatic encephalopathy sometimes present with subtle psychiatric and behavioral manifestations that may be missed on routine clinical examination. To detect subclinical hepatic encephalopathy, detailed psychometric testing is necessary. Features of hepatic encephalopathy not seen in patients with metabolic encephalopathies include extrapyramidal signs such as muscular rigidity, hypokinesia, tremor, and dyskinesia.

Young patients with neuropsychiatric or neurologic manifestations must be screened for Wilson's disease, a disorder of copper metabolism. Patients with Wilson's disease present with hepatic dysfunction or neurologic dysfunction or both, usually between the ages of 5 and 30 years. Initial symptoms may include a subtle change in behavior or poor performance in school. Overt neurologic manifestations are characterized predominantly by extrapyramidal features such as incoordination, dysarthria, tremor, ataxia, dystonia, spasticity, and grand mal seizures. Hepatic manifestations include fulminant hepatic failure, chronic active hepatitis, and cirrhosis. The diagnosis can be made by demonstrating a combination of findings including the Kayser–Fleischer ring, low serum ceruloplasmin concentrations, and elevated concentrations of urinary copper and hepatic copper. Early, accurate diagnosis is essential because chelating therapy can reverse or substantially improve the manifestations of the disease.

4. CONCLUSION

A detailed history and physical examination are essential to recognize liver disease in an asymptomatic patient. With advances in diagnostic testing, early diagnosis of liver disease enables the physician to effectively treat these diseases and prevent the development of cirrhosis of the liver.

REFERENCES

[1] Budillon, G., Cuomo, R., Taccone, W., Panico, G., Pumpo, R., Iaquinto, G. and Manzillo, G. (1996) Gastrointestinal peptide hormones in acute viral hepatitis. *Ital. J. Gastroenterol.* **28**, 86–90.

[2] Mendenhall, C.L., Anderson, S., Weesner, R.E., Goldberg, S.J. and Crolic, K.A. (1984) Protein-calorie malnutrition associated with alcoholic hepatitis. Veterans Administration Cooperative Study Group on Alcoholic Hepatitis. *Am. J. Med.* **76**, 211–222.

[3] Cauch-Dudek, K., Abbey, S., Stewart, D.E. and Heathcote, E.J. (1998) Fatigue in primary biliary cirrhosis. *Gut* **43**, 705–710.

[4] Goldblatt, J., Taylor, P.J., Lipman, T., Prince, M.I., Baragiotta, A., Bassendine, M.F., James, O.F. and Jones, D.E. (2002) The true impact of fatigue in primary biliary cirrhosis: a population study. *Gastroenterology* **122**, 1235–1241.

[5] Barkhuizen, A., Rosen, H.R., Wolf, S., Flora, K., Benner, K. and Bennett, R.M. (1999) Musculoskeletal pain and fatigue are associated with chronic hepatitis C: a report of 239 hepatology clinic patients. *Am. J. Gastroenterol.* **94**, 1355–1360.

[6] Swain, M.G., Patchev, V., Vergalla, J., Chrousos, G. and Jones, E.A. (1993) Suppression of hypothalamic–pituitary–adrenal axis responsiveness to stress in a rat model of acute cholestasis. *J. Clin. Invest.* **91**, 1903–1908.

[7] Wilson, W.M. and Maughan, R.J. (1992) Evidence for a possible role of 5-hydroxytryptamine in the genesis of fatigue in man: administration of paroxetine, a 5-HT re-uptake inhibitor, reduces the capacity to perform prolonged exercise. *Exp. Physiol.* **77**, 921–924.

[8] Laurin, J.M., DeSotel, C.K., Jorgensen, R.A., Dickson, E.R. and Lindor, K.D. (1994) The natural history of abdominal pain associated with primary biliary cirrhosis. *Am. J. Gastroenterol.* **89**, 1840–1843.

[9] Bergasa, N.V. and Jones, E.A. (1995) The pruritus of cholestasis: potential pathogenic and therapeutic implications of opioids. *Gastroenterology* **108**, 1582–1588.

[10] Chuang, T.Y., Stitle, L., Brashear, R. and Lewis, C. (1999) Hepatitis C virus and lichen planus: a case-control study of 340 patients. *J. Am. Acad. Dermatol.* **41**, 787–789.

[11] Belghiti, J. and Durand, F. (1997) Abdominal wall hernias in the setting of cirrhosis. *Semin. Liver Dis.* **17**, 219–226.

[12] Runyon, B.A., Montano, A.A., Akriviadis, E.A., Antillon, M.R., Irving, M.A. and McHutchison, J.G. (1992) The serum-ascites albumin gradient is superior to the exudate–transudate concept in the differential diagnosis of ascites. *Ann. Intern. Med.* **117**, 215–220.

[13] Castro, M., Krowka, M.J., Schroeder, D.R., Beck, K.C., Plevak, D.J., Rettke, S.R., Cortese, D.A. and Wiesner, R.H. (1996) Frequency and clinical implications of increased pulmonary artery pressures in liver transplant patients. *Mayo Clin. Proc.* **71**, 543–551.

[14] Krowka, M.J., Porayko, M.K., Plevak, D.J., Pappas, S.C., Steers, J.L., Krom, R.A. and Wiesner, R.H. (1997) Hepatopulmonary syndrome with progressive hypoxemia as an indication for liver transplantation: case reports and literature review. *Mayo Clin. Proc.* **72**, 44–53.

[15] Kirsch, C.M., Chui, D.W., Yenokida, G.G., Jensen, W.A. and Bascom, P.B. (1991) Case report: hepatic hydrothorax without ascites. *Am. J. Med. Sci.* **302**, 103–106.

[16] Rubinstein, D., McInnes, I.E. and Dudley, F.J. (1985) Hepatic hydrothorax in the absence of clinical ascites: diagnosis and management. *Gastroenterology* **88**, 188–191.

[17] Eriksson, S., Carlson, J. and Velez, R. (1986) Risk of cirrhosis and primary liver cancer in alpha 1-antitrypsin deficiency. *N. Engl. J. Med.* **314**, 736–739.

[18] Lee, W.M. (1993) Acute liver failure. *N. Engl. J. Med.* **329**, 1862–1872.

[19] Williams, R. and Gimson, A.E. (1991) Intensive liver care and management of acute hepatic failure. *Dig. Dis. Sci.* **36**, 820–826.

Hepatology: A Practical Approach
B. Al Knawy, M.L. Shiffman, R.H. Wiesner (editors)

Chapter 2
Interpretation and Evaluation of Liver Chemistries

Andrea Gossard and Keith Lindor

Division of Gastroenterology/Hepatology, Department of Internal Medicine, Mayo Clinic Rochester, 200 First Street SW, Rochester, MN 55905, USA

1. Introduction 11
2. Liver Chemistries 11
  2.1 Measures of liver injury 11
    2.1.1 Aminotransferases 12
    2.1.2 Alkaline phosphatase 12
    2.1.3 Gamma-glutamyltransferase 12
    2.1.4 Lactate dehydrogenase 12
  2.2 Measures of synthetic function 13
    2.2.1 Prothrombin time 13
    2.2.2 Albumin 13
  2.3 Measures of clearance of metabolites 13
    2.3.1 Bilirubin 13
    2.3.2 Ammonia 14
3. Interpretation 14
  3.1 Hepatocellular disease 14
  3.2 Cholestatic diseases 16
4. Evaluation 16
  4.1 Abnormal liver tests 16
  4.2 Evaluating jaundice 17
  4.3 The role of liver biopsy 17
  4.4 Algorithms for patients with abnormal liver tests 17
5. Summary 17
References 19

1. INTRODUCTION

The incidental discovery of elevated liver enzymes is relatively common in clinical practice. In addition, many patients are referred for further evaluation of elevated liver tests noted at the time of blood donation or during an assessment for insurance purposes. This further evaluation may be confined to simply repeating basic blood tests in 3–6 months, or may involve more extensive evaluation including more specific blood tests, radiologic evaluation and more invasive studies. This chapter will discuss the blood tests often used to evaluate liver injury and function, as well as review interpretation and recommendation for further evaluation based on the results of the tests.

2. LIVER CHEMISTRIES

2.1 Measures of liver injury

These tests, which include aspartate aminotransferase, alanine aminotransferase, alkaline phosphatase, gamma-glutamyl transpeptidase, and lactate dehydrogenase may be elevated for a variety of reasons, some of which may not be related to the liver.

These tests are commonly called "liver function tests". The tests themselves do not actually measure liver function, but rather are measures of liver injury or inflammation.

2.1.1 Aminotransferases

The aminotransferases (previously known as transaminases) are enzymes found in hepatocytes and are therefore markers of liver cell injury or hepatocellular disease when released into the serum. Hepatocyte membrane injury allows these enzymes to "leak" out of liver cells and increases in serum are seen within a few hours after liver injury [1]. Aspartate aminotransferase (AST), formerly known as serum glutamic oxaloacetic transaminase (SGOT) and alanine aminotransferase (ALT), formerly known as serum glutamic pyruvic transaminase (SGPT), catalyze the transfer of amino groups from aspartic acid or alanine to ketoglutaric acid to produce oxaloacetic acid and pyruvic acid, respectively [2]. Isoenzymes of AST are present in mitochondria and liver cell cytoplasm whereas isoenzymes of ALT are present only in the cytoplasm of the liver [3]. Therefore, ALT is specific to the liver whereas AST is found in cardiac muscle, brain, pancreas and kidney cells as well as the liver. Typically, serum levels of aminotransferases are below 40 IU/l but may be elevated to 10,000 IU/l or more in acute viral, toxic, or ischemic injury. These enzymes can be useful in monitoring disease activity once the presence of liver disease has been established, however, they correlate poorly with the extent of liver injury at presentation.

2.1.2 Alkaline phosphatase

Alkaline phosphatase is an enzyme that is found on the hepatocyte membrane bordering bile canaliculi (the smallest branches of the bile ducts). Serum alkaline phosphatase is the name applied to a group of enzymes that catalyze the hydrolysis of phosphate esters at an alkaline pH [4]. These enzymes are widely distributed throughout tissue including the liver, bone, intestine, kidney, placenta, leukocytes, and in various neoplasms [2]. The normal serum activity in adults is 25–85 IU/l but may be much higher in children and during pregnancy. Normally, serum alkaline phosphatase activity reflects primarily the hepatic and bone isozymes, although the intestinal form may account for 20–60% of the total after a fatty meal, particularly in subjects with blood groups O and B [3]. The serum alkaline phosphatase test is most useful in detecting cholestasis. Serum alkaline phosphatase activity may be increased in bone disorders, later stages of pregnancy, during periods of rapid bone growth, chronic renal failure and occasionally malignancy not involving the bones or liver. Determination of alkaline phosphatase isoenzymes is one way to identify if the elevation is from liver or bone. Another is the determination of gamma-glutamyltransferase (GGT), an enzyme not found in bone. Other than to confirm the hepatic origin of an elevated alkaline phosphatase, the GGT has little use (see below).

Slight to moderate increases in serum alkaline phosphatase activity may occur in many parenchymal disorders of the liver. Elevations of a greater degree (10 times normal) often indicate intrahepatic or extrahepatic obstruction of bile flow. Up to 33% of patients with isolated elevations of alkaline phosphatase will have no demonstrable liver or biliary disease [3].

2.1.3 Gamma-glutamyltransferase

Similar to the alkaline phosphatase, this enzyme is found in many different tissues including the kidney, spleen, heart, lung, and brain. There are a variety of etiologies for elevations of this test including myocardial infarction, neuromuscular disease, pancreatic disease, pulmonary disease, diabetes, and ingestion of ethanol. It is not found, however, in appreciable quantities in bone and therefore, as mentioned previously, may be helpful in corroborating the hepatic origin of alkaline phosphatase. It is a sensitive test for liver disease but not specific. Many who have elevations will have no identifiable liver disease upon further study.

2.1.4 Lactate dehydrogenase

Again, this enzyme is found in a number of tissues other than the liver including red blood cells, cardiac muscle, and kidney. Unfortunately, it lacks both sensitivity and specificity and as a result, is of little value in the evaluation of liver disease. An exception may be in the evaluation of ischemic hepatitis or malignant infiltration of the liver. Significant but transient elevations of the lactate dehydrogenase (LDH) are seen in ischemic hepatitis whereas more persistent LDH elevations in conjunction with elevations in the alkaline phosphatase may suggest malignant infiltration of the liver [2].

2.2 Measures of synthetic function

True markers of hepatic synthetic function include the prothrombin time (PT) and serum albumin. Both prothrombin and albumin are synthesized exclusively by hepatocytes and the immunoglobulins.

2.2.1 Prothrombin time

PT measures proteins produced by the liver which are involved in clotting of blood. Production of prothrombin is dependent on adequate vitamin K intake and absorption as well as liver function. The PT measures the activity of coagulation factors II, V, VII, and X. These are involved in the extrinsic coagulation pathway and are dependent on vitamin K for synthesis. In general, a prolongation of two or more seconds is considered abnormal. The PT is not, however, a sensitive index of chronic liver disease because it may be normal even in patients with cirrhosis.

The differential diagnosis of an elevated PT includes vitamin K deficiency due to malnutrition, malabsorption, or antibiotic use; warfarin administration; consumptive coagulopathy such as disseminated intravascular coagulation; and liver disease [2]. Prolongation of the PT may occur both in decompensated parenchymal disease with hepatocellular dysfunction and in chronic cholestatic disease with concomitant fat malabsorption and vitamin K deficiency. Vitamin K replacement by either 5–10 mg/day orally or 10 mg given subcutaneously should reduce a prolonged PT secondary to vitamin K deficiency by at least 30% within 24 h [2].

2.2.2 Albumin

Albumin is quantitatively the most important protein synthesized by the liver. It has a half-life of 21 days; so, decreases due to liver dysfunction do not occur acutely. Normal values range from 3.5 to 4.5 g/dl. The average adult synthesizes 12–15 g/day. Albumin synthesis is regulated by changes in nutritional status, osmotic pressure, systemic inflammation, and thyroid and glucocorticoid hormones. Plasma albumin concentration is decreased in severe acute and chronic liver disease. Hypoalbuminemia is more common in individuals with chronic liver disorders, such as cirrhosis, and usually reflects severe liver damage and decreased albumin synthesis. One exception is the patient with ascites, in whom synthesis may be normal or even increased but serum levels are low because of the increased volume of distribution [6,7]. Hypoalbuminemia may also occur in patients without liver disease but with protein malnutrition such as with a protein losing enteropathy or severe bacteremia.

2.3 Measures of clearance of metabolites

The liver is strategically placed to remove various metabolites and ingested toxins from the blood. In the setting of liver disease, this function may be compromised due to loss of parenchymal cells, obstruction of bile flow, impaired cellular uptake or metabolism, or reduced hepatic blood flow.

2.3.1 Bilirubin

Bilirubin is an endogenous organic anion that is derived primarily from the degradation of hemoglobin released from the red blood cells [8]. The normal value for serum bilirubin is less than 1 mg/dl and it is largely unconjugated in the circulation. The value reflects a balance between rate of production and hepatobiliary excretion. Hyperbilirubinemia is classified as either unconjugated (indirect bilirubin), which is protein bound, or conjugated (direct bilirubin). Unconjugated bilirubin circulates bound to protein in the blood until it reaches the liver. Here, it is conjugated with glucuronic acid by glucuronide transferase to form monoglucuronides and diglucuronides. Conjugation makes bilirubin water soluble, allowing it to be excreted into the bile.

A primarily conjugated hyperbilirubinemia is more typical for patients with hepatocellular dysfunction or cholestasis. Hepatocyte dysfunction or bile flow impairment will produce hyperbilirubinemia that is usually <50% conjugated. The degree of elevation of bilirubin is of important prognostic value in primary biliary cirrhosis (PBC), alcoholic hepatitis, and fulminant hepatic failure [5,9]. Furthermore, recent studies of liver transplant recipients have suggested that marked and transient hyperbilirubinemia is common after hepatitis C reinfection of the allograft and that the level of hyperbilirubinemia may again be important prognostically [10].

Unconjugated hyperbilirubinemia results from either increased bilirubin production, as with hemolysis, or from inherited or acquired defects in hepatic uptake or conjugation. Of note, chronic hemolysis cannot produce elevations of serum bilirubin above 5 mg/dl in the absence of liver disease. Furthermore, these processes are typically characterized by hyperbilirubinemia that is <20% conjugated.

2.3.2 Ammonia

Ammonia is a potentially toxic substance that is produced by colonic bacteria and by deamination of glutamine in the small bowel. It is absorbed into the portal circulation and must be removed from the circulation by the liver, metabolized, and secreted by the kidneys. There are two main pathways for this process to occur. The major pathway is urea synthesis by means of the Krebs–Henseleit cycle. The minor pathway is glutamine synthesis. In the setting of severe liver disease or portosystemic shunting, serum ammonia levels rise. Often, this level is used to diagnose or confirm the presence of hepatic encephalopathy. In addition, it may be used to monitor the success of therapy for hepatic encephalopathy, however, this correlation is only approximate [3]. Elevated ammonia levels may also be seen when ammonia production is increased by intestinal flora such as after a high protein meal or with gastrointestinal bleeding, by the kidney as in response to metabolic alkalosis or hypokalemia, or in rare genetic disease which affect the pathway of urea synthesis.

3. INTERPRETATION

When a patient presents with abnormal liver tests, it may be helpful to put the patient into a clinical scenario as outlined in Table 1.

Table 1. Abnormal liver tests: clinical scenarios.

"First-time" elevations
Acute hepatitis
Chronic hepatitis
Cholestasis without hepatitis or jaundice
Jaundice
Cirrhosis or portal hypertension

Patients with "first-time" elevations are generally asymptomatic and the liver test abnormalities are found incidentally. As long as no risk factors for liver disease are identified, liver enzymes are less than three times normal, liver function is preserved, and the patient feels well, observation with repeat tests in a few months is reasonable. If the tests are still abnormal, then the patient fits into a chronic hepatitis or cholestasis category and appropriate evaluation can then be initiated.

Incidental discovery of elevated liver tests, usually aminotransferases, is not uncommon particularly amongst blood donors. Screening of healthy, asymptomatic individuals has revealed that at least 6% have abnormal liver tests [8] and some have suggested this may be as high as 25% [11]. The prevalence of established liver disease in the general population, however, is significantly lower. Often, no significant disease is found despite extensive evaluation. A systemic inflammatory process such as infection or an immune disorder may produce mild nonspecific abnormalities of liver tests. Usually, the abnormalities are a mixed cholestatic (alkaline phosphatase) and hepatocellular (ALT or AST) pattern. In general, the higher the aminotransferase elevation, the less likely it is to represent a nonspecific response and the more likely it is to reflect underlying liver disease. Causes of elevated "liver" enzymes include medications, alcohol use, bone disease, and muscle injury as well as liver disease itself.

3.1 Hepatocellular disease

Diseases primarily affecting hepatocytes are termed hepatocellular disorders and are characterized by predominant elevations of aminotransferases. The disorders are best characterized as acute (generally less than 3 months) or chronic. Acute hepatitis may

Table 2. Common causes of acute hepatitis.

Disease	Clinical clues	Diagnostic tests
Hepatitis A	Exposure history	IgM anti-HAV
Hepatitis B	Risk factors	HBsAg, IgM anti-HBc
Hepatitis C	Risk factors	Anti-HCV, HCV-PCR
Drug induced	Compatible medication	Improvement after withdrawal from agent
Alcoholic hepatitis	History of alcohol excess, AST:ALT > 2, AST < 400	Liver biopsy; improvement with abstinence
Ischemic hepatitis	History of severe hypotension	Rapid improvement of aminotransferases

be accompanied by malaise, anorexia, abdominal pain and jaundice. Common causes of acute hepatitis are listed in Table 2.

The pattern of aminotransferase elevation may also be helpful. Acute hepatitis due to ischemic viruses or drugs generally produces marked elevations of aminotransferases, often in the thousands. In general, ALT is more elevated than AST. Ischemia, acetaminophen hepatotoxicity and herpes simplex hepatitis result in the highest levels of aminotransferases. Alcoholic hepatitis is characterized by more modest aminotransferase elevations, almost always less than 400 IU and at times near normal. In addition, patients with alcoholic hepatitis usually have an AST:ALT ratio greater than 1 and sometimes greater than 2:1. Finally, patients with alcoholic hepatitis frequently will have a markedly elevated bilirubin out of proportion to the aminotransferase elevations. Ischemic hepatitis occurs in patients after an episode of hypotension during which the aminotransferases may become extremely high but then improve within a few days. Another cause of transient elevations of aminotransferases is bile duct obstruction, usually due to a stone. These elevations can be as high as several thousand U/l but improve within 24–48 h. In patients with pancreatitis, a transient elevation of AST or ALT suggests gallstone pancreatitis.

Diseases producing sustained (<3 months) elevations of aminotransferases are put in the category of chronic hepatitis. In general, aminotransferase elevations are more modest than those seen in acute hepatitis, usually 2–5 times normal but at times over 10 times normal. Patients may be entirely asymptomatic or may complain of fatigue and right upper quadrant pain. The differential diagnosis of a chronic hepatitis is relatively lengthy. The most important and common disorders are found in Table 3.

Table 3. Common causes of chronic hepatitis.

Disease	Clinical clues	Diagnostic tests
Hepatitis A	Risk factors	Anti-HAV
Hepatitis B	Risk factors	HbsAg, HbeAg, Anti-Hbe, HBcAb
Hepatitis C	Risk factors	Anti-HCV, HCV-PCR
Hemochromatosis	Arthritis, diabetes, family history	Iron studies, gene test, biopsy
Wilson's disease	Neurologic symptoms, hemolysis	Ceruloplasmin, urine copper
Alpha-1 antitrypsin deficiency	None	Alpha-1antitrypsin level and phenotype
Autoimmune hepatitis	ALT 200–1500, usually female, other autoimmune disease	Antinuclear or antismooth muscle antibody, biopsy
Alcoholic liver disease	History, AST:ALT > 2	Liver biopsy
Nonalcoholic fatty liver disease	Obesity, diabetes, hyperlipidemia	Ultrasound, liver biopsy

Table 4. Common causes of cholestasis.

Disease	Clinical clues	Diagnostic tests
Primary biliary cirrhosis	Middle-aged female	Antimitochondrial antibody
Primary sclerosing cholangitis	Association with ulcerative colitis	Cholangiography
Large bile duct obstruction	Jaundice and pain common	Ultrasound, cholangiography
Drug induced	Compatible medication/timing	Improvement after withdrawal of the agent
Intrahepatic mass lesions	History of malignancy	Ultrasound, CT
Inflammation associated	Symptoms of underlying inflammatory disorder	Blood cultures, appropriate antibodies

3.2 Cholestatic diseases

Diseases that predominantly affect the biliary system are termed cholestatic diseases. These can affect the microscopic ducts (e.g., PBC), large bile ducts (e.g., pancreatic cancer causing common bile duct obstruction), or both (e.g., primary sclerosing cholangitis). In general, the predominant abnormality in these disorders is in alkaline phosphatase levels. Although diseases that produce elevations in bilirubin are often called "cholestatic", it is important to remember that severe hepatocellular injury, such as that occurs with an acute hepatitis, will also produce hyperbilirubinemia because of hepatocellular dysfunction and cholestatic disease, but may have normal bilirubin levels. Common causes of cholestasis are illustrated in Table 4.

PBC is common in middle-aged women who may complain of fatigue or pruritus. Primary sclerosing cholangitis (PSC) has a strong association with ulcerative colitis. Patients with PSC are often asymptomatic but may have jaundice, fatigue, or pruritus. Large bile duct obstruction is often due to stones or benign or malignant strictures and may produce marked alkaline phosphatase elevations. Intrahepatic mass lesions should be considered in a patient with cholestatic liver test abnormalities and a history of malignancy.

4. EVALUATION

Evaluation of patients with abnormal liver tests hinges on many clinical factors including the chief complaints of the patient, patient age, risk factors for liver disease, personal or family history of liver disease, medications, and physical examination findings. Furthermore, elevation of liver enzymes in the absence of positive clinical findings is not uncommon and further evaluation is probably only necessary in those individuals in which the elevations persist.

4.1 Abnormal liver tests

Approximately one-third of patients will have normal enzyme levels on follow-up testing. Initial evaluations should include careful screening for exposure to hepatotoxic agents such as alcohol, prescription drugs, over the counter medications such as acetaminophen, herbs, chemicals, and occupational exposures. Hepatic origin should be confirmed by determining the ALT if only the AST was initially screened. If the ALT was indeed abnormal, viral serologies should be performed to rule out hepatitis A, B, C, or E. Older individuals should also be screened for hemochromatosis by evaluating iron levels and transferrin saturation. Wilson's disease, a metabolic disorder that affects primarily younger individuals, may be ruled out by evaluating the ceruloplasmin and urine copper. Malaria (which can be seen in southeast Asia and South America) and schistosomiasis should be considered for patients who have compatible travel histories. An alpha-1 antitrypsin level and phenotype may also be performed to rule out the metabolic disorder alpha-1 antitrypsin deficiency. Autoimmune markers should be checked, particularly in women. These include an antinuclear antibody and antismooth muscle antibody. In addition, an antimitochondrial antibody (AMA) test should be conducted, particularly if there is an elevation of the alkaline phosphatase as 95% of patients with PBC will have a positive AMA. AST elevations caused by alcohol-induced steatosis should normalize several weeks after discontinuation of alcohol. Elevations of the AST and ALT in a patient with no history of alcohol abuse may be due to nonalcoholic fatty liver disease (NAFLD).

This is a relatively common diagnosis, particularly if the patient is diabetic or obese. Often, an abdominal ultrasound will corroborate the diagnosis by revealing fatty infiltration of the liver. A diagnosis of exclusion, NAFLD, may respond to weight loss or improved diabetic control.

4.2 Evaluating jaundice

Evaluation of the jaundiced patient is an important diagnostic skill. Jaundice is due to visibly evident hyperbilirubinemia and is seen only with a bilirubin above 2.5 mg/dl. As noted previously, it is important to note whether the bilirubin elevation is predominantly conjugated or unconjugated. A common disorder that will produce an unconjugated hyperbilirubinemia (although not usually jaundice) is Gilbert's syndrome. The total bilirubin is generally less than 3.0 mg/dl while the direct will be 0.3 mg/dl or less. The bilirubin is generally higher in the fasting state or when the patient is ill. A presumptive diagnosis of Gilbert's can be made in an otherwise well patient with unconjugated hyperbilirubinemia, normal hemoglobin (to exclude hemolysis), and normal liver enzymes (to exclude liver disease), especially if the bilirubin level is lower in the nonfasting state.

More common in the jaundiced patient is direct hyperbilirubinemia. One way to categorize such patients is by those with nonobstructive conditions and those with obstruction. Abdominal pain, fever, and/or a palpable gallbladder are suggestive of obstruction. Risk factors for viral hepatitis, a bilirubin greater than 15 mg/dl, and persistently high aminotransferases suggest that the jaundice is due to hepatocellular dysfunction and not obstruction. A sensitive, specific, and noninvasive test to exclude obstructive causes of jaundice is hepatic ultrasonography. Diseases characterized by large duct obstruction will generally exhibit intrahepatic bile duct dilatation, especially if the bilirubin is greater than 10 mg/dl and the patient has been jaundiced for more than 2 weeks. Acute large duct obstruction, usually from a stone, may not produce bile duct dilatation and if the clinical suspicion for bile duct obstruction remains strong despite a normal ultrasound, endoscopic retrograde cholangiography should be considered.

Patients may also present with cirrhosis or portal hypertension. Most patients with portal hypertension have cirrhosis although occasionally patients present with noncirrhotic portal hypertension that is idiopathic or due to portal vein thrombosis. The evaluation of a patient with cirrhosis is similar to that of chronic hepatitis and cholestasis (as described above). Alpha-1-antitrypsin deficiency, genetic hemochromatosis, and alcoholic liver disease patients frequently present with cirrhosis with or without portal hypertension as the first manifestation of liver disease.

4.3 The role of liver biopsy

The role of liver biopsy for the evaluation of asymptomatic liver test elevations is limited. It may, however, be an important component in establishing a definitive diagnosis, assessing therapeutic response, or when staging a disease. Even when used for these particular purposes, the role of liver biopsy is controversial particularly in settings in which therapy is unavailable [12].

4.4 Algorithms for patients with abnormal liver tests

Algorithms for abnormal liver tests are at best guidelines for management. The patient's clinical presentation should always be considered when evaluating (or not evaluating) abnormal liver tests. In general, abnormalities of liver tests that are less than three times normal may be followed by repeat testing in several months as long as the patient is asymptomatic and the albumin, PT, or bilirubin are normal. If these are persistent abnormalities, then they should be evaluated. Algorithms for an elevated ALT, alkaline phosphatase, and conjugated bilirubin are shown in Figures 1–3.

5. SUMMARY

The interpretation of abnormal liver tests typically requires additional information which may be obtained through a detailed interview with the patient, additional blood tests, imaging, and occasionally other more invasive studies. Deciding which to pursue involves complex decision making

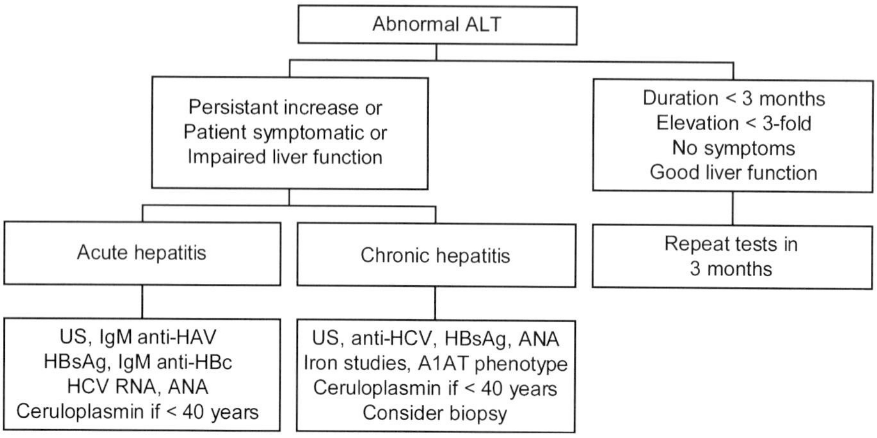

Figure 1. Evaluation of abnormal ALT.

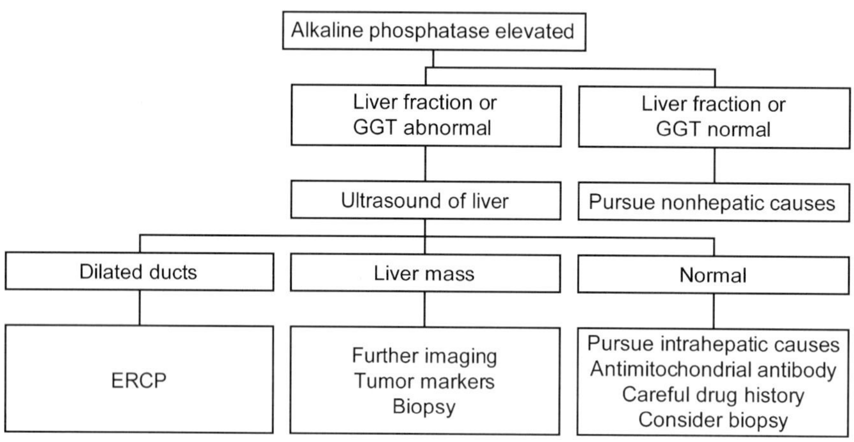

Figure 2. Evaluation of elevated alkaline phosphatase.

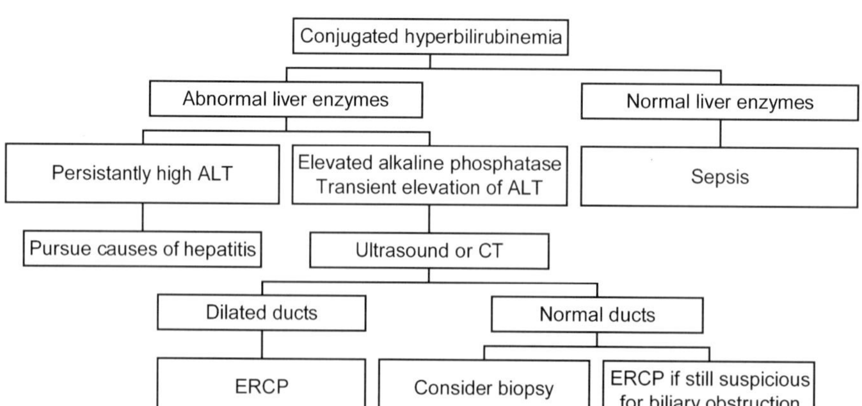

Figure 3. Evaluation of conjugated hyperbilirubinemia.

and an appreciation of the classic patterns of blood test abnormalities. Limitations of each of the blood tests, including problems with specificity and sensitivity, always need to be taken into account.

REFERENCES

[1] Pratt, D.S. and Kaplan, M.M. (1999) Evaluation of the liver, A: laboratory tests, in *Diseases of the Liver*, eds. Schiff, E.R., Sorrell, M.F. and Maddrey, W.C. (Lippincott–Raven, Philadelphia, PA) pp. 205–244.

[2] Davern, T.J. and Scharschmidt, B.F. (1998) Biochemical liver tests, in *Gastrointestinal and Liver Disease*, eds. Sleisinger, M.H., Feldman, M. and Scharschmidt, B.F. (W.B. Saunders, Philadelphia, PA) pp. 1112–1122.

[3] Weisiger, R.A. (2000) Laboratory tests in liver disease and approach to the patient with abnormal tests, in *Textbook of Medicine*, eds. Goldman, L. and Bennet, J.C. (W.B. Saunders, Philadelphia, PA) pp. 775–779.

[4] Baker, A.L. (1996) Liver chemistry, in *Liver and Biliary Disease*, ed. Kaplowitz, N. (Williams & Wilkins, Baltimore, MD) pp. 207–220.

[5] O'Grady, J.G., Alexander, G.J., Hayller, K.M. and Williams, R. (1989) Early indicators of prognosis in fulminant hepatic failure. *Gastroenterology* **97**, 439.

[6] Rothschild, M.A., Oratz, M., Zimmon, D., Schreiber, S.S., Weiner, I. and Van Caneghem, A. (1969) Albumin synthesis in cirrhotic subjects studied with carbonate 14C. *J. Clin. Invest.* **48**, 344.

[7] Hasch, E., Jarnum, S., Tygstrup, N. (1967) Albumin synthesis rate as a measure of liver function in patients with cirrhosis. *Acta. Med. Scand.* **182**, 83–92.

[8] Rosen, H.R. and Keefe, E.B. (2000) Evaluation of abnormal liver enzymes, use of liver tests and the serology of viral hepatitis, in *Liver Disease: Diagnosis and Management*, eds. Bacon, B.R. and Di Bisceglie, A.M. (Churchill Livingstone, New York) pp. 24–35.

[9] Shapiro, J.M., Smith, H. and Shaffner, F. (1979) Serum bilirubin: a prognostic factor in primary biliary cirrhosis. *Gut* **20**, 137–140.

[10] Rosen, H.R., Martin, P., Goss, J., Donovan, J., Melinek, J., Rudich, S., Imagawa, D.K., Kinkhabwala, M., Seu, P., Busuttil, R.W. and Shackleton, C.R. (1998) Significance of early aminotransferase elevation after liver transplantation. *Transplantation* **65**, 68–72.

[11] Clark, J.M., Brancati, F.L. and Diehl, A.M. (2001) Nonalcholic fatty liver disease: the most common cause of abnormal liver enzymes in the U.S. population. *Gastroenterology* **120**(5), A344.

[12] Sorbi, D., McGill, D.B., Thistle, J.L., Therneau, T.M., Henry, J. and Lindor, K.D. (2000) An assessment of the role of liver biopsies in asymptomatic patients with chronic liver test abnormalities. *Am. J. Gastroenterol.* **95**(11), 3206–3210.

Hepatology: A Practical Approach
B. Al Knawy, M.L. Shiffman, R.H. Wiesner (editors)

Chapter 3

Imaging the Liver

Robert A. Halvorsen

Radiology Department, Medical College of Virginia Hospitals & Physicians, Virginia Commonwealth University Health System, Main Building, 3rd Floor, Room 3-407B, 1250 East Marshall Street, P.O. Box 980615, Richmond, VA 23298-0615, USA

1. Introduction 21
2. Cirrhosis 22
3. Hepatocellular Carcinoma 23
4. Liver Metastases 24
5. Cavernous Hemangioma 25
6. Hepatocellular Adenoma 26
7. Focal Nodular Hyperplasia 26
8. Hepatic Cysts 26
9. Regenerative and Dysplastic Nodules 27
10. Fatty Liver 28
11. Incidental Liver Lesions 28
12. An Algorithmic Approach 29
References 31

1. INTRODUCTION

There are four primary imaging modalities widely used for detection of liver pathology: sonography, computed tomography (CT), magnetic resonance (MR), and nuclear medicine studies. The most cost-effective imaging strategy to diagnose a potential liver problem varies from patient to patient, depending not only on the strengths and weaknesses of the various imaging techniques but also on their cost.

Sonographic examination of the liver and bile ducts is a useful tool in the work-up of many patients with right upper quadrant pathology. Ultrasound excels in the detection of dilated intra- and extra-hepatic bile ducts, as well as gall bladder pathology. In North America the use of ultrasound in the detection of hepatic parenchymal disease is somewhat limited, but sonography is frequently used in Europe for the detection of liver masses.

CT has been a mainstay in the evaluation of the liver and bile ducts for years. Recent advances in CT technology include helical CT scanners with multiple detectors that allow improved spatial resolution and 3D imaging now allowing CT angiography, which can replace hepatic arteriography in many cases. CT is widely used as the primary screening tool for liver metastases from GI tract malignancies and is also frequently used as the tool for the detection of hepatocellular carcinoma (HCC) in patients with cirrhosis.

The role of magnetic resonance imaging (MRI) has evolved gradually over the last two decades. Contemporary MR devices provide fast imaging making possible the scanning of the entire liver during a single breath hold, markedly diminishing respiratory motion artifacts. And with the introduction of routine use of intravenous contrast media during MR, the applicability of MR for evaluation of hepatic and biliary abnormalities has improved.

Even more dramatic than the increased utility of abdominal MRI is the development of magnetic resonance cholangiopancreatography (MRCP), which in some institutions has replaced the routine use of endoscopy retrograde cholangiopancreatography. MRCP is an excellent tool for the evaluation of intra- and extra-hepatic bile ducts, as well as the pancreatic duct.

In the past, MR of the liver and bile ducts was generally reserved as a problem-solving tool when CT or ultrasound was non-diagnostic. In some academic centers, MR is replacing CT for the detection of liver pathology. Nationwide, the number of abdominal MR procedures doubled from 1996 to 1999 [1]. While MR is still utilized at 1/10th the frequency of abdominal CT for evaluation of the abdomen, the usage of MR is increasing in some areas more than others. In a Northeastern state, abdominal MR studies were performed five times more frequently in urban than rural hospitals [1]. Also, teaching hospitals utilized abdominal MR at twice the rate of non-teaching hospitals. MR can be especially useful in patients who cannot have a contrast enhanced CT examination. For instance, if a patient has an intravenous contrast media allergy or renal failure, MR is the procedure of choice as the contrast media given for MR is not cross-reactive with the contrast media used for CT.

Problems still limiting the widespread utilization of MR include the high cost compared to CT and the more widespread availability of CT scanners.

The role of nuclear medicine in the evaluation of liver and biliary disease is also evolving, especially with the introduction of positron emission tomography (PET). PET is a nuclear medicine imaging technique that uses radiopharmaceuticals. Typically, a radionuclide-labeled analog of glucose, fluorodeoxyglucose (FDG) is used to detect abnormal metabolic activity. Since malignant tumors usually have increased cellular metabolism resulting in increased glucose metabolism, PET is able to localize malignant tissue [2]. PET scanning is an effective tool for the detection of liver metastases. Hepatobiliary nuclear medicine agents are still widely used for evaluation of the biliary tree and gallbladder. The role of the traditional technetium sulfur colloid liver spleen scan has diminished over recent years with the increased use of CT and MR.

In the choice of an imaging test, cost must be considered. PET scans are the most expensive with a Medicare reimbursement rate of $1764 for oncology patients in 2002. In comparison, the global Medicare rate for inpatient MR of the abdomen is $925, $570 for abdominal and pelvic CT, and $104 for ultrasound. Depending upon an individual patient's situation, a more costly test may be the most cost-effective, if the test leads to avoidance of surgery or a shortened hospital stay. A single definitive test is often preferable to a series of inconclusive or "suggestive but not diagnostic" studies.

The following sections will discuss the strengths and weaknesses of various imaging modalities in the work-up of patients with potential pathology.

2. CIRRHOSIS

Cirrhosis produces changes in the morphology of the liver that can be detected by CT or MR. In many patients with cirrhosis, there is atrophy of the right lobe of the liver and hypertrophy of the caudate lobe and lateral segment of the left lobe. When the caudate enlarges and the right lobe atrophies, a simple measurement can be performed which is diagnostic of cirrhosis. When the width of the caudate lobe is more than two-thirds the width of the right lobe on the same CT section, cirrhosis can be predicted with 97% accuracy [3]. Another easily applied and highly reliable sign of cirrhosis on either CT or MR is the expanded gallbladder fossa sign [4]. In the normal, non-cirrhotic patient the gallbladder extends between the right lobe and the medial segment of the left lobe. With cirrhosis, the medial segment atrophies. If the medial segment is not visible at the level of the gallbladder on CT or MR, there is an "expanded gallbladder fossa", which has a reported specificity and positive predictive value of 98% for the diagnosis of cirrhosis [4] (Figure 1).

Not all livers in patients with cirrhosis will have an abnormal size or configuration. In a series of 508 pretransplant cirrhotic patients with pathologic proof, approximately 25% of patients with end-stage cirrhosis had livers that were normal in size and configuration. Another 36% of these patients had a diffusely atrophic liver, while the remainder

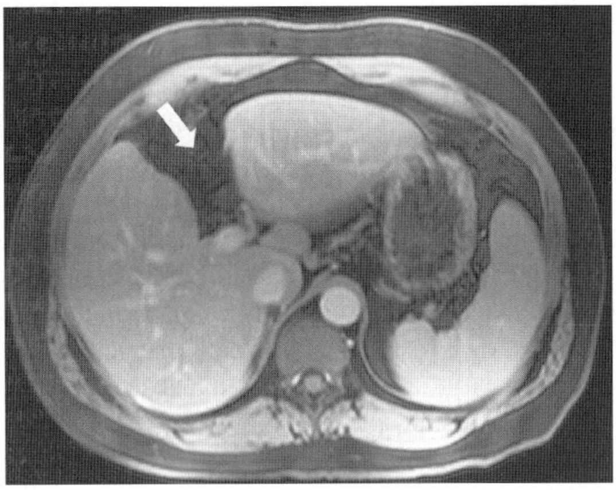

Figure 1. Enlarged gallbladder fossa sign of cirrhosis. Note the fat replacing the medial segment of the left lobe (arrow) with no medial segment of left lobe visible in this patient with cirrhosis.

showed a combination of segmental atrophy and hypertrophy [5].

Another finding detectable on CT ultrasound or MR highly suggestive of cirrhosis is the presence of a recanalized periumbilical vein. The umbilical and periumbilical veins normally atrophy after birth. In a patient with portal hypertension, these vessels recanalize providing a portosystemic shunt drainage pathway via the periumbilical veins, to a caput medusa at the umbilicus. These recanalized periumbilical veins are often detectable on imaging modalities in patients with late stage cirrhosis.

When cirrhosis has progressed to end-stage liver disease, the liver surface, as seen on CT or MR, is smooth in 37%, nodular in 48%, and lobular in 15% [5]. The nodularity of the liver in cirrhosis is due to either micronodular or macronodular disease. A lobular contour is present when there is subsegmental atrophy of portions of the liver and occasionally hypertrophy of other subsegmental areas. Nodularity is caused by a variety of entities, but a lobular contour is more frequent in patients with biliary cirrhosis, such as primary sclerosis cholangitis.

On unenhanced CT and T2-weighted MRI, there is often diffuse heterogeneity within the liver parenchyma in patients with end-stage liver disease. This heterogeneity can be due to fibrosis, fat deposition, or iron within regenerating nodules [6].

3. HEPATOCELLULAR CARCINOMA

The early detection of primary HCC is the impetus behind screening programs of patients at high risk for the development of HCC. Patients with hepatitis B or C induced chronic active hepatitis and cirrhotic patients are often screened with sonography, triple phase CT or contrast enhanced MR. There is no consensus yet achieved on which imaging test is superior in the detection of HCC. Ultrasound is a less costly examination and more widely available than CT or MR, but some studies have reported a lower detection rate with sonography than with CT. In a study of 200 patients who underwent pre-liver transplantation sonography, the sensitivity of sonography in the detection of HCC of any size was low (30%) [7]. Sonography only detected three (75%) of four HCCs larger than 5 cm in diameter and only 14% of tumors 1–2 cm in diameter. The authors concluded that sonography should not be the sole imaging modality used for lesion detection before liver transplantation. As an alternative to sonography, some proponents recommend MR over CT, but in academic institutions in North America at this time, CT is more widely utilized in liver screening. In a small prospective study of patients imaged with sonography, helical CT and contrast enhanced MR, the detectability of 13 HCCs was evaluated [8]. The sensitivity for these tumors was the lowest with sonography (46%), slightly better with CT (54%) and best with MR (77%).

Regardless of whether CT or MR is performed, the use of intravenous contrast media is considered essential. As hepatomas are fed by the hepatic artery and are hypervascular, they are best detected with intravenous contrast media administration, especially during the hepatic arterial phase of contrast enhancement (Figure 2). Modern MR breath hold scanning is capable of obtaining images during both the hepatic arterial phase and the portal venous phase of enhancement with a single bolus of contrast. In a similar fashion helical CT scanners can obtain dual phase studies of the liver, including both hepatic arterial and portal venous phases images. Hepatomas are demonstrated on CT and MR as enhancing masses within the liver parenchyma during the hepatic arterial phase of enhancement. If scanning is delayed by 30 s into the portal venous phase of

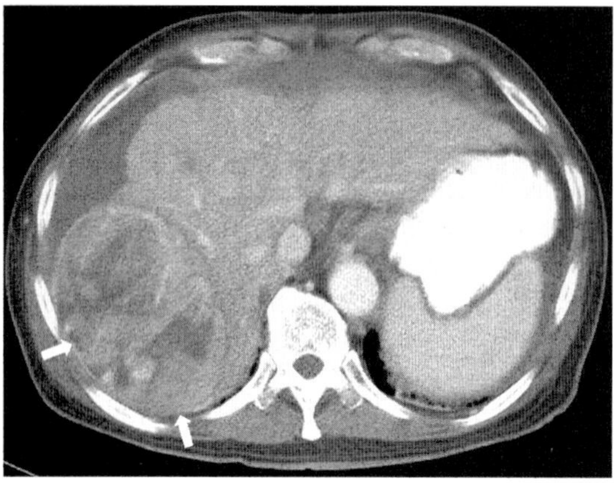

Figure 2. Rupturing hepatoma: large oval mass (arrows) in posterior segment of right lobe. Perihepatic blood in this patient with a rupturing hepatoma.

enhancement, the ability of either CT or MR to detect HCC diminishes significantly. Therefore, technique is important.

A typical patient who is screened for hepatoma is 45–65 years old with chronic hepatitis B, hepatitis C infection, or is an alcoholic. Primary HCCs are solitary in about one-half of patients and multiple in the other 50%. The CT and MR appearance of an HCC is a non-specific heterogeneous mass. Less than 10% of these tumors will have a tumor capsule. Fat also is detectable within the mass in less than 10% cases.

There are some specific findings that are highly suggestive of HCCs and help to differentiate them from metastases from extra-hepatic sites. With hepatoma, the presence of portal vein thrombosis is quite frequent, and very infrequent with liver metastases. Segmental or global portal vein thrombosis occurs in as many as 30% of patients with HCC [9]. Hepatic vein thrombosis is about 1/10 as frequent as portal vein thrombosis but is still detectable by CT in 3–5% of patients with hepatoma. If a liver mass bleeds, it is much more likely to be an HCC than a metastasis.

The detection of HCC or its predecessor, the dysplastic nodule, is difficult, especially in cirrhotic livers. And size matters. In a study that determined the sensitivity of MR for detection of HCC and dysplastic nodules, Krinsky *et al.* reported that MR had an overall lesion sensitivity of 55% in patients undergoing liver transplantation [10]. Only 47% of small lesions (less than 2 cm in diameter) were detected by MR.

A variant type of hepatoma is the fibrolamellar hepatoma. This is a different pathological entity than ordinary hepatoma and occurs in young to middle age patients and is usually solitary. These lesions are frequently large at the time of diagnosis averaging 13 cm in diameter and are well defined on CT and MR [11]. The characteristic appearance on imaging is the detection of a large central or eccentric scar that is visible on CT or MRI. The central scars may or may not demonstrate delayed contrast media enhancement. These fibrolamellar tumors often contain calcification.

4. LIVER METASTASES

Each year more than 59,000 patients in the United States will be diagnosed with hepatic metastases from gastrointestinal tract cancers [12].

Liver metastases are the most frequently encountered liver masses on imaging and most metastases are hypovascular compared to normal liver. The imaging strategy required to detect liver metastases differs from that of an HCC. Hypovascular metastases are best seen during the portal venous phase of contrast enhancement on either CT or MR. Since the metastases are hypovascular, and the surrounding liver has normal vascularity, obtaining CT or MR when normal liver is maximally enhanced increases the detectability of metastases. Since approximately 80% of the normal blood flow to the liver comes through the portal vein, obtaining images during the portal venous phase of enhancement is most efficacious.

With MRI, not only is contrast enhancement useful but also unenhanced T1- and T2-weighted pulse sequences can detect metastases. In general, pathology on MR produces low signal on T1-weighted images and high signal on T2-weighted images often described as a "flip-flop" appearance. Metastases are visualized as dark lesions on T1-weighted images and bright on T2-weighted pulse sequences.

Non-invasive tests that can detect hepatic metastases include liver function tests, carcinoembryonic antigen (CEA) and imaging tests. While the reported sensitivity of CEA measurements is low (56–59%), sensitivities of imaging tests vary widely, ranging 57–100% for ultrasound, 36–94% for CT, 69–96% for MR and 86–99% for PET using the tracer fluorine 18 (18F) FDG [12].

While the most cost-effective test or combination of laboratory and imaging tests is unclear, and may vary between patients, there is growing documentation of the effectiveness of individual tests. Kinkel *et al.* performed a meta-analysis of studies of imaging modalities in the detection of hepatic metastases from colorectal, gastric and esophageal cancer [12]. They included series with histopathologic correlation or at least 6 months of patient follow-up. Among 111 data sets in studies with a reported specificity higher than 85%, the mean reported sensitivity was 55% for ultrasound, 72% for CT, 76% for MR and 90% for FDG PET.

The role of PET in the detection of hepatic metastases is still unclear. While the cost of PET is high, if it can provide enough information to avoid other tests, then PET may be cost-effective. However, a major drawback of PET is the lack of detailed anatomic information that it provides clinical decision making may require more spatial resolution than possible with PET.

For instance, another imaging test such as CT may be required to confirm that an area of increased uptake on PET is intra-hepatic, or to determine which hepatic segment is involved or wherever the lesion is located in relationship to hepatic vessels. Therefore, in some patients, a positive PET study will require a subsequent CT, increasing the total cost of imaging.

5. CAVERNOUS HEMANGIOMA

The most frequent benign hepatic mass is the hemangioma reported to occur in 1–20% of the population. The later figure is from a prospective autopsy study in which a dedicated search for hemangiomas was made [13]. There is a strong female preponderance with 70–95% of hemangiomas occurring in women [14].

The hemangioma, which is defined microscopically as a tumor composed of multiple vascular channels supported by thin fibrous stroma, demonstrates its vascularity with characteristic vascular enhancement on CT or MRI. Hemangiomas contain vascular spaces that fill from the periphery toward the center of the mass, producing a peripheral globular enhancement pattern. In one study, a 100% positive

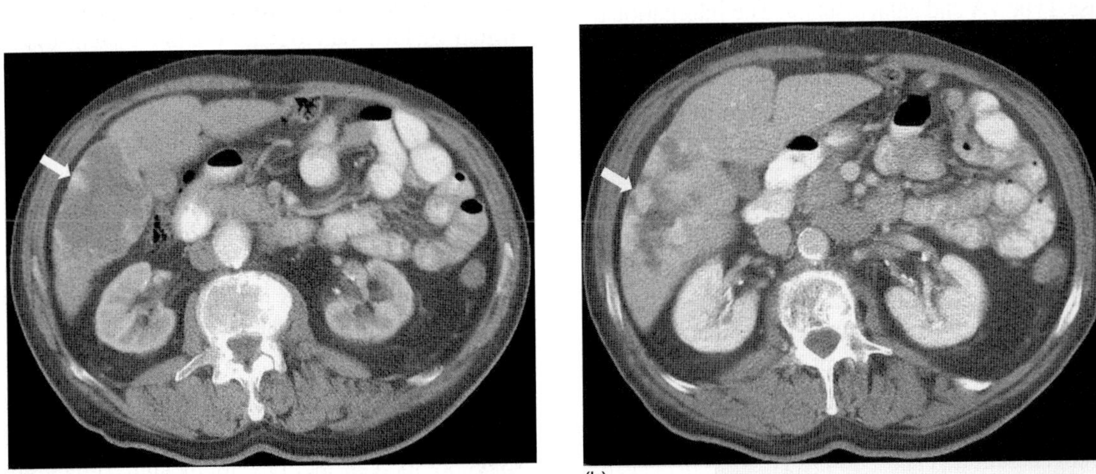

(a) (b)

Figure 3. (a) Cavernous hemangioma demonstrating globular enhancement. Peripheral enhancing nodules (arrow) with contrast enhancement equal to or greater than that of aorta are considered diagnostic of hemangioma. (b) Delayed scan demonstrates progressive enhancement (arrow) of central portions of hemangioma.

predictive value was reported for hemangioma if a liver lesion demonstrated a globule of peripheral enhancement that enhanced equal to or greater than the aorta [15] (Figure 3).

The nuclear medicine technetium-99m red-blood-cell scan is an excellent confirmatory test for cavernous hemangiomas. A red-blood-cell scan is especially useful in patients with liver masses that are suggestive but not diagnostic of hemangioma on MR or CT. Labeled red blood cells are injected intravenously and scans are obtained immediately as well as after a short delay. Hemangiomas demonstrate a "flip-flop" appearance of isointensity with the liver on dynamic early scanning and a hot spot on delayed blood pool images. The delay in uptake demonstrated by hemangiomas reflects the delayed fill in seen on CT and MR.

6. HEPATOCELLULAR ADENOMA

The hepatocellular adenoma is defined as a benign neoplasm composed of hepatocytes occurring in a liver that is otherwise histologically normal or nearly normal [16]. As the definition implies, the clinical setting is critical for the diagnosis of adenoma. Almost all examples of adenoma occur in a setting of hepatocellular stimulation, typically all contraceptive or anabolic steroid use. Less frequently, adenomas are associated with diabetes, glycogen storage disease Type 1A and galactosemia. The International Working Party on nodular hepatocellular lesions suggest that if none of these conditions are present, the diagnosis is doubtful and other diagnostic possibilities should be considered.

Hepatic adenomas have a relatively characteristic appearance on imaging studies, especially multi-phase CT. Adenomas are normally isoattenuating to normal liver on non-enhanced, portal venous phase and delayed images, but are hyperattenuating to normal liver during hepatic arterial phase. Lesions enhance completely and are nearly homogeneous except for areas of necrosis, hemorrhage or focal fatty degeneration [17].

With MR adenomas frequently contain demonstrable fat or hemorrhage within the mass and have inhomogeneous contents. Adenomas do not have a central artery or central scar, a useful distinguishing characteristic from focal nodular hyperplasia (FNH).

7. FOCAL NODULAR HYPERPLASIA

FNH is an uncommon benign tumor of the liver that is more frequently diagnosed today due to improved imaging techniques. In a study of 2500 consecutive autopsies, the prevalence of FNH was found to be 0.9%. Because FNH is benign and usually asymptomatic, and because fine-needle aspiration cytology is usually non-diagnostic, accurate diagnosis of FNH is important to preclude invasive and expensive evaluation.

With multi-phase helical CT, FNH is somewhat similar to adenoma in appearance. Both FNH and adenomatous lesions are typically undetectable on non-contrast examinations and portal venous phase images. Both lesions typically are seen well only during hepatic arterial phase scans. The FNH appears as a homogenous, markedly enhancing hypervascular mass, with a central scar that is hypoattenuating on early scans. On delayed imaging the central scar enhances brightly but the mass itself disappears. A central scar with a central artery within the scar is probably the most reliable CT feature for distinguishing FNH from hepatic adenoma [17]. Delayed, persistent enhancement of the central scar is typically seen in both CT and MRI of FNH. Hepatic adenoma demonstrates very different MRI characteristics, which include heterogeneity and frequent evidence of fat or hemorrhage content within in the adenoma.

Hepatic scintigraphy using 99m-technetium sulfur colloid can be useful in difficult cases. If a mass that is detected on CT or MR shows normal or increased uptake with sulfur colloid, then a diagnosis of FNH can be made with certainty (Figure 4). HCC or hepatic metastasis would show no uptake with sulfur colloid and therefore demonstrate a defect in the liver.

8. HEPATIC CYSTS

Liver cysts can be developmental, infectious or traumatic. Congenital liver cysts are thought to arise from bile duct epithelium. They are usually unilocular and are often multiple. They have been reported to occur between 5 and 14% of

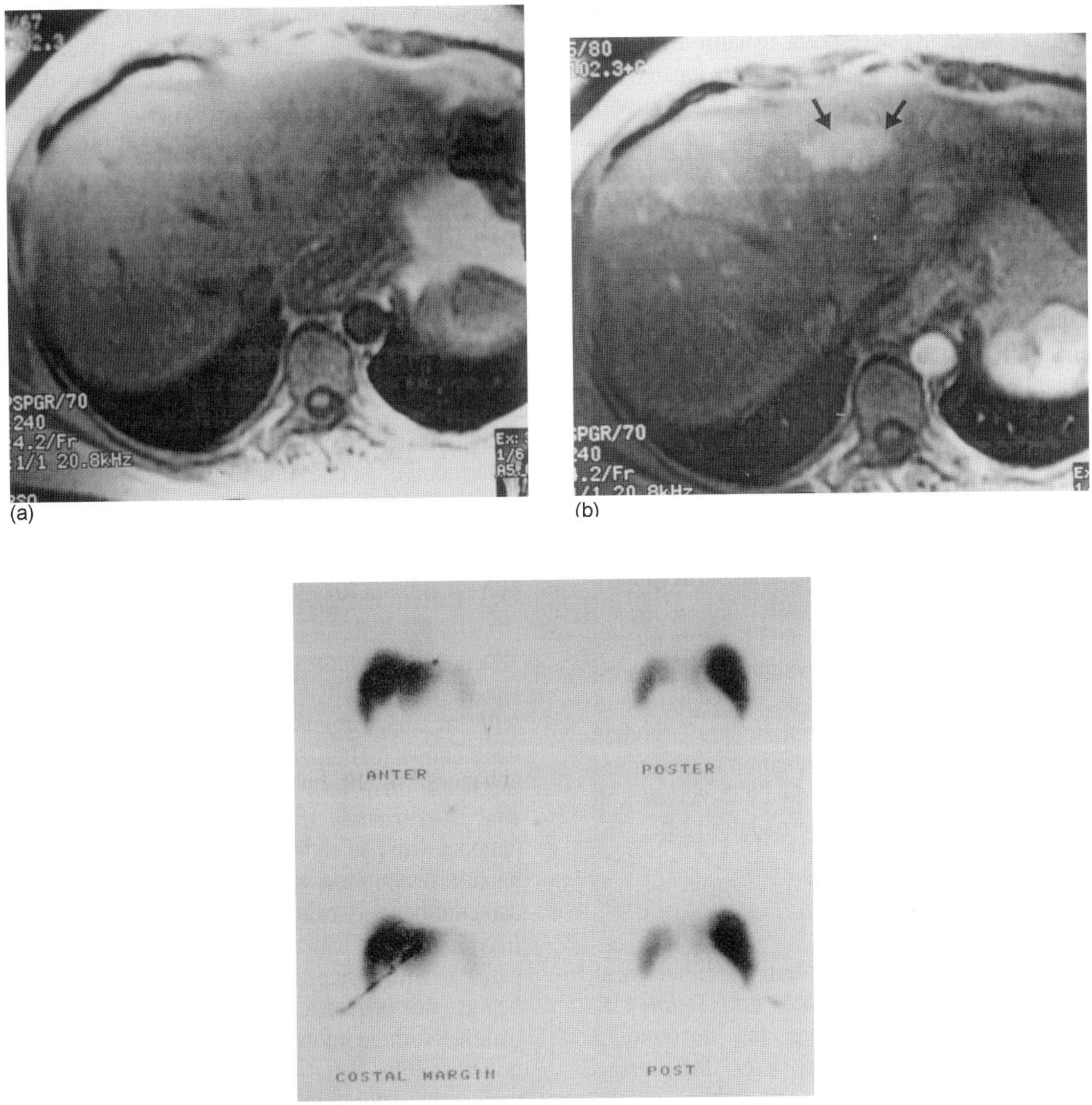

(a) (b) (c)

Figure 4. Focal nodular hyperplasia. (a) Precontrast T1-weighted image is normal. (b) Postcontrast T1-weighted sequence obtained during hepatic arterial phase of enhancement (note that hyperintense lesion (arrows) in left lobe). (c) Liver–spleen scan demonstrates normal uptake.

the population, and are more prevalent in women (4.5 to 1) [18].

The imaging diagnosis of simple liver cysts is not difficult. With ultrasound, hepatic cysts are anechoic. Because they do not attenuate the ultrasound beam, the posterior wall is well seen and distinct, and there is enhanced through transmission. On CT scans, liver cysts are thin-walled, sharply marginated lesions of water density that do not show a change in density with intravenous contrast. On MR, cysts have low signal on T1 and high signal on T2-weighted sequences with a "light-bulb" appearance [19].

9. REGENERATIVE AND DYSPLASTIC NODULES

Parenchymal nodular lesions in cirrhotic patients can be separated into two broad categories, regenerative vs. dysplastic nodules. Regenerative nodules can be thought of a parenchymal response to harmful stimuli, contain more than one portal tract and are located in a liver that is otherwise abnormal, usually with cirrhosis [16]. Dysplastic nodules are premalignant.

Regenerative nodules are better visualized on MRI than CT. In end-stage cirrhotic patients who all have regenerative nodules in pathologic specimens, CT detects nodules in about 25% of patients, while they are detected with MRI in about 50% of patients. MR best detects regenerative nodules on T2-weighted sequences or on post-contrast T1-weighted images. Nodules that are visualized on CT are visible because of high iron content and are therefore seen on unenhanced CT.

Dysplastic nodules may not be detected on CT or MR until they have become large. These larger dysplastic nodules have a characteristic combination of signal intensity, brightly hyperintense on T1 and markedly hypointense to liver on T2-weighted sequences. When malignant transformation occurs, signal intensity changes can be seen on MR producing a "nodule in a nodule" appearance. Dynamic gadolinium contrast imaging may show marked enhancement in the portions of frank HCC in the nodules [20].

10. FATTY LIVER

Hepatic steatosis or fatty liver can be either focal or diffuse and is easily detectable on CT. On CT, an area of lower density than the surrounding normal liver characterizes fatty liver. MRI using fat suppression techniques is also useful in the diagnosis of fatty liver.

Fatty liver can mask masses. Because liver metastases are detectable on CT as areas of lower density than normal liver, and fatty liver is also lower density than normal liver, liver metastases and fatty liver may be isodense-making metastases undetectable on CT. In a similar fashion, when a patient has fatty liver with a density approaching that of water, dilated intra-hepatic bile ducts may not be detectable because the surrounding liver is of identical density. Using fat suppression techniques, MR can be especially helpful in order to distinguish fatty liver from tumor or dilated bile ducts.

A concept that is useful in the differentiation of fatty liver from solid neoplasm is that fatty liver is not a mass and does not produce mass effect or displace adjunct structures [21]. Fatty liver has an infiltrative appearance, without mass effect. Liver metastases or primary HCC are masses which deform the contour of the liver or displace intra-hepatic vessels, while focal fatty liver does not.

11. INCIDENTAL LIVER LESIONS

Benign liver lesions may be encountered as an incidental finding during routine imaging of the abdomen. The cavernous hemangioma of the liver is the second most common liver mass after metastases and the most frequently encountered benign lesion. Benign hepatic cysts also occur in 1–14% of the population and also occur more frequently in women (5:1) than in men [14].

When a liver mass is encountered on an imaging study, it is helpful to integrate the clinical history with the imaging findings. For instance, if a patient has a known malignancy, a liver mass is more likely a metastasis than in a patient with no known malignancy. In a study from Emory University of outpatients who had abdominal CT that detected a small hepatic lesion (less than or equal to 15 mm), they detected hepatic lesions in 254 patients (17%) [22]. In 51% of these patients, the lesions were benign. In patients with cancer, half of the liver lesions were benign, not metastatic lesions. Most importantly, in patients with no known cancer at the time of the CT, none of the hepatic lesions turned out to be malignant. Therefore, if a patient has a small liver lesion detected during a CT examination, the work-up should depend upon the patient's history. If the patient has no known history of cancer, the lesion is highly likely to be benign and no further work-up warranted. However, if the patient has a known malignancy about half of the lesions will be malignant and further imaging studies or biopsy will be necessary.

The appearance of hepatic lesions is specific in certain circumstances. In a detailed analysis of the CT appearance of benign and malignant liver lesions studies with spiral CT, van Leeuwen *et al.* describe five characteristic or "pathognomonic" patterns [23].

First, a cavernous hemangioma can be diagnosed if the entire mass enhances to the same degree as arteries. Second, if a lesion demonstrates peripheral globular enhancement, it also represents a cavernous hemangioma. Third, a continuous rim of enhancement that is less than arterial always indicates malignancy. Fourth, all lesions with inhomogeneous areas of enhancement less than the arterial system also were malignant. Fifth, if the lesion is water density and does not enhance, it is a cyst.

12. AN ALGORITHMIC APPROACH

The work-up of a liver lesion should depend upon the individual patient's history. Patients can be grouped into three major categories: (1) cancer; (2) cirrhosis; (3) no known cancer or cirrhosis.

Cancer: In a patient with a known extra-hepatic malignancy, liver metastases are a concern and based on the Emory study [22], about half of liver lesions will be malignant. Therefore, any mass detected in the liver needs to be categorized. An algorithm for such patients is found in Figure 5. If the liver lesions are new, growing or multiple large lesions, then they can be assumed to represent metastases and no biopsy or further imaging test is warranted. Multiple small lesions could represent "micro-abscesses", typically due to fungal infection and cannot be assumed to represent metastases. Also, if the lesion demonstrates a continuous rim of enhancement (less than arterial in degree) or demonstrates internal inhomogeneous enhancement, it can be considered malignant and no further work-up warranted. If it meets criteria for a cyst, an ultrasound should be performed to ensure that it represents a simple cyst and not a cystic metastasis. If globular enhancement is detected at the periphery of the lesion, then it likely represents a cavernous hemangioma. When the globular enhancement equals that of arteries, then the appearance is pathognomonic of cavernous hemangioma. If the degree of enhancement approaches arterial or is difficult to quantify, then a 99m-Tc-RBC study can be performed. If the mass has an infiltrating appearance, focal fatty liver needs to be differentiated from an infiltrating tumor such as lymphoma and either liver MR with fat suppression or a 99m-Tc-sulfur colloid liver spleen scan should be performed. Small lesions (<5 mm) that are too small to characterize or biopsy should have a follow-up study in 3–6 months.

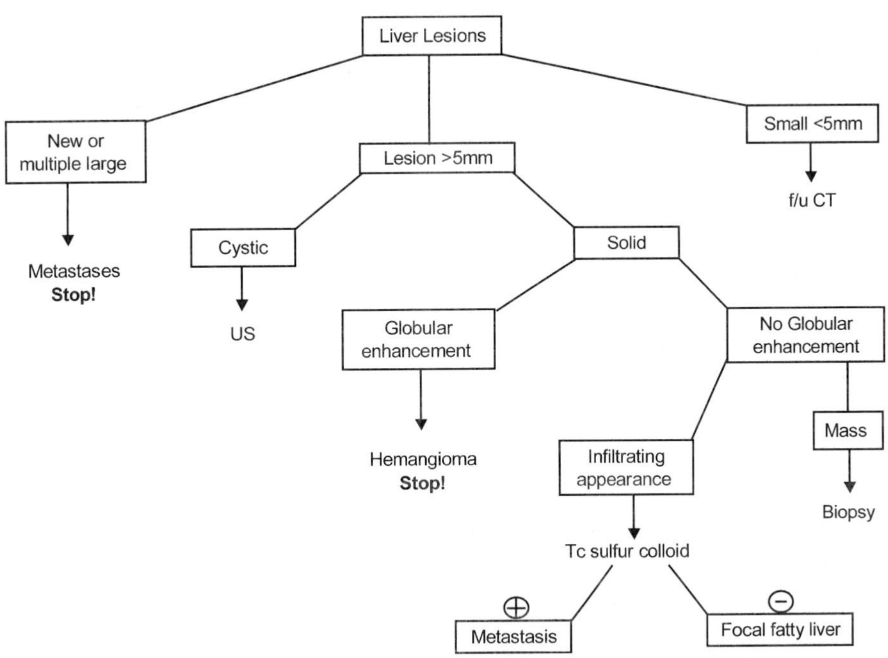

Figure 5. Known malignancy.

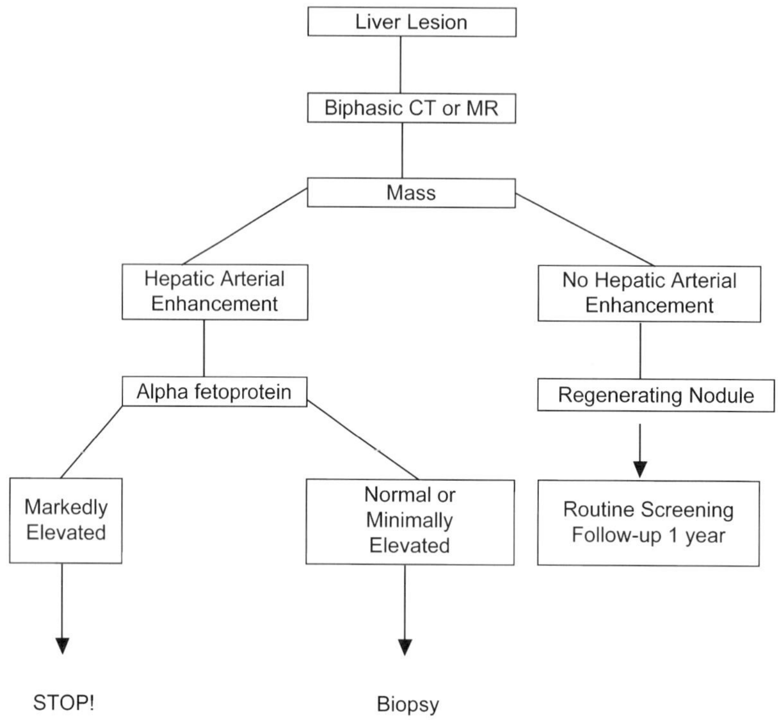

Figure 6. Cirrhotic patient.

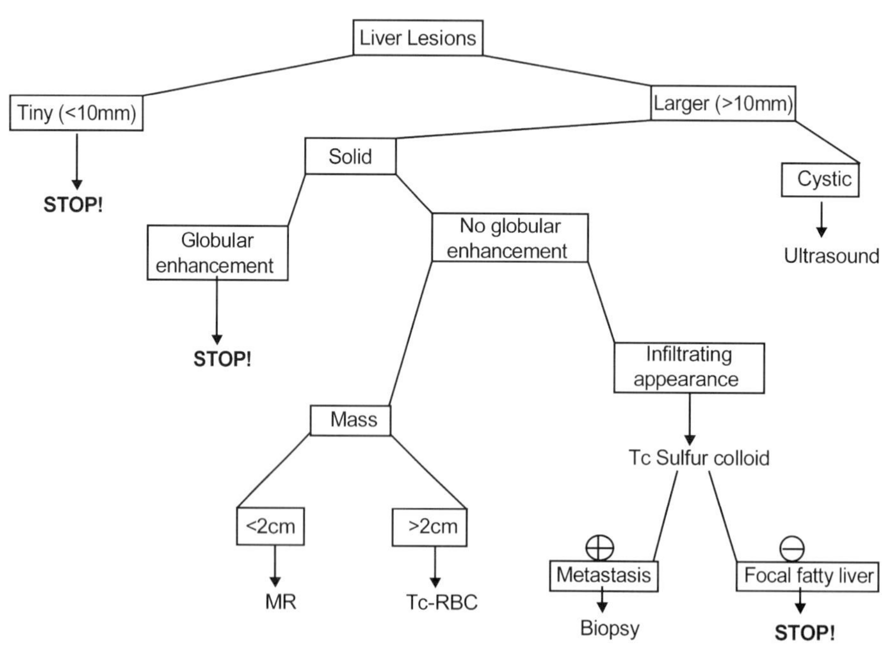

Figure 7. No known malignancy or cirrhosis.

Cirrhosis: In a patient with known or suspected cirrhosis, HCC or its predecessor, the dysplastic nodule, needs to be excluded. Cavernous hemangiomas are infrequently encountered in cirrhotics, possibly because they are obliterated by the fibrosis laid down in cirrhosis. Therefore, any enhancing mass in a patient with cirrhosis is suspicious for hepatoma and no mass should be assumed to represent a hemangioma unless rigorously proved to be so.

The imaging algorithm for cirrhotics starts with a biphasic contrast enhanced study (either CT or MR) that includes hepatic arterial phase enhancement (Figure 6). Any nodule that enhances during the hepatic arterial phase is either an HCC or a dysplastic nodule. Lesions that demonstrate "arterial enhancement" either in the periphery or throughout should be considered likely to be malignant, even though they would have been considered pathognomonic of cavernous hemangioma in the non-cirrhotic patient.

Small lesions, too small to characterize or biopsy (<5 mm) should be monitored closely with follow-up examinations and alpha-fetoprotein every 3–6 months.

No known cancer or cirrhosis: Hepatic lesions encountered in patients with no known malignancy or cirrhosis can be assumed to have benign disease. Unless a mass demonstrates atypical findings worrisome for malignancy, no further work-up is warranted (Figure 7).

REFERENCES

[1] Mitchell, D.G., Parker, L., Sunshine, J.H. and Levin, D.C. (2002) Body MR imaging and CT volume: variations and trends based on an analysis of medicare and fee-for-service health insurance databases. *AJR* **179**, 27–31.

[2] Balk, E. and Lau, J. (2001) PET scans and technology assessment. *JAMA* **285**, 936–937.

[3] Harbin, W.P., Robert, N.J. and Ferrucci, Jr., J.T. (1980) Diagnosis of cirrhosis based on regional changes in hepatic morphology: a radiologic and pathological analysis. *Radiology* **135**, 273–283.

[4] Ito, K., Mitchell, D.G., Grabata, T. and Hussain, S.M. (1999) Expanded gallbladder fossa: simple MR imaging sign of cirrhosis. *Radiology* **211**, 723–726.

[5] Dodd, G.D., Baron, R.L., Oliver, J.H. and Federle, M.P. (1999) Spectrum of imaging findings of the liver in end-stage cirrhosis: Part I, gross morphology and diffuse abnormalities. *AJR* **173**, 1031–1036.

[6] Dodd, G.D., Baron, R.L., Oliver, J.H. and Federle, M.P. (1999) Spectrum of imaging findings of the liver in end-stage cirrhosis: Part II, focal abnormalities. *AJR* **173**, 1185–1192.

[7] Bennett, G.L., Krinsky, G.A., Abitbol, R.J., Kim, S.Y., Theise, N.D. and Teperman, L.W. (2002) Sonographic detection of hepatocellular carcinoma and dysplastic nodules in cirrhosis: correlation of pretransplantation sonography and liver explant pathology in 200 patients. *AJR* **179**, 75–80.

[8] Rode, A., Bancel, B., Douek, P., Chevallier, M., Vilgrain, V., Picaud, G., Henry, L., Berger, F., Bizollon, T., Gaudin, J.-L. and Ducerf, C. (2001) Small nodule detection in cirrhotic livers: evaluation with US, spiral CT, and MRI and correlation with pathologic examination of explanted liver. *J. Comput. Assist. Tomogr.* **25**(3), 327–336.

[9] Novick, S.L. and Fishman, E.K. (1998) Portal vein thrombosis: spectrum of helical CT and CT angiographic findings. *Abdom. Imaging* **23**, 505–510.

[10] Krinsky, G.A., Lee, V.S., Theise, N.D., Weinreb, J.C., Rofsky, N.M., Diflo, T. and Teperman, L.W. (2001) Hepatocellular carcinoma and dysplastic nodules in patients with cirrhosis: prospective diagnosis with MR imaging and explantation correlation. *Radiology* **219**, 445–454.

[11] Brant, D.J., Johnson, C.D., Stephens, D.H. and Weiland, L.H. (1988) Imaging of fibrolamellar planocellular carcinoma. *AJR* **151**, 295–299.

[12] Kinkel, K., Lu, Y., Both, M., Warren, R.S. and Thoeni, R.F. (2002) Detection of hepatic metastases from cancers of the gastrointestinal tract by using noninvasive imaging methods (US, CT, MR imaging, PET): a meta-analysis. *Radiology* **224**, 748–756.

[13] Karhumen, P.J. (1986) Benign hepatic tumors and tumor-like conditions in men. *J. Clin. Pathol.* **39**, 183–188.

[14] Ros, P.R. and Taylor, H.M. (2000) Benign tumors of the liver, in *Textbook of Gastrointestinal Radiology*, eds. Gore, R.M. and Levine, M.S., 2nd edition (W.B. Saunders, Philadelphia, PA) pp. 1487–1522.

[15] Leslie, D.F., Johnson, C.D., Johnson, C.M., Ilstrup, D.M. and Harmsen, W.S. (1995) Distinction

between cavernous hemangiomas of the liver and hepatic metastases on CT: value of contrast enhancement patterns. *AJR* **164**, 625–629.

[16] International Working Party (1995) Terminology of nodular hepatic lesions. *Hepatology* **22**, 983–993.

[17] Ichikawa, T., Federly, M.P., Grazioli, L. and Nalesnik, M. (2000) Hepatocellular adenoma: multifaceted CT and histopathologic findings in 25 patients. *Radiology* **214**, 861–868.

[18] Craig, J.R., Peters, R.L. and Edmondson, H.A. (1989) *Tumors of the Liver and Enteropathic Bile Ducts, Second Series, FASC 26* (Armed Forces Institute of Pathology, Washington, DC).

[19] Wanless, I.R., Albrecht, S., Bilbao, J., Frei, J.V., Heathcote, E.J., Roberts, E.A. and Chiasson, D. (1989) Multiple focal nodular hyperplasia of the liver associated with vascular malformations of various organs and neoplasia of the brain: a new syndrome. *Mod. Pathol.* **2**, 456–462.

[20] Barren, R.L. and Peterson, M.S. (2001) Screening the cirrhotic liver for hepatocellular carcinoma with CT and MR imaging: opportunities and pitfalls. *RadioGraphics* **21**, 117–132.

[21] Halvorsen, R.A., Korobkin, M., Ram, P.C. and Thompson, W.M. (1982) CT appearance of focal fatty infiltration of the liver. *AJR* **139**, 277–281.

[22] Jones, E.C., Chezmar, J.L., Nelson, R.C. and Burnedino, M.E. (1992) The frequency and significance of small (less than or equal to 15 mm) hepatic lesions detected by CT. *AJR* **158**, 535–539.

[23] van Leeuwn, M.S., Noordzij, J., Feldberg, M.A.M., Hennipman, A.H. and Doornewaard, H. (1996) Focal liver lesions: characterization with triphasic spiral CT. *Radiology* **201**, 327–336.

Hepatology: A Practical Approach
B. Al Knawy, M.L. Shiffman, R.H. Wiesner (editors)

Chapter 4
Diagnostic Laparoscopy

Javier Parra[a] *and K. Rajender Reddy*[b]

[a] Albert Einstein Medical Center, Philadelphia, PA, USA

[b] University of Pennsylvania, 3 Ravdin, 3400 Spruce Street, Philadelphia, PA 19104, USA

1. Introduction 33
2. Indications 34
  2.1 Chronic hepatitis and cirrhosis 34
  2.2 Hepatocellular carcinoma 35
  2.3 Ascites of unknown origin 36
  2.4 Staging of intra-abdominal malignancies 37
  2.5 Other indications 39
3. Contraindications 40
  3.1 Preparation of the patient 40
  3.2 Methods and techniques 41
4. Complications 42
References 43

1. INTRODUCTION

The history of laparoscopy dates back to the early 19th century when Phillip Bozzini invented the "Lichtleiter", a hollow instrument that used a candle as its source of light. Antoine Jean Desormeaux used it in a human patient in 1857 and, as expected, burns were the major complications. In 1876, Maximilian Nitzke modified Edison's light bulb, adding it to the instrument and using it mainly for urologic procedures. Mikulicz and Leiter modified Nitzke's principle and invented the first rigid gastroscope, which was used as a diagnostic tool at Billroth's clinic in Vienna. In 1901, Dimitri Von Ott first explored the abdominal cavity of a pregnant woman, and in the same year Georg Kelling described the use of "koelioskopie", an examination of dogs' abdominal cavities performed with a cystoscope. One of Kelling's main interests was in stopping intraperitoneal bleeding by insufflating extreme amounts of air into the peritoneum thus creating a tamponade effect. During the first decade of the 20th century, Hans Christian Jacobaeus performed and published "laparothorakoskopie" and coined the term laparoscopy. He also suggested that this diagnostic modality could be used to confirm the diagnosis of cirrhosis, metastatic malignancies and tuberculous peritonitis [1,2].

Bertram Bernheim performed the first laparoscopy in the United States in 1911 at Johns Hopkins University. He stated "In cases of ordinary exploratory operation for carcinoma, before having recourse to the usual large incision, the cystoscope introduced through a very small and relatively unimportant incision, possibly made with cocaine, may reveal general metastases or a secondary nodule in the liver, thus rendering further procedures unnecessary and saving the patient a rather prolonged convalescence. In other obscure conditions of the upper abdomen, possibly the abdomen in general, the diagnosis might be cleared up by this simple method" [1].

Fervers' description of the creation of a pneumoperitoneum and Veress' development of a spring-loaded needle followed in the evolution and aided in the safety of the procedure.

By 1929, Heinz Kalk, the father of the German school of laparoscopy, used a 135° lens and described a dual trocar approach, and in 1939 published a series of 2000 liver biopsies without mortality [2].

Initially, mainly gastroenterologists performed laparoscopy, but with the advent of less invasive diagnostic procedures such as CT scan with its ability to do an imaging study guided biopsy, it fell out of favor. Since the mid-1980s, with the advent of the videolaparoscope in 1982 and the first laparoscopic cholecystectomy by Phillipe Mouret from France in 1987, laparoscopy has had a resurgence and has become one of the preferred tools for minimally invasive procedures in general and gynecological surgery [2–5].

Mainly, the difference in the use of laparoscopy by various specialists lies in its use for therapeutics by surgeons and as a diagnostic modality by gastroenterologists/hepatologists. Recently, the indications for surgical laparoscopy have expanded to include blunt abdominal trauma and evaluation of bowel ischemia and chronic abdominal pain.

In the era of resource rationalization, laparoscopy can be used as a day-case procedure, since, as proven for decades, it can be done under local anesthesia and conscious sedation with minimal complications. This and the recent introduction of mini-laparoscopes, has called again the attention of gastroenterologists and hepatologists alike to the use of this procedure for liver biopsies, staging of intra-abdominal malignancies, diagnosis of ascites, treatment of hepatocellular carcinoma (HCC) and even biopsy of intra-abdominal allografts. However, this procedure, despite its great utility, has had a declining interest among gastroenterologists and is not formally integrated as a part of training in all gastroenterology and hepatology programs [2–5].

In regards to the evaluation of liver disease, laparoscopy is underused. Blind or US-guided liver biopsy will fail to detect 10–25% of patients with cirrhosis, mainly due to the fact that even the widest needle may not be able to encompass a complete cirrhotic nodule. Therefore, the false negative rate of histology alone can be reduced by macroscopically evaluating the liver. Also, the direct observation of biopsy sites heightens the degree of safety of the procedure and offers the use of therapy for control of bleeding [6,7,9–11].

With the increasing body of evidence and the number of alternatives in cancer management, it is necessary to properly stage malignancies for either dissemination or regression. This has to be done in a way that offers minimal morbidity and acceptable cost-effectiveness. Laparoscopic staging meets these conditions in patients with a spectrum of malignancies [17,19].

2. INDICATIONS

2.1 Chronic hepatitis and cirrhosis

Many studies have been done to compare the overall sensitivity and specificity of both ultrasonography and laparoscopy in the diagnosis of chronic hepatitis (Table 1).

Various parameters such as the ability to detect the presence of inflammation when compared to histology as the "gold standard" have been used. In evaluating for chronic hepatitis, the sensitivity and specificity of ultrasonography have been around 67 and 72%, respectively [9]. Features suggestive of chronic hepatitis are: increased liver size, abnormal echogenicity, outline and shape [9]. In assessing the degree of inflammation, false-positive

Table 1. Indications for diagnostic laparoscopy.

Chronic liver disease
Hepatocellular carcinoma
Benign hepatic tumors
Staging of gastrointestinal malignancies
Metastatic liver disease
Ascites of unclear cause
Peritoneal infection
Lymphoma
FUO
Abdominal mass evaluation
Chronic abdominal pain
Hepatosplenomegaly of unclear cause
Liver disease in renal failure
Assessment for liver transplantation
Subfulminant hepatic failure

and false-negative rates of 6% have each been observed for laparoscopy, while ultrasonography has a false-negative rate of up to 33%. Although it is rather difficult to control inter-observer variability, the appearance of the surface of the liver as revealed by laparoscopy has been correlated with the histologic stage of inflammation and stage of fibrosis [9, 12]. Laparoscopic and histological identifications of liver diseases were compared in 145 patients. For fatty change, the sensitivity and specificity of laparoscopy have been 96 and 100%, respectively, for fibrosis 100 and 95% and for inflammation 94 and 95%, respectively. For cirrhosis, laparoscopy has been 100% sensitive and 97% specific [10,12].

Differences in staging and grading of inflammation have been observed between right and left biopsies obtained laparoscopically. A 24% difference of at least one grade of inflammation and a 33% difference of at least one stage of fibrosis between biopsy samples obtained from either the left or right lobes of the liver have been observed. In addition, diagnosis of cirrhosis may be under-represented if only one lobe is biopsied and this difference is evident in approximately 15% of patients [10]. A sonographic staging system that closely correlates with laparoscopic and histologic findings has been proposed. The system involves six different sonographic stages. The staging involves observation of the liver surface (smooth, to slightly, moderately or severely irregular) and evaluation for the presence of echogenic bands, which in turn can be anywhere from absent to diffusely present with an irregular liver texture. The reproducibility of this sonographic staging is unknown but inter-observer variability and feasibility of this system could be issues of concern [21].

For the follow-up of patients with hepatitis C, laparoscopic and histologic findings have been compared in patients undergoing treatment with interferon, finding weak correlations between laparoscopic appearances and both inflammation and fibrosis scores. The presence of early disease (demonstrated by a smooth liver surface as opposed to a granular or frankly nodular surface) and early histologic degree were correlated with a higher degree of sustained response to therapy, but were not strong predictors when compared to genotype 2a/2b and viral load [22].

The prevalence of hepatic dysfunction and, in general, the presence of chronic hepatitis is higher in patients with end-stage renal disease (ESRD) than in the general population. Underlying liver dysfunction in patients with ESRD may increase surgical risk and adversely affect patient and graft survival. The prevalence of hepatitis C in the ESRD population receiving hemodialysis varies between 12 and 20%. Prior to renal transplantation, the evaluation of chronic liver disease can be done with laparoscopy. The procedure can be performed with DDAVP administration and only minor complications should be expected. In patients undergoing peritoneal dialysis, the Tenckoff catheter can be used for the insufflation of pneumoperitoneum, thus obviating the need for the Veress needle [8].

Comparing the accuracy of laparoscopy-guided vs. US-guided or blind biopsy, the false negative rate of percutaneous liver biopsy, for the diagnosis of cirrhosis, ranges from 20 to 30%. Laparoscopy has been found to be superior to ultrasonography with a reported specificity of 95–100 vs. 89% in the diagnosis of cirrhosis. More studies are warranted to compare the accuracy of the newer radiologic diagnostic modalities (CT, MRI) in the assessment and diagnosis of cirrhosis [9]. Accurate staging of the severity of liver disease is likely to then lead to addressing relevant issues of surveillance for HCC and endoscopic screening for identification of large varices, which, if present, should lead to the use of beta-blocker prophylaxis. It has also been suggested that the appearance of the liver during laparoscopy, namely macronodular cirrhosis, and degree of atrophy may serve as prognostic features in cirrhosis [7,13].

2.2 Hepatocellular carcinoma

Laparoscopy can be used both as a diagnostic and therapeutic tool in the management of HCC. Changes on the liver surface, such as yellow and hypervascular nodules, as well as hyperemic lesions differing from other nodules, are suggestive of HCC (Figure 1). Seeding of the needle biopsy track is controversial; nevertheless, biopsy of a suspicious lesion should be

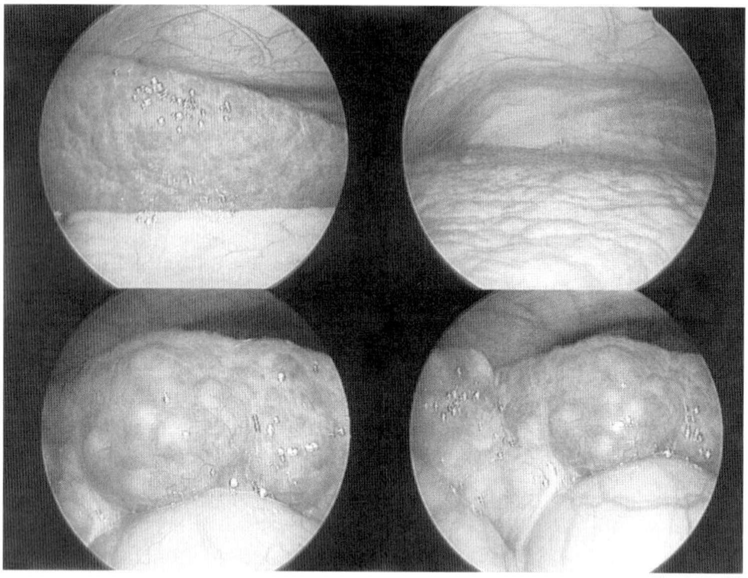

Figure 1. Cirrhotic appearing liver with a relatively hypervascular and nodular lesion anterior to the gallbladder which was a biopsy-proven HCC. (*For colored version, see Plate I on page 563 at the end of the book.*)

avoided particularly if liver transplantation is a therapeutic consideration. Aggressive biopsy techniques should be avoided while sampling hypervascular lesions for fear of bleeding, and since the less invasive modality of aspiration cytology can successfully confirm the diagnosis of HCC in most cases. Since HCC can be multicentric, laparoscopy can assess the extent of the primary lesion and evaluate for synchronous tumors. Rising levels of α-fetoprotein with negative or indeterminate imaging studies should prompt a laparoscopic evaluation, as in experienced hands it can detect lesions as small as 1 mm in diameter. Further, the addition of laparoscopic ultrasound and its use as a diagnostic tool for HCC has been proven to impact on treatment selection by defining the presence of multicentric HCC [15]. Although still in preliminary stages of investigation, the diagnosis of HCC can also be aided by the administration of 5-aminolevulinic acid (5-ALA) and the use of D-light AF systems during laparoscopy [14,15].

Laparoscopy is being increasingly used for purposes of therapeutic interventions in HCC [16]. Although long-term survival is affected by local recurrence in the cirrhotic liver, modalities such as microwave coagulation, local therapy with ethanol injection and radiofrequency ablation have been applied laparoscopically for control of disease. These techniques are especially helpful for palliative therapy in cases for which neither resection nor transplantation is suitable. Although rare, the complication of seeding at the port site has been reported [23]. Laparoscopic liver resection is a rapidly evolving field. Both benign and malignant liver and biliary tract diseases have been treated laparoscopically. Large tumors of greater than 5 cm have been resected successfully. In experienced hands, laparoscopic resection has failed infrequently. Although preliminary and in small number of patients, a possible survival benefit with *in situ* ablation and with resection of various types of primary and metastatic liver tumors has been observed [23].

2.3 Ascites of unknown origin

Diagnostic evaluation of ascites of unknown origin can be a challenging process. Whenever clinical history, physical examination and ancillary testing are unrevealing, laparoscopy is an invaluable tool, revealing an etiologic diagnosis in up to 86% in this subgroup of patients. Etiologies include: peritoneal carcinomatosis (up to 60%) from adenocarcinoma, lymphoma and mesothelioma, tuberculous peritonitis (up to 20%), and cirrhosis (6%) [24].

2.4 Staging of intra-abdominal malignancies

Thorough staging of tumors proves critical in the development of treatment strategies for malignancy. Accuracy, cost-effectiveness and acceptable morbidity are issues to consider when choosing the appropriate diagnostic tool.

The presence of inflammatory processes, anatomic variation, and benign tumors of the liver can complicate the staging of malignancies. Staging of malignancies often relies on non-invasive techniques such as MRI, CT and, more recently, PET scanning. The preoperative findings provided by such studies are often inaccurate leading to understaging, which can then lead to a failed attempt at a curative resection when intra-operative findings differ; this not only inflicts physical, but also psychological stress on the patient.

The current technological status of laparoscopy makes it an ideal tool for accurately diagnosing, staging and treating intra-abdominal malignancies in a palliative or curative manner. With the recent addition of laparoscopic ultrasound to the overall armamentarium, laparoscopy is now able to detect intrahepatic and lymph node metastases [17].

Meticulous evaluation of the abdominal cavity, gastrohepatic, gastrocolic attachments, retroduodenal spaces and their associated lymph nodes as well as saline solution lavage for cytology should be routinely performed during staging laparoscopy [17].

Esophageal cancer prognosis is independently affected by lymph node metastases. Similar diagnostic accuracy has been observed in a comparison between thoracoscopy and laparoscopy staging modalities. For the detection of hepatic metastases (Figure 2), another unfavorable prognostic factor in esophageal cancer, the sensitivity, specificity and accuracy of laparoscopy when compared to CT and ultrasonography are 88, 100 and 96%, respectively. Similarly, the detection of peritoneal metastases is more often made reliably with laparoscopy as compared with imaging studies. The ultimate benefit of laparoscopy is enabling the clinician to make a tissue diagnosis.

The sensitivity of laparoscopy for the detection of hepatic metastases and peritoneal spread in patients with gastric cancer is 87 and 83%, respectively [17].

Pancreatic cancer is the fourth leading cause of cancer-related deaths in the United States. Five-year survival rates are estimated to be around 2–3%. Recent surgical advances for the palliation of pancreatic cancer and the superiority of laparoscopy compared to high-resolution dynamic CT scan make it a valuable procedure for patients with this malignancy. Laparoscopy has helped in better staging of these tumors and thus has avoided unnecessary surgery. False-negative rates for CT scans, when compared to laparoscopy in detecting liver or peritoneal metastases in pancreatic carcinoma, are around 20% (Figure 3). When combined with laparoscopy, both modalities achieve a 94% negative predictive value for metastatic disease to the liver, peritoneum or mesentery, while the positive predictive value of laparoscopy alone to detect these metastases is around 88%. In predicting resectability, laparoscopy has a reported specificity of 50% and an accuracy of 65%. Laparoscopic ultrasound adds to the specificity and accuracy of laparoscopy making them 88 and 89%, respectively. For the detection of metastatic disease, most enlarged lymph nodes reveal reactive hyperplasia and some normal lymph nodes can harbor micrometastatic disease. Such characteristics warrant lymph node biopsies during the staging procedure [17–19].

Short-term outcomes for benign colorectal lesions resected through laparoscopy have been reported as being similar to those treated with open resection. Trials are being conducted to compare and standardize the use of laparoscopic colorectal cancer resection. In conventional surgery, palpation of the liver and periaortic tissues is carried to detect metastatic disease. The use of intra-operative laparoscopic ultrasound for the detection of liver metastases may compensate for the inability to palpate and has been shown to change the initial ultrasound or CT staging of the disease in approximately 10–15% of patients. However, preoperative staging of colorectal

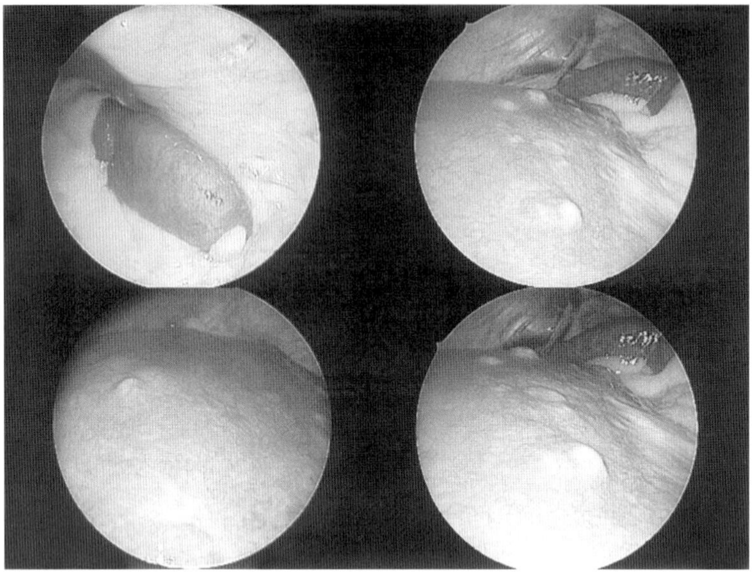

Figure 2. Laparoscopy demonstrating raised, partly whitish areas, on the surface of the liver which, on biopsy, proved to be metastatic liver disease. (*For colored version, see Plate II on page 563 at the end of the book.*)

cancer with laparoscopy is not as beneficial as for other cancers since most patients require resection, even with metastatic disease to the liver or other organs [17].

An issue of great interest and current research is that of trocar site seeding from malignancies. The use of gasless laparoscopy as well as the use of wall-lift devices may prove beneficial in decreasing the risk of this complication.

The introduction of laparoscopy for the staging of lymphomas has led to a decreasing use of laparotomy. The use of laparoscopic staging of Hodgkin's disease

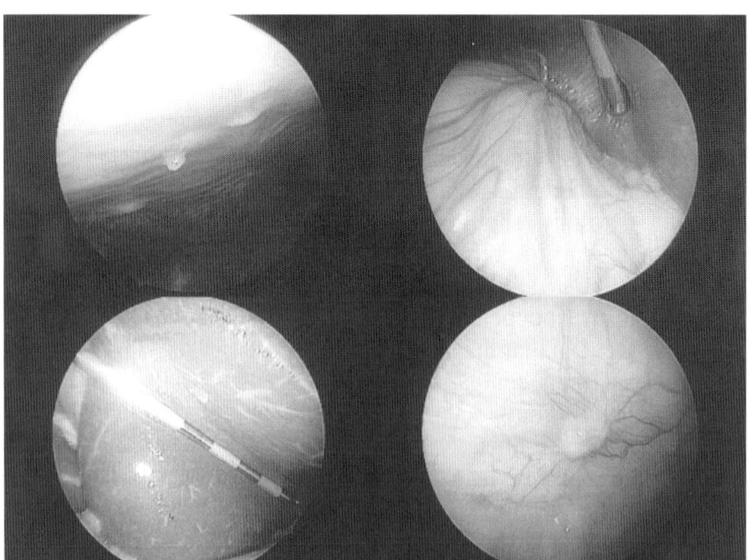

Figure 3. Tiny white implants on the peritoneal surface consistent with peritoneal metastasis. (*For colored version, see Plate III on page 564 at the end of the book.*)

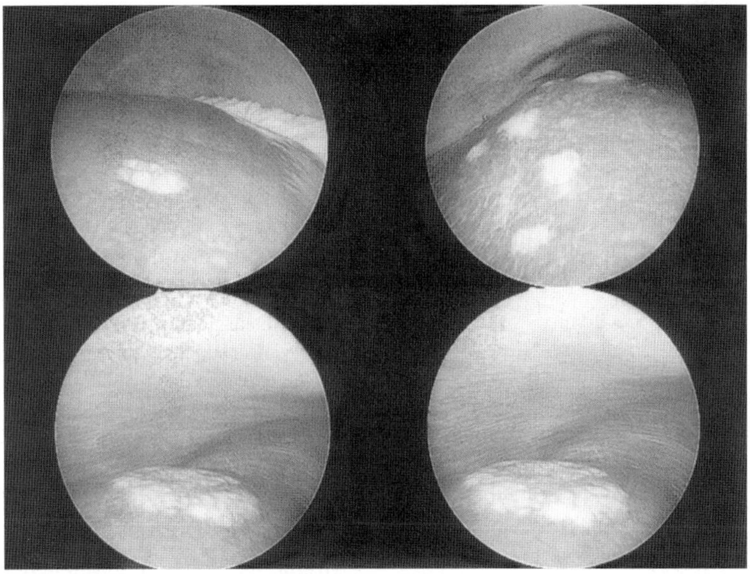

Figure 4. Large white, circumscribed areas over the liver which were due to a lymphoma on biopsy. (*For colored version, see Plate IV on page 564 at the end of the book.*)

may reveal unsuspected hepatic involvement mainly seen as white spots or nodules, or occult splenic involvement that helps upstage the disease (Figure 4). Such benefit is also seen in the staging of non-Hodgkin's lymphomas. In the staging and treatment of gynecological malignancies, the advantages of laparoscopy are proven in endometrial cancer and there is a growing body of evidence for cervical cancer [20].

For ovarian cancer, a high false-negative rate of up to 55% with imaging studies makes laparotomy preferable [17].

The development and use of laparoscopic techniques have largely been confined to gastroenterologists and general surgeons, but with conclusive data demonstrating its usefulness in staging malignancies, it is likely to become a tool in the armamentarium of surgical oncologists [2].

2.5 Other indications

Laparoscopy has been used to aid in the diagnosis of acute abdomen and in the identification of injuries from abdominal trauma. 120 patients with acute abdomen were compared to 310 patients treated without laparoscopy. In the group in which acute appendicitis was suspected ($n = 42$), laparoscopy avoided non-therapeutic laparotomies in 2%, corrected the diagnosis in 19% and changed treatment in 2% of cases. From the groups with acute abdomen of uncertain etiology ($n = 54$) and abdominal trauma ($n = 24$), laparotomy was avoided in 13 and 38%, respectively and the diagnosis was changed in 48 and 75%, respectively. The reported sensitivity, specificity and accuracy of laparoscopy were 99, 83 and 89%, respectively. Not only was laparoscopy shown to avoid unnecessary procedures, but it also helped in decreasing hospital stay, and also in reducing morbidity and mortality by avoiding therapeutic delays [25].

Diagnostic laparoscopy has also reduced appendectomy rates from 49 to 14% in women and from 22 to 11% in men.

The feasibility and 100% overall accuracy of laparoscopy have been also reported for the investigation of the source of sepsis in critically ill patients, especially those with abnormal chemistries or physical signs of an intra-abdominal process [26].

In terms of abdominal trauma, laparoscopy is advocated for the diagnosis and treatment of missed diaphragmatic rupture. The overall benefits include avoiding double lumen intubation, ease of release of adhesions and the ability to repair even large diaphragmatic defects [25].

Laparoscopic resection of hydatid cysts has been proven safe and effective, although the technique itself is yet to be standardized. Forty-eight patients from a series experienced morbidity in 6% and no mortality. Laparoscopy was successful in 96% of patients in achieving complete removal of the hydatid cysts [27].

In the work-up of patients with fever of unknown origin (FUO), laparoscopy can provide the diagnosis in up to 68% of cases, providing a diagnosis in 44% and contributing to establishing a diagnosis in 24%. Laparoscopy is especially useful when the patient in question has biochemical or physical signs of an intra-abdominal process [28].

Due to the high degree of postoperative complications, surgical procedures are usually avoided in patients with cirrhosis. Child's class A and B patients can safely undergo laparoscopic cholecystectomy with significantly less morbidity and mortality than those who undergo open cholecystectomy [29].

Laparoscopy has been used successfully in neonates with prolonged jaundice, helping to distinguish between extrahepatic biliary atresia and neonatal hepatitis. It can avoid as many as 42% of unnecessary surgical procedures [30].

In summary, laparoscopy can be of help in establishing diagnoses and in treating a wide range of intra-abdominal diseases seen in both surgical and non-surgical environment.

3. CONTRAINDICATIONS

With the accumulated experience over the past several decades, contraindications once thought to be absolute are now relative (Table 2). For example, in patients with history of abdominal surgery, the Hasson procedure is useful. This technique involves the creation of a small incision just under the umbilicus and into the peritoneum, allowing the operator to see the path of the trocar as it is passed through the incision. A blunt trocar is used with this technique and then the skin and subcutaneous tissue around the trocar are tightened around the trocar with sutures; then gas insufflation can begin [2–4].

Table 2. Contraindications to diagnostic laparoscopy.

Absolute
Severe/decompensated cardiopulmonary failure
Acute myocardial infarction
Intestinal obstruction
Bacterial peritonitis
Abdominal wall infection
Relative
Uncooperative patient
Severe coagulopathy
Previous abdominal surgery
Non-reducible external hernia
Morbid obesity
Large ventral hernia
Diaphragmatic hernia

Although preliminary, for patients with coagulopathy secondary to liver disease, the use of factor VIIa has been proven safe and effective [31]. To date, relative contraindications are mostly patient dependent.

3.1 Preparation of the patient

It is essential to obtain a detailed history with particular attention given to previous surgeries and physical examination, and documentation of scars in the anterior abdominal wall.

Before obtaining consent, the operator should explain the procedure to the fasted patient along with its possible complications. Before starting the procedure, it has proven helpful to have the patient practice abdominal distention in order to facilitate placement of the Veress needle and trocar.

When scheduling the procedure, the patient should be told to avoid NSAIDs and salicylate compounds for at least 1 week before the procedure. Coagulation guidelines are similar to those of percutaneous blind or US-guided biopsy. After obtaining informed consent, testing of all equipment is recommended before starting sedation.

Gastroenterologists and hepatologists may choose to perform diagnostic laparoscopies in an outpatient-based environment, along with procedures such as colonoscopies and upper endoscopies, but in a dedicated laparoscopy room within the gastroenterology suite.

3.2 Methods and techniques

The procedure starts with placement of an intravenous line and preprocedure medication with approximate doses of meperidine HCl 50 mg IM and promethazine 50 mg IM and IM atropine 0.6 mg. During the procedure, varying amounts of IV meperidine HCl and IV midazolam are administered to achieve appropriate sedation and patient cooperation. Electrocardiographic, blood pressure and pulse-oximetry monitoring should be followed throughout the procedure. To avoid desaturation, it is recommended that oxygen supplementation be given via nasal cannula.

The patient is placed in a supine position and the anterior abdominal wall is scrubbed with povidone-iodine, or non-iodine solutions for iodine-allergic patients, and then covered with sterile drapes, exposing the anterior abdominal wall.

The chosen entry point for the Veress needle is identified. Usually, a point to the left of the paramedian area is used. However, a right paramedian or sub-umbilical approach may be necessary in patients with an enlarged left hepatic lobe, marked splenomegaly, or previous splenectomy.

A local anesthetic (1% lidocaine) is injected at the chosen point of entry with a 22-gauge needle, forming a 1 cm wheal. Then, a 16-gauge needle is inserted perpendicularly into the center of the wheal to reach the parietal peritoneum, at which point the patient usually acknowledges pain. All layers of subcutaneous tissue should be anesthetized within a 2 cm radius and in a 360° fashion. For obese patients, a spinal needle may be needed to anesthetize the parietal peritoneum. A total of 15–20 ml of 1% lidocaine or a maximum of 300 mg is used. This step is of utmost importance as insufficient anesthesia can lead to patient discomfort when the Veress needle is inserted or the laparoscope is manipulated.

The most critical part of the procedure is the placement of the Veress needle. A small incision is made in the center of the wheal and the patient is asked to distend the abdominal wall without arching his/her back. Then, the Veress needle is inserted into the abdominal cavity and two distinct "pops" are heard. After the needle is inserted into the abdominal cavity, aspiration with a 10 cm^3 syringe will evaluate for an inadvertent entry into a blood vessel and thus avoid an air embolism, or recognize inadvertent intestinal perforation, both rare complications in laparoscopy. Attaching the insufflator's tubing to the Veress needle starts gas insufflation. Correct placement of the needle can be determined with the assistance of the insufflator's gauges. Generally, pressures above 20 mmHg indicate wedging of the needle in the subcutaneous fat, fascia or in the omentum. When the pressure gauge is at about 10–15 mmHg, the gas is delivered at approximately 1 l/min.

The choice of gas is usually nitrous oxide. Carbon dioxide is a peritoneal irritant, so that increasing sedation is required. It also has important physiologic effects in patients with previous or recent history of trauma, particularly head trauma, as it may elevate intracerebral pressure (ICP), and also in patients with lung disease as it may worsen retention and cause acidosis. Helium and nitrous oxide have been compared with carbon dioxide for pneumoperitoneum and have been shown to increase ICP to a lesser degree.

Normally, a total of 3–6 l, depending on the capacity of the abdominal cavity, are insufflated to achieve pressures in the range of 20 mmHg. Once this is achieved, manual insufflation is converted to an automatic mode. After the Veress needle is removed, a 20 ml half-filled syringe is introduced into the abdominal cavity and rotated 360°, while aspirating, in order to test for equal distribution of N_2O. Gas bubbles within the syringe help identify a free and unobstructed area for placement of the trocar. A second operator can check for the disappearance of hepatic dullness to indicate adequate insufflation. An incision is made within the wheal and blunt dissection is carried to reach the fascial planes. Then the patient is asked again to distend the abdomen and a 5 mm disposable trocar is inserted with a semicircular motion. Two distinct "pops" are again heard to confirm the adequate placement of the trocar. A 30 or 45° oblique view videolaparoscope is then inserted into the abdominal cavity through the trocar.

During recent years, there has been an increase in the use of mini-laparoscopes. These devices allow the creation of pneumoperitoneum through a 2.3 mm trocar bearing a Veress cannula inside. The 2.3 mm trocar is also used for the insertion of the 1.9 mm of an end viewing mini-laparoscope. The disadvantage of an end viewing laparoscope is that it does not allow for a good visualization of the superior aspects of the right lobe and thus may be an ideal tool for staging laparoscopy. Contrary to first impressions, this device is associated with a lower complication rate, given its greater flexibility. Some of the limitations of this technique (easy to overcome) are the limited visualization by the available lenses, and the need of a second access for biopsy because the reduction in size does not allow an instrument channel. Once 30 and 45° lenses become available and instrument channels develop the technological advance of a biopsy channel, it may be favored and reintroduced for diagnostic uses because it minimizes patient discomfort and is even less invasive than conventional laparoscopy.

The area perpendicular to the scope is then examined for bleeding, or damage to intra-abdominal structures. With the patient in Trendelenburg position, the bladder and pelvic structures are visualized. Then the patient is placed in reverse Trendelenburg position and a thorough inspection of the right and left upper quadrants is done. Both upper and lower quadrants can be visualized with movement of the laparoscope.

A second trocar is often then placed into the right mid-clavicular line at the right lower quadrant following the local anesthesia technique previously described. This trocar site will allow inspection of the superior aspect of the right lobe of the liver and delivery of a palpating probe or a biopsy needle. In addition, the primary entry site can be visualized.

A liver biopsy is obtained from the left lobe with the use of a 14-, 16- or 18-gauge biopsy gun or less frequently with a Tru-Cut needle. The recommended approach is tangential and to the left of the falciform ligament in order to avoid large intrahepatic vessels.

For patients with massive ascites, the Veress needle must be placed tangentially in order to avoid contact with the ascitic fluid during insufflation of nitrous oxide because bubble formation may be a limiting factor to adequate visualization of intra-abdominal organs. Others advocate placing the patient in a reverse Trendelenburg position in patients with ascites such that hollow viscera and fluid accumulate in the pelvis while the Veress needle is placed. Several liters of ascites should be removed during the procedure. This can avoid the dissection of fluid into the scrotum and subcutaneous tissues. Placement of chromic sutures of the deep planes, following the procedure, may also aid to avoid such complications. Albumin replacement should be carried as necessary to avoid circulatory collapse and renal failure in patients with cirrhosis and ascites.

After the procedure is completed the second trocar is removed under direct visualization while assessing for trocar site bleeding complications and then the original trocar is removed after evacuation of the pneumoperitoneum. The incision sites are sutured and then covered with sterile bandages.

Post-procedure observation periods have varied from 3 to 24 h and complication rates appear to be comparable.

4. COMPLICATIONS

Careful patient selection and proper training in the performance of the procedure training can help avoid or minimize the rate of complications (Table 3). Anatomic variations can lead to bleeding or perforation. Frail patients and those with extensive comorbidities may not withstand a minor complication. Generally, complications are related to inexperience of the operator, anesthesia/sedation-related issues, placement of the Veress needle or trocar, and liver biopsy related bleeding. Minor complications include vasovagal reactions, subcutaneous emphysema, abdominal pain, nausea and vomiting [10,11].

Table 3. Frequency of complications in laparoscopy.

Series (year)	Total procedures	Minor	Major	Mortality, %
Bruehl (1966)	63,845	590 (1)	174 (0.3)	18 (0.03)
Barry *et al.* (1978)	238	3 (1.2)	3 (1.2)	1 (0.4)
Kane and Krejs (1984)	603	31 (5.1)	14 (2.3)	3 (0.49)
Henning (1985)	11,017	NA	3 (0.03)	1 (0.01)
DeGroen *et al.* (1987)	1121	105 (9.4)	20 (1.8%)	1 (0.04)
Phillips *et al.* (1987)	313	9 (2.9)	3 (0.09)	0
Herrera *et al.* (1989)	100	2 (2.0)	1 (1)	0
Crantock *et al.* (1994)	200	1 (0.5)	2 (1)	0
Vargas *et al.* (1995)	1794	31 (1.7)	8 (0.45)	1 (0.06)

Veress needle insertion may cause bleeding or perforation of intra-abdominal structures. Liver biopsy site bleeding can be controlled with local tamponade with a probe, or heater or bicap application, or it can also be controlled with the topical application of thrombin. Caution is needed with coagulation devices if nitrous oxide is the insufflating gas because of the risk of an explosion. Hemobilia as a result of liver biopsy is mainly seen in patients with portal hypertension. In patients with multiple surgeries, bacterial peritonitis or tuberculous peritonitis, there is a risk of bowel perforation, primarily because of the likelihood of multiple adhesions. In case a bowel perforation is identified, the trocar should be left in place until a surgical assessment has been completed. In case bleeding is visualized from the trocar insertion site while withdrawing it, Avitene plugs can be placed within the trocar's track and/or the site can be surgically intervened to close the bleeding epigastric vessel [10,11].

A modest degree of shoulder-tip pain in the postoperative period occurs in 50–60%. A trial with low-pressure CO_2 pneumoperitoneum of 9 mmHg compared to 13 mmHg of regular pneumoperitoneum demonstrated benefits in the incidence of postoperative shoulder-tip pain. In the lower pressure group 11% of patients reported pain vs. 32% in the normal pressure group. The length of the procedure did not differ when both groups were compared [11].

If the pneumoperitoneum volume exceeds 2 l, cardiovascular complications may arise due to decreased venous return. Hypoventilation may also be caused by over-insufflation.

REFERENCES

[1] http://www.laparoscopy.com/shows/lapstry2.htm, History of Laparoscopy Website, Last accessed 6/19/03.

[2] Karnam, U.S. and Reddy, K.R. (2002) Diagnostic laparoscopy: an update. *Endoscopy* **34**(2), 146–153.

[3] Haydon, G.H. and Hayes, P.C. (1997) Diagnostic laparoscopy by physicians: we should do it. *Q. J. Med.* **90**, 297–304.

[4] Schneider, A.R.J., Eickhoff, A. and Riemann, J.C. (2001) Diagnostic laparoscopy. *Endoscopy* **33**(1), 55–59.

[5] Boyd, W.P. and Nord, H.J. (1998) Diagnostic laparoscopy. *Endoscopy* **30**, 189–197.

[6] Schneider, A.R. and Benz, C. (2001) Minilaparoscopy versus conventional laparoscopy in the diagnosis of hepatic diseases. *Gastrointest. Endosc.* **53**, 771–775.

[7] Crantock, L.R.F., Dillon, J.F. and Hayes, P.C. (1994) Diagnostic laparoscopy and liver disease: experience of 200 cases. *Aust. NZ Med.* **24**, 258–262.

[8] Ribeiro, A., Reddy, R., Bernstein, D.E., Roth, D., Jeffers, L. and Schiff, E.R. (1997) Laparoscopic evaluation of liver disease in chronic renal failure prior to renal transplantation. *Gastrointest. Endosc.* **45**(6), 503–507.

[9] Cardi, M., Muttillo, I.A., Amadori, L., Petroni, R., Mingazzini, P., Barillari, P., Lisi, D. and Bolognese, A. (1997) Superiority of laparoscopy compared to ultrasonography in diagnosis of widespread liver diseases. *Dig. Dis. Sci.* **42**(3), 546–548. Study of 210 patients with chronic liver diseases.

[10] Vargas, C., Jeffers, L.J., Bernstein, D., Reddy, K.R., Munnangi, S., Behar, S., Scott, C., Parker, T. and

Schiff, E.R. (1995) Diagnostic laparoscopy: a 5-year experience in a hepatology training program. *Am. J. Gastroenterol.* **90**(8), 1258–1262.

[11] Reddy, K.R., Mallat, D. and Jeffers, L.J. (1999) *Evaluation of the Liver: Liver Biopsy and Laparoscopy*. Schiff's Diseases of the Liver, 8th edition (Lippincott Williams & Wilkins, Philadelphia, PA).

[12] Poniachik, J., Bernstein, D.E., Reddy, K.R., Jeffers, L.J., Coelho-Little, M.E., Civantos, F. and Schiff, E.R. (1996) The role of laparoscopy in the diagnosis of cirrhosis. *Gastrointest. Endosc.* **43**, 568–571.

[13] Jalan, R., Harrison, D.J., Dillon, J.F., Elton, R.A., Finlayson, N.D. and Hayes, P.C. (1995) Laparoscopy and histology in the diagnosis of chronic liver disease. *Q. J. Med.* **88**, 559–564.

[14] Shiraki, K., Shimizu, A., Takase, K., Suzuki, A., Tameda, Y. and Nakano, T. (2001) Prospective study of laparoscopic findings with regard to the development of hepatocellular carcinoma in patients with hepatitis C virus-associated cirrhosis. *Gastrointest. Endosc.* **53**, 449–455.

[15] Ido, K., Nakazawa, Y., Isoda, N., Kawamoto, C., Nagamine, N., Ono, K., Hozumi, M., Sato, Y., Kimura, K. and Sugano, K. (1999) The role of laparoscopic US and laparoscopic US-guided aspiration biopsy in the diagnosis of multicentric hepatocellular carcinoma. *Gastrointest. Endosc.* **50**, 523–526.

[16] Seki, S., Sakaguchi, H., Kadoya, H., Morikawa, H., Habu, D., Nishiguchi, S., Shiomi, S., Kitada, T. and Kuroki, T. (2000) Laparoscopic microwave coagulation therapy for hepatocellular carcinoma. *Endoscopy* **32**(8), 591–597.

[17] Pratt, B.L. and Greene, F.L. (2000) Role of laparoscopy in the staging of malignant disease. *Surg. Clin. N. Am.* **80**(4), 1111–1126.

[18] Jimenez, R.E., Warshaw, A.L., Rattner, D.W., Willett, C.G., McGrath, D. and Fernandez-del Castillo, C. (2000) Impact of laparoscopic staging in the treatment of pancreatic cancer. *Arch. Surg.* **135**, 409–415.

[19] Reddy, K.R., Levi, J., Livingstone, A., Jeffers, L., Molina, E., Kilgerman, S., Bernstein, D., Kodali, V.P. and Schiff, E.R. (1998) Experience with staging laparoscopy in pancreatic malignancy. *Gastrointest. Endosc.* **49**(4) Part 1, 498–503. Superiority of laparoscopy to CT scan.

[20] Sans, M., Andreu, V., Bordas, J.M., Llach, J., Lopez-Guillermo, A., Cervantes, F., Bruguera, M., Mondelo, F., Montserrat, E., Teres, J. and Rodes, J. (1998) Usefulness of laparoscopy with liver biopsy in the assessment of liver involvement at diagnosis of Hodgkin's and non-Hodgkin's lymphomas. *Gastrointest. Endosc.* **47**(5), 391–395.

[21] Khan, K.N., Yamasaki, M., Yamasaki, K., Inoue, O., Yatsuhashi, H., Koga, M. and Yano, M. (2000) Proposed abdominal sonographic staging to predict severity of liver diseases: analysis with peritoneoscopy and histology. *Dig. Dis. Sci.* **45**(3), 554–564.

[22] Ohkawa, K., Hayashi, N., Yuki, N., Kasahara, A., Oshita, M., Mochizuki, K., Katayama, K., Fusamoto, H., Kato, M., Masuzawa, M., Yoshihara, H., Mukuda, T. and Kamada, T. (1997) Disease stage of chronic hepatitis C assessed by both peritoneoscopic and histologic findings and its relationship with response to interferon therapy. *Gastrointest. Endosc.* **45**(2), 168–175.

[23] Gigot, J.F., Glineur, D., Santiago Azagra, J., Goergen, M., Ceuterick, M., Morino, M., Etienne, J., Marescaux, J., Mutter, D., van Krunckelsven, L., Descottes, B., Valleix, D., Lachachi, F., Bertrand, C., Mansvelt, B., Hubens, G., Saey, J.P. and Schockmel, R. (2002) Laparoscopic liver resection for malignant liver tumors: preliminary results of a multicenter European study. *Ann. Surg.* **236**(1), 90–97.

[24] Chu, C.M., Lin, S.M., Peng, S.M., Wu, C.S. and Liaw, Y.F. (1994) The role of laparoscopy in the evaluation of ascites of unknown origin. *Gastrointest. Endosc.* **40**(3), 285–289.

[25] Majewski, W. (2000) Diagnostic laparoscopy for the acute abdomen and trauma. *Surg. Endosc.* **14**(10), 930–937.

[26] Gagne, D.J., Malay, M.B., Hogle, N.J. and Fowler, D.L. (2002) Bedside diagnostic minilaparoscopy in the intensive care patient. *Surgery* **131**(5), 491–496.

[27] Ertem, M., Karahasanoglu, T., Yavuz, N. and Erguney, S. (2002) Laparoscopically treated liver hydatid cysts. *Arch. Surg.* **137**(10), 1170–1173.

[28] Arch-Ferrer, J.E., Velazquez-Fernandez, D., Sierra-Madero, J., Lopez-Karpovitch, X., Angeles-Angeles, A., Gamino, R. and Herrera, M.F. (2003) Laparoscopic approach to fever of unknown origin. *Surg. Endosc.* **17**(3), 494–497. Equb 2002 Nov 20.

[29] Tuech, J.J., Pessaux, P., Regenet, N., Rouge, C., Bergamaschi, R. and Arnaud, J.P. (2002) Laparoscopic cholecystectomy in cirrhotic patients. *Surg. Laparosc. Endosc. Percutan. Tech.* **12**(4), 227–231.

[30] Senyuz, O.F., Yesildag, E., Emir, H., Tekant, G., Bozkurt, P., Sarimurat, N. and Soylet, Y. (2001) Diagnostic laparoscopy in prolonged jaundice. *J. Pediatr. Surg.* **36**(3), 463–465.

[31] Jeffers, L., Chalasani, N., Balart, L., Pyrsopoulos, N. and Erhardtsen, E. (2002) Safety and efficacy of recombinant factor VIIa in patients with liver disease undergoing laparoscopic liver biopsy. *Gastroenterology* **123**(1), 118–126.

Hepatology: A Practical Approach
B. Al Knawy, M.L. Shiffman, R.H. Wiesner (editors)

Chapter 5

Liver Biopsy – A Pathologist's Perspective

J. Craig

Department of Pathology, St Jude Medical Center, 101 E Valencia mesa Drive, Fullerton, CA 92835, USA

1. Types of Liver Biopsy and Complications 45
2. Indications for Liver Biopsy 47
    2.1 Diagnosis of liver biopsy at large US community hospital 22 months – 195 procedures 48
        2.1.1 Contraindications for liver biopsy 48
3. Processing of Tissue and Adequacy 48
4. Light Microscopy 49
5. Special Procedures 50
6. Interpretation Challenges in Hepatic Histopathology 50
References 53

Study of the liver corresponded with the general advances in microscopic anatomy during the 18th and 19th centuries. Although needle biopsy of the liver was promoted by the availability of the Vim-Silverman needle in 1938, the report by Menghini of a one-second needle biopsy technique in 1958 increased utilization of the technique. Furthermore, the widespread application of serum tests for liver evaluation (due to automation) and multiple biopsies in the same patient allowed more accurate correlation of hepatic histopathology and clinical diagnosis of acute and chronic hepatic disorders [1]. Intravenous drug use in the 1960s aided the rapid spread of hepatitis viruses and many liver units had opportunities to see multiple jaundice episodes in the same patient. Subsequent development of serologic tests for several hepatitis agents were widely applied after 1970 and the histologic features of the multiple agents in time lead to a number of proposals for nomenclature of chronic hepatic conditions. These classifications have undergone revision as new viruses and patterns have been recognized. For example, the term "unresolved viral hepatitis" was applied to hepatitis B virus infection that some authorities considered chronic persistent hepatitis. However, both terms are now replaced by newer diagnostic categories. The recent measurement of hepatitis C virus (by PCR) and the evolution of effective drug treatment have also stimulated a resurgence in the use of liver biopsy as a means to stage the degree of fibrosis and measure the drug treatment effect. There have been many drug company sponsored treatment trials in which the liver biopsy has served a critical part of the staging process and a central pathology review has indicated some variation in application of the histologic criteria for staging and scoring these needle biopsies. With a variety of drug treatment regimes available, the histologic scoring of liver biopsies is commanding a greater interest by clinicians. Whether all patients with chronic hepatitis C warrant biopsy is a subject of considerable debate [2]. Repeated biopsies may demonstrate histologic improvement even without biochemical evidence of response and cirrhotic patients may benefit from treatment of hepatitis C [3].

1. TYPES OF LIVER BIOPSY AND COMPLICATIONS

Although the percutaneous needle biopsy of liver is commonly performed in tertiary liver units, and in general hospitals by radiologists, there are several other options to consider for liver biopsy [4]. These multiple biopsy techniques include operative biopsy (wedge and needle at surgery often for nonhepatic reasons and performed to classify an incidental finding), directed needle biopsy utilizing ultrasound or CT scanning, transvenous access (transjugular needle biopsy), and fine needle aspiration (for focal lesions). Also, survey of endoscopic ultrasound centers has indicated a growing application of ultrasound guided endoscopic liver biopsy (i.e., left sided liver mass lesions biopsied through the stomach) [5]. Historically, many percutaneous liver needle biopsies were performed at the bedside of hospitalized patients. However, outpatient needle biopsy has become widespread because of improved biopsy needles, numerous outpatient centers with postoperative monitoring devices, and concern to reduce hospitalization costs. As this transition to outpatient biopsy occurred, reports described the safety and cost issues [6,7]. Complications of the percutaneous needle biopsy included pain or hypotension (6%), and are usually recognized within 3 h of the procedure. Cirrhosis accounted for an increased number of complications. One large series from a survey of many Italian centers reported that the complication rate of liver needle biopsy correlated with the type of liver disease and needle used [8]. Hemoperitoneum led to death only in patients with cirrhosis or malignant disease and the frequency was 9/100,000. The Tru-Cut needle was associated with three times the complication rate of the Menghini needle. Most complications were discovered within 2 h of the biopsy and nearly all complications were detected within 1 day. Complications reported in this large series included pleural effusion, pneumothorax, biliary peritonitis, and shock. A large series from the Mayo Clinic of 9212 biopsies revealed a mortality of 0.11% and the risk of bleeding was 10 times higher in the group with malignancy compared to benign liver disorders [9]. The Tru-Cut needle is preferred for cirrhotic liver biopsies [10]. Pain is also a common complication and a scoring system for this pain has been described which may serve to guide analgesia [11]. Guidelines for outpatient liver biopsy have been published [12]. A rare and unusual complication of needle aspiration is seeding of the needle tract with malignant cells [13]. Fortunately, this is rare and many needle biopsies have been performed in the setting of malignant tumor (both primary and metastatic) without apparent spread of tumor.

As additional radiographic procedures became implemented including CT scan, many patients were discovered to have focal hepatic lesions that included benign and malignant nodules. To reduce the complications and to increase accuracy of the biopsy procedure (for focal lesions), laparoscopic directed needle biopsy and percutaneous ultrasound directed needle biopsy were popularized. Furthermore, some patients have abnormal bleeding risks (low platelets or prolonged bleeding tests) and the transjugular needle biopsy technique was introduced [14]. Adequate tissue retrieval is a concern with the transjugular approach and in a large series of 200 patients over a 5-year period, 77% of the procedures yielded diagnostic tissue (see Figure 1 for comparison of needle biopsy fragments in the two procedures). In another series, the automated (transjugular) Tru-Cut needle was used with multiple passes, and the mean number of portal triads per patient exceeded 6 [15]. Because many liver diseases are generalized and affect the entire liver uniformly, the blind needle biopsy is appropriate. However, the biopsy needle diameter and type may

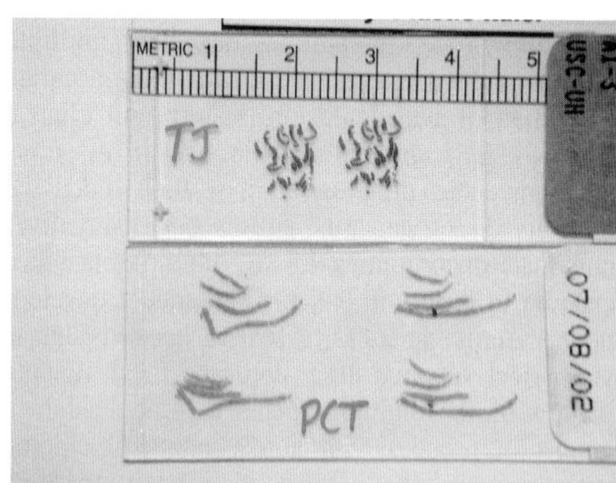

Figure 1. Needle biopsy yield requires multiple "sticks" to provide adequate tissue and enough portal areas to evaluate for chronic hepatitis. TJ is for transjugular entry and PCT is for percutaneous entry. Fragmentation in part is due to breakage after placing in formalin but transjugular biopsies are usually small fragments and multiple samples are needed for histology.

influence the amount of tissue removed. Aspiration needles may remove liver tissue but leave fibrous tissue behind and thus for the patient with cirrhosis, the cutting needle may be more reliable in obtaining the fibrous component needed for diagnosis. Needle bore size may also be important but some authorities recognize higher bleeding tendency with larger bore needles.

Ultrasound guidance of focal lesions has been a standard practice in many centers. An aspiration needle may reduce complications (compared to cutting needle) and the evaluation of smears obtained from the needle may allow justification to obtain more tissue or consider the specimen adequate (especially if cancer is suspected) [16]. Laparoscopic liver needle biopsy may occur during routine laparoscopy performed to assess the liver (and often associated with cholecystectomy). Small miliary lesions may be detected by viewing the liver surface and these may be small Meyenberg complexes or culture may prove the presence of tuberculosis. Thus, multiple small liver lesions must be considered as potential infectious granulomata and thus culture can be important. The sequence of additional radiographic tests and ultimate needle biopsy and timing of the biopsy are the subject of considerable debate and discussion [17]. Sensitivity and accuracy of these radiographic tests requires continued study and validation by pathologic confirmation. Unfortunately, needle biopsy may also be limited as small biopsies of focal nodular hyperplasia can be nondiagnostic and some hepatic nodules are not typical (or classifiable) with all radiographic and pathologic features of a known entity. In a recent large series based on pathologic examination, 20% of focal nodular hyperplasia lesions were nonclassical [18]. A combination of scoring radiographic and histologic features was suggested and this process may preclude the surgical removal of some atypical but benign lesions [19].

The indications for biopsy are described in numerous sources and depend in part on the nature of the clinical service. Major liver centers tend to list medical purposes and major transplant centers recognize the need to document the liver status with posttransplant biopsies. Cancer centers often recognize liver lesions due to staging procedures that require a biopsy to classify a nondiagnostic radiographic finding. After review of the indications, discussion of risks and benefits with a patient, and selection of the optimal technique (blind needle biopsy vs. directed biopsy), the consent must be completed and the procedure performed. The operator will help the pathologist by also providing key clinical data (such as purpose of the biopsy), and considering alternative uses of the tissue such as culture, and saving some tissue for metal analysis. Iron quantitation can also be determined from paraffin tissue as well [20].

2. INDICATIONS FOR LIVER BIOPSY

1. Evaluation of chronic liver disease (e.g., known hepatitis B or C).
2. Evaluation of abnormal liver tests after clinical assessment.
3. Evaluation of treatment of chronic liver disease (progression of cirrhosis).
4. Measurement of metals (iron or copper) in part of biopsy and diagnosis of hemachromatosis or Wilsons disease.
5. Diagnosis of focal defect (radiographic or visual at surgery).
6. Diagnosis of systemic disorder (sarcoidosis, etc.).
7. Obtain tissue for culture (TB, etc.).
8. Assessment of hepatomegaly.
9. Staging of systemic disease including cancer (metastatic colon, etc.).
10. Evaluation of posttransplant hepatic conditions.
11. Assessment of liver injury from drugs (e.g. methotrexate treatment).

Indications for liver biopsy vary with the nature of the hospital and medical group practice. A large nationwide survey of liver centers in university and referral centers revealed that the purpose of the biopsy in 1997 was primarily chronic hepatitis C evaluation (54%) in France [21]. Ultrasound guidance was utilized in 56% of the 2084 biopsies. In the western US, most centers perform outpatient liver needle biopsies in contrast to the 27% of procedures in the report from France. Indications for the liver biopsy performed in a large community general medical hospital are given below.

2.1 Diagnosis of liver biopsy at large US community hospital 22 months – 195 procedures

(1) Liver needle biopsy 51% (99/195)
  (a) Benign changes 30% (29/99)
  (b) Chronic hepatitis C 55% (55/99)
    (i) Cirrhosis in 16 of 55
  (c) Cirrhosis (not HCV) 5% (10/99)
  (d) Chronic hepatitis B 1% (2/99)
    (i) Cirrhosis in 1 of 2
  (e) Autoimmune hepatitis with cirrhosis 1% (1/99)
  (f) Malignant tumor 3%
    (i) lymphoma in 1
    (ii) metastatic ca in 2 (unsuspected)
(2) Fine needle aspiration of liver 15% (29/195)
  (i) Benign changes 24% (7/29)
  (ii) Metastatic cancer 76% (22/29)
(3) Liver biopsy during surgery 34% (67/195)
  (a) Cancer surgery 22% (15/67)
    (i) Bladder surgery 3/15 (HCC, metastatic bladder ca, negative)
    (ii) Colon cancer surgery 11/15 (9 with metastatic ca; 2 negative)
    (iii) Gastric cancer surgery 1/15 (metastatic ca)
  (b) Liver biopsy other noncancer surgery 78% (52/67)
    (i) Gall bladder surgery 29/52; 3 with incidental cancer
    (ii) Gyn surgery 3/52 (1 with metastatic cancer)
    (iii) Colon surgery, benign 2/52 (cirrhosis in 1)
    (iv) Peritoneal bx 1/52 (cirrhosis unsuspected)
    (v) Gastric resection (benign) 1/52 (cirrhosis discovered)
    (vi) Hernia repair 1/52 (incidental liver bx)
(4) Radiographic directed procedure biopsy for cyst or mass lesion 7% (14/195)
  (a) Benign cyst 4/14
  (b) Metastatic Ca (10/14)

In the community hospital setting (US), malignant tumors lead to liver biopsy and may account for up to 26% of the procedures in contrast to tertiary liver centers that encounter metastatic tumors less frequently. In a large national audit of 1500 liver biopsies in England performed in 1991, 38% of these biopsies were for malignant tumor (suspected or part of staging process) [22]. Liver biopsies (and fine needle aspirations) performed for tumor identification can be aided by pathology processing for immediate smear interpretation in order to guide confirmation of adequate tissue. Thus, additional passes for aspiration or biopsy as well as clinical history may enhance the interpretation.

Contraindications for liver biopsy have not been subjected to rigorous controlled trials and considerable clinical judgment is required to assess the risk vs. benefit. Some contraindications are listed below.

2.1.1 Contraindications for liver biopsy

1. Prolonged bleeding time or low platelets.
2. Uncooperative patient.
3. Lack of monitoring postprocedure.
4. Lack of blood for transfusion.
5. Suspected echinococcal cyst.
6. Suspected hemangioma.

There is limited data to indicate the safe range of specific values for platelets and coagulation times for liver biopsy. Relative contraindications for the liver biopsy include the presence of ascites because the liver fibrosis may not yield tissue by a cutting needle. Morbid obesity is a relative contraindication for percutaneous needle biopsy due to the long distance to the liver below the thick fat pad. Surprisingly, needle biopsy of hemangioma and angiosarcoma may be performed with no apparent clinical problem but these biopsies are unintentional.

3. PROCESSING OF TISSUE AND ADEQUACY

Routine needle biopsies are usually performed at the bedside (inpatient within a hospital), in a radiology suite, or outpatient surgical center, or within the surgical operating room (as part of a larger procedure such as colectomy or hysterectomy). The tissue is submitted in formalin (or other fixative such as B5) but in some settings, the fresh tissue may be submitted to pathology for analysis (such as rapid smear to determine if tumor is present) and possible subdivision of tissue for culture (especially if the patient has a fever), or metal analysis (iron quantitation).

Routine histopathologic processing is typically done overnight and a series of levels and stains is examined. We cut a long ribbon of paraffin and make 10 slides with several levels (cuts) on each blank. Different blanks (numbered in order) are submitted for routine hematoxylin and eosin (such as blanks 1, 5, and 10) and the other blank slides are utilized for iron, orcein, PAS with and without diastase, and trichrome. A typical needle biopsy of liver may yield 50–100 thin paraffin cuts that are mounted on glass. Most laboratories cut about half way through the block for routine work and then as recuts are requested, the block is refaced and more cuts are made. A continuing problem in nationwide trials is that the block is requested for additional cuts, and the originating laboratory will cut more sections and these additional blank slides may be incomplete since the block may be cut nearly through. Although, the clinician (operator) submits a single or multiple long cores of liver tissue in formalin, during transport to the pathology laboratory, many of these cores break apart and the final slides may have numerous fragments (especially if from a cirrhotic liver).

What is an adequate biopsy? Clearly, a biopsy that yields the correct diagnosis is adequate. With more complete information and progress in classification and staining techniques, some old needle or wedge biopsies become adequate. In general for needle biopsy of the liver, at least four portal areas are preferred for review. But defining a portal area (especially at the edge of the needle fragment) may be difficult and careful systematic search of all levels is required. A careful study of the normal liver has indicated that 38% of portal areas did not contain a portal vein, 7% did not contain a bile duct, and 9% did not contain a hepatic artery [23]. Portal dyads (which lack one of the three structures, bile duct, portal vein, or hepatic arteriole) are common. The smallest portal area may be a bile duct part, some fibrous tissue, a few lymphocytes, and perhaps a vascular structure. Some studies have required a certain length for adequacy (such as 1.5 cm) but this is not always reliable as the complete portal areas are preferred for scoring of many chronic disease patients.

4. LIGHT MICROSCOPY

A systematic review of the histologic features is critical in order to be complete. One approach is to follow the blood flow and count the portal areas, describe the portal components in sequence (bile ducts, vascular structures, limiting plate, lymphocytes, and other cells), and then the lobule and terminal hepatic venule. Within the lobule several changes are important such as appearance of hepatocytes, sinusoidal lining cells (Ito cells), and presence or absence of sinusoidal collagen. Various terms may be applied to the liver lobule and the microanatomy [24]. The typical Menghini needle biopsy is 1.8 cm (±0.8) long and has an average of seven fragments (range 2–13) in normal patients without the contribution of liver disease or fibrosis that would likely increase the fragmentation. Serial sections and staining (with keratin markers) of a single biopsy indicates the canals of Hering extend into part way into the lobule from biliary connections in the portal area [25]. Polarized light may also detect crystals in portal macrophages and this is a result of prior intravenous drug use (talc) [26].

Interpretation and description of the biopsy without reference to clinical data is desirable for the first impression and then after referring to the clinical details, a more astute analysis may be rendered. However, because many biopsy procedures are performed by radiologists without contact with clinical details and the history and laboratory data provided to the pathologist is minimal.

Diagnosis of cirrhosis on a needle biopsy is a recurring challenge as the small fragments may be from separate cirrhotic nodules and the dense fibrous tissue may not be removed during the biopsy process (see Figure 2b). If cirrhosis is present, about 80% of the needle biopsies will reflect diagnostic tissue. Furthermore, there is recent concern for regression of cirrhosis especially following drug treatment [27].

Wedge biopsies may be subject to difficulties in interpretation due to subcapsular fibrosis. The inferior border of the liver is a favorite location for the surgeon

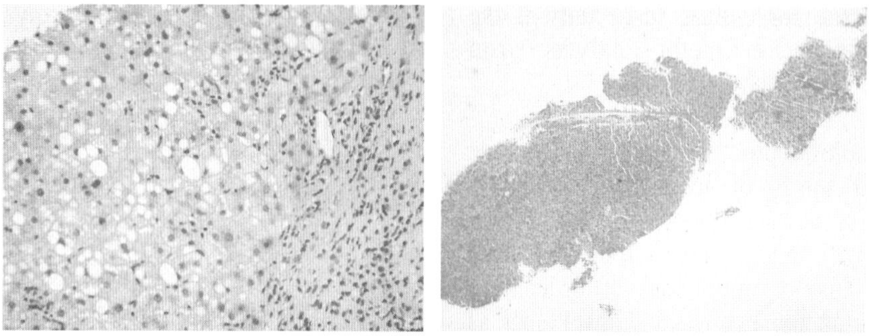

(a) (b)

Figure 2. (a) Interface hepatitis in chronic hepatitis C: there is near continuous lymphocytic spread beyond limiting plate into the adjacent lobule. × 400. (b) Trichrome stain of possible regenerative nodule. The upper end of the central fragment has a rim of collagen around one half the nodule. This is likely a true regenerative nodule in contrast to a tangential section of a portal area. Deeper sections may help resolve the issue (with more evident fibrosis or only a few bile ducts to indicate a tangential section of a large portal area). × 150.

and occasionally the fibrosis appears more dramatic than a needle biopsy of the same liver. The degree of subcapsular fibrosis has been debated [28]. Surgical retraction of the liver region may produce a prominent acute inflammatory reaction within the sinusoids and must not be misinterpreted. Furthermore, the wedge biopsy may be performed for scattered small nodules that on microscopic examination are von Meyenburg complexes. Such small nodules are easily mistaken as metastatic carcinoma by both surgeon and pathologist (at the time of frozen section).

5. SPECIAL PROCEDURES

Immunohistochemical staining is available for many hepatic related antigens but may not be needed if the clinical history and test results are provided. For example, staining for hepatitis B surface antigen is readily performed and is a reliable marker for chronic hepatitis B, and the cytoplasmic staining is abundant in scattered cells (see Figure 3). However, this immunotest result is not needed if the serum hepatitis B surface antigen is already measured.

Distinction of hepatocellular adenoma from carcinoma can be very difficult on histologic grounds alone. Adequate sampling of the tumor is essential and thus a needle biopsy may provide a bland tumor and other techniques may be applied. Comparative genomic hybridization has been applied to this problem and well-differentiated HCC may contain chromosomal alterations diagnostic of carcinoma [29]. This technique has not be accepted or widely applied.

Treatment of focal hepatic lesions (such as hepatocellular carcinoma or metastatic carcinoma) by radiofrequency ablation may be assessed by needle biopsy and performance of histochemical staining [30]. Routine stains are unreliable for recognition of cell death in the early phases of such treatment and the enzyme histochemical reactions reveal cell viability. Typically additional radiographic study and follow-up of serum markers may help assess treatment as histochemical staining is not widely available.

6. INTERPRETATION CHALLENGES IN HEPATIC HISTOPATHOLOGY

Common interpretative problems in histopathology include: (1) scoring of chronic hepatitis; (2) distinction of hepatocellular proliferation (as focal nodular hyperplasia vs. adenoma vs. hepatocellular carcinoma); (3) diagnosis of adenocarcinoma in liver (hepatocellular carcinoma vs. cholangiocarcinoma vs. metastatic adenocarcinoma); (4) recognition of benign lesions such as angiomyolipoma.

Chronic hepatitis C is the major reason for liver biopsy in many liver centers and the main purpose is to determine the stage of fibrosis and the necrotizing activity. Repeated liver biopsy in chronic hepatitis C may help to identify the rate of fibrosis [31].

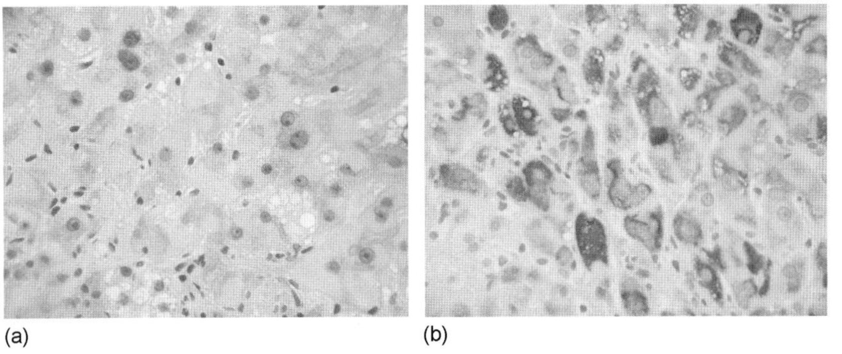

Figure 3. (a) Ground glass cells containing abundant Hbs Antigen (homogeneous lighter cytoplasmic change involving about 1/2 of cells). H & E × 400. (b) Immunoperoxidase stain with anti-HBs: Dark cytoplasmic staining of cells with HBs (ground glass cells) indicating chronic hepatitis B infection. × 400.

Even normal transaminase values in chronic hepatitis C may lead over time to cirrhosis and hepatocellular carcinoma [32]. To guide interpretation of the spectrum of histological changes, several scoring systems have been proposed including Knodell, Ishak, and the French Metavir. Although these systems have widespread application in clinical research trials, application to routine liver biopsy interpretation may not be warranted [33]. As the recent trials for chronic hepatitis C have progressed and been completed by several pathologists at major tertiary centers, it is clear that there is considerable opinion about how to apply these descriptive terms and systems. In general, most pathologists are scoring low compared to the "trial center" pathologists. As a general rule, review of all prior biopsies and re-scoring at the same time is advised as the individual pathologist threshold for the scoring will change in time. Thus, re-scoring will assist the clinician in evaluating the benefit of therapy. A popular system introduced in 1980, the Knodell system has four components (periportal inflammation, lobular inflammatory activity, portal inflammation, and fibrosis) [34]. Some criteria for each category were included in the initial description but application of these criteria has not been widely practiced. The first category is nonlinear (in scores, as there is no 2) and includes bridging necrosis. The first category is interface hepatitis or piecemeal necrosis. To apply the score to piecemeal necrosis, one reviews all portal areas (at least 4 needed) and a score of one is for minimal changes in a few areas (in contrast to 0), a score of 3 (there is no 2) for moderate activity with several portal areas with less than 1/2 the circumference altered by lymphocytes exuding into the adjacent cords, and a score of 4 if more than 50% of the portal areas have more than 50% of the circumference activated. Thus, with partial portal areas, there is considerable judgment required (see Figure 2). Similarly with the second category of lobular inflammation, one counts the number of small aggregates of mononuclear cells that reflect cell necrosis. If there are multiple areas in a single lobule, then this is scored as marked. The fibrosis score requires judgment for the presence of regenerative nodules or bridging fibrosis. Fragmentation interferes with the accuracy of this score and deeper cuts and review of all special stains is critical (such as iron stain to see another level of the same marginal "nodule"). Other systems for scoring are the Ishak and Metavir [35,36].

Hepatocellular proliferations may include focal nodular hyperplasia as well as hepatocellular adenoma. This distinction may be challenging because of sampling variation as well as incomplete development of the lesion [37]. Distinction of well-differentiated hepatocellular carcinoma from a macroregenerative nodule (with or without dysplasia) may be very difficult in minute samples and sampling may also play a role. Cytologic criteria for this distinction are fairly reliable (especially with experience) and many fine needle aspiration samples include microfragments that may be diagnostic in up to 75% of lesions [38]. For the diagnosis of focal hepatocellular lesions, it may be helpful to obtain a separate needle core biopsy from a nonlesion area as a control for staining and hepatocytes cell size.

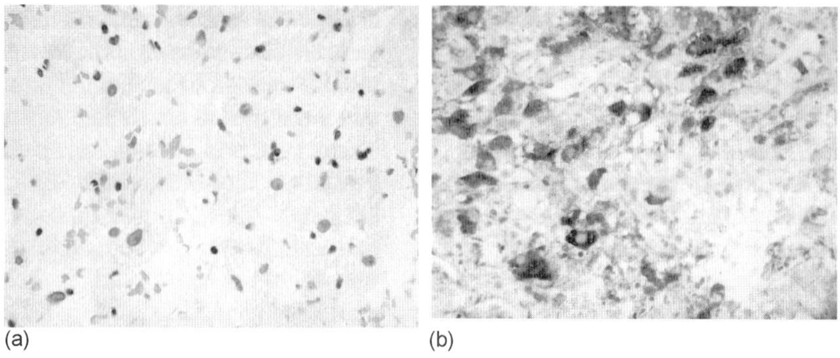

Figure 4. (a) A 3 cm solitary lesion by CT scan with FNA showing small clusters of vacuolated large cells with some features of hepatocellular carcinoma. H & E × 300. (b) HMB-45 immunostain with dramatic strong staining of cytoplasm indicating the diagnosis is angiomyolipoma (benign). × 200.

Although multiple biopsies are not obtained in many such situations, the ultimate interpretation of the small fragments may be aided by a separate fragment of "normal" nonlesional tissue. Many liver biopsies include portions of a malignant neoplasm and often these are easily classified to a primary site if such a site is already known. However, the distinction of primary hepatocellular carcinoma from benign and metastatic tumor can be very difficult. Development of a specific hepatocyte marker (HepPar 1) has greatly aided recognition of hepatocellular carcinoma and its distinction from metastatic carcinoma [39]. Although the canalicular staining pattern by CEA has been useful to recognize hepatocellular carcinoma, the diffuse cytoplasmic staining by HepPar1 is very useful. Primary liver tumors that mimic hepatocellular carcinoma include angiomyolipoma and inflammatory pseudotumor [40]. Staining for HMB 45 is important in identification of large cells from angiomyolipoma and this staining pattern may be diagnostic in fine needle aspiration samples (see Figure 4) [41]. Cytokeratin 7, 19, and 20 staining patterns are used to separate various metastatic and primary liver tumors [42]. Poorly differentiated hepatocellular carcinoma may mimic many other tumors and the HepPar1 is useful. Metastatic adenocarcinoma may also be identical in appearance to cholangiocarcinoma. Metastatic neuroendocrine carcinoma to the liver may produce a very similar pattern by routine H & E staining. Careful search for the trabecular growth pattern with the wrapping layer of endothelium around small nests of cells (with prominent nucleoli) is necessary to diagnose the hepatocellular carcinoma whereas the neuroendocrine carcinoma lack nucleoli and the endothelial wrapping around the nests of cells. A question of neuroendocrine differentiation should prompt a chromogranin and synaptophysin immunostain that are strikingly positive. Diagnosis of fibrolamellar carcinoma is also easy if the needle sample includes both the large eosinophilic hepatocytes and the lamellar fibrosis [43]. This tumor has a distinctive histologic appearance and better outcome than usual hepatocellular carcinoma. Fibrotic nodules may be sclerosed hemangiomas but careful search of the sclerotic tissue for small clusters of malignant cells is critical as epithelioid hemangioendothelioma and metastatic carcinoma can produce large fibrotic areas that at first glance seem benign (see Figure 5).

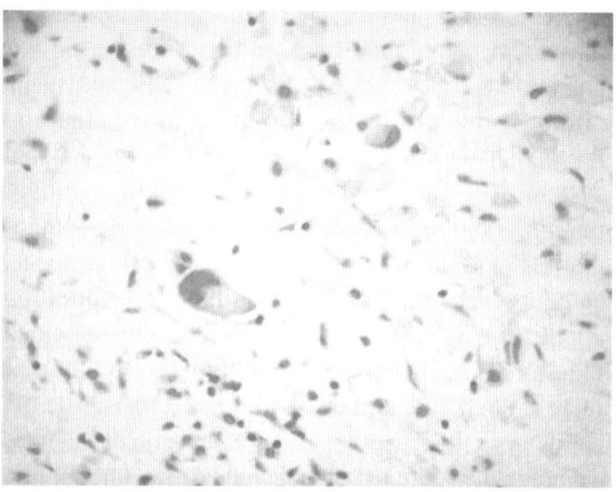

Figure 5. Sclerotic nodule with a few rare metastatic carcinoma cells. Careful search and deeper sections of a block are needed to find the small foci of cancer clusters in this biopsy that may otherwise resemble a sclerotic hemangioma. H & E × 400.

REFERENCES

[1] Menghini, G. (1958) One-second needle biopsy of the liver. *Gastroenterology* **35**, 190–199.

[2] Saadeh, S., Cammell, G., Carey, W.D. *et al.* (2001) The role of liver biopsy in chronic hepatitis C. *Hepatology* **33**, 196–200.

[3] Heathcote, E.J., Shiffman, M.L., Cooksleyl, G.E. *et al.* (2000) Peg interferon α-2a in patients with chronic hepatitis C and cirrhosis. *N. Engl. J. Med.* **343**, 1673–1680.

[4] Bravo, A.A., Sheth, S.G. and Chopra, S. (2001) Current concepts: liver biopsy. *N. Engl. J. Med.* **344**, 495–500.

[5] TenBerge, J., Hoffman, B.J., Hawes, R.H. *et al.* (2002) EUS-guided fine needle aspiration of the liver: indications, yield, and safety based on an international survey of 167 cases. *Gastrointest. Endosc.* **55**, 859–862.

[6] Perrault, J., McGill, D.B., Ott, B.J. *et al.* (1978) Liver biopsy: complications in 1000 patients and outpatients. *Gastroenterology* **74**, 103–106.

[7] Garcia-Tsao, G. and Boyer, J.L. (1993) Outpatient liver biopsy: how safe is it? *Ann. Intern. Med.* **118**, 150–153.

[8] Piccinino, F., Sagnelli, E., Pasquale, G. *et al.* (1986) Complications following percutaneous liver biopsy. A multicentre retrospective study on 68276 biopsies. *J. Hepatol.* **2**, 165–172.

[9] McGill, D.B., Rakela, J., Zinsmeister, A.R. *et al.* (1990) A 21 year experience with major hemorrhage after percutaneous liver biopsy. *Gastroenterology* **99**, 1396–1400.

[10] Colombo, M., Del Ninno, E., de Franchis, R. *et al.* (1988) Ultrasound-assisted percutaneous liver biopsy: superiority of the Tru-Cut over the Menghini needle for diagnosis of cirrhosis. *Gastroenterology* **95**, 487–489.

[11] Castrea, L., Negre, I., Samii, K. *et al.* (1999) Pain experienced during percutaneous liver biopsy. *Hepatology*, 1529–1530.

[12] Jacobs, W.H. and Goldberg, S.B. (1989) Statement on outpatient percutaneous liver biopsy. *Dig. Dis. Sci.* **34**, 322–323.

[13] Hamazaki, K., Matsubara, N., Mori, M. *et al.* (1995) Needle tract implantation of hepatocellular carcinoma after ultrasonically guided needle liver biopsy: a case report. *Hepatogastroenterology* **42**, 601–606.

[14] Corr, P., Beningfield, S.J. and Davey, N. (1992) Transjugular liver biopsy: a review of 200 biopsies. *Clin. Radiol.* **45**, 238–239.

[15] De Hoyos, A., Loredo, M.L., Martinez-Rios, M.A. *et al.* (1999) Transjugular liver biopsy in 52 patients with an automated Trucut-type needle. *Dig. Dis. Sci.* **44**, 177–180.

[16] Buscarini, L., Fornari, F., Bolondi, L. *et al.* (1990) Ultrasound-guided fine-needle biopsy of focal liver lesions: techniques, diagnostic accuracy and complications. A retrospective study on 2091 biopsies. *J. Hepatol.* **11**, 344–348.

[17] Ros, P.R. and Davis, G.L. (1998) The incidental focal liver lesion: photon, proton, or needle? *Hepatology* **27**, 1183–1191.

[18] Nguyen, B.N., Flejou, J., Terris, B. *et al.* (1999) Focal nodular hyperplasia. A comprehensive pathologic study of 305 lesions and recognition of new histologic forms. *Am. J. Surg. Pathol.* **23**, 1441–1454.

[19] Fabre, A., Audet, P., Vilgrain, V. *et al.* (2002) Histologic scoring of liver biopsy in focal nodular hyperplasia with atypical presentation. *Hepatology* **35**, 414–420.

[20] Olynyk, J.K., O'Neill, R., Britton, R.S. *et al.* (1994) Determination of hepatic iron concentration in fresh and paraffin-embedded tissue: diagnostic implications. *Gastroenterology* **106**, 674–677.

[21] Cadranel, J., Rufat, R., Degos, F. *et al.* (2000) Practice of liver biopsy in France: results of a prospective nationwide survey. *Hepatology* **32**, 477–481.

[22] Jenkins, D., Gilmore, I.T., Doel, C. *et al.* (1995) Liver biopsy in the diagnosis of malignancy. *Q. J. Med.* **88**, 819–825.

[23] Crawford, A., Lin, X. and Crawford, L.M. (1998) The normal adult human liver biopsy: a quantitative reference standard. *Hepatology* **28**, 323–331.

[24] Saxena, R., Theise, N.D. and Crawford, J.M. (1999) Microanatomy of the human liver – exploring the hidden interfaces. *Hepatology* **30**, 1340–1346.

[25] Theise, N.D., Saxena, R., Portmann, B.C. *et al.* (1999) The canals of Hering and hepatic stem cells in humans. *Hepatology* **30**, 1425–1433.

[26] Allaire, G.S., Goodman, Z.D., Ishak, K.G. *et al.* (1989) Talc in liver tissue of intravenous drug abusers withchronic hepatitis. *Am. J. Clin. Pathol.* **92**, 583–588.

[27] Wanless, I.R., Nakashima, E. and Sherman, M. (2000) Regression of human cirrhosis. *Arch. Pathol. Lab. Med.* **124**, 1599–1607.

[28] Petrelli, M. and Scheuer, P.J. (1967) Variation in subcapsular liver structure and its significance in the interpretation of wedge biopsies. *J. Clin. Pathol.* **20**, 743–748.

[29] Wilkens, L., Bredt, M., Flemming, P. *et al.* (2001) Differentiation of liver cell adenomas from well-differentiated hepatocellular carcinomas by comparative genomic hybridization. *J. Pathol.* **193**, 476–482.

[30] Morimoto, M., Sugimori, K., Shirato, K. *et al.* (2002) Treatment of hepatocellular carcinoma with radiofrequency ablation: radiologic–histologic correlation during follow-up periods. *Hepatology* **35**, 1467–1475.

[31] Poynard, T., Bedossa, P., Opolonn, P. *et al.* (1997) Natural history of liver fibrosis progression in patients with chronic hepatitis C. *Lancet* **349**, 825–832.

[32] Civiidini, A., Rebucci, C., Sillini, E. *et al.* (2001) Is the natural history of hepatitis C virus carriers with normal aminotransferase really benign? *Gastroenterology* **121**, 1526–1527.

[33] Brunt, E. (2000) Grading and staging the histopathological lesions of chronic hepatitis: the Knodell histology activity index and beyond. *Hepatology* **31**, 241–246.

[34] Knodell, R.G., Ishak, K.G., Black, W.C. *et al.* (1981) Formulation and application of a numerical scoring system for assessing histological activity in asymptomatic chronic active hepatitis. *Hepatology* **1**, 431–435.

[35] Ishak, K., Baptista, A., Bianchi, L. *et al.* (1995) Histological grading and staging of chronic hepatitis. *Hepatology* **22**, 696–699.

[36] French METAVIR Cooperative Study Group (1994) Intraobserver and interobserver variations in liver biopsy interpretation in patients with chronic hepatitis C. *Hepatology* **20**, 15–20.

[37] Biolac-Sage, P., Balabaud, C. and Wanless, I. (2001) Diagnosis of focal nodular hyperplasia. Not so easy. *Am. J. Surg. Pathol.* **25**, 1322–1325.

[38] Longchampt, E., Patriarche, C. and Fabre, M. (2000) Accuracy of cytology vs. microbiopsy for the diagnosis of well-differentiated hepatocellular carcinoma and macroregenerative nodule. *Acta Cytol.* **44**, 515–523.

[39] Leong, A.S.-Y., Sormunen, R.T., Tsui, W.M.S. *et al.* (1998) HepPar 1 and selected antibodies in the immunohistological distinction of hepatocellular carcinoma from cholangiocarcinoma, combined tumours and metastatic carcinoma. *Histopathology* **33**, 318–324.

[40] Craig, J.R. (1994) Mesenchymal tumors of the liver. Diagnostic Problems for the surgical pathologist. *Pathol. State Art Rev.* **3**, 141–160.

[41] Blasco, A., Vargas, J., de Agustin, P. *et al.* (1995) Solitary angiomyolipoma of the liver. Report of a case with diagnosis by fine needle aspiration biopsy. *Acta Cytol.* **39**, 813–816.

[42] Maeda, T., Kajiyama, K., Adachi, E. *et al.* (1996) The expression of cytokeratins 7, 19 and 20 in primary and metastatic carcinoma of the liver. *Mod. Pathol.* **9**, 901–909.

[43] Craig, J.R., Peters, R.L., Edmondson, H.A. *et al.* (1980) Fibrolamellar carcinoma of the liver: a tumor of adolescents and young adults with distinctive clinico-pathologic features. *Cancer* **46**, 372–379.

Section II

Acute and Chronic Liver Disease

Section Editor – M. Shiffman

Hepatology: A Practical Approach
B. Al Knawy, M.L. Shiffman, R.H. Wiesner (editors)

Chapter 1

Hepatitis A

Raymond S. Koff

University of Massachusetts Medical School, 55 Lake Avenue North, Worcester, MA 01655, USA

1. Introduction 57
   1.1 Definition 57
   1.2 Prevalence and incidence 58
   1.3 General demographics and epidemiology 58
2. Pathophysiology 59
3. Clinical Features 59
   3.1 Typical hepatitis A 59
   3.2 Relapsing hepatitis A 60
   3.3 Cholestatic hepatitis A 60
   3.4 Acute liver failure 60
   3.5 Unusual associations 61
4. Diagnosis 61
   4.1 Serologic tests 61
   4.2 Biochemical tests 61
   4.3 Imaging studies 62
   4.4 Pathological studies 62
5. Management 62
   5.1 Medical therapeutics 62
      5.1.1 Typical hepatitis A 62
      5.1.2 Relapsing hepatitis A 62
      5.1.3 Cholestatic hepatitis A 62
      5.1.4 Acute liver failure 62
6. Prevention 63
   6.1 General measures 63
   6.2 Immune globulin 63
   6.3 Hepatitis A vaccines 63
      6.3.1 Indications 64
      6.3.2 Dose and vaccination schedules 65
      6.3.3 Adverse effects 65
References 65

1. INTRODUCTION

1.1 Definition

Hepatitis A is an acute, necroinflammatory disease of the liver resulting from the immunological response to infection by the hepatitis A virus (HAV), a non-enveloped, enterically transmitted RNA-containing virus. HAV is the only member of the *Hepatovirus* genus within the Picornaviridae family of small RNA viruses. Only one serotype of human HAV has been identified although four distinct genotypes are recognized. Genotype I strains are predominant, accounting for about 80%

of worldwide isolates [1]. Although of no clinical utility, genotyping and nucleotide sequencing may be used epidemiologically to identify sources of outbreaks [2]. A single infection with any strain provides lifelong immunity to reinfection against all strains. HAV has been experimentally transmitted to non-human primates and its propagation in tissue culture has resulted in the development of inactivated, whole-virus particle vaccines. In infected human beings, replication of HAV occurs in the liver and possibly at low levels in intestinal epithelium [3]. Extrahepatic and extraintestinal sites of replication have not been identified. Because hepatitis A is not associated with a human intestinal carrier state or prolonged viremia, transmission from acutely infected individuals to susceptibles is required for its maintenance in nature. Chronic forms of HAV infection are unknown. As a consequence, eradication of hepatitis A by vaccination seems feasible.

1.2 Prevalence and incidence

Over several decades and well before the availability of inactivated vaccines, the incidence of hepatitis A has been declining in the United States. This may be a result of a general improvement in sanitary and hygienic standards, socioeconomic levels, and a reduction in household size. Nonetheless, hepatitis A still accounts for more than half of all reported cases of acute viral hepatitis and in some regions of the United States, attack rates remain high, occasionally reaching levels seen in developing countries where the disease is endemic. Nationwide attack rates, estimated at 9–10 cases per 100,000 persons in the mid-1990s, are now lower, probably closer to 4–5 cases per 100,000. The decline in incidence is reflected in national surveillance data as well as in a reduction of the seroprevalence of antibodies to HAV, an indicator of past infection. Currently, no more than 30% of the US population is anti-HAV positive and therefore immune to reinfection [4]. The age-specific anti-HAV seroprevalence for the civilian population of the United States in the period between 1988 and 1994 is shown in Table 1.

Table 1. Age-specific seroprevalence of anti-HAV (United States) (adapted from Ref. [4]).

Age group (years)	Seroprevalence (%)
6–11	9
12–19	12
20–29	19
30–39	25
40–49	33
50–59	47
≥60	63

The reduction in incidence and prevalence coupled with only limited vaccine use in the general population suggests that an increasing proportion of individuals is now susceptible to infection. Because disease severity increases with increasing age, hepatitis A will continue to be a clinically important problem until vaccination is more widely utilized.

Hepatitis A is widely distributed throughout the world. In many developing countries, the disease is endemic with very high infection rates beginning early in life and continuous circulation of the infection from infected individuals to susceptibles. Travelers to these areas from non-endemic regions are at high risk. With improvements in hygiene and sanitary standards, infection rates decline among children but the virus continues to circulate. As a consequence, older susceptible children and young adults are at risk and the proportion of symptomatic cases rises markedly. Furthermore, sudden outbreaks may emerge in these populations.

1.3 General demographics and epidemiology

Hepatitis A can present sporadically or in the form of mini-outbreaks, or large community-wide epidemics lasting months to years. Because it is shed in the feces of infected individuals in large amounts and because it demonstrates remarkable chemical and thermal resistance, HAV may survive in domestic sewage and sewage-contaminated river water. Fecal–oral spread is the predominant mode of transmission [5]. When transmitted by this route, the incubation period is about 30 days with a range of 15–50 days. HAV is shed in the feces as early as 2 weeks after exposure, reaches peak levels at the onset of symptoms, and then declines rapidly during the first 10 days of illness. Low, presumably non-infectious levels may continue to be shed for months. Viremia also tends to be short-lived but may persist for 1–3 months at levels detectable by highly sensitive techniques. This extended viremia after the acute illness may be responsible for the occasional bloodborne infection.

No risk factor can be identified in nearly half of reported cases in the US. Person-to-person contact involving young children, in whom infection may be asymptomatic, is often the most likely source of infection. In fact, young children and their older siblings generally have the highest attack rates in most but not all community-wide outbreaks. They are responsible for household spread and spread in day-care centers. The probability of infection within the household in the presence of one infected individual is estimated to be about 23% for transmission to a susceptible child and 15% for transmission to a susceptible adult [4]. Other risk factors include international travel to developing countries, injection and other illicit drug use, high-risk behaviors in men who have sex with men, and receipt of clotting factor concentrates, especially Factor VIII and IX. Common-source outbreaks have been linked to contamination of domestic drinking water, fruits, vegetables, and inadequately cooked or raw bivalve mollusks.

2. PATHOPHYSIOLOGY

Little is known about the entry of HAV into the liver following transport from the intestine into the bloodstream. Recent studies have suggested that intestinal IgA may serve as a carrier of HAV with uptake of the virus at the asialoglycoprotein receptor on the hepatocytes [6]. The virus is not thought to be directly cytopathic while replicating in the cytoplasm. Hepatocyte injury appears to be mediated by cellular immune mechanisms and release of cytokines. CD8+ T-lymphocytes, natural killer cells, and cytokines, including gamma-interferon, and possibly nitric oxide may contribute. Both hepatocyte necrosis and apoptosis with portal and lobular lymphocytic infiltration are evident in biopsy specimens.

3. CLINICAL FEATURES

The spectrum of illness in acute viral hepatitis is broad and highly variable. Young children may have no jaundice, no symptoms, no recognized illness, and therefore do not come to medical attention. Some patients (older children and young adults) with anicteric infection may have an abbreviated course characterized by transient gastrointestinal or upper respiratory symptoms with a day or two of fever, resembling a non-specific flu-like viral infection. In the absence of testing for liver chemistry abnormalities or serologic markers, these infections also may fail to be recognized.

3.1 Typical hepatitis A

Among patients with jaundice, the clinical presentation is often dramatic. The illness may begin with an abrupt prodromal constellation of symptoms which include malaise, fatigue, low-grade fever, anorexia, and nausea and vomiting. Arthalgias and myalgias may be present during this period which may last for a few days to a week or so. Rarely, the occurrence of fever, rash, and arthritis in hepatitis A may resemble juvenile rheumatoid arthritis.

With the onset of jaundice, which is almost invariably preceded by darkening of the urine, the prodrome resolves, although malaise and right upper quadrant discomfort may remain prominent. Non-specific, constitutional and gastrointestinal and hepatic symptoms and their reported frequencies are shown in Tables 2 and 3. In some patients distressing pruritus accompanies the development of jaundice.

Table 2. Non-specific, constitutional symptoms reported by adult patients with acute hepatitis A.

Symptom	Frequency (%)
Fatigue or lassitude	50–90
Fever or chilly sensation	30–75
Headache	25–75
Myalgias	15–50
Arthralgias	10–40
Sore throat	0–20

Table 3. Gastrointestinal and hepatic symptoms reported by adult patients with acute hepatitis A.

Symptom	Frequency (%)
Dark urine	70–95
Anorexia	40–90
Jaundice	40–80
Nausea or vomiting	25–90
Abdominal discomfort	35–65
Light colored stools	50–60

Physical examination may reveal minimal hepatomegaly, often with mild punch tenderness over the liver. The spleen may become palpable in no more than 20% of patients and posterior cervical lymphadenopathy is occasionally observed. Jaundice may deepen for several days but usually peaks during the second week and disappears slowly, together with pruritus, over the ensuing 2–8 weeks, except in the variant called cholestatic hepatitis A. For most patients with typical icteric hepatitis A, symptomatic recovery occurs as jaundice diminishes and before the complete resolution of biochemical abnormalities. Most infections run their course with full biochemical recovery anticipated within 3 months of the onset of symptoms in about 85% [7].

3.2 Relapsing hepatitis A

Between 3 and 20% of patients with apparently typical hepatitis A may experience a relapse during the recovery phase. This variant appears to be more common in children than in adults and, in the former, more than one relapse may occur. Because HAV again may be shed in the feces and viremia may be present during the relapse, affected patients may spread infection to others. Relapses typically occur within 18 weeks of the initial episode but may be seen as early as within 2 weeks of apparent recovery. Symptoms may closely resemble those of the initial episode and biochemical abnormalities may be similar. Occasionally, laboratory abnormalities may be either more severe or milder. Symptomatic relapses are variable in duration and their accompanying laboratory abnormalities may persist for weeks after clinical remission.

In a few patients with relapsing hepatitis A, a self-limited syndrome of transient arthritis, vasculitis, and cryoglobulinemia has been observed. Complete symptomatic, biochemical, and histologic recovery may be expected in all patients with relapsing hepatitis A.

3.3 Cholestatic hepatitis A

Cholestatic hepatitis A is an uncommon variant in which jaundice and pruritus are prolonged, lasting for 2–8 months. Serum bilirubin levels may exceed 20 mg/dl but rarely rise above 30 mg/dl. The serum aminotransferase levels are initially similar to those seen in typical hepatitis A and they may decline despite the prolonged jaundice. Serum alkaline phosphatase and serum cholesterol levels are variably elevated, and striking elevations of the former may be seen. Anorexia, diarrhea, and malaise may persist throughout the period of jaundice in some patients while in others jaundice and pruritus are the only symptoms. Complete recovery is to be expected in all patients.

3.4 Acute liver failure

Acute liver failure is the most dreaded complication of hepatitis A. It is most commonly seen in middle-aged and older patients, but it is also known to afflict children. Case-fatality rates are highest in patients over 50 years old. Acute liver failure also appears to be more common when hepatitis A superinfection occurs in the setting of pre-existing chronic liver disease, e.g., chronic hepatitis C [8]. Although less certain, it is also more likely to occur in hepatitis A patients with other co-morbid diseases, such as diabetes, and chronic cardiac and pulmonary diseases.

The predominant features of acute liver failure due to hepatitis A include progressive jaundice, alterations in mental status, and extensive prolongation of the prothrombin time, occurring within 2–8 weeks of the onset of the illness as defined by symptoms or jaundice. Serum aminotransferase levels may be strikingly elevated at the onset but typically decline despite disease progression. Serum albumin levels decline and Factor VII levels may be dramatically reduced. Life-threatening complications of acute liver failure include cerebral edema (typically without papilledema or specific computer-tomographic findings), renal failure with hypotension, metabolic abnormalities, sepsis, gastrointestinal bleeding, and the development of multi-organ system failure (respiratory and cardiac). Cerebral edema with uncal herniation appears to be the single most common cause of death in acute liver failure. Other characteristic metabolic features include hypoglycemia, hypokalemia, respiratory alkalosis, and hyponatremia, with a terminal lactic acidosis.

3.5 Unusual associations

Rarely, features of acute cholecystitis and pancreatitis have been reported in hepatitis A. Although renal failure is a characteristic feature of acute liver failure, in a few instances hepatitis A has been linked with transient renal failure that may require hemodialysis in the absence of evidence of acute liver failure. Another distinctly unusual phenomenon is the development of a transient, sensory neuropathy during the prodrome, acute phase, or recovery period of hepatitis A. The mechanisms underlying each of these phenomena are unknown.

4. DIAGNOSIS

4.1 Serologic tests

The diagnosis of HAV infection is based on serologic testing which is routinely available. As shown in Table 4, diagnosis of current or recent infection requires the detection in serum of anti-HAV of the IgM class. This antibody is often present during the week preceding the onset of symptoms and is almost invariably present during the acute phase of illness. Hence, a single serum sample obtained after the onset of symptoms should be diagnostic and repeated testing is unnecessary. The assay for IgM anti-HAV has been designed so that a positive test may remain positive for about 3–6 months. In rare instances, positive tests have been reported to persist for 1 year after the acute infection. Concomitantly with IgM anti-HAV, anti-HAV of the IgG class also may be present early in the acute phase of infection. This antibody persists for decades after recovery.

Table 4. Serologic tests of HAV infection.

Test	Interpretation
Total anti-HAV-negative	No HAV infection
Total anti-HAV-positive	Past or present HAV infection
IgM anti-HAV-positive	Present or recent (within 6 months) HAV infection
IgM anti-HAV-negative	Past infection, receipt of HAV immunoglobulin within past 2–3 months, or vaccination

The detection of IgG anti-HAV in the absence of the IgM anti-HAV is consistent with past infection, recent administration of immunoglobulin, or previous vaccination. However, it should be noted that detection of IgG anti-HAV following vaccination requires more specialized testing than routinely performed. In a patient with biochemical evidence of acute hepatitis, the presence of IgG anti-HAV without IgM anti-HAV strongly suggests that another disorder is responsible for the hepatitis.

Detection of HAV RNA in blood or stool by polymerase chain reaction is not widely available. It remains a research tool, too expensive and cumbersome for use in diagnosis.

4.2 Biochemical tests

The most prominent laboratory abnormality in hepatitis A is elevation of the serum aminotransferase levels. Although both enzyme levels are usually elevated, the alanine aminotransferase (ALT) is often slightly higher than the aspartate aminotransferase (AST). Peak levels for both are often between 400 and 5000 U/ml. Serum total bilirubin levels are also variably elevated, with a predominance of the direct (conjugated) fraction. In most jaundiced patients, total serum bilirubin levels do not exceed 10 mg/dl. When bilirubin levels are higher, the development of cholestatic hepatitis or acute liver failure should be considered. The latter is usually heralded by prolongation of the prothrombin time beyond 4–6 s over control values. However, striking elevations of total bilirubin and the unconjugated fraction of bilirubin may also be seen as a consequence of hemolysis in hepatitis A patients with underlying glucose-6-phosphate dehydrogenase deficiency or other disorders predisposed to hemolysis.

In most patients with uncomplicated hepatitis A, serum albumin levels are normal or only slightly depressed and prothrombin times are either normal or prolonged by no more than 1–3 s. Serum alkaline phosphatase levels are usually normal or mildly elevated to less than twice the upper limits of normal. Mild leukopenia and atypical lymphocytes may be present but hemoglobin levels are usually normal unless the illness is complicated by hemolysis. Thrombocytopenia is not expected. Although rarely encountered, aplastic anemia is a reported sequel in resolving hepatitis A. Hence, a late decline in hemoglobin, white cell count, or platelet counts is an ominous finding.

4.3 Imaging studies

As in other forms of acute viral hepatitis, imaging studies are usually unrevealing and generally unrewarding. The principal use of imaging studies, including ultrasound and CT examinations, is to exclude extrahepatic biliary obstruction in patients with cholestasis hepatitis A in whom a co-incidental obstructive disorder might be considered. The finding of a co-incidental disorder, e.g., choledocholithiasis, in this setting is exceedingly unusual. In acute liver failure, imaging studies may confirm a shrinking liver size but the absence of this finding should not exclude that diagnosis from consideration.

4.4 Pathological studies

With the development of sensitive and specific serologic testing for HAV infection, liver biopsy is not necessary for diagnosis.

5. MANAGEMENT

5.1 Medical therapeutics

5.1.1 Typical hepatitis A

Antiviral therapy for hepatitis A is not available. Inhibitors of the only proteinase known to be encoded by the virus, cysteine proteinase 3C, may have antiviral activity *in vitro*, but clinical studies of therapeutic efficacy are not yet available. Management is largely symptomatic, supportive, and almost always undertaken at home. Hospitalization is reserved for patients with refractory vomiting or severe anorexia resulting in dehydration and hypoglycemia or in whom features of acute liver failure are evident. No specific dietary restrictions are helpful and no recommendations other than to attempt to maintain adequate fluid and calorie intake can be made. Shifting the bulk of calories to breakfast and lunch may prove helpful since nausea usually progresses during the day. Alcohol and non-essential drugs are best avoided during the acute phase of illness with the exception of oral contraceptives, which may be continued without concern. Extreme physical activity should be avoided during the acute phase but mild exercise is not contraindicated. Enforced bed rest is not beneficial; the need for rest should be determined by the patient based on the severity of experienced weakness and fatigue. In general, patients return to their usual daily activities of work or school within several weeks of the onset of symptoms, when they feel ready to do so. It is not essential that all biochemical tests have returned to normal.

5.1.2 Relapsing hepatitis A

No specific therapy for relapsing hepatitis is available. Each episode is managed as in typical hepatitis A, with the expectation of full recovery.

5.1.3 Cholestatic hepatitis A

Although prospective, randomized, placebo-controlled clinical trials of treatment with corticosteroids or ursodeoxycholic acid are not available, anecdotal experiences suggest that the former may shorten the duration of symptoms and the latter may accelerate resolution of laboratory abnormalities. Whether or not intervention is used, all patients recover fully.

5.1.4 Acute liver failure

No specific treatment is available. Despite early hospitalization and prompt admission to an intensive care unit, survival rates have been as low 30% with only supportive management. Early referral to a center with a liver transplantation unit and with extensive experience in treating acute liver failure may permit survival in as many as 65%.

6. PREVENTION

6.1 General measures

In endemic regions of the developing world, improvements in economic conditions and sanitary standards, and the assurance of safe, potable water and food supplies are likely to reduce the risk of HAV infection. The use of immunoprophylaxis in these regions will become increasingly important as a concomitant control measure as the incidence of infection declines and disease severity increases. Until the risk declines, travelers to developing regions can be protected by pre-travel immunoprophylaxis and the avoidance of drinking water or ice of uncertain origin. Inadequately cooked bivalve mollusks and uncooked fruits and vegetables are also best avoided in such regions. In developed countries, such as the United States, with lower endemicity, further reductions in the frequency of outbreaks and the elimination of HAV will become feasible once universal early childhood immunization is implemented. This will not be achieved until HAV vaccines are combined with other pediatric vaccines in polyvalent preparations suitable for routine pediatric immunization. A combined HAV/HBV vaccine is currently available but in the United States it has yet to be approved for immunization of children.

6.2 Immune globulin

Immunoprophylaxis of hepatitis A may be achieved by passive transfer via intramuscular injection of anti-HAV in the form of human immune globulin (IG). IG preparations contain HAV-neutralizing IgG antibodies (IgG anti-HAV). Circulating levels of anti-HAV in the range of 10–20 mIU/ml, which are thought to be seroprotective, appear within 1–2 days after injection. Peak circulating levels of about 100 mIU/ml are reached within a few days. Protective efficacy against clinical disease may be achieved in 75–90% of immunized individuals for a period of 2–5 months, depending on the dose of IG administered. Thereafter, antibody levels decline and immunity wanes.

IG for intramuscular administration produced in the United States has a superb safety record but has been in short supply for a number of years. The availability of effective and safe inactivated HAV vaccines has reduced the need for IG in pre-exposure immunoprophylaxis. Pre-exposure prophylaxis with IG is still necessary for children less than 2 years of age (the vaccines are not approved for children under 2 years of age) and for travelers leaving shortly for endemic regions because vaccine-induced immunity may not be reached until 2 weeks after vaccine inoculation. Further studies are needed to determine whether vaccine alone will be sufficient in this setting. Until this is clarified, travelers may be given both IG and HAV vaccine concurrently at different deltoid sites; while peak anti-HAV titers may be slightly lower than after HAV vaccine alone, levels are sufficiently high to provide adequate protection and titers of anti-HAV after the second HAV vaccine dose are similar to those seen in individuals receiving two doses of vaccine alone [9].

IG is also indicated for post-exposure prophylaxis of household or sexual contacts of acutely infected index cases. The current recommendation is intramuscular administration of IG in a dose of 0.02 ml/kg body weight given as soon as possible after exposure. Protective efficacy is thought to decline if IG is given more than 2 weeks after exposure.

Use of IG in the control of community-wide outbreaks is likely to be wasteful of this product and is invariably ineffective. In fact, IG use may extend the duration of fecal excretion of virus and enhance transmission. IG is also likely to be ineffective in the control of common-source outbreaks.

6.3 Hepatitis A vaccines

Although a number of live and inactivated HAV vaccines are available elsewhere, the only two United States FDA-approved HAV vaccines comprise attenuated human HAV strains adapted to cell culture and then inactivated with formaldehyde. The close genetic relatedness of human HAV isolates suggests that all HAV infections should be preventable with vaccine [1] and, at least thus far, these whole-virus HAV vaccines have provided protection against infection by all recognized strains of human HAV.

The inactivated HAV vaccines (Havrix and Vaqta) are highly stable, have nearly similar immunogenicity [10], are likely to have similar effectiveness, and each has an excellent safety record. The major adverse event associated with vaccination has been transient pain and tenderness at the deltoid injection site. Headache and fever occur in no more than 15% of vaccinated subjects. Switching between vaccines does not impair immunogenicity [11] and HAV vaccines do not impair the immune response to other vaccines given concurrently [12].

Peak circulating anti-HAV levels following two vaccine doses approach those seen in natural infection and may be 100- to 300-fold higher than those observed following IG administration. Within a month after a single intramuscular dose, nearly 100% of vaccinees develop protective levels of antibody and circulating anti-HAV is detectable as early as 15 days in 70–98% of vaccinees. The inactivated HAV vaccines are highly immunogenic in children, adolescents, and adults, including those who are middle-aged and overweight [13]. However, as might be anticipated, HIV-positive individuals and other immunocompromised patients are less responsive than those who are immunocompetent.

Patients with advanced liver disease or recipients of liver transplants on immunosuppressing regimens are also less responsive [14,15]. As a consequence, immunization should be undertaken early following the diagnosis of chronic liver disease. In patients with milder disease, the anti-HAV immune response to vaccination appears adequate to provide protection from infection in nearly 95% of vaccinated individuals.

Although intradermal vaccine injection elicits anti-HAV, it is not generally recommended. Subcutaneous vaccine administration appears to be safe in children with hemophilia but antibody levels may be lower than in non-hemophilia siblings vaccinated by the intramuscular route. Jet injection of HAV vaccine provides adequate seroconversion rates but more local reactivity.

Based on studies of the rate of decline in circulating anti-HAV levels over time, it would appear that vaccine-induced humoral immunity following two doses may persist for 20–50 years. In individuals who lose detectable vaccine-induced anti-HAV, a rapid anamnestic response has been observed on re-exposure. HAV vaccine induction of specific memory B cells and a proliferative T-cell response [16] suggests that vaccine-induced protection may persist even after loss of antibody and may be lifelong.

HAV vaccine may be useful for post-exposure immunoprophylaxis but definitive, controlled clinical trials comparing vaccine to IG are not yet available. IG remains the standard in this setting.

6.3.1 Indications

Current recommendations of the Advisory Committee on Immunization Practices in the US call for vaccination of high-risk individuals (see Table 5) [17]. Other groups probably at increased risk for whom vaccination may be reasonable are listed in Table 6.

Table 5. High-risk populations recommended for HAV vaccination (adapted in part from Ref. [17]).

High-risk populations
Children in communities with HAV attack rates twice the national average or those experiencing periodic outbreaks
Children in communities with HAV attack rates above the national average (for consideration by responsible public health officials)
Travelers to endemic regions
Individuals from non-endemic regions working in HAV endemic countries
Individuals with chronic liver disease or recipients of liver transplants
Recipients of solvent/detergent treated clotting factor concentrates
Men who have sex with men
Injecting and non-injecting illicit drug users
Individuals who work with HAV or HAV-infected non-human primates
Food handlers, depending on local conditions (at discretion of local public health officials)

Table 6. Populations in whom HAV vaccination might be considered.

Sewage and waste-water treatment plant workers
Employees of day-care centers, pre-school centers, institutions for developmentally disadvantaged children and adults
Health care workers in neonatal intensive care units

Testing for susceptibility by pre-vaccination screening for anti-HAV should be considered in individuals who have lived in an endemic region, those with a probable history of hepatitis A, and those over 55 years of age.

6.3.2 Dose and vaccination schedules

The HAV vaccines are available in both adult and pediatric dose forms. While the pediatric formulations are FDA approved for use in children aged 2 years through 17 or 18 years, in Europe and other parts of the world they are licensed for use in children over 12 months of age. Available data indicate that their immunogenicity is good and they are well tolerated in toddlers between 12 and 24 months of age [18]. Although limited studies indicate that a single dose of the inactivated hepatitis A vaccines may confer detectable anti-HAV for at least 1 year in about 95% of vaccinated subjects, the vaccines are only FDA approved in a two-dose schedule with intervals between the first and second doses of 6–18 months.

For individuals 18 years of age or older who require protection against both hepatitis A and hepatitis B, a three-dose (0, 1, and 6 months) combined HAV/HBV vaccine (Twinrix) is FDA approved. It is highly immunogenic and well tolerated. A combined higher dose HAV/HBV vaccine, given in a two-dose schedule to children, adolescents, and adults appears to induce a similar immune response as the approved three-dose vaccine but remains in development [19,20].

6.3.3 Adverse effects

Inactivated HAV vaccines are well tolerated. Short-lived soreness, erythema, or swelling at the injection site is seen in about 50%. Side effects reported in less than 15% of vaccinated individuals include transient malaise, fatigue, headache, fever, anorexia, and nausea and vomiting. HAV use during pregnancy is unlikely to carry any specific risk for the developing fetus but should be reserved for situations in which the risk of acquisition of HAV infection is increased.

REFERENCES

[1] Robertson, B.H., Jansen, R.W., Khanna, B., Totsuka, A., Nainan, O.V., Siegl, G., Widell, A., Margolis, H.S., Isomura, S. and Ito, K. (1992) Genetic relatedness of hepatitis A virus strains recovered from different geographical regions. *J. Gen. Virol.* **73**, 1365–1377.

[2] Arauz-Ruiz, P., Sundqvist, L., Garcia, Z., Taylor, L., Visona, K., Norder, H. and Magnius, L.O. (2001) Presumed common source outbreaks of hepatitis A in an endemic area confirmed by limited sequencing within the VP1 region. *J. Med. Virol.* **65**, 449–456.

[3] Blank, C.A., Anderson, D.A., Beard, M. and Lemon, S.M. (2000) Infection of polarized cultures of human intestinal cells with hepatitis A virus: vectorial release of progeny virions through apical cellular membranes. *J. Virol.* **74**, 6476–6484.

[4] Meyerhoff, A.S. and Jacobs, R.J. (2001) Transmission of hepatitis A through household contact. *J. Viral Hepat.* **8**, 454–458.

[5] Koff, R.S. (1998) Hepatitis A. *Lancet* **351**, 1643–1649.

[6] Dotzauer, A., Gebhardt, U., Bieback, K., Gottke, U., Kracke, A., Mages, J., Lemon, S.M. and Vallbracht, A. (2000) Hepatitis A virus-specific immunoglobulin A mediates infection of hepatocytes with hepatitis A virus via the asialoglycoprotein receptor. *J. Virol.* **74**, 10950–10957.

[7] Koff, R.S. (1992) Clinical manifestations and diagnosis of hepatitis A virus infection. *Vaccine* **10**(Suppl. 1), S15–S17.

[8] Vento, S., Garofano, T., Renzini, C., Cainelli, F., Casali, F., Ghironz, G., Ferraro, T. and Concia, E. (1998) Fulminant hepatitis associated with hepatitis A virus superinfection in patients with chronic hepatitis C. *N. Engl. J. Med.* **338**, 286–290.

[9] Walter, E.B., Hornick, R.B., Poland, G.A., Tucker, R., Bland, C.L., Clements, D.A., Rhamstine, C.C., Jacobson, R.M., Brown, L., Giess, J.O., Harris, K.E., Wiens, B.L. and Nalin, D.R. (1999) Concurrent administration of inactivated hepatitis A vaccine with immune globulin in healthy adults. *Vaccine* **17**, 1468–1473.

[10] Ashur, Y., Adler, R., Rowe, M. and Shouval, D. (1999) Comparison of immunogenicity of two hepatitis A vaccines – VAQTA and HAVRIX – in young adults. *Vaccine* **17**, 2290–2296.

[11] Bryan, J.P., Henry, C.H., Hoffman, A.G., South-Paul, J.E., Smith, J.A., Creuss, D., Spieker, J.M. and de Medina, M. (2000) Randomized, cross-over, controlled comparison of two inactivated hepatitis A vaccines. *Vaccine* **19**, 743–750.

[12] Bock, H.L., Kruppenbacher, J.P., Bienzle, U., De Clercq, N.A., Hofmann, F. and Clemens, R.L. (2000) Does the concurrent administration of an inactivated hepatitis A vaccine influence the immune response to other travelers vaccines. *J. Travel Med.* **7**, 74–78.

[13] Bertino, J.S., Thoelen, S., Van Damme, P., Bryan, J.P., Becherer, P.R., Frey, S., Hayden, F.G., Marcus, L.C., Parenti, D.M., Sperling, M., Chan, I.S., Brown, L. and Nalin, D. (1998) A dose response study of hepatitis A vaccine in healthy adults who are ≥ 30 years old and weigh ≥ 77 kg. *J. Infect. Dis.* **178**, 1181–1184.

[14] Dumot, J.A., Barnes, D.S., Younossi, Z., Gordon, S.M., Avery, R.K., Domen, R.E., Henderson, J.M. and Carey, W.D. (1999) Immunogenicity of hepatitis A vaccine in decompensated liver disease. *Am. J. Gastroenterol.* **94**, 1601–1604.

[15] Arslan, M., Wiesner, R.H., Poterucha, J.J. and Zein, N.N. (2001) Safety and efficacy of hepatitis A vaccination in liver transplantation recipients. *Transplantation* **72**, 272–276.

[16] Cederna, J.B., Klinzman, D. and Stapleton, J.T. (2000) Hepatitis A virus-specific humoral and cellular immune responses following immunization with a formalin-inactivated hepatitis A vaccine. *Vaccine* **18**, 893–898.

[17] Centers for Disease Control and Prevention (1996) Prevention of hepatitis A through active or passive immunization: recommendations of the Advisory Committee on Immunization Practices (ACIP). *MMWR* **45**(RR-15), 1–30.

[18] Abarca, K., Ibanez, I., Flores, J., Vial, P.A., Safary, A. and Potin, M. (2001) Efficacy of hepatitis A vaccination in children aged 12–24 months. *Arch. Med. Res.* **32**, 468–472.

[19] Burgess, M.A., Rodger, A.J., Waite, S.A. and Collard, F. (2001) Comparative immunogenicity and safety of two dosing schedules of a combined hepatitis A and B vaccine in healthy adolescent volunteers: an open, randomised study. *Vaccine* **19**, 4835–4841.

[20] Greub, G., Genton, B., Safary, A., Thoelen, S. and Frei, P.C. (2001) Comparison of the reactogenicity and immunogenicity of a two injection combined high-dose hepatitis A and hepatitis B vaccine to those of Twinrix. *Vaccine* **19**, 1113–1117.

Hepatology: A Practical Approach
B. Al Knawy, M.L. Shiffman, R.H. Wiesner (editors)

Chapter 2
Hepatitis B Virus Infection

Philippe Merle, Fabien Zoulim and Christian Trepo

Service d'Hépato-Gastroentérologie, Hôpital de l'Hôtel-Dieu, 1 Place de l'Hôpital, 69288 Lyon Cedex 02, France

1. Introduction 68
2. Epidemiology 68
3. Natural History of Hepatitis B Virus Infection 69
4. Physiopathology of Hepatitis B Virus Infection 71
5. Serologic Testing and Diagnosis 72
6. Special Forms of Chronic Hepatitis: Viral Coinfections and Extrahepatic Manifestations 74
7. Chronic Hepatitis B Therapy 74
   7.1 Interferon-alpha 74
      7.1.1 Interferon-alpha therapy for HBeAg-positive chronic hepatitis B 74
      7.1.2 Interferon-alpha therapy for HBeAg-negative pre-C mutant-related chronic hepatitis B 75
      7.1.3 Interferon-alpha therapy for HBV-related cirrhosis 75
      7.1.4 Interferon-alpha therapy prior to liver transplantation for HBV-related decompensated liver disease 75
      7.1.5 Peginterferon-alpha therapy 75
   7.2 Lamivudine 76
      7.2.1 Lamivudine therapy for chronic hepatitis B 76
      7.2.2 Special populations 76
         7.2.2.1 Pre-C mutants 76
         7.2.2.2 Decompensated HBV-related cirrhosis 77
         7.2.2.3 Viral recurrence after liver transplantation 77
      7.2.3 Viral resistances to lamivudine 77
   7.3 Adefovir dipivoxil 77
8. Special Therapeutic Indications 78
   8.1 Acute hepatitis B 78
   8.2 Human immunodeficiency virus coinfection 78
   8.3 Hepatitis delta virus coinfection 79
9. Therapeutic Indications for Chronic Hepatitis B 79
10. Prevention or Infection Control Measures 80
11. Conclusion 81
References 81

Hepatitis B virus (HBV) infection is a major public health problem worldwide. Infections acquired early in life at birth or in infancy progress most often to chronicity. The virus is noncytopathic, and hepatic and extrahepatic manifestations are immunologically mediated. The natural history of chronic infection can be divided in three phases: immunotolerance, immune clearance which is responsible for chronic liver inflammation which may progress to cirrhosis and HCC and resolution. Extrahepatic manifestations include vasculitis and glomerulonephritis. Treatment of chronic hepatitis B should be started as early as possible during the natural course of HBV-related liver disease to prevent its evolution toward cirrhosis, liver failure, and hepatocellular carcinoma (HCC). Interferon-alpha was previously the only available therapy, leading to anti-HBe seroconversion for 30–50% of patients. An oral nucleoside analogue, lamivudine, does provide an interesting alternative therapeutic approach, leading to viral replication inhibition for more than 90% of patients. However, this immediate benefit should be weighed against the probability of resistant mutants selection (about 50% of patients after 3 years of treatment). Adefovir dipivoxil, a recently registered nucleoside analogue, has shown *in vitro* and *in vivo* efficacy against lamivudine-resistant strains, providing a new therapeutic option for chronic hepatitis B. In the future, combinations of nucleoside analogues and immunotherapy will certainly be desirable to ensure complete viral replication recovery.

1. INTRODUCTION

More than 300 million people are chronically infected worldwide by the hepatitis B virus (HBV) [1]. In Asian and African countries, contamination occurs mostly in childhood through perinatal transmission or close family contact. In western countries, the infection is mainly sexually transmitted in adulthood or through blood exposure [2]. Liver cirrhosis is a common outcome of HBV-related chronic hepatitis, leading in a substantial percentage of patients to portal hypertension, hepatic insufficiency, and hepatocellular carcinoma (HCC) [3]. Therapeutic strategies aim to control HBV infection at an early stage of the natural history of the disease, to prevent such complications and improve prognosis.

2. EPIDEMIOLOGY

Despite the availability of efficient vaccines, HBV continues to pose a serious global health problem [1,4]. The World Health Organization (WHO) estimates that hepatitis B is the ninth leading cause of death worldwide. Of the 2 billion people who have been infected with HBV worldwide, more than 350 million are chronically infected. These chronic carriers are exposed to a high risk of life-threatening progressive chronic hepatitis, liver cirrhosis, and HCC. The distribution of HBV infection varies greatly throughout the world. HBV incidence remains particularly high in developing countries of Asia, Africa, the Amazon, the Middle East, and the Pacific Islands where vaccination programs are either not available, being installed or too recently introduced to measure their impact and where perinatal or child-to-child transmission is still important. Infection is less common in Western Europe and North America where less than 1% of the population is infected. For instance, in the United States there are approximately 1.25 million HBV carriers and the number of new infections per year has declined from an average of 450,000 in the 1980s to about 80,000 in 1999 (Center for Disease Control data). However, worldwide, it is estimated that more than 50 million new infections with HBV occur yearly, and as many as 1 million deaths annually can be attributed to the effects of this infection.

HBV is transmitted by contact with blood or body fluids of an infected person. Worldwide, most infections occur from infected mother to child, from child-to-child contact in household settings, from unprotected sexual activity, from blood transfusion, and from reuse of unsterilized needles and syringes. In many developing countries, almost all children born from infected mothers become infected with the virus. About 90% of infants infected at birth or during their first year of life, and 30–50% of children infected between 1 and 4 years of age, develop a chronic infection. This risk of chronic infection declines to ~5% for older children and adults. The risk of death from HBV-related cirrhosis or liver cancer is estimated at 25% for persons who become chronically infected during childhood. In industrialized countries, the pattern of transmission is different. The primary risk factors for HBV infection include (i) unprotected sexual activity which represents the most frequent route of infection, (ii) sharing needles for injection of drugs, (iii) hemodialysis, and (iv) contacts with contaminated sharp instruments during tattooing or body piercing (CDC data). Transmission of HBV through needle-stick injuries has declined since the establishment of a vaccination program for hospital personnel. Perinatal transmission of the virus from HBsAg-positive mothers to their newborns has also declined with the introduction of screening programs for HBV infection and immune prophylaxis for the newborn. HBV infection from blood transfusion has been almost completely eradicated by routine screening and the use of volunteer blood donors. It is worth noting that a study realized by the CDC in 1992 has shown that approximately 30% of patients with chronic hepatitis do not have any identifiable risk factors (CDC data).

3. NATURAL HISTORY OF HEPATITIS B VIRUS INFECTION

The consensus definition and diagnostic criteria for clinical terms relating to HBV infection adopted at the National Institutes of Health (NIH) workshop on Management of Hepatitis B 2000 are summarized in Table 1 [4]. Although most of the patients remain symptom free, a wide clinical and histopathological heterogeneity bears witness to complex interactions between the virus, the immune response and other factors (i.e., hepatitis C or delta or human immunodeficiency virus coinfections; consumption of cytotoxic, immunosuppressive or glucocorticoid medicines, or alcohol abuse) (Figure 1).

In acute primary HBV infection, in adults almost 75% of patients remain symptom free. Fortunately about 90–95% of patients recover spontaneously. However, the prognosis can be worsened by: (1) fulminant hepatitis with extended liver parenchyma necrosis leading to liver failure (about 1% of acutely infected patients); or (2) absence of HBsAg clearance and evolution to chronic infection (about 5–10% of acutely infected patients in adulthood). In acute primary infection acquired in childhood, most of the patients will not clear HBV and remain chronically infected.

Chronic HBV infection affects 350 million people in the World, and 25–40% will eventually die of either cirrhosis-related complications or HCC. The natural history of chronic HBV infection is of major importance with regard to the strategy for its treatment. In chronic HBV infections, patients can either develop chronic hepatitis leading to liver lesions or be in an "inactive carrier" state. The change from chronic hepatitis to the "inactive carrier" state is accompanied by the loss of HBeAg, the normality of alanine aminotransferases (ALT) levels, the absence of HBV-DNA (using hybridization DNA assays with a cut-off of 10^5 copies), the normality (or minimal abnormality) of liver biopsies and mostly integration of HBV-DNA in the liver. The "inactive" HBV HBsAg carriers usually do not experience progressive liver disease [2]. By contrast, chronically HBV-infected patients may develop necroinflammatory and fibrosing lesions of the liver parenchyma characteristic of chronic hepatitis whose evolution can be divided in three different steps (Figure 2) [2]:

(1) The first prolonged step (1–15 years) with high levels of viral replication, immune inactivity, and low level hepatic necroinflammatory activity corresponding to immune tolerance.

Table 1. Glossary and clinical terms used in HBV infection.

Definitions

Chronic hepatitis B: Chronic necroinflammatory disease of the liver caused by persistent infection with hepatitis B virus. Chronic hepatitis B can be subdivided into HBeAg-positive and HBeAg-negative chronic hepatitis B

Inactive HBsAg carrier state: Persistent HBV infection of the liver without significant, ongoing necroinflammatory disease

Resolved hepatitis B: Previous HBV infection without further virologic, biochemical, or histologic evidence of active virus infection or disease

Acute exacerbation or flare of hepatitis B: Intermittent elevations of aminotransferase activity to more than 10 times the upper limit of normal and more than twice the baseline value

Reactivation of hepatitis B: Reappearance of active necroinflammatory disease of the liver in a person known to have the inactive HBsAg carrier state or resolved hepatitis B

HBeAg clearance: Loss of HBeAg in a person who was previously HBeAg positive

HBeAg seroconversion: Loss of HBeAg and detection of anti-HBe in a person who was previously HBeAg positive and anti-HBe negative, associated with decrease in serum HBV DNA to $< 10^5$ copies/ml

HBeAg reversion: Reappearance of HBeAg in a person who was previously HBeAg negative, anti-HBe positive

Diagnostic criteria

Chronic hepatitis B

- HBsAg positive >6 months
- Serum HBV DNA $> 10^5$ copies/ml
- Persistent or intermittent elevation in ALT/AST levels
- Liver biopsy showing chronic hepatitis

Inactive HBsAg carrier state

- HBsAg positive >6 months
- HBeAg negative, anti-HBc positive
- Serum HBV DNA $< 10^5$ copies/ml
- Persistently normal ALT/AST levels
- Liver biopsy confirms absence of significant hepatitis

Resolved hepatitis B

- Previous known history of acute or chronic hepatitis B or the presence of anti-HBc ± anti-HBs
- HBsAg negative
- Undetectable serum HBV DNA
- Normal ALT levels

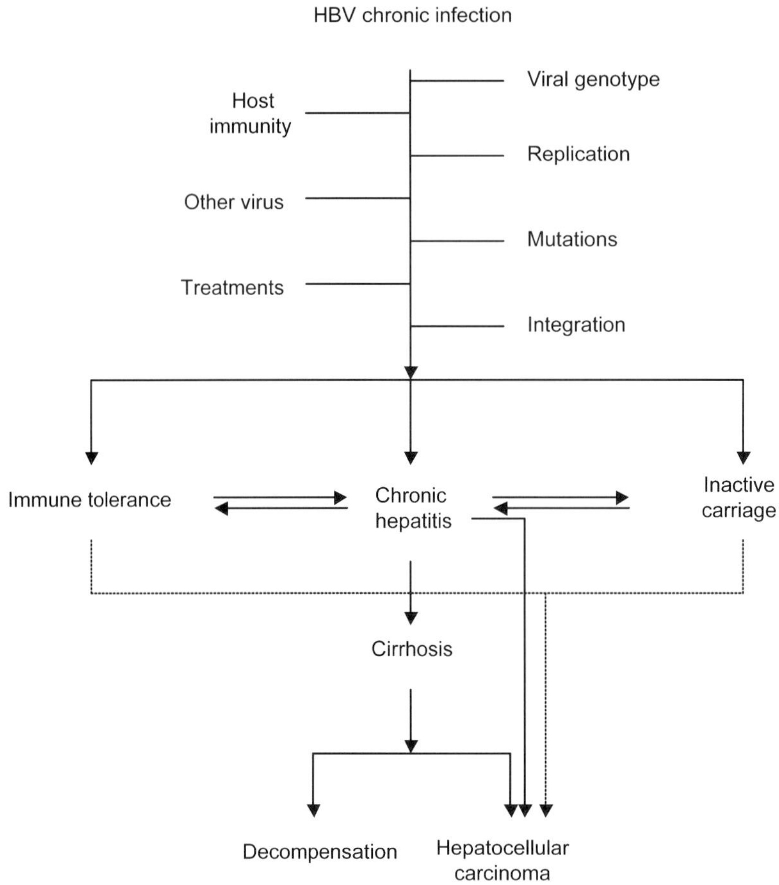

Figure 1. Host and viral determinants involved in the evolution of the different forms of hepatitis B virus infection.

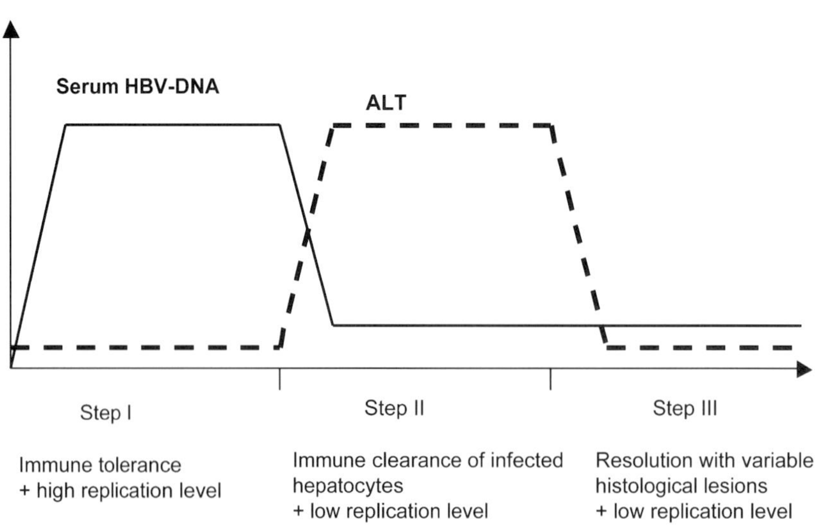

Figure 2. Steps of hepatitis B virus chronic infection. At the third step, a reactivation may occur (increase of HBV-DNA and ALT levels) with a wild type strain (HBeAg reversion) or a pre-C mutant strain (persistence of anti-HBe antibodies).

In Asian HBV patients, because the infection is acquired during early childhood, the immunotolerance phase usually lasts for two or more decades. In contrast, Caucasians who acquire the infection during adolescence or adulthood do not really have an immunotolerance phase.

(2) A second step (very variable in duration) reflects the immune-mediated clearance of infected hepatocytes leading to hepatic necroinflammatory activity with rises in serum ALT, decrease of viral replication, disappearance of HBeAg, and anti-HBe seroconversion. Clinically, HBeAg seroconversion may lead although rarely (<3% of patients) to hepatic decompensation and death [5]. Under the anti-HBe immune pressure, pre-core/core mutated HBV strains (pre-C mutants) may develop subsequently to anti-HBe seroconversion (15–80% of patients according to genotypes) [6]. Pre-C mutant infections carry a more severe prognosis and are mainly characterized by low levels of replication, fluctuating values of HBV-DNA and ALT, absence of HBeAg and persistence of anti-HBe [7,8].

(3) The third step is characterized by low levels of viral replication (HBV-DNA detectable by PCR-based techniques only), high frequency of integration of viral DNA in the hepatocyte host genome, disappearance of necroinflammatory lesions but with a spectrum of complications including fibrosis and cirrhosis possibly leading to HCC later on. In an Asian study, the annual incidence for the occurrence of cirrhosis was found to be 2.4 and 1.3% for HBsAg-positive and anti-HBe-positive patients, respectively (difference statistically nonsignificant) [9]. Cirrhosis is significantly more frequent in patients with episodes of hepatic decompensation.

In summary, the processes of immune clearance and HBeAg seroconversion cause hepatic damage, but the damage can continue after HBeAg seroconversion, with the development of cirrhosis in patients who are anti-HBe positive. Although severe, repeated exacerbations with persistent ALT elevation are known risk factors for the development of cirrhosis, these probably account for only a proportion of the cirrhosis cases. In others, the progression to cirrhosis can be relatively silent.

Despite development of cirrhosis, the prognosis still remains relatively good in compensated patients: 84% survival at 5 years and 68% at 10 years; 23% hepatic decompensation (including ascitis, variceal bleeding, and encephalopathy) probability at 5 years and 37% at 10 years. Inhibition of viral replication and/or normalization of ALT levels are associated with a better prognosis [10]. However, complications of cirrhosis can develop even after spontaneous loss of HBsAg in cirrhotic patients [11]. Prognosis is much worse in decompensated cirrhosis: 25% survival 5 years after the first decompensation course [12].

HCCs develop mostly in cirrhotic livers although noncirrhotic chronic infections may also give rise to liver cancer [13]. Recommendations for HCC screening by alpha-fetoprotein (AFP) monitoring and liver ultrasound (US) examination should involve HBV carriers with high risks for HCC such as men over 45 years, patients with cirrhosis, and with a family history of HCC [14]. There is considerable evidence that HCC can be detected early when chronic HBV carriers undergo periodic screening. In clinic-based periodic screening studies involving both AFP and US, small tumors (<5 cm) can be detected in 57 and 83%, respectively, of HCC cases [13,15]. Effective treatment modalities for small HCC have resulted in successful ablation of tumor and reports of long-term tumor-free survival [16].

4. PHYSIOPATHOLOGY OF HEPATITIS B VIRUS INFECTION

HBV virions target mostly hepatocytes. After interaction with a still poorly known cell membrane receptor complex, virions enter the cytoplasm and lose their capsid (Figure 3). The viral genome is carried towards the nucleus and transformed into supercoiled DNA, so-called covalently closed circular DNA (cccDNA). This extrachromosomal viral DNA serves as transcription matrix for viral messenger RNAs subsequently translated into viral proteins. However one of these RNAs, the so-called pregenomic RNA, is encapsidated with the viral polymerase in the cytoplasm and reverse transcribed into negative polarity DNA strand. The DNA-dependent DNA-polymerase activity of the viral polymerase allows synthesis of the complementary

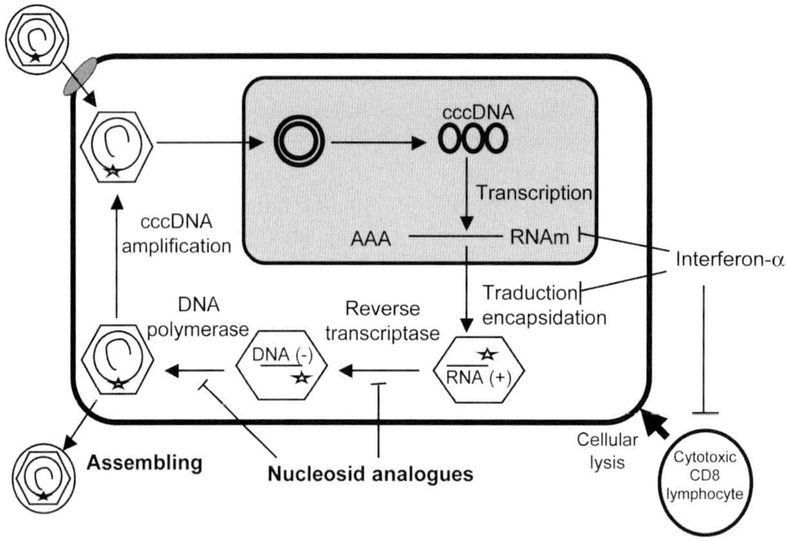

Figure 3. Hepatitis B virus replication cycle and antiviral drugs targets.

positive polarity DNA strand. Mature nucleocapsids can follow two different pathways: (1) recycling towards the nucleus for amplification of the initial cccDNA; or (2) envelopment and secretion of infectious virions targeting new hepatocytes [17]. The viral reverse transcription step is devoid of proofreading and is responsible for spontaneous mistakes leading to a diversification of the viral genome. This phenomenon gives rise to selection of mutant viral strains varying in terms of viral replication levels and immunogenicity through the natural history of HBV chronic infection [18].

HBV replication does not lead to a direct cytopathic effect. In absence of immune response, the half-life of infected hepatocytes is not shortened and is about 100 days. At the cellular level, persistence of HBV infection is due to cccDNA. The different *in vitro* systems and *in vivo* animal models have shown that several mechanisms are needed for complete viral clearance: (1) cytotoxic T-lymphocyte mediated lysis of infected hepatocytes; (2) antiviral activity of the TH1 pathway-related cytokines (interferon-gamma, TNF-alpha and interleukin 12); and (3) hepatocyte renewal, the division of infected hepatocytes probably leading to the disintegration of nucleocapsids and cccDNA during mitosis [17].

Once equilibrium between viral replication (allowing *de novo* infection of other hepatocytes) and immune response (implicated in clearance of infected hepatocytes) is established, chronic liver lesions do develop which characterize chronic hepatitis [19]. These data do suggest that antiviral treatments are likely to be most efficient in patients with low-level viral replication and strong immune response. However, antiviral therapies induce a selection pressure on the virus, triggering the emergence of resistant mutant strains [17].

5. SEROLOGIC TESTING AND DIAGNOSIS

Because the clinical symptoms of HBV infection are indistinguishable from other forms of viral hepatitis, definitive diagnosis is dependent on serologic testing [20]. Acute HBV infection is characterized by the presence of HBsAg in serum and the development of IgM class antibody (IgM anti-HBc) (Figure 4). Detection of HBsAg has evolved to sensitive enzyme immunoassays which can detect HBsAg at concentrations of ≥ 0.1 ng/ml. HBeAg is also detectable during acute infection. During convalescence, HBsAg and HBeAg are cleared, and anti-HBe and anti-HBs develop. Anti-HBs is a protective antibody that neutralizes the virus. The presence of anti-HBs following acute infection indicates recovery and immunity from reinfection. Anti-HBs is also detected among persons who have received hepatitis

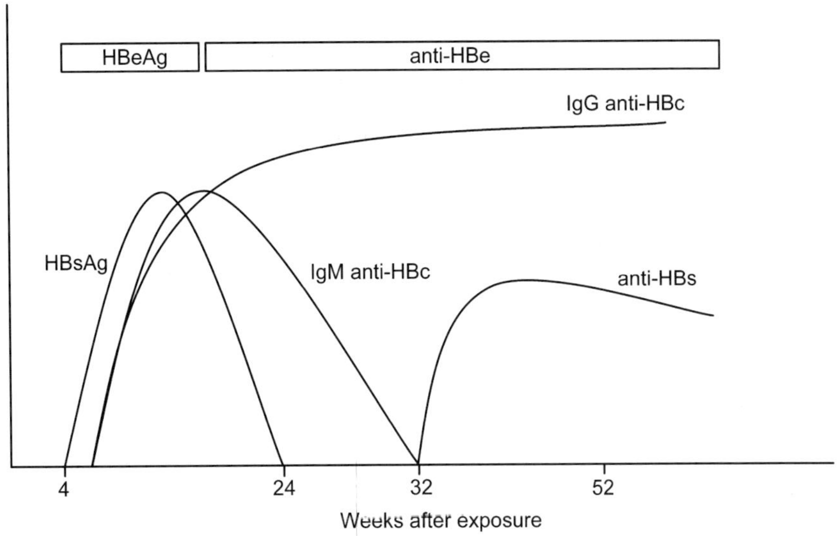

Figure 4. Profile of acute hepatitis B with recovery.

B vaccine. Immunoassays for the detection of total anti-HBc involve both IgM and IgG class antibody to the core protein and indicate current or past exposure to the virus. IgG anti-HBc appears shortly after HBsAg among persons with acute disease and generally persists for life. The detection of IgM anti-HBc allows the diagnosis of acute HBV infection.

In chronic HBV infections, HBsAg remains persistently detectable (Figure 5). Generally, HBeAg reflects a persistent replicative state of wild-type HBV while it is absent for patients infected with a pre-core/core mutant HBV strain. HBV-DNA is detectable in the serum of persons with acute and chronic HBV infection. Most hybridization assays

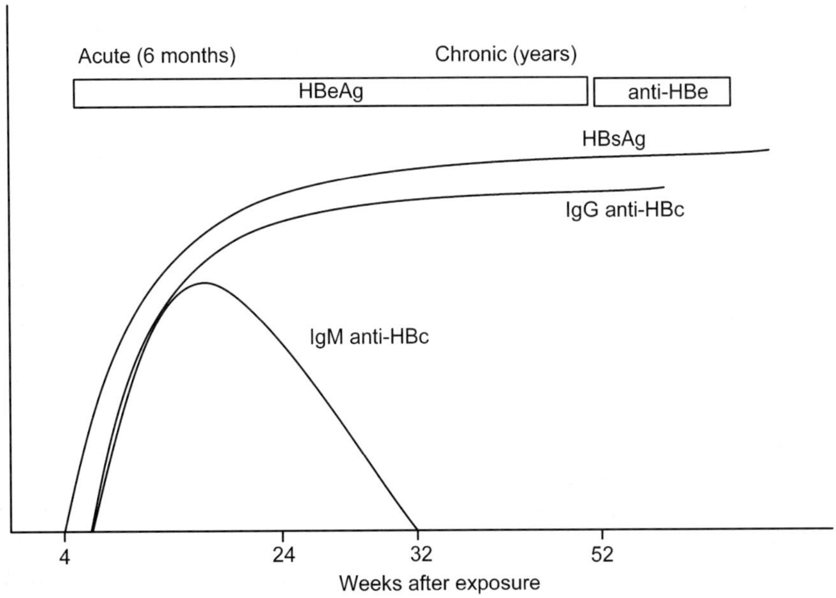

Figure 5. Profile of chronic wild type HBV infection. In pre-core/core HBV mutant infected patients, HBeAg is not detectable.

liquid or dot blot can detect HBV-DNA levels as low as 5 pg/ml, which corresponds to 1.5×10^6 genomes per ml. The branched-DNA hybridization assay detects 2.5 pg of HBV-DNA per ml. PCR is much more sensitive than direct hybridization and detects HBV-DNA levels of 0.001 pg/ml (approximately 100–1000 genomes) [21].

The clinical significance of detecting HBV-DNA by hybridization and by PCR is quite different. Generally, detection by PCR has the same significance as detection of HBsAg and indicates current HBV infection. In contrast, detection by hybridization indicates significant viral replication and a high probability of active liver disease (similar to HBeAg). In pre-core/core HBV-mutant infected patients, HBeAg remains absent while the active replication state is reflected by presence of significant HBV-DNA levels only.

6. SPECIAL FORMS OF CHRONIC HEPATITIS: VIRAL COINFECTIONS AND EXTRAHEPATIC MANIFESTATIONS

Persons who are chronically infected with both HBV and HCV may have more rapid progression of liver disease and a higher risk of developing HCC than patients with HBV infection only [22]. Individuals with HBV and HIV coinfection tend to have higher levels of HBV-DNA, lower rates of spontaneous HBeAg seroconversion, and more severe liver disease [23].

Hepatitis D virus (HDV) is a satellite virus, which is dependent on HBV for the production of envelope proteins. HBV/HDV coinfection mostly occurs in the Mediterranean area and parts of South America. HDV infection can occur in two forms. The first form is caused by the simultaneous coinfection of HBV and HDV; this usually results in a more severe acute hepatitis with a higher mortality than acute hepatitis B alone, but rarely results in chronic infection [24]. A second form is a result of a superinfection of HDV in an HBV carrier. HDV superinfection can manifest as a severe acute hepatitis in previously asymptomatic HBV carriers or exacerbations of underlying chronic hepatitis B. Unlike coinfection, HDV superinfection in HBV carriers almost always results in chronic infection with both viruses. Although persons with chronic HBV/HDV infection can exhibit a wide spectrum of liver pathology, a higher proportion develops cirrhosis, hepatic decompensation, and HCC compared with those with chronic HBV infection alone [25].

Several extrahepatic pathologies have been reported in HBV chronically infected patients, mainly special types of glomerulopathies and periarteritis nodosa (PAN). High and prolonged levels of HBV replication may allow formation of soluble immune complexes HBsAg/anti-HBs with excess of HBsAg. These complexes can precipitate into the endothelium of small and middle size arteries, leading to a multisystemic necrosing vasculitis [26].

7. CHRONIC HEPATITIS B THERAPY

7.1 Interferon-alpha

Recombinant interferon-alpha (IFN-α) 2a or 2b is a cytokine with both antiviral and immunostimulatory properties. Only HBV chronically infected patients with ongoing viral replication, high levels of ALT and histological aggressiveness are considered as candidates for IFN-α therapy. Efficacy is dose-dependent and the most commonly used schedules range from 4.5 to 5.0 million unit injection thrice weekly for 6 months, or a daily 5 million unit injection or a 10 million unit injection thrice weekly for 4 months. Pretreatment predictive factors of favorable therapeutic response include: (1) elevated ALT level between 2- and 4-fold the upper limit of the normal; (2) low HBV-DNA levels (<50 pg/ml); (3) genotype A virus and absence of pre-C gene mutation; (4) absence of immune suppression; and (5) absence of cirrhosis and/or of liver decompensation [27,28].

7.1.1 Interferon-alpha therapy for HBeAg-positive chronic hepatitis B

Several clinical trials have shown that IFN-α therapy can achieve the clearance of HBeAg in 30–50% of patients (versus 5–10% for nontreated patients) [29,30]. Anti-HBe seroconversion is frequently associated with a normalization of ALT levels and a nondetection of serum HBV-DNA (by the poorly sensitive molecular hybridization tests). Longitudinal long-term studies have shown that IFN-α-induced HBeAg clearance is associated with: (1) a low risk of viral reactivation; (2) an improvement of symptoms and survival; and (3) an improvement of histological lesions with lower risk of liver cancer. Later on, patients may even lose HBsAg and clear HBV-DNA (by sensitive PCR-based tests) [31,32]. However, this IFN-α-induced anti-HBe seroconversion is usually preceded by an ALT flare that reflects immune clearance of infected hepatocytes and may abruptly worsen HBV-related chronic liver disease. Sometimes this may even trigger liver decompensation in advanced cases (hepatic encephalopathy, ascitis, digestive bleeding, ...). This transient hepatitis exacerbation is fortunately most often better tolerated and typically elevation of ALT parallels a decrease of HBV-DNA titers which become undetectable (by molecular hybridization tests).

7.1.2 Interferon-alpha therapy for HBeAg-negative pre-C mutant-related chronic hepatitis B

Core promoter and pre-C gene mutations either down-regulate or abolish the production of HBeAg and may lead to the synthesis of a mutated capsid protein interfering with T-lymphocyte activity and decreasing IFN-α therapy efficiency [33]. HBeAg-negative chronic hepatitis B shows typically alternative exacerbation and remission steps. Controlled clinical trials have shown that although prolonged IFN-α administration (6–24 months) is able to inhibit viral replication and normalize ALT levels, subsequent reactivation of the disease will occur sooner or later after discontinuation of therapy [34–36] while HBV replication universally resumes in the long term. Although the common development of cirrhosis does worsen prognosis prolonged IFN-α therapy does seem to improve survival of patients, delay the need for liver transplantation, and decrease the risk of liver decompensation or liver cancer [37].

7.1.3 Interferon-alpha therapy for HBV-related cirrhosis

In HBeAg-positive compensated cirrhosis, several randomized studies have shown that IFN-α therapy is able to promote the clearance of HBeAg, although at lower frequency and with higher risks than for non-cirrhotic patients. Longitudinal studies have confirmed that anti-HBe seroconversion in this setting shares the same features between cirrhotic and non-cirrhotic patients: (1) low frequency of viral recurrences; (2) normalization of ALT levels; and (3) reduction of liver inflammatory activity, clinical, and survival improvement [29,32,38–40]. Some studies also suggested that IFN-α therapy might decrease the incidence of liver cancer (31 versus 17% after a 10-year follow-up; $p < 0.05$) [41]. However, the high frequency and severity of complications (digestive bleeding, worsening of ascitis and encephalopathy, ascitis fluid infection or pneumopathy) in cirrhotic patients forced to decrease the dosage of IFN-α (below 3 MU thrice weekly) especially in decompensated chronic liver diseases [42–45]. Although administered at low doses in the later studies, IFN-α therapy might still induce a clearance of HBV-DNA (by molecular hybridization tests), a decrease of ALT levels and an anti-HBe seroconversion.

7.1.4 Interferon-alpha therapy prior to liver transplantation for HBV-related decompensated liver disease

The main risk after liver transplantation for HBV liver disease remains HBV infection recurrence on the graft, with accelerated deterioration of liver parenchyma and decreased survival of the transplanted patients due to immunosuppression. Although post-transplantation passive immunotherapy with high-dose anti-HBs immunoglobulins (Ig) can reduce the risk of HBV recurrence on the graft, this therapy is not efficient when transplantation is performed for patients with HBV-DNA levels higher than 10^5 copies/ml (positivity by hybridization tests). Some studies showed that combined pre-transplant IFN-α-induced HBV-DNA clearance and post-transplant anti-HBs Ig immunoprevention could reduce the risk of HBV recurrence in high-level replicating patients prior to transplantation [46,47].

7.1.5 Peginterferon-alpha therapy

The attachment of a polyethylene glycol (PEG) molecule to a therapeutic protein has a marked effect on the potency and pharmacodynamic–pharmacokinetic characteristics of that protein.

Pegylation has been used in the development of pegylated IFN-α. Cooksley *et al.* conducted a phase II study, randomizing peginterferon alpha-2a versus conventional IFN-α2a for HBeAg positive patients, and showed that the combined response (HBeAg loss, HBV-DNA suppression, and ALT normalization) of peginterferon alpha 2-a was twice that achieved with conventional IFN-α2a (24% vs 12%; $p = 0.036$) [48]. Another study tested peginterferon alpha 2-a versus lamivudine or the two in combination, for 48 weeks in HBeAg-negative patients plus a 24 weeks follow-up. In study, it was shown that peginterferon alpha 2-a alone led to higher rates of sustained suppression of HBV DNA (19%) after cessation of therapy than with lamivudine alone (7%), and the addition of lamivudine to peginterferon alpha 2-a did not improve post-therapy response rates (20%) [49].

7.2 Lamivudine

Lamivudine is a nucleoside analogue inhibiting both the HBV reverse transcriptase and the DNA-dependent DNA-polymerase activities [50]. Furthermore, lamivudine may allow to restore the specific anti-HBV CD4- and CD8-cell mediated immune responses [51]. However, lamivudine does not prevent initial cccDNA formation and is not capable to eradicate cccDNA from the nucleus. Kinetic studies have also indicated that prolonged lamivudine therapy is very likely required (1–5 years) for complete viral clearance. Lamivudine is commonly used orally at a daily dose of 100–150 mg and its tolerance is excellent [28].

7.2.1 Lamivudine therapy for chronic hepatitis B

Lamivudine therapy leads to viral replication inhibition in 90–95% of patients (viremia undetectable by molecular hybridization tests), anti-HBe seroconversion rates ranging from 16 to 18% (versus 19% under IFN-α therapy and 4–6% for placebo-treated patients) and normalization of ALT levels occurring in 40–72% of patients (versus 15–17% under IFN-α therapy and 5–24% for placebo-treated patients) [52–54]. Histological liver lesions also improve under lamivudine therapy: (1) decrease of necroinflammation (50 versus 25% for placebo); and (2) reduction of both fibrosis and evolution to cirrhosis (1.8 versus 7.1% for placebo) [52,53]. Anti-HBe seroconversion rates do increase with duration of lamivudine therapy: 22, 29, 40, and 47% at 1, 2, 3, and 4 years, respectively [53,55,56]. A pre-treatment high-level of ALT (>2 times upper range of normal) is a predictive factor of lamivudine-induced anti-HBe seroconversion [57]. After lamivudine therapy discontinuation, most of the patients remain anti-HBe positive as for IFN-α treated patients (83% versus 87%) while a few others may revert to HBeAg (anti-HBe clearance and HBeAg appearance) [6]. These data must call for caution before interruption of lamivudine therapy which should be allowed only in the following conditions: (1) effective and stable (6-month interval) anti-HBe seroconversion; (2) normality of ALT levels; and (3) absence of detectable viremia (by PCR-based tests) or viral load below 10^3 copies/ml.

The efficacy of the combination of lamivudine and IFN-α is still open to debate. Early clinical trials did not show any advantage of the combination by comparison with either IFN-α or lamivudine monotherapy for anti-HBe seroconversion [54,58]. However, other studies showed that the combination therapy provided higher rates of anti-HBe seroconversion and viral clearance by comparison to lamivudine monotherapy (33 versus 15%; $p = 0.014$), and improvement of histological inflammatory lesions (46 versus 27%; $p = 0.021$) [59]. Furthermore, other combination regimens including sequential administration of lamivudine and IFN-α might induce durable normalization of ALT levels and even HBsAg clearance without selection of lamivudine-resistant HBV strains [60].

7.2.2 Special populations

7.2.2.1. Pre-C mutants. Lamivudine seems to induce both normalization of ALT levels and HBV-DNA clearance (hybridization tests) in two-thirds of pre-C mutant HBV infected patients [61]. Unfortunately, recurrence is a common event after discontinuation of therapy (85–88% of patients) [62,64]. Furthermore selection of drug resistant mutants may be associated with severe acute exacerbation of liver disease [64,65].

7.2.2.2. Decompensated HBV-related cirrhosis. Lamivudine has substantially improved the treatment of decompensated HBV-related cirrhosis [66]. Although a few patients developing leucopenia under lamivudine therapy have been reported, this drug is very well tolerated [28]. Viral replication inhibition is usually associated with either improvement or at least a stabilization of liver functions. Under these conditions, improvement in liver function occurs after 6 months of therapy [67–69].

7.2.2.3. Viral recurrence after liver transplantation. Preliminary studies suggested that pre-transplant lamivudine therapy (for 1–8 months) could promote HBV-DNA clearance (hybridization tests) in most patients. Furthermore, in combination with lamivudine HBs-Ig long-term post-transplant administration (18–90 weeks), it could maintain negativity of HBsAg (6-month follow-up) [70,71]. The long-term outcome of these patients, however, remains to be further evaluated.

For patients with HBV post-transplant reinfection, some studies showed that a 1-year course of lamivudine therapy was able to induce HBV-DNA clearance (60% of patients), normalization of ALT levels (71% of patients), HBeAg clearance (31% of patients), loss of HBsAg (6% of patients), and significant improvement of histological lesions. However, 27% of patients developed resistance to lamivudine, leading to clinical deterioration for half of them [72,73].

7.2.3 Viral resistances to lamivudine

Lamivudine administration gives rise to a selection pressure on the HBV replication. The onset of resistant strains is characterized by an increase of HBV-DNA levels. In phase III clinical trials, resistant strains may develop after 6 months of therapy and their frequency increases with the duration of treatment: 16, 42, and 53% at 1, 2, and 3 years, respectively. In spite of the phenotypic resistance, HBV-DNA and ALT levels remain commonly lower than the pre-therapeutic values, and liver disease may not worsen in all patients [52,53,55,61,74,75]. The viral resistance is due to the occurrence of mutations of the viral polymerase gene located in the reverse transcriptase YMDD motif within the catalytical site of the enzyme [75]. Recently, it was shown that: (1) viral mutations can be detected about 5 months prior to HBV-DNA recurrence by quantitative PCR; (2) high levels of HBV-DNA and ALT prior to therapy are associated with faster development of resistance; and (3) viral resistance might be more severe in pre-C mutant HBV strain infected patients [64,65,76,77].

7.3 Adefovir dipivoxil

PMEA [9-(2-phosphonylmethoxyethyl)adenine] or adefovir, and its prodrugs adefovir dipivoxil, belong to a new antiviral drug family: the acyclic nucleoside phosphonates [78]. *In vitro* studies have shown that adefovir dipivoxil is efficient against both wild type and lamivudine-resistant HBV polymerases [79–81]. Clinical studies have confirmed *in vivo* that adefovir dipivoxil is able to inhibit HBV replication and does improve biochemical parameters for patients chronically infected by either wild type or lamivudine-resistant HBV strains [82,83]. In a few cases, adefovir dipivoxil proved life saving for patients with fulminant hepatitis after renal transplantation [84], or fibrosing cholestatic hepatitis after liver transplantation [85].

In phase II studies, adefovir dipivoxil was shown to be efficient at a 10 mg daily dose for the inhibition of lamivudine-resistant HBV strain replication. Resistances to adefovir were not reported. Higher dosages (30, 60, or 120 mg daily) may, however, lead to severe renal toxicity [81,86–88], calling for caution especially in decompensated cirrhotic patients prone to the hepato-renal syndrome.

Large phase III trials were conducted to study the efficacy of adefovir dipivoxil. In one trial, 515 *HBeAg positive patients* with compensated liver function were enrolled at 78 international sites. A low number of patients (2%) discontinued study medication for an adverse event: pharyngitis (32%), headache (25%), asthenia (25%), abdominal pain (21%), and flu syndrome (19%). Significant histologic improvements were noted in a higher percentage of the adefovir dipivoxil cohort compared with the placebo group. Ranked assessment of necroinflammatory activity and fibrosis also showed improvement compared with placebo. In the assessment of virologic response, serum HBV-DNA became undetectable by polymerase chain reaction (PCR) assay in approximately one-fourth of the patients treated with adefovir dipivoxil 10 mg/day and in none of the patients treated with placebo. Overall, a substantial reduction of serum HBV-DNA levels was seen in the adefovir dipivoxil group. Assessment of biochemical response revealed reduced levels of serum ALT and a higher proportion of patients achieving normalized ALT levels in the adefovir dipivoxil group compared with placebo recipients. Furthermore, sequencing of the HBV polymerase gene and *in vitro* phenotypic analysis revealed no adefovir-resistant mutations during the 48 weeks of treatment, emphasizing the therapeutic benefit in the long-term treatment of HBeAg positive patients [88].

In another phase III trial the efficacy of adefovir dipivoxil versus placebo was evaluated in HBeAg negative chronic hepatitis B (so-called pre-core mutants infection); 185 patients enrolled at 28 sites. More patients in the adefovir dipivoxil group exhibited improvement in liver histology compared with the placebo group. Treatment with adefovir dipivoxil also resulted in improvements in ranked necroinflammatory and fibrosis scores compared with placebo. Worsening of necroinflammatory activity was significantly greater in the placebo group. Virologic assessment demonstrated undetectable HBV-DNA in more than half of patients receiving adefovir dipivoxil compared with none in the placebo group. Serum HBV-DNA levels decreased in patients receiving adefovir dipivoxil by comparison with the placebo group ($p < 0.0001$). HBV-DNA became undetectable by PCR (<400 copies/ml, Roche Amplicor PCR) in 51% of the ADV group versus 0% of the placebo group. Assessment of the biochemical response showed more patients in the adefovir dipivoxil group with normalized ALT levels than in the placebo group. These results underlined the clinical benefit of adefovir dipivoxil in the therapy of pre-core mutant infections [90]. Furthermore additional studies showed that no HBV polymerase mutations associated with adefovir resistance could be identified for patients receiving approximately 2 years (72–136 weeks) of adefovir dipivoxil therapy at 10 or 30 mg. A recent study showed that long-term adefovir therapy significantly decreased the HBV covalently closed circular DNA (cccDNA) levels, strengthening the powerful antiviral effect of adefovir [91].

In light of all these results, adefovir dipivoxil obtained recently a favorable assessment by the FDA and will be registered soon for the therapy of chronic hepatitis B worldwide.

8. SPECIAL THERAPEUTIC INDICATIONS

8.1 Acute hepatitis B

Therapeutic management of acute hepatitis B remains mainly symptomatic as 90–95% of patients will spontaneously recover, while 5–10% will further progress to chronicity. Patients with prolonged hepatitis (high ALT levels and detectable HBV-DNA 6 weeks after the beginning of the disease) are inevitably exposed to chronicity. For these patients, an early IFN-α therapy can eradicate HBV infection and prevent chronic hepatitis progression in up to 30–75% of cases [92].

In fulminant hepatitis, IFN-α is contraindicated and liver transplantation is presently the only rescuer therapy. No study has evaluated extensively the efficacy of lamivudine although a few case reports highlighted its helpful use in severe acute hepatitis: (1) after liver transplantation [93]; (2) after cardiac transplantation [94]; (3) severe and prolonged acute hepatitis [95]; and (4) HBV-related life threatening PAN [96].

8.2 Human immunodeficiency virus coinfection

One-year lamivudine therapy was shown beneficial as compared with placebo in HIV/HBV coinfected patients with 45% HBV-DNA clearance (by PCR-based tests), 55% normalization of ALT levels, 22% negativation of HBeAg, and 12% clearance of HBsAg [97]. However, viral escape is common and may occur as early as 2 months after therapy onset [98]. Adefovir was shown to provide an effective alternative to rescue HBV resistance to lamivudine [99] as well as the newly available reverse transcriptase inhibitor, Tenofovir.

8.3 Hepatitis delta virus coinfection

Small size studies suggested a possible efficiency of trisodic phosphonoformate (Foscarnet) in severe forms associated with HDV superinfection [100].

In chronic HBV/HDV coinfections, treatments are of limited efficacy. IFN-α therapy showed that prolonged high doses (9–10 million units thrice weekly for 12 months) could normalize ALT levels, induce HBV-DNA clearance (hybridization tests), and improve histological parameters. However, relapse is a most common event [101–103]. IFN-α impacts mainly on the HBV replication while HDV does not seem affected. The HDV-RNA and HDAg disappearance does not always reflect the HDV clearance and IFN-α therapy should be interrupted with caution [100].

Lamivudine administered alone or in association with IFN-α in small size studies showed a decrease of HBV-DNA levels but unfortunately with persistence of HDV-RNA, HBsAg and absence of histological improvement [104,105].

9. THERAPEUTIC INDICATIONS FOR CHRONIC HEPATITIS B

Therapeutic management of HBV chronically infected patients must take account of ALT levels, HBV levels and histological examination to establish the prognosis of the infection (Figure 6); the simple virus chronic carrier state associated with immune tolerance requires a mere follow-up while aggressive chronic hepatitis calls for specific therapeutic management. IFN-α therapy still represents an interesting approach in patients with high ALT levels and low HBV-DNA levels. In other patients, nucleoside analogues are a more attractive therapeutic option (Figure 7). In cirrhotic patients, IFN-α is usually poorly tolerated and therapeutic schedules largely depend on the severity of the disease (Figure 7). In decompensated cirrhosis and transplanted patients, lamivudine or adefovir is the only current therapeutic option. Therapeutic indications in patients awaiting liver transplantation have to be chosen in coordination with the transplantation staff to reduce the risk of viral escape prior to transplantation. In pre-C mutant infected patients, data are still limited and further clinical studies are needed to specify therapeutic schedules.

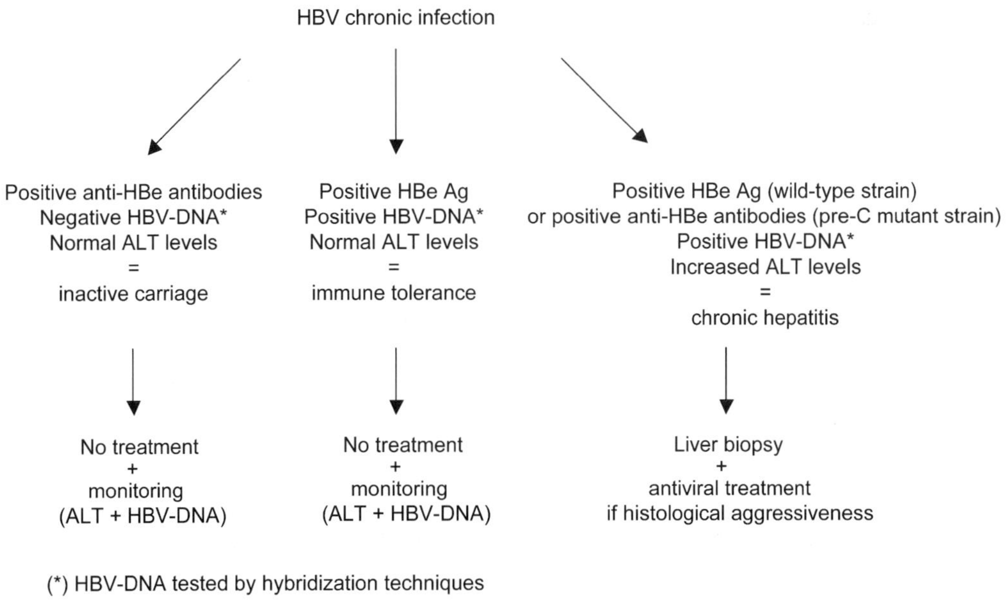

Figure 6. Therapeutic indications in the different forms of hepatitis B virus chronic infections.

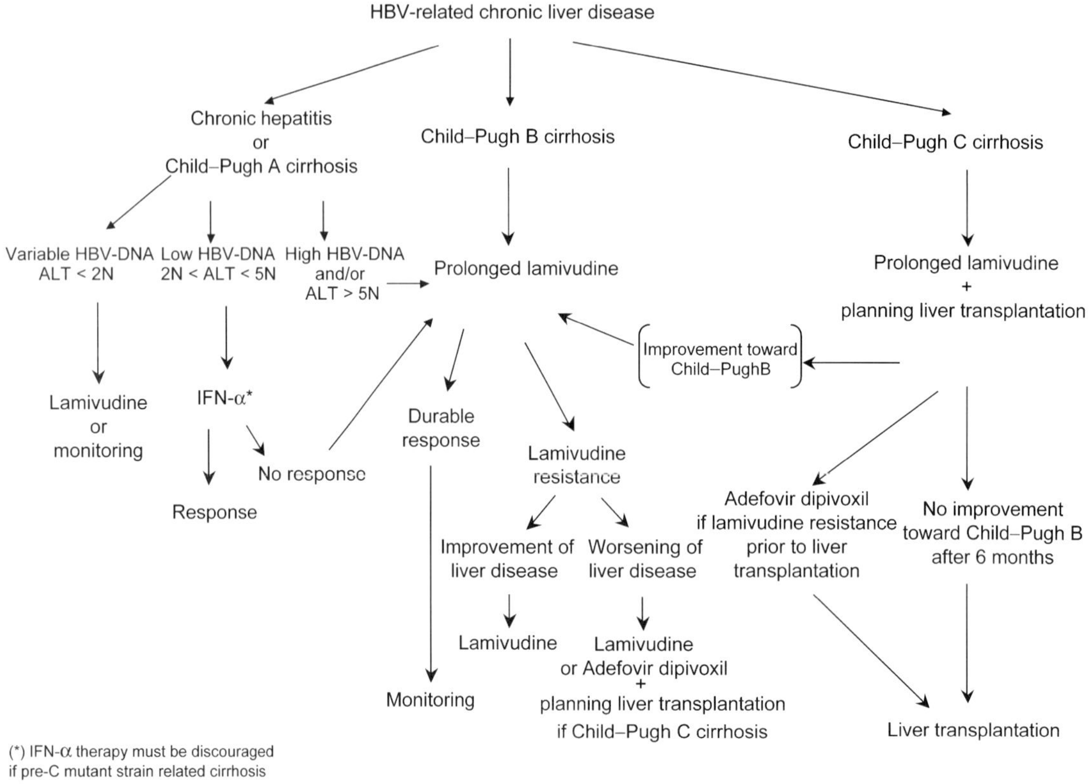

Figure 7. Algorithms of therapeutic management of the different forms of hepatitis B virus-related chronic liver disease.

10. PREVENTION OR INFECTION CONTROL MEASURES

Even though a vaccine for hepatitis B has been available since the early 1980s, and WHO has made recommendation for a large-scale vaccination program, there is still a need to generalize these programs to eradicate this ubiquitous infection. It was clearly shown that the initial vaccination program targeting only high-risk groups failed to affect the overall HBV carrier rate. As the risk of chronicity of viral infection is higher in young children and the efficacy of the hepatitis B vaccine is usually greater in children, it was therefore recommended by WHO to target the population of newborns and children for mass vaccination.

In Taiwan, a large-scale vaccination of all newborns, regardless of the status of their mother, started in 1985 [106]. In 10 years, this program was able to decrease the prevalence of HBsAg carriage from 8 to 0.8% in Taiwanese children. Moreover, this was associated with the decrease in HCC incidence in children while the incidence of other cancers remained stable over time. The results of this study clearly demonstrated the benefit of HBV vaccination at the scale of a country.

In Italy, a campaign for hepatitis B immunization of children and teenagers started in 1991. Its impact was determined by the incidence of hepatitis B. It was shown that the hepatitis B incidence declined from 10.4/100,000 in 1987 to 2.9/100,000 in 1997. The drop in hepatitis B incidence was even more significant after the introduction of mass vaccination [107].

The results of these different studies confirm the prediction that universal immunization of the total world population could bring hepatitis B to a clinically nonrelevant disease within a predictable time frame. Different models have also confirmed the cost-effectiveness of universal infant immunization against hepatitis B.

Beside large-scale vaccination programs, infection control measures should include the implementation of routine screening for blood donors, pregnant women and health-care workers, and should rely on general population counseling to decrease exposure to HBV. Both non-carriers and HBV-carriers should be widely informed about the disease and its transmissions and therefore should be expected to have a responsible behavior (e.g., use of condoms) with respect to the spread of infection. Finally, close contacts of HBV-carriers should be tested for HBV infection. If they have not developed HBV infection or immunity to HBV, they should receive HBIg and/or HBV vaccine.

11. CONCLUSION

HBV chronic infection is a major problem of public health worldwide. While IFN-α had remained the only therapeutic option for many years, its efficacy and tolerance limit its widespread use. Lamivudine has substantially revolutionized the treatment of HBV infection. Unfortunately, genome variability of HBV in polymerase sequences allows virus escape leading to drug resistance. New therapeutic strategies with other nucleoside analogues such as adefovir dipivoxil allow to circumvent resistance to lamivudine. Future perspectives including associations of antiviral drugs and immunotherapy should allow inhibition of viral replication and the clearance of infected hepatocytes. Finally, enforcement of universal vaccination programs against HBV should not be neglected since it remains the best option to reduce HBV-related morbidity and mortality [106].

REFERENCES

[1] Lee, W.M. (1997) Hepatitis B virus infection. *N. Engl. J. Med.* **337**, 1733–1745.

[2] Hoofnagle, J.H., Shafritz, D.A. and Popper, H. (1987) Chronic type B hepatitis and the healthy HBs Ag carrier state. *Hepatology* **7**, 758–763.

[3] Beasley, R.P. (1988) Hepatitis B: the major etiology of hepatocellular carcinoma. *Cancer* **61**, 1942–1956.

[4] Lok, A.S., Heathcote, E.J. and Hoofnagle, J.H. (2001) Management of Hepatitis B 2000, Summary of a Workshop. *Gastroenterology* **120**, 1828–1853.

[5] Sheen, I.S., Liaw, Y.F., Tai, D.I. and Chu, C.M. (1985) Hepatic decompensation associated with hepatitis B e antigen clearance in chronic type B hepatitis. *Gastroenterology* **89**, 732–735.

[6] Pichoud, C., Berby, F., Stuyver, L., Petit, M.A. and Trepo, C. and Zoulim, F. (2000) Persistence of viral replication after anti-HBe seroconversion during antiviral therapy for chronic hepatitis B. *J. Hepatol.* **32**, 307–316.

[7] Li, J., Tong, S., Vitvitski, L., Zoulim, F. and Trepo, C. (1990) Rapid detection and further characterization of infection with hepatitis B virus variants containing a stop codon in the distal pre-C region. *J. Gen. Virol.* **71**, 1993–1998.

[8] Grandjacques, C., Pradat, P., Stuyver, L., Chevallier, M., Chevallier, P., Pichoud, C., Maisonnas, M., Trepo, C. and Zoulim, F. (2000) Rapid detection of genotypes and mutations in the pre-core promoter and the pre-core region of hepatitis B virus genome: correlation with viral persistence and disease severity. *J. Hepatol.* **33**, 430–439.

[9] Liaw, Y.F., Tai, D.I., Chu, C.M. and Chen, T.J. (1988) The development of cirrhosis in patients with chronic type B hepatitis: a prospective study. *Hepatology* **8**, 493–496.

[10] Fattovich, G., Giustina, G., Schalm, S.W., Hadziyannis, S., Sanchez-Tapias, J., Almasio, P., Christensen, E., Krogsgaard, K., Degos, F. and Carneiro de Moura, M. (1995) Occurrence of hepatocellular carcinoma and decompensation in Western patients with cirrhosis type B. *Hepatology* **21**, 77–82.

[11] Huo, T.I., Wu, J.C., Lee, P.C., Chau, G.Y., Lui, W.Y., Tsay, S.H., Ting, L.T., Chang, F.Y. and Lee, S.D. (1998) Sero-clearance of hepatitis B surface antigen in chronic carriers does not necessarily imply a good prognosis. *Hepatology* **28**, 231–236.

[12] Liaw, Y.F., Lin, D.Y., Chen, T.J. and Chu, C.M. (1989) Natural course after the development of cirrhosis in patients with chronic hepatitis B: a prospective study. *Liver* **9**, 235–241.

[13] Sherman, M., Peltekian, K.M. and Lee, C. (1995) Screening for hepatocellular carcinoma in chronic carriers of hepatitis B virus: incidence and prevalence of hepatocellular carcinoma in a North American urban population. *Hepatology* **22**, 432–438.

[14] Lok, A.S. and McMahon, B.J. (2001) Chronic hepatitis B. *Hepatology* **34**, 1225–1241.

[15] Sheu, J.C., Sung, J.L., Chen, D.S., Lai, M.Y., Wang, T.H., Yu, J.Y., Yang, P.M., Chuang, C.N., Yang, P.C. and Lee, C.S. (1985) Early detection of hepatocellular carcinoma by real-time ultrasonography. A prospective study. *Cancer* **56**, 660–666.

[16] Dusheiko, G.M., Hobbs, K.E., Dick, R. and Burroughs, A.K. (1992) Treatment of small hepatocellular carcinomas. *Lancet* **340**, 285–288.

[17] Zoulim, F. (1999) Therapy of chronic hepatitis B virus infection: inhibition of the viral polymerase and other antiviral strategies. *Antiviral Res.* **44**, 1–30.

[18] Hadziyannis, S.J. (1995) Hepatitis B e antigen negative chronic hepatitis B: from clinical recognition to pathogenesis and treatment. *Viral Hepat. Rev.* **1**, 7–36.

[19] Chisari, F. (1995) Hepatitis B virus transgenic mice: insights into the virus and the disease. *Hepatology* **22**, 1316–1325.

[20] Hoofnagle, J.H. and Di Bisceglie, A.M. (1991) Serologic diagnosis of acute and chronic viral hepatitis. *Semin. Liver Dis.* **11**, 73–83.

[21] Mahoney, J.F. (1999) Update on diagnosis, management, and prevention of hepatitis B virus infection. *Clin. Microbiol. Rev.* **12**, 351–366.

[22] McMahon, B.J. (1997) Hepatocellular carcinoma and viral hepatitis, in *Viral Hepatitis*, ed. Wilson, R.A. (Marcel Dekker, New York) pp. 315–330.

[23] Housset, C., Pol, S., Carnot, F., Dubois, F., Nalpas, B., Housset, B., Berthelot, P. and Brechot, C. (1992) Interactions between human immunodeficiency virus-1, hepatitis delta virus and hepatitis B virus infections in 260 chronic carriers of hepatitis B virus. *Hepatology* **15**, 578–583.

[24] Caredda, F., Rossi, E., d'Arminio Monforte, A., Zampini, L., Re, T., Meroni, B. and Moroni, M. (1985) Hepatitis B virus-associated coinfection and superinfection with delta agent: indistinguishable disease with different outcome. *J. Infect. Dis.* **151**, 925–928.

[25] Fattovich, G., Giustina, G., Christensen, E., Pantalena, M., Zagni, I., Realdi, G. and Schalm, S.W. (2000) Influence of hepatitis delta virus infection on morbidity and mortality in compensated cirrhosis type B. The European concerted action on viral hepatitis (Eurohep). *Gut* **46**, 420–426.

[26] Trepo, C. and Guillevin, L. (2001) Polyarteritis nodosa and extrahepatic manifestations of HBV infection: the case against autoimmune intervention in pathogenesis. *J. Autoimmun.* **16**, 269–274.

[27] Perrillo, R.P. (1993) Interferon in the management of chronic hepatitis B. *Dig. Dis. Sci.* **38**, 577–593.

[28] Merle, P., Trepo, C. and Zoulim, F. (2001) Current management strategies for hepatitis B in the elderly. *Drugs and Aging* **10**, 725–735.

[29] Tine, F., Liberati, A., Craxi, A., Almasio, P. and Pagliaro, L. (1993) Interferon treatment in patients with chronic hepatitis B: a meta-analysis of the published literature. *J. Hepatol.* **18**, 154–162.

[30] Wong, D.K., Cheung, A.M., O'Rourke, K., Naylor, C.D., Detsky, A.S. and Heathcote, J. (1993) Effect of alpha-interferon treatment in patients with hepatitis B e antigen-positive chronic hepatitis B. A meta-analysis. *Ann. Intern. Med.* **119**, 312–323.

[31] Lok, A.S., Chung, H.T., Liu, V.W. and Ma, O.C. (1993) Long-term follow-up of chronic hepatitis B patients treated with interferon alfa. *Gastroenterology* **105**, 1833–1838.

[32] Perrillo, R.P. and Brunt, E.M. (1991) Hepatic histologic and immunohistochemical changes in chronic hepatitis B after prolonged clearance of hepatitis B e antigen and hepatitis B surface antigen. *Ann. Intern. Med.* **115**, 113–115.

[33] Naoumov, N.V., Thomas, M.G., Mason, A.L., Chokshi, S., Bodicky, C.J., Farzaneh, F., Williams, R. and Perrillo, R.P. (1995) Genomic variations in the hepatitis B core gene: a possible factor influencing response to interferon alfa treatment. *Gastroenterology* **108**, 505–514.

[34] Brunetto, M., Giarin, M., Saracco, G., Oliveri, F., Calvo, P., Capra, G., Randone, A., Abate, M.L., Manzini, P. and Capalbo, M. (1993) Hepatitis B virus unable to secrete e antigen and response to interferon in chronic hepatitis B. *Gastroenterology* **105**, 845–850.

[35] Alberti, A. and Fattovich, G. (1994) Interferon therapy for the anti-HBe positive form of chronic hepatitis B. *Antiviral Res.* **24**, 145–153.

[36] Lampertico, P., Del Ninno, E., Manzin, A., Donato, M.F., Rumi, M.G., Lunghi, G., Morabito, A., Clementi, M. and Colombo, M. (1997) A randomized, controlled trial of a 24-month course of interferon alfa 2b in patients with chronic hepatitis B who had hepatitis B virus DNA without hepatitis B e antigen in serum. *Hepatology* **26**, 1621–1625.

[37] Papatheodoridis, G.V., Manesis, E. and Hadziyannis, S.J. (2001) The long-term outcome of interferon-α treated and untreated patients with HBeAg-negative chronic hepatitis B. *J. Hepatol.* **34**, 306–313.

[38] Korenman, J., Baker, B., Waggoner, J., Everhart, J.E., Di Bisceglie, A.M. and Hoofnagle, J.H. (1991) Long-term remission of chronic hepatitis B after interferon therapy. *Ann. Intern. Med.* **114**, 629–634.

[39] Niederau, C., Heintges, T., Lange, S., Goldmann, G., Niederau, C.M., Mohr, L. and Haussinger, D. (1996) Long-term follow-up of HBeAg-positive patients treated with interferon alfa for chronic hepatitis B. *N. Engl. J. Med.* **334**, 1422–1427.

[40] Lin, S.M., Sheen, I.S., Chien, R.N., Chu, C.M. and Liaw, Y.F. (1999) Long-term beneficial effect of interferon therapy in patients with chronic hepatitis B virus infection. *Hepatology* **29**, 971–975.

[41] Ikeda, K., Saitoh, S., Suzuki, Y., Kobayashi, M., Tsubota, A., Fukuda, M., Koida, I., Arase, Y., Chayama, K., Murashima, N. and Kumada, H. (1998) Interferon decreases hepatocellular carcinogenesis in patients with cirrhosis caused by the hepatitis B virus. *Cancer* **82**, 827–835.

[42] Hoofnagle, J.G., Di Bisceglie, A.M., Waggoner, J.G. and Park, Y. (1993) Interferon alfa for patients with clinically apparent cirrhosis due to chronic hepatitis B. *Gastroenterology* **104**, 1116–1121.

[43] Nevens, F., Goubau, P., Van Eyken, P., Desmyter, J., Desmet, V. and Fevery, J. (1993) Treatment of hepatitis B-induced cirrhosis with low doses of interferon alpha. *Liver* **13**, 15–19.

[44] Perrillo, R.P., Tamburro, C., Regenstein, F., Balart, L., Bodenheimer, H., Silva, M., Schiff, E., Bodicky, C., Miller, B. and Denham, C. (1995) Low-dose titratable alpha interferon in decompensated liver disease due to chronic infection with hepatitis B virus. *Gastroenterology* **109**, 908–916.

[45] Marcellin, P., Giuily, N., Loriot, M.A., Durand, F., Samuel, D., Bettan, L., Degott, C., Bernuau, J., Benhamou, J.P. and Erlinger, S. (1997) Prolonged interferon-alpha therapy of hepatitis B virus-related decompensated cirrhosis. *J. Viral Hepat.* **4**(Suppl. 1), 21–26.

[46] Marcellin, P., Samuel, D., Areias, J., Loriot, M.A., Arulnaden, J.L., Gigou, M., David, M.F., Bismuth, A., Reynes, M. and Brechot, C. (1994) Pretransplantation interferon treatment and recurrence of hepatitis B virus infection after liver transplantation for hepatitis B-related end-stage liver disease. *Hepatology* **19**, 6–12.

[47] Tchervenkov, J.I., Tector, A.J., Barkun, J.S., Sherker, A., Forbes, C.D., Elias, N., Cantarovich, M., Cleland, P., Metrakos, P. and Meakins, J.L. (1997) Recurrence-free long-term survival after liver transplantation for hepatitis B using interferon-alpha pretransplant and hepatitis B immune globulin posttransplant. *Ann. Surg.* **226**, 356–365.

[48] Cooksley, W.G., Piratvisuth, T., Lee, S.D., Mahachai, V., Chao, Y.C., Tanwandee, T., Chutaputti, A., Chang, W.Y., Zahm, F.E. and Pluck, N. (2003) Peginterferon alpha-2a (40 kDa): an advance in the treatment of hepatitis B e antigen-positive chronic hepatitis B. *J. Viral Hepat.* **4**, 298–305.

[49] Marcellin, P., Lau, G.K., Bonino, F., Farci, P., Hadziyannis, S., Jin, R., Lu, Z.M., Piratvisuth, T., Germanidis, G., Yurdaydin, C., Diago, M., Gurel, S., Lai, M.Y., Button, P. and Pluck, N. (2004) Peginterferon Alfa-2a HBeAg-Negative Chronic Hepatitis B Study Group. Peginterferon alfa-2a alone, lamivudine alone, and the two in combination in patients with HBeAg-negative chronic hepatitis B. *N. Engl. J. Med.* **351**, 1206–1217.

[50] Severini, A., Liu, X.Y., Wilson, J.S. and Tyrrell, D.L. (1995) Mechanism of inhibition of duck hepatitis B virus polymerase by (−)-β-L-2′,3′-dideoxy-3′-thyacytidine. *Antimicrob. Agents Chemother.* **39**, 1430–1435.

[51] Boni, C., Penna, A., Ogg, G.S., Bertoletti, A., Pilli, M., Cavallo, C., Cavalli, A., Urbani, S., Boehme, R., Panebianco, R., Fiaccadori, F. and Ferrari, C. (2001) Lamivudine treatment can overcome cytotoxic T-cell hyporesponsiveness in chronic hepatitis B: new perspectives for immune therapy. *Hepatology* **33**, 963–971.

[52] Dienstag, J.L., Schiff, E.R., Wright, T.L., Perrillo, R.P., Hann, H.W., Goodman, Z., Crowther, L., Condreay, L.D., Woessner, M., Rubin, M. and Brown, N.A. (1999) Lamivudine as initial treatment for chronic hepatitis B in the United States. *N. Engl. J. Med.* **341**, 1256–1263.

[53] Lai, C.L., Chien, R.W., Leung, N.W., Chang, T.T., Guan, R., Tai, D.I., Ng, K.Y., Wu, P.C., Dent, J.C., Barber, J., Stephenson, S.L. and Gray, D.F. (1998) A one year trial of lamivudine for chronic hepatitis B. *N. Engl. J. Med.* **339**, 61–68.

[54] Heathcote, J., Schalm, S.W. and Cianciara, J. (1998) Lamivudine and intron A combination treatment in patients with chronic hepatitis B infection. *J. Hepatol.* **28**(Suppl. 1), 43.

[55] Dienstag, J.L., Schiff, E.R., Mitchell, M., Casey, D.E. Jr., Gitlin, N., Lissoos, T., Gelb, L.D., Condreay, L., Crowther, L., Rubin, M. and Brown, N. (1999) Extended lamivudine retreatment for chronic hepatitis B: maintenance of viral suppression after discontinuation of therapy. *Hepatology* **30**, 1082–1087.

[56] Liaw, Y.F., Leung, N.W., Chang, T.T., Guan, R., Tai, D.I., Ng, K.Y., Chien, R.N., Dent, J., Roman, L., Edmundson, S. and Lai, C.L. (2000) Effects of extended lamivudine therapy in Asian patients with chronic hepatitis B. Asia hepatitis lamivudine study group. *Gastroenterology* **119**, 172–180.

[57] Chien, R.N., Liaw, Y.F. and Atkins, M. (1999) Pretherapy alanine transaminase level as a determinant for hepatitis B e antigen seroconversion during lamivudine therapy in patients with chronic

hepatitis B. Asian hepatitis lamivudine trial group. *Hepatology* **30**, 770–774.

[58] Schalm, S.W., Heathcote, J., Cianciara, J., Farrell, G., Sherman, M., Willems, B., Dhillon, A., Moorat, A., Barber, J. and Gray, D.F. (2000) Lamivudine and alpha interferon combination treatment of patients with chronic hepatitis B infection: a randomized trial. *Gut* **46**, 562–568.

[59] Barbaro, G., Zechini, F., Pellicelli, A.M., Francavilla, R., Scotto, G., Bacca, D., Bruno, M., Babudieri, S., Annese, M., Matarazzo, F., Di Stefano, G. and Barbarini, G. (2001) Lamivudine Italian Study Group Investigators. Long-term efficacy of interferon alpha-2b and lamivudine in combination compared to lamivudine monotherapy in patients with chronic hepatitis B. An Italian multicenter, randomized trial. *J. Hepatol.* **3**, 406–411.

[60] Serfaty, L., Thabut, D., Zoulim, F., Andreani, T., Chazouilleres, O., Carbonell, N., Loria, A. and Poupon, R. (2001) Sequential treatment with lamivudine and interferon monotherapies in patients with chronic hepatitis B not responding to interferon alone: results of a pilot study. *Hepatology* **34**, 573–577.

[61] Tassopoulos, N.C., Volpes, R., Pastore, G., Heathcote, J., Buti, M., Goldin, R.D., Hawley, S., Barber, J., Condreay, L. and Gray, D.F. (1999) Efficacy of lamivudine in patients with hepatitis B e antigen-negative/hepatitis B virus DNA-positive (precore mutant) chronic hepatitis B. *Hepatology* **29**, 889–896.

[62] Tassopoulos, N.C., Volpes, R. and Pastore, G. (1999) Post lamivudine treatment follow up of patients with HBeAg negative chronic hepatitis B. *J. Hepatol.* **30**(Suppl. 1), 117 abstract.

[63] Santantonio, T., Mazzola, M., Iacovazzi, T., Miglietta, A., Guastadisegni, A. and Pastore, G. (2000) Long-term follow-up of patients with anti-HBe/HBV DNA-positive chronic hepatitis B treated for 12 months with lamivudine. *J. Hepatol.* **32**, 300–306.

[64] Hadziyannis, S.J., Papatheodoridis, G.V., Dimou, E., Laras, A. and Papaioannou, C. (2000) Efficacy of long-term lamivudine monotherapy in patients with hepatitis B e antigen-negative chronic hepatitis B. *Hepatology* **32**(4 Pt 1), 847–851.

[65] Si Ahmed, S., Tavan, D., Pichoud, C., Berby, F., Stuyver, L., Johnson, M., Merla, P., Abidi, H., Trepo, C. and Zoulim, F. (2000) Early detection of viral resistance by determination of HBV polymerase mutations in patients treated by lamivudine for chronic hepatitis B. *Hepatology* **32**, 1078–1088.

[66] Merle, P. and Trepo, C. (2001) Therapeutic management of hepatitis B related cirrhosis. *J. Viral Hepat.* **6**, 391–399.

[67] Villeneuve, J.P., Condreay, L.D., Willems, B., Pomier-Layrargues, G., Fenyves, D., Bilodeau, M., Leduc, R., Peltekian, K., Wong, F., Margulies, M. and Heathcote, E.J. (2000) Lamivudine treatment for decompensated cirrhosis resulting from chronic hepatitis B. *Hepatology* **31**, 207–210.

[68] Yao, F.Y. and Bass, N.M. (2000) Lamivudine treatment in patients with severely decompensated cirrhosis due to replicating hepatitis B infection. *J. Hepatol.* **33**, 301–307.

[69] Kapoor, D., Guptan, R.C., Wakil, S.M., Kazim, S.N., Kaul, R., Agarwal, S.R., Raisuddin, S., Hasnain, S.E. and Sarin, S.K. (2000) Bcncficial effects of lamivudine in hepatitis B virus-related decompensated cirrhosis. *J. Hepatol.* **33**, 308–312.

[70] Grellier, L., Multimer, D., Ahmed, M., Brown, D., Burroughs, A.K., Rolles, K., McMaster, P., Beranek, P., Kennedy, F., Kibbler, H., McPhillips, P., Elias, E. and Dusheiko, G. (1996) Lamivudine prophylaxis against reinfection in liver transplantation for hepatitis B cirrhosis. *Lancet* **348**, 1212–1215.

[71] Yao, F.Y., Osorio, R.W., Roberts, J.P., Poordad, F.F., Briceno, M.N. Garcia-Kennedy, R. and Gish, R.R. (1999) Intramuscular hepatitis B immune globulin combined with lamivudine for prophylaxis against hepatitis B recurrence after liver transplantation. *Liver Transpl. Surg.* **5**, 491–496.

[72] Perrillo, R., Rakela, J., Dienstag, J., Levy, G., Martin, P., Wright, T., Caldwell, S., Schiff, E., Gish, R., Villeneuve, J.P., Farr, G., Anschuetz, G., Crowther, L. and Brown, N. (1999) Multicenter study of lamivudine therapy for hepatitis B after liver transplantation. Lamivudine transplant group. *Hepatology* **29**, 1581–1586.

[73] Perrillo, R.P., Wright, T., Rakela, J., Levy, G., Schiff, E., Gish, R., Martin, P., Dienstag, J., Adams, P., Dickson, R., Anschuetz, G., Bell, S., Chondreay, L. and Brown, N. (2001) A multicenter United States–Canadian trial to assess lamivudine monotherapy before and after liver transplantation for chronic hepatitis B. *Hepatology* **33**, 424–432.

[74] Liaw, Y.F., Chien, R.N., Yeh, C.T., Tsai, S.L. and Chu, C.M. (1999) Acute exacerbation and hepatitis B virus clearance after emergence of YMDD motif mutation during lamivudine therapy. *Hepatology* **30**, 567–572.

[75] Allen, M.I., Deslauriers, M., Andrews, C.W., Tipples, G.A., Walters, K.A., Tyrrell, D.L., Brown, N. and Condreay, L.D. (1998) Identification and

characterization of mutations in hepatitis B virus resistant to lamivudine. Lamivudine clinical investigation group. *Hepatology* **27**, 1670–1677.

[76] Lau, D.T., Khokhar, M.F., Doo, E., Ghany, M.G., Herion, D., Park, Y., Kleiner, D.E., Schmid, P., Condreay, L.D., Gauthier, J., Kuhns, M.C., Liang, T.J. and Hoofnagle, J.H. (2000) Long-term therapy of chronic hepatitis B with lamivudine. *Hepatology* **32**(4 Pt 1), 828–834.

[77] Lok, A.S., Hussain, M., Cursano, C., Margotti, M., Gramenzi, A., Grazi, G.L., Jovine, E., Benardi, M. and Andreone, P. (2000) Evolution of hepatitis B virus polymerase gene mutations in hepatitis B e antigen-negative patients receiving lamivudine therapy. *Hepatology* **32**, 1145–1153.

[78] Balzarini, J., Hao, Z., Herdewijn, P., Johns, D.G. and De Clercq, E. (1991) Intracellular metabolism and mechanism of anti-retrovirus action of 9-(2-phosphonylmethoxyethyl)adenine, a potent anti-human immunodeficiency virus compound. *Proc. Natl Acad. Sci. USA* **88**, 1499–1503.

[79] Ono-Nita, S.K., Kato, N., Shiratori, Y., Lan, K.H., Yoshida, H., Carrilho, F.J. and Omata, M. (1999) Susceptibility of lamivudine-resistant hepatitis B virus to other reverse transcriptase inhibitors. *J. Clin. Invest.* **103**, 1635–1640.

[80] Fu, L., Liu, S.H. and Cheng, Y.C. (1999) Sensitivity of L-(−)2,3-dideoxythiacytidine resistant hepatitis B virus to other antiviral nucleoside analogues. *Biochem. Pharmacol.* **57**, 1351–1359.

[81] Xiong, X., Flores, C., Yang, H., Toole, J.J. and Gibbs, C.S. (1998) Mutations in hepatitis B DNA polymerase with resistance to lamivudine do not confer resistance to adefovir *in vitro*. *Hepatology* **28**, 1669–1673.

[82] Peters, M.G., Hann, H.H., Martin, P., Heathcote, E.J., Buggisch, P., Rubin, R., Bourliere, M., Kowdley, K., Trepo, C., Gray, Df.D., Sullivan, M., Kleber, K., Ebrahimi, R., Xiong, S. and Brosgart, C.L. (2004) Adefovir dipivoxil alone or in combination with lamivudine in patients with lamivudine-resistant chronic hepatitis B. *Gastroenterology* **126**, 91–101.

[83] Perrillo, R., Hann, H.W., Mutimer, D., Willems, B., Leung, N., Lee, W.M., Moorat, A., Gardner, S., Woessner, M., Bourne, E., Brosgart, C.L. and Schiff, E. (2004) Adefovir dipivoxil added to ongoing lamivudine in chronic hepatitis B with YMDD mutant hepatitis B virus. *Gastroenterology* **126**, 81–90.

[84] Peters, M.G., Singer, G., Howard, T., Jacobsmeyer, S., Xiong, X., Gibbs, C.S., Lamy, P. and Murray, A. (1999) Fulminant hepatic failure resulting from lamivudine-resistant hepatitis B virus in a renal transplant recipient: durable response after orthotopic liver transplantation on adefovir dipivoxil and hepatitis B immune globulin. *Transplantation* **68**, 1912–1914.

[85] Walsh, K.M., Woodall, T., Lamy, P., Wight, D.G., Bloor, S. and Alexander, G.J. (2001) Successful treatment with adefovir dipivoxil in a patient with fibrosing cholestatic hepatitis and lamivudine resistant hepatitis B virus. *Gut* **49**, 436–440.

[86] Heathcote, E.J., Jeffers, L. and Wright, T. (1998) Loss of serum HBV DNA and HBeAg and seroconversion following short-term (12 weeks) adefovir dipivoxil therapy in chronic hepatitis B: two placebo controlled phase II studies. *Hepatology* **28**, 317A (abstract).

[87] Gilson, R.J., Chopra, K.B., Newell, A.M., Murray-Lyon, I.M., Nelson, M.R., Rice, S.J., Tedder, R.S., Toole, J., Jaffe, H.S. and Weller, I.V. (1999) A placebo-controlled phase I/II study of adefovir dipivoxil in patients with chronic hepatitis B virus infection. *J. Viral Hepat.* **6**, 387–395.

[88] Perrillo, R., Schiff, E.R. and Magill, A. (1999) *In vivo* demonstration of sensitivity of YMDD mutants to adefovir. *Gastroenterology* **116**, L0356.

[89] Marcellin, P., Chang, T.T., Lim, S.G., Tong, M.J., Sievert, W., Shiffman, M.L., Jeffers, L., Goodman, Z., Wulfsohn, M.S., Xiong, S., Fry, J. and Brosgart, C.L. (2003) Adefovir Dipivoxil 437 Study Group. Adefovir dipivoxil for the treatment of hepatitis B e antigen-positive chronic hepatitis B. *N. Engl. J. Med.* **348**, 808–816.

[90] Hadziyannis, S.J., Tassopoulos, N.C., Heathcote, E.J., Chang, T.T., Kitis, G., Rizzetto, M., Marcellin, P., Lim, S.G., Goodman, Z., Wulfsohn, M.S., Xiong, S., Fry, J. and Brosgart, C.L. (2003) Adefovir Dipivoxil 438 Study Group. Adefovir dipivoxil for the treatment of hepatitis B e antigen-negative chronic hepatitis B. *N. Engl. J. Med.* **348**, 800–807.

[91] Werle-Lapostolle, B., Bowden, S., Locarnini, S., Wursthorn, K., Petersen, J., Lau, G., Trepo, C., Marcellin, P., Goodman, Z., Delaney, W.E. 4th, Xiong, S., Brosgart, C.L., Chen, S.S., Gibbs, C.S. and Zoulim, F. (2004) Persistence of cccDNA during the natural history of chronic hepatitis B and decline during adefovir dipivoxil therapy, *Gastroenterology* **126**, 1750–1758.

[92] Trepo, C., Chemin, I., Petit, M.A., Chossegros, P., Zoulim, F., Chevallier, P. and Sepetjan, M. (1990) Possible prevention of chronic hepatitis B by early interferon therapy. *J. Hepatol.* **11**, S95–S99.

[93] Andreone, P., Caraceni, P., Grazi, G.L., Belli, L., Milandri, G.L., Ercolani, G., Jovine, E., D'Errico, A., Dal Monte, P.R., Ideo, G., Forti, D., Mazziotti, A., Cavallari, A. and Bernardi, M. (1998) Lamivudine treatment for acute hepatitis B after liver transplantation. *J. Hepatol.* **29**, 985–989.

[94] Perrillo, R., Rakela, J. and Martin, P. (1996) Lamivudine for hepatitis B after liver transplantation (OLT). *Hepatology* **24**(Suppl.), 182A abstract.

[95] Reshef, R., Sbeit, W. and Tur-Kaspa, R. (2000) Lamivudine in the treatment of acute hepatitis B. *N. Engl. J. Med.* **343**, 1123–1124.

[96] Gupta, S., Piraka, C. and Jaffe, M. (2001) Lamivudine in the treatment of polyarteritis nodosa associated with acute hepatitis B. *N. Engl. J. Med.* **344**, 1645–1646.

[97] Dore, G.J., Cooper, D.A., Barrett, C., Goh, L.E., Thakrar, B. and Atkins, M. (1999) Dual efficacy of lamivudine treatment in human immunodeficiency virus/hepatitis B virus-coinfected persons in a randomized, controlled study (CAESAR). The CAESAR coordinating committee. *J. Infect. Dis.* **180**, 607–613.

[98] Benhamou, Y., Bochet, M., Thibault, V., Di Martino, V., Caumes, E., Bricaire, F., Opolon, P., Katlama, C. and Poynard, T. (1999) Long-term incidence of hepatitis B virus resistance to lamivudine in human immunodeficiency virus-infected patients. *Hepatology* **30**, 1302–1306.

[99] Benhamou, Y., Bochet, M., Thibault, V., Calvez, V., Fievet, M.H., Vig, P., Gibbs, C.S., Brosgart, C., Fry, J., Namini, H., Katlama, C. and Poynard, T. (2001) Safety and efficacy of adefovir dipivoxil in patients co-infected with HIV-1 and lamivudine-resistant hepatitis B virus: an open-label pilot study. *Lancet* **358**, 718–723.

[100] Merle, P., Chossegros, P. and Trepo, C. (1999) Management of chronic hepatitis delta. *Medical Management of Liver Disease* (Marcel Dekker, New York) pp. 89–98.

[101] Rosina, F. and Cozolongo, R. (1994) Interferon in HDV infection. *Antiviral Res.* **24**, 165–174.

[102] Farci, P., Mandas, A., Coiana, A., Lai, M.E., Desmet, V., Van Eyken, P., Gibo, Y., Caruso, L., Scaccabarozzi, S. and Criscuolo, D. (1994) Treatment of chronic hepatitis D with interferon alfa-2a. *N. Engl. J. Med.* **330**, 88–94.

[103] Gaudin, J.L., Faure, P., Godinot, H., Gerard, F. and Trepo, C. (1995) The French experience of treatment of chronic type D hepatitis with 12-months course of interferon alpha-2b. Results of a randomized controlled trial. *Liver* **15**, 45–52.

[104] Lau, D.T., Doo, E., Park, Y., Kleiner, D.E., Schmid, P., Kuhns, M.C. and Hoofnagle, J.H. (1999) Lamivudine for chronic delta hepatitis. *Hepatology* **30**, 546–549.

[105] Wolters, L.M., van Nunen, A.B., Honkoop, P., Vossen, A.C., Niesters, H.G., Zondervan, P.E. and de Man, R.A. (2000) Lamivudine-high dose interferon combination therapy for chronic hepatitis B patients co-infected with the hepatitis D virus. *J. Viral Hepat.* **7**, 428–434.

[106] Chang, M.H., Chen, C.J., Lai, M.S., Hsu, H.M., Wu, T.C., Kong, M.S., Liang, D.C., Shau, W.Y. and Chen, D.S. (1997) Universal hepatitis B vaccination in Taiwan and the incidence of hepatocellular carcinoma in children. *N. Engl. J. Med.* **336**, 1855–1859.

[107] Stroffolini, T., Mele, A., Tosti, M.E., Gallo, G., Balocchini, E., Ragni, P., Santonastasi, F., Marzolini, A., Ciccozzi, M. and Moiraghi, A. (2000) The impact of the hepatitis B mass immunisation campaign on the incidence and risk factors of acute hepatitis B in Italy. *J. Hepatol.* **33**, 980–985.

Hepatology: A Practical Approach
B. Al Knawy, M.L. Shiffman, R.H. Wiesner (editors)

Chapter 3

Hepatitis C

Steven L. Zacks, Mark W. Russo and Michael W. Fried[1]

Division of Gastroenterology and Hepatology, University of North Carolina at Chapel Hill, Chapel Hill, NC, USA

1. Introduction 87
2. Epidemiology 87
3. Natural History of HCV Infection 88
   3.1 Acute hepatitis C infection 88
   3.2 Chronic hepatitis C 89
4. Diagnosis of HCV Infection 90
5. Risk Factors for HCV Infection 91
6. Diagnostic Tests for Hepatitis C 92
   6.1 Anti-HCV antibody 92
   6.2 Supplemental assays 93
   6.3 Nucleic acid testing 93
   6.4 HCV genotype 93
   6.5 Liver biopsy 95
7. Counseling of the HCV-Infected Individual 95
8. Therapy for HCV 95
9. Summary 98
References 98

1. INTRODUCTION

Hepatitis C (HCV), a significant cause of liver disease throughout the world, is unique among hepatotropic viruses because of its propensity to develop into a chronic infection. It has been estimated that at least 170 million people, including 4 million in the United States, have been infected with HCV. Individuals with chronic hepatitis C are at risk for the development of cirrhosis, portal hypertension, liver failure, and hepatocellular carcinoma. Because hepatitis C is a slowly progressive disease, clinical manifestations of advanced liver injury may not be apparent for decades after the initial infection. An understanding of the epidemiology, natural history, diagnostic algorithms, and management of chronic hepatitis C will allow clinicians to intervene in a timely manner and, hopefully, prevent complications of the disease.

2. EPIDEMIOLOGY

The epidemiology of chronic hepatitis C infection has been well defined in a number of studies that have analyzed populations around the world. Globally, it is estimated that 170 million people are infected with hepatitis C, although it is acknowledged that reporting from many countries is incomplete [1,2]. The prevalence of HCV infection varies geographically and ranges from a low prevalence of 1% in Europe to 5.6% in Africa. Certain countries are noted to have an extremely high prevalence of hepatitis C. In Egypt, prevalence of HCV is reported as high as 20%, apparently due to parenteral antischistosomal therapy programs that utilized reusable syringes [3] (Figure 1).

[1] Present address: University of North Carolina, CB# 7080, Room 1111 Bioinformatics, Chapel Hill, NC 27599, USA.

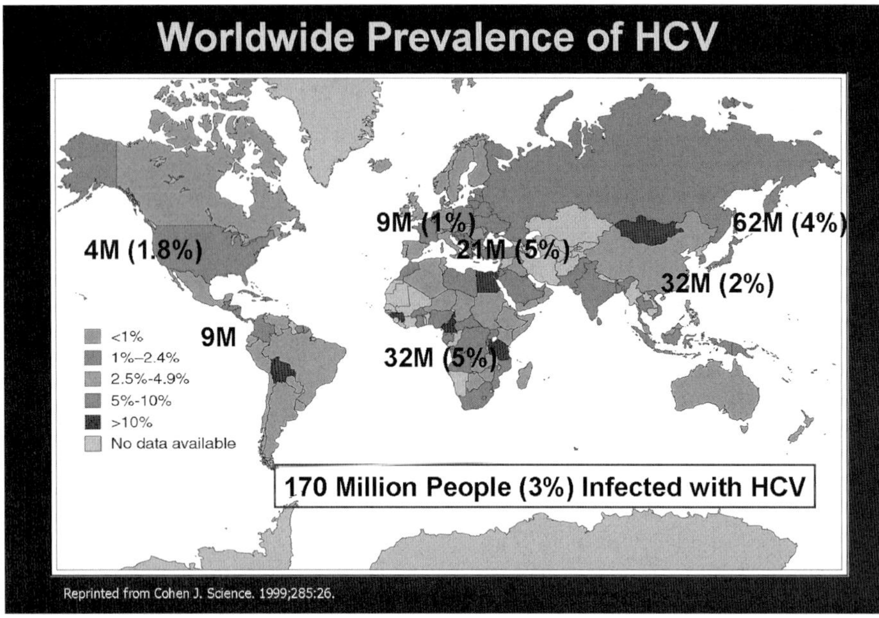

Figure 1. Worldwide prevalence of HCV. (*For colored version, see Plate V on page 565 at the end of the book.*)

The prevalence of hepatitis C in the United States is 1.8% among individuals above the age of 6 years [4]. The actual prevalence is probably somewhat higher since institutionalized people, such as prison inmates, were excluded from this landmark study performed between 1988 and 1994 by the Centers for Disease Control and Prevention (NHANES II). Numerically, 4 million people in the US have been infected with HCV and of these, almost 3 million, are believed to be chronically infected and remain at risk for progressive liver disease.

The prevalence of hepatitis C is also affected by age, gender, and race. Among all participants aged 30–49, the prevalence of HCV infection was ~4% (Figure 2). Among all age groups males are more commonly infected than females and increased prevalence rates were found in non-Hispanic blacks (3.2%) compared to non-Hispanic whites (1.8%). The highest prevalence rate of 9.8% was found in non-Hispanic black males between the ages of 30 and 49 years [4]. These differences in HCV prevalence across racial groups do not persist after adjustments for risk factors and other confounding variables.

3. NATURAL HISTORY OF HCV INFECTION

3.1 Acute hepatitis C infection

Identification of a person with acute hepatitis C is not common unless they are part of a systematic surveillance program. The majority of acute HCV infections have relatively mild, self-limited systemic symptoms that usually go undiagnosed [5]. Recent studies support earlier results that only 25–30% of individuals developing HCV infection after needle-stick injuries or other percutaneous exposures develop icteric hepatitis. Therefore, data concerning this interesting group of patients are somewhat limited. The diagnosis of acute HCV relies on a clinical history compatible with recent exposure, abnormal ALT > 10 times the upper limit of normal, seroconversion for anti-HCV, and detectable HCV RNA in sera (both discussed below). After a direct occupational needlestick injury from an HCV-positive source, it is estimated that 3–5% of patients will become infected with HCV. Overall, as many as 50% of those who develop acute hepatitis C after a known exposure will spontaneously resolve the

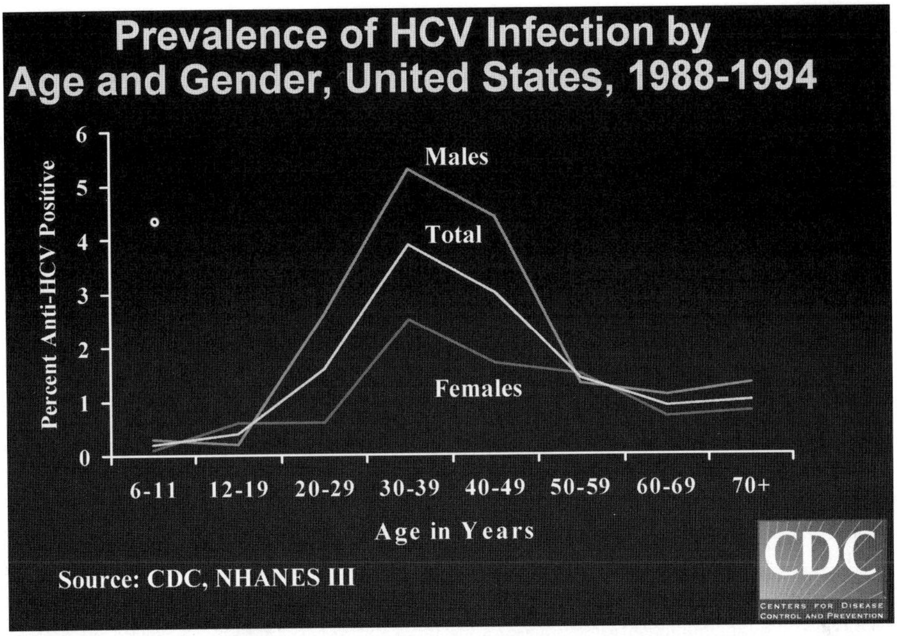

Figure 2. Age adjusted prevalence of hepatitis C infection in the United States. (*For colored version, see Plate VI on page 565 at the end of the book.*)

infection without treatment. Interestingly, individuals with icteric hepatitis at presentation are more likely to spontaneously clear their HCV than those with asymptomatic acute HCV infection. It should be stressed that spontaneous clearance occurs exclusively at the time of initial infection, rather than after chronic infection is established. This has important implications for counseling patients about treatment options. Although beyond the scope of this volume, treatment of acute hepatitis C within 4–6 months after exposure (after spontaneous clearance has been excluded) is almost universally successful in preventing chronicity [6].

3.2 Chronic hepatitis C

Although it is still accepted that most patients develop chronic infection after HCV exposure, recent data indicate that certain populations may be at greater, or lesser, risk for persistent infections. In a study of injection drug users, black subjects who were positive for anti-HCV were less likely to have spontaneously cleared virus than were whites (33 versus 67%, $p = 0.004$), a finding that remained significant in a multivariate analysis (Odds ratio = 4.8) [7]. In contrast, spontaneous HCV clearance has been reported in up to 50% of children infected at the time of cardiac surgery or chemotherapy and in young women infected with anti-D immunoglobulin during childbirth [8,9].

The clinical course of HCV liver disease is variable and difficult to predict for an individual patient (Figure 3). Progression to cirrhosis heralds the development of complications of portal hypertension and hepatocellular carcinoma. The estimates of the likelihood of developing cirrhosis after 20 years of HCV infection vary between 2 and 4% from studies in children and young women, to up to 20–30% among older males infected through blood transfusions [10]. Studies that have attempted to define the natural history of hepatitis C have yielded conflicting results. In an early study of transfusion associated non-A, non-B hepatitis, there was a small, but significant, increase of liver related mortality, particularly among those who drank alcohol [11]. At a tertiary referral center, a high incidence of cirrhosis (51%) and death from liver failure or HCC (15%) was found in patients with post-transfusion hepatitis [12]. Similarly, end-stage liver disease due to hepatitis C is the most common indication for liver transplantation in the United States [13].

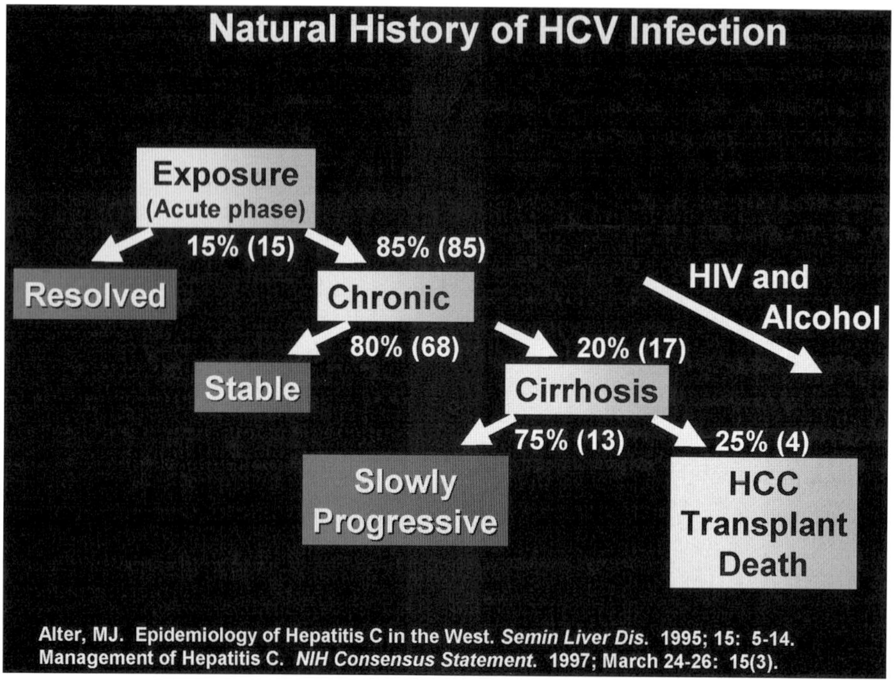

Figure 3. Natural history of chronic hepatitis C. (*For colored version, see Plate VII on page 566 at the end of the book.*)

The former results were undoubtedly biased by the nature of the referral population although they still indicate that hepatitis C can be a progressive, deadly liver disease in some patients.

In contrast, studies of Irish and German women who were infected with hepatitis C from anti-D immunoglobulin identified fewer than 10% who progressed to cirrhosis after 20 years and the majority had mild chronic hepatitis [8,9]. A more benign course to HCV infection is also suggested in a study of well-compensated patients whose 10-year survival probability was 79%, despite the presence of established cirrhosis [14]. Thus, these studies indicate that the clinical course of hepatitis C infection may not be uniformly relentless across all patient populations.

Certain co-factors will accelerate disease progression. Three independent risk factors, older age at acquisition, alcohol consumption greater than 50 g/day, and male gender, were associated with more rapid progression of fibrosis [15]. Concomitant alcohol use, in the setting of HCV infection, has repeatedly been implicated as a promoter for fibrogenesis leading to more advanced liver disease in many patients. Additional characteristics that are associated with more rapid disease progression include co-infection with human immunodeficiency virus (HIV) or hepatitis B virus (HBV), the presence of hepatic steatosis, hepatic schistosomiasis, and a predisposition to hepatic iron overload. Interestingly, virological factors such as HCV genotype and levels of HCV RNA in sera have not been consistently associated with poorer outcomes.

4. DIAGNOSIS OF HCV INFECTION

Most patients with chronic hepatitis C are asymptomatic. When symptoms are present they are rather non-specific including fatigue, malaise, mild abdominal discomfort in the right upper quadrant, and arthralgias. Occasionally, the initial presentation can be associated with signs and symptoms of portal hypertension (thrombocytopenia, esophageal variceal hemorrhage, ascites), reinforcing the generally insidious nature of this disease.

Hepatitis C has been associated with a number of extrahepatic manifestations, usually immune mediated, that can be the dominant clinical features

Table 1. Extrahepatic manifestations of chronic hepatitis C.

Cryoglobulinemia
Glomerulonephritis
B-cell lymphoma
Porphyria cutanea tarda
Thyroidoitis
Lichen planus
Sialadenitis
Mooren corneal ulcer

leading to the diagnosis of hepatitis C [16] (Table 1). The most widely characterized extrahepatic manifestation is mixed cryoglobulinemia. Cryoglobulins are serum immunoglobulins that precipitate with cooling. The presence of rheumatoid factor in this setting should not be confused with a diagnosis of rheumatoid arthritis. Clinical manifestations of cryoglobulins include leukocytoclastic vasculitis, characterized by palpable purpura, most commonly on the lower extremities, membrano-proliferative glomerulonephritis, and neuropathy. Numerous other extrahepatic manifestations have been reported including porphyria cutanea tardae, B-cell lymphoma, Lichen planus, thyroiditis, and corneal ulcer.

Since, symptoms are unreliable for the early diagnosis of chronic hepatitis C, the first step in diagnosis of HCV is identifying individuals at increased risk for HCV infection so that they can be appropriately tested. It is imperative that primary healthcare providers become familiar with the potential risk factors for acquisition of HCV infection and actively elicit this information from their patients during a thorough medical history [17]. Because of the sensitive nature of some of the inquiries, direct face-to-face questioning may be more fruitful compared to completing a written questionnaire.

5. RISK FACTORS FOR HCV INFECTION

Epidemiologic studies have identified a number of risk factors that are associated with HCV infection. Approximately 60% of HCV infections were acquired as a result of injection drug use while blood transfusions were the second leading cause of HCV infection, responsible for approximately 10% of infections. The most striking prevalence of HCV infection (approximately 90%) is found in hemophilics, who were exposed to non-inactivated factor replacement prior to 1987. Since, adequate screening of blood products for HCV began in the early 1990s, the risk of HCV infection from transfusions is rare (Figure 4).

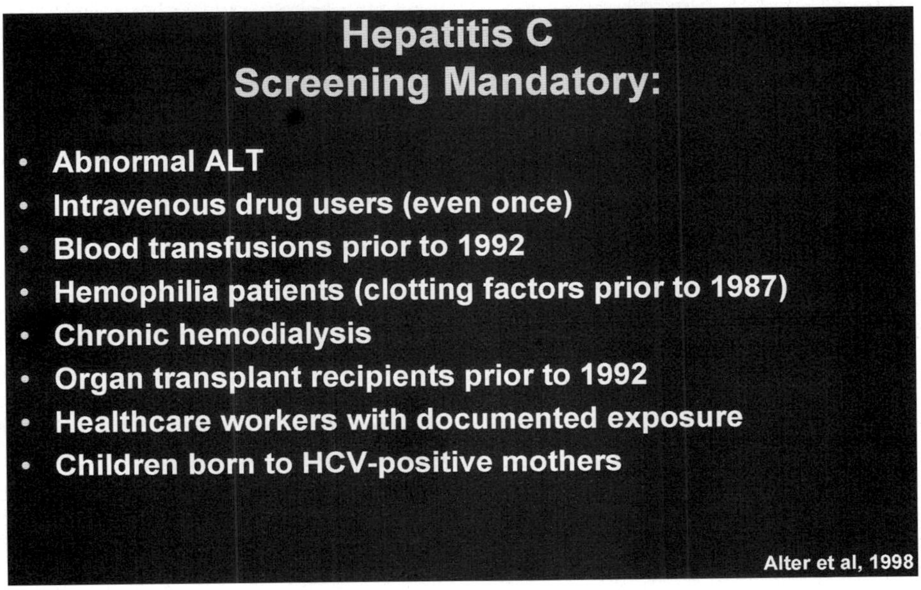

Figure 4. Risk factors for HCV acquisition. (*For colored version, see Plate VIII on page 566 at the end of the book.*)

The CDC has recommended routine screening for HCV for any individuals with the following risk factors for exposure [17]:

- injection drug use at any time;
- history of blood transfusions or solid organ transplant prior to 1992;
- history of chronic hemodialysis; and
- persistently abnormal serum alanine aminotransferase (ALT) activity.

Testing for hepatitis C is also recommended for healthcare workers exposed to HCV-positive blood through needlesticks or mucosal routes, although the risk of infection is low (<2%). Similarly, children born to HCV-positive mothers should be tested for hepatitis C at a point beyond the passive transfer of maternal antibodies, and when blood sampling is more convenient. Perinatal transmission is an uncommon mode of transmission (approximately 5% in non-HIV infected women), such that the presence of maternal HCV infection should not affect decisions concerning pregnancy, breastfeeding, or mode of delivery. The roles of tattoos and body piercing in HCV transmission remain poorly defined.

6. DIAGNOSTIC TESTS FOR HEPATITIS C

Once an individual is identified as having an increased risk for HCV infection, clinicians should embark on a thorough, cost-effective evaluation. Numerous assays are available for the diagnosis and monitoring of patients with chronic hepatitis C; however, they should be applied to specific clinical situations.

6.1 Anti-HCV antibody

Anti-HCV antibody (anti-HCV) is an enzyme immunoassay (EIA) that is the best screening test when HCV infection is suspected [10,18] (Figure 5). They are inexpensive and easy to perform. Anti-HCV seroconversion occurs 3–8 weeks after acute infection and usually remains positive indefinitely, even in patients who spontaneously recover. Thus, the presence of anti-HCV indicates exposure to HCV but does not differentiate between an acute, a chronic, or a resolved infection. It does not confer immunity to hepatitis C. Current versions of EIA anti-HCV

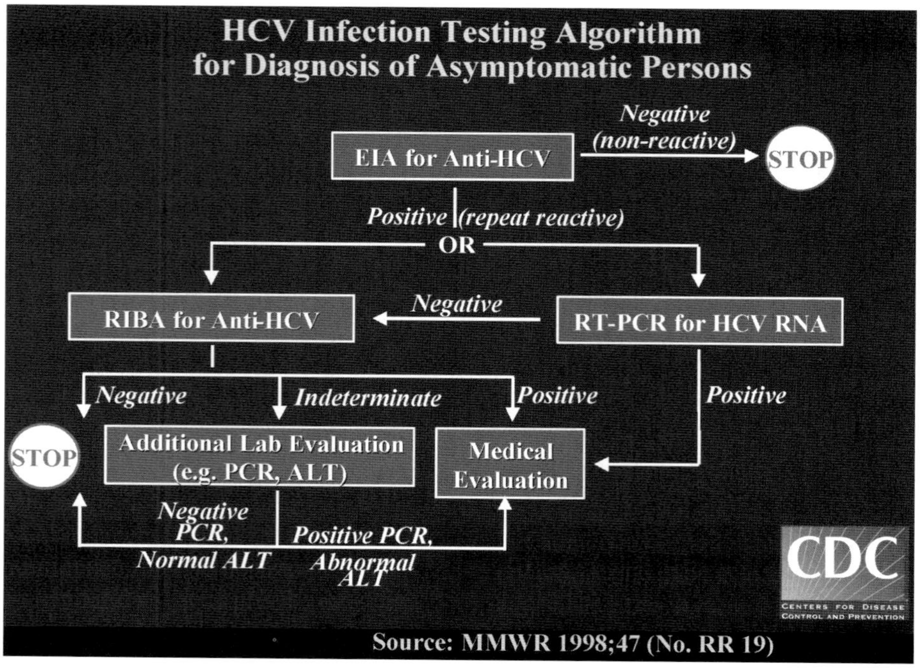

Figure 5. CDC recommendations for HCV serologic testing. *(For colored version, see Plate IX on page 567 at the end of the book.)*

assays detect antibodies to epitopes from multiple regions of the HCV genome, yielding a highly sensitive and specific assay (>95%). A positive anti-HCV in an individual with risk factors for HCV infection and an abnormal ALT is virtually diagnostic of HCV infection. Rarely, false negative anti-HCV antibody can occur in patients who are immunosuppressed such as those on renal dialysis, undergoing chemotherapy, or coinfected with HIV. In these circumstances, a sensitive and specific nucleic acid test to detect HCV RNA should be used (discussed below).

6.2 Supplemental assays

False positive anti-HCV results can occur, particularly in low-risk (no identified risk factors) individuals with normal ALT. In this setting, supplemental assays should be considered to verify the results of the anti-HCV antibody. Recombinant immunoblot assay (RIBA) is a serological assay utilizing recombinant antigens derived from different regions (structural and non-structural) of the HCV genome [18]. RIBAs may be interpreted as positive, negative, or indeterminate. A positive RIBA indicates true exposure to HCV, while a negative RIBA indicates a false positive EIA assay. Indeterminate results require additional evaluation with nucleic acid testing. Although the RIBA assay is regularly used in blood banking, the role of RIBA in clinical practice for routine diagnosis has diminished, due to the excellent sensitivity and specificity of anti-HCV antibody tests. RIBA is useful for confirming true HCV exposure in low-risk populations (i.e., absent of identifiable HCV risk factors) who test positive for anti-HCV antibody. However, in most clinical situations direct tests of HCV viremia (discussed below) may be more appropriate.

6.3 Nucleic acid testing

Nucleic acid testing (NAT) for HCV RNA is the most specific test for the diagnosis of current HCV infection. Virologic testing relies on target amplification techniques [polymerase chain reaction (PCR) or transcription mediated amplification (TMA)] or a signal amplification technique (branched DNA assay) [19]. NAT is performed to confirm viremia in a patient with a positive anti-HCV. NAT is mandatory before considering anyone for antiviral therapy and it is also used to monitor therapeutic response.

Qualitative assays detect only the presence, or absence, of HCV RNA, while *quantitative* assays provide a measurement of HCV RNA levels in international units. Quantitative assays vary in their sensitivities and dynamic ranges at which they are able to quantify HCV RNA (Figure 6). Highly sensitive assays are important for detecting low levels of viremia during therapy, while assays with a broad dynamic range allow for accurate quantitation of HCV RNA at high levels of viremia [19]. It should be noted that neither levels of HCV RNA nor HCV genotype (discussed below) correlate with rates of disease progression. Despite standardization of quantitative assays to the international unit (IU), there is some inherent variability and care should be taken to avoid switching to different assays during an individual treatment course in order to avoid confusion while interpreting therapeutic response.

NAT is the initial test of choice in the occasional patient in whom acute hepatitis C is suspected. In acute HCV, EIA anti-HCV may be negative in the early weeks of infection while HCV RNA may be detectable within the first 7 days after exposure. Testing for HCV RNA is also important to define spontaneous clearance of HCV infection. In this situation, anti-HCV and RIBA are positive but HCV RNA is repeatedly negative (on at least two occasions), in the absence of antiviral therapy.

6.4 HCV genotype

Hepatitis C is a heterogeneous RNA virus with great variability in its genetic sequence. Six major genotypes and multiple subtypes of HCV have been recognized. Genotypes have a geographic distribution (Figure 7). In the United States, genotype 1 (1a or 1b) is found in approximately 75% of patients with the remainder being genotype 2 or 3. In Europe and Japan, genotype 1b is the predominant strain, while genotype 4 appears to be unique to Egypt.

HCV RNA Assays
Performance Characteristics

Assay	Type	Lower Limit Detection	Dynamic Range
Amplicor HCV v2.0	Qual	50 IU/ml	N/A
Versant HCV RNA	Qual	10 IU/ml	N/A
Monitor HCV v2.0	Quant	600 IU/ml	600-500,000
Versant v3.0	Quant	615 IU/ml	615-7,700,000
SuperQuant	Quant	30 IU/ml	30-1,470,000

Adapted from Pawlotsky, 2002

Figure 6. HCV RNA assays. *(For colored version, see Plate X on page 567 at the end of the book.)*

Obtaining HCV genotype is mandatory before beginning therapy for hepatitis C. Hepatitis C genotype has been shown to be the single most predictive factor of treatment response to all approved antiviral agents. Patients with genotype 1 have decreased response rates to therapy than patients with genotypes 2 or 3 [10,20]. Recent data indicate that patients with genotypes 2 or 3 can be treated with a lower dose of ribavirin for a shorter duration without compromising efficacy, when compared with more aggressive regimen [21]. Thus, knowledge of genotype can help tailor the treatment regimen for a specific patient.

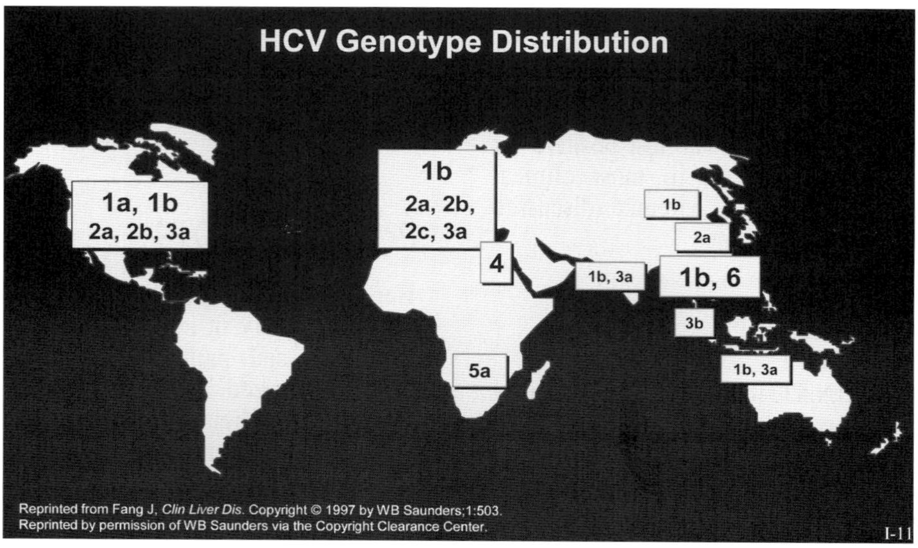

Figure 7. Geographic distribution of HCV genotypes. *(For colored version, see Plate XI on page 568 at the end of the book.)*

6.5 Liver biopsy

The role of liver biopsy in the management of HCV patients is evolving. Specific serological tests for HCV obviate the need for liver biopsy solely for diagnosis of chronic hepatitis C. However, liver biopsy remains the only tool that provides prognostic information regarding hepatic inflammation and fibrosis; laboratory data is insufficiently sensitive or specific, except in the most advanced cases. Multiple scoring system has been developed that describe the grade (inflammatory score) and the stage (fibrosis score). Prognosis is directly related to the stage of the liver biopsy. Those with increased fibrosis on liver biopsy have an increased risk of disease progression over time. Recent attention has focused on the association of HCV and hepatic steatosis which can have some impact on prognosis and, possibly, on response to therapy. Therefore, liver biopsy is important in advising the patient about the extent of liver injury that has occurred since infection and also provides some insights into the likelihood of progression in the future, although with less certainty. Cirrhosis can be diagnosed without a liver biopsy in individuals with obvious hepatic decompensation and evidence of portal hypertension.

7. COUNSELING OF THE HCV-INFECTED INDIVIDUAL

Many patients recently diagnosed with chronic hepatitis C are bewildered that they have chronic liver disease. This is particularly true in the asymptomatic patient who was tested for HCV at the time of blood donation or coincidentally during an annual medical check-up. It is important that the primary healthcare practitioner provides some basic information that will set the proper tone as the patient begins processing the implications of this unexpected diagnosis.

- Reinforce the generally slow progression of hepatitis C while stressing the importance of being fully evaluated.
- Hepatitis C is treatable and can be cured in over 50% of those treated.
- Discuss modes of transmission and dispel myths about casual contact, sharing food utensils, etc.
- Reassure about the low risk to sexual partners but inform that the risk is measurable; there are no specific CDC recommendations for altering sexual practices.
- Reassure that vertical transmission occurs infrequently. The CDC has no specific recommendations concerning altering birthing practices or breastfeeding.
- Discuss avoidance of alcohol.

Written materials from reputable agencies such as the Centers for Disease Control and Prevention and the American Liver Foundation should be freely distributed.

8. THERAPY FOR HCV

Treatment of chronic hepatitis C has improved greatly since the identification of HCV in 1989 (Figure 8). The recent NIH Consensus Statement on hepatitis C noted that all patients with chronic hepatitis C are potential candidates for therapy with peginterferons and ribavirin [10]. Before embarking on therapy, however, healthcare providers must thoroughly examine the risks and benefits to therapy within the context of the medical history of their patient.

Several absolute contraindications to therapy exist and, in these situations, therapy should never be initiated:

- pregnancy, pregnancy in the partner of a patient, contemplating pregnancy, unwillingness to use adequate contraception, or breast feeding (due to effects of ribavirin on the fetus);
- poorly controlled psychiatric disease, including recent history of suicide attempt (due to psychiatric effects of interferon); and
- symptomatic coronary artery disease (due to ribavirin-induced anemia).

Numerous other contraindications and cautions to therapy are noted in the product inserts of these antiviral agents. Some of the cautions may be considered as relative, rather than absolute, contraindications to therapy such that decisions concerning treatment must be individualized.

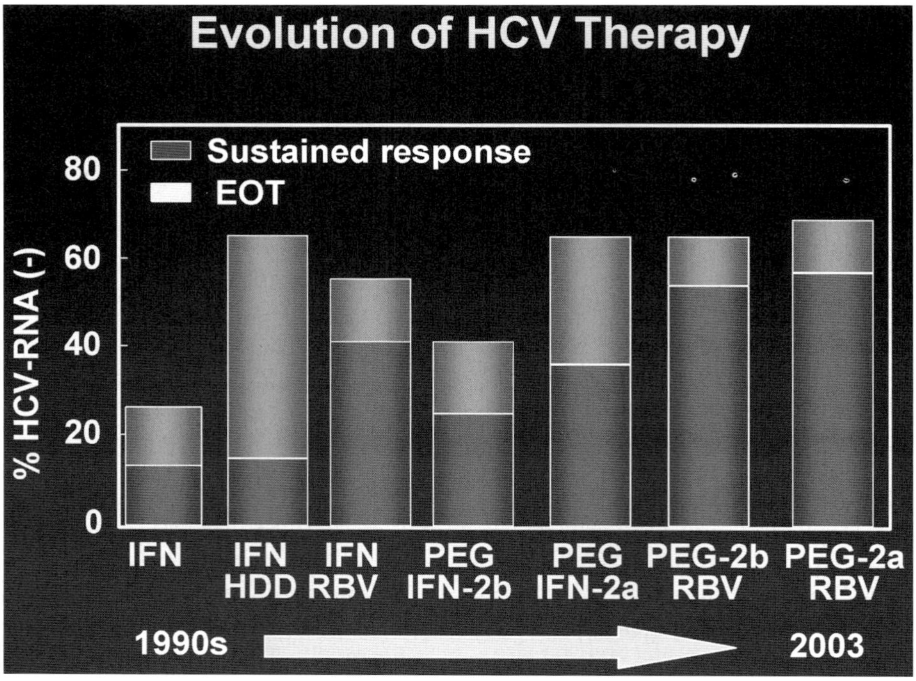

Figure 8. Improvement in antiviral therapy for chronic hepatitis C over the last decade (EOT = End of treatment response). (*For colored version, see Plate XII on page 568 at the end of the book.*)

The goal of treatment is permanent eradication of the virus, which can now be achieved in more than half of the patients undergoing therapy. Sustained virological response (SVR) is defined as having undetectable HCV RNA in serum, 6 months *after* antiviral therapy has been completed (Figure 9). Patients achieving SVR are essentially cured of hepatitis C; long-term follow-up studies have shown that the likelihood of relapse beyond this time point rarely occurs [22]. Furthermore, HCV RNA is no longer detectable in liver tissue of individuals with SVR [23]. Multiple studies have also demonstrated improvement in hepatic histological scores for necroinflammatory activity and for fibrosis [24].

The newest drugs to treat hepatitis C are pegylated interferons (peginterferon alfa-2a and peginterferon alfa-2b). The addition of a polyethylene glycol moiety to an interferon molecule alters the pharmacokinetic properties of the native protein resulting in a prolonged serum half-life and the ability to dose once weekly as a subcutaneous injection rather than thrice weekly. Peginterferon alfa-2a utilizes a branched, 40 kDa PEG while peginterferon alfa-2b encompasses a linear 12 kDa PEG molecule. Differences in pharmacokinetic properties of peginterferons, such as serum half-life, are dependent upon the size and configuration of the attached PEG molecule. Both of these agents have demonstrated superiority in achieving SVR as monotherapy compared to standard interferon [25,26]. Combination therapy with peginterferon and ribavirin, a nucleoside analogue, has been established as the standard of care for patients with chronic hepatitis C [10].

Sustained virologic response rates for patients treated with peginterferon (2a or 2b) and ribavirin range from 54 to 56% by intention to treat analyses [20,27] (Figure 10). For patients with genotype 1, considered more resistant to therapy, SVR was achieved in 42% (peginterferon alfa-2b) to 51% (peginterferon alfa-2a) of patients treated for 48 weeks [20,21,27]. Patients with genotype 2 or 3, recognized as more responsive to treatment, had uniformly favorable response to treatment with SVR in approximately 80% of individuals who received treatment for 24 weeks using a lower dose of ribavirin in combination

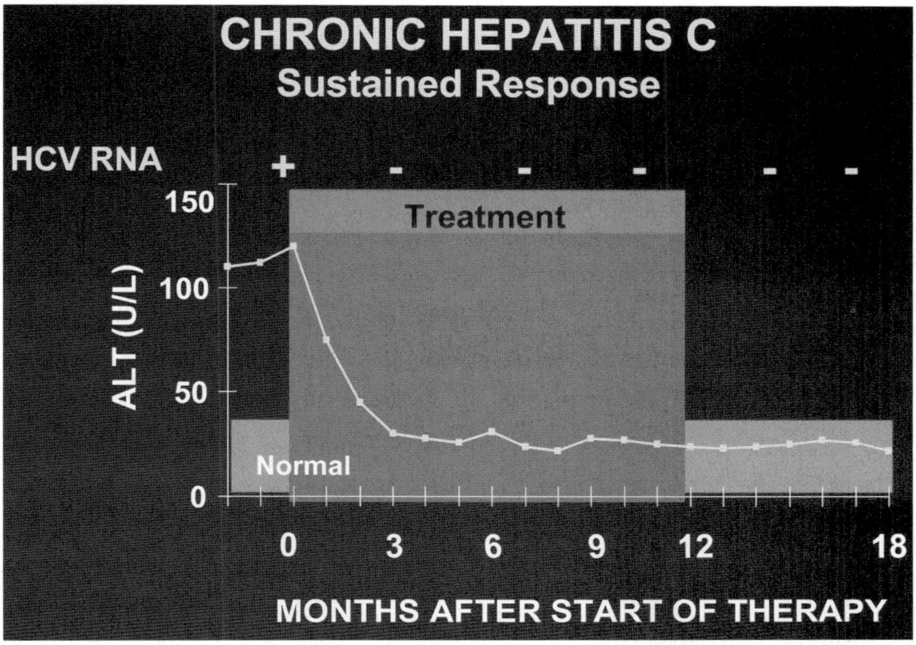

Figure 9. Schematic of sustained virological response (SVR). (*For colored version, see Plate XIII on page 569 at the end of the book.*)

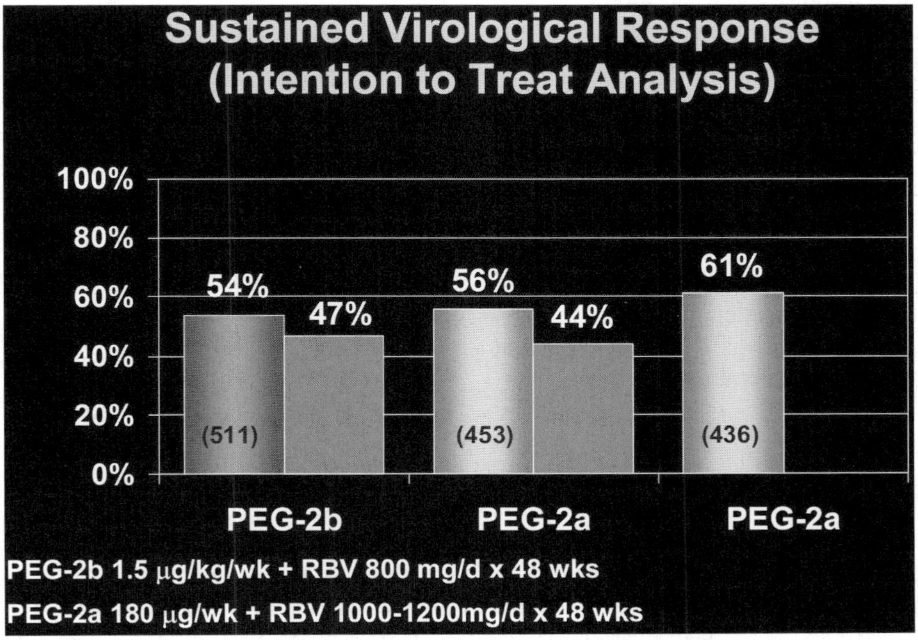

Figure 10. Sustained virological response using peginterferon alfa-2a or peginterferon alfa-2b in combination with ribavirin [20,21,27]. (*For colored version, see Plate XIV on page 569 at the end of the book.*)

with peginterferon alfa-2a [21]. Thus, genotype is very important for tailoring the course of treatment to the individual patient.

Peginterferons and ribavirin have significant side effects that require close monitoring and frequent interventions to maintain patient safety and efficacy [28]. All patients experience increased fatigue and influenza-like symptoms during the early phase of treatment. Depression and other neuropsychiatric side effects have been reported in 20–30% of patients on therapy. Peginterferons regularly cause reversible neutropenia while ribavirin universally causes hemolytic anemia with an average decrease in hemoglobin of approximately 2.5 g. Despite these side effects, most patients complete the treatment regimen. Excessive dose reductions or premature discontinuations due to adverse events are associated with decreased therapeutic response. Therefore, only healthcare providers comfortable with the use of these agents should manage patients on antiviral therapy.

9. SUMMARY

Hepatitis C is a global health problem. Chronic hepatitis C is a leading cause of morbidity and mortality from end-stage liver disease and its complications of portal hypertension and hepatocellular carcinoma. Most individuals are asymptomatic so that primary healthcare providers should actively question their patients about behaviors and any past medical history that places them at increased risk for HCV infection. Appropriate serological screening is then mandatory. Patients should be encouraged about the natural history of chronic hepatitis C and informed about the availability of excellent treatments that can permanently eradicate hepatitis C virus and prevent complications of chronic liver disease.

REFERENCES

[1] Kim, W.R. (2002) Global epidemiology and burden of hepatitis C. *Microbes Infect.* **4**, 1219–1225.

[2] Wasley, A. and Alter, M.J. (2000) Epidemiology of hepatitis C: geographic differences and temporal trends. *Semin. Liver Dis.* **20**, 1–16.

[3] Frank, C., Mohamed, M.K., Strickland, G.T., Lavanchy, D., Arthur, R.R., Magder, L.S., El Khoby, T. *et al.* (2000) The role of parenteral antischistosomal therapy in the spread of hepatitis C virus in Egypt. *Lancet* **355**, 887–891.

[4] Alter, M.J., Kruszon-Moran, D., Nainan, O.V., McQuillan, G.M., Gao, F., Moyer, L.A., Kaslow, R.A. and Margolis, H.S. (1999) The prevalence of hepatitis C virus infection in the United States, 1988 through 1994. *N. Engl. J. Med.* **341**, 556–562.

[5] Gordon, S.C. (2003) New insights into acute hepatitis C. *Gastroenterology* **125**, 253–256.

[6] Gerlach, J.T., Diepolder, H.M., Zachoval, R., Gruener, N.H., Jung, M.C., Ulsenheimer, A., Schraut, W.W., Schirren, C.A., Waechtler, M., Backmund, M. and Pape, G.R. (2003) Acute hepatitis C: high rate of both spontaneous and treatment-induced viral clearance. *Gastroenterology* **125**, 80–88.

[7] Thomas, D.L., Astemborski, J., Rai, R.M., Anania, F.A., Schaeffer, M., Galai, N., Nolt, K., Nelson, K.E., Strathdee, S.A., Johnson, L., Laeyendecker, O., Boitnott, J., Wilson, L.E. and Vlahov, D. (2000) The natural history of hepatitis C virus infection: host, viral, and environmental factors. *J. Am. Med. Assoc.* **284**, 450–456.

[8] Wiese, M., Berr, F., Lafrenz, M., Porst, H. and Oesen, U. (2000) Low frequency of cirrhosis in a hepatitis C (genotype 1b) single-source outbreak in Germany: a 20-year multicenter study. *Hepatology* **32**, 91–96.

[9] Kenny-Walsh, E. (1999) Clinical outcomes after hepatitis C infection from contaminated anti-D immune globulin. Irish Hepatology Research Group. *N. Engl. J. Med.* **340**, 1228–1233.

[10] National Institutes of Health Consensus Development Conference Statement (2002) Management of hepatitis C 2002 (June 10–12, 2002). *Gastroenterology* **123**, 2082–2099.

[11] Seeff, L.B., Buskell-Bales, Z., Wright, E.C., Durako, S.J., Alter, H.J., Iber, F.L., Hollinger, F.B., Gitnick, G., Knodell, R.G., Perrillo, R.P. (1992) Long-term mortality after transfusion-associated non-A, non-B hepatitis. The National Heart, Lung, and Blood Institute Study Group. *N. Engl. J. Med.* **327**, 1906–1911.

[12] Tong, M.J., el-Farra, N.S., Reikes, A.R. and Co, R.L. (1995) Clinical outcomes after transfusion-associated hepatitis C. *N. Engl. J. Med.* **332**, 1463–1466.

[13] Kim, W.R. (2002) The burden of hepatitis C in the United States. *Hepatology* **36**, S30–S34.

[14] Fattovich, G., Giustina, G., Degos, F., Tremolada, F., Diodati, G., Almasio, P., Nevens, F., Solinas, A., Mura, D., Brouwer, J.T., Thomas, H., Njapoum, C.,

Casarin, C., Bonetti, P., Fuschi, P., Basho, J., Tocco, A., Bhalla, A., Galassini, R., Noventa, F., Schalm, S.W. and Realdi, G. (1997) Morbidity and mortality in compensated cirrhosis type C: a retrospective follow-up study of 384 patients. *Gastroenterology* **112**, 463–472.

[15] Poynard, T., Bedossa, P. and Opolon, P. (1997) Natural history of liver fibrosis progression in patients with chronic hepatitis C. The OBSVIRC, METAVIR, CLINIVIR, and DOSVIRC groups. *Lancet* **349**, 825–832.

[16] Mehta, S., Levey, J.M. and Bonkovsky, H.L. (2001) Extrahepatic manifestations of infection with hepatitis C virus. *Clin. Liver Dis.* **5**, 979–1008.

[17] Centers for Disease Control and Prevention (1997) Transmission of hepatitis C virus infection associated with home infusion therapy for hemophilia. *J. A. Med. Assoc.* **278**, 1057–1058.

[18] Alter, M.J., Kuhnert, W.L. and Finelli, L. (2003) Guidelines for laboratory testing and result reporting of antibody to hepatitis C virus. Centers for Disease Control and Prevention. *MMWR Recomm. Rep.* **52**, 1–13. 15; quiz CE11-14.

[19] Pawlotsky, J.M. (2002) Use and interpretation of virological tests for hepatitis C. *Hepatology* **36**, S65–S73.

[20] Fried, M.W., Shiffman, M.L., Reddy, K.R., Smith, C., Marinos, G., Goncales, F.L., Haussinger, D., Diago, M., Carosi, G., Dhumeaux, D., Craxi, A., Lin, A., Hoffman, J. and Yu, J. (2002) Peginterferon alfa-2a plus ribavirin for chronic hepatitis C virus infection. *N. Engl. J. Med.* **347**, 975–982.

[21] Hadziyannis, S., Cheinquer, H., Morgan, T., Diago, M., Jensen, D.M., Sette, H., Jr., Ramadori, G., Bodenheimer, H.C., Marcellin, P., Lee, S.-D., Roberts, P.J. and Ackrill, A.M. (2002) Peginterferon alfa-2a (PEGASYS) in combination with ribavirin: efficacy and safety results from a phase III randomized, double-blind, multicenter trial examining effect of duration of treatment and ribavirin dose. *J. Hepatol.* **36**(Suppl. 1), 3 (abstract).

[22] Lau, D.T., Kleiner, D.E., Ghany, M.G., Park, Y., Schmid, P. and Hoofnagle, J.H. (1998) 10-Year follow-up after interferon-alpha therapy for chronic hepatitis C. *Hepatology* **28**, 1121–1127.

[23] McHutchison, J.G., Poynard, T., Esteban-Mur, R., Davis, G.L., Goodman, Z.D., Harvey, J., Ling, M.H., Garaud, J.J., Abrecht, J.K., Patel, K. and Dienstag, J.L., for the International Hepatitis Interventional Therapy Group. (2002) Hepatic HCV RNA before and after treatment with interferon alone or combined with ribavirin. *Hepatology* **35**, 688–693.

[24] Poynard, T., McHutchison, J., Davis, G.L., Esteban-Mur, R., Goodman, Z., Bedossa, P. and Albrecht, J. (2000) Impact of interferon alfa-2b and ribavirin on progression of liver fibrosis in patients with chronic hepatitis C. *Hepatology* **32**, 1131–1137.

[25] Zeuzem, S., Feinman, S.V., Rasenack, J., Heathcote, E.J., Lai, M.Y., Gane, E., O'Grady, J., Reichen, J., Diago, M., Lin, A., Hoffman, J. and Brunda, M.J. (2000) Peginterferon alfa-2a in patients with chronic hepatitis C. *N. Engl. J. Med.* **343**, 1666–1672.

[26] Lindsay, K.L., Trepo, C., Heintges, T., Shiffman, M.L., Gordon, S.C., Hoefs, J.C., Schiff, E.R., Goodman, Z.D., Laughlin, M., Yao, R., Albrecht, J.K., Hepatitis Interventional Therapy Group. (2001) A randomized, double-blind trial comparing pegylated interferon alfa-2b to interferon alfa-2b as initial treatment for chronic hepatitis C. *Hepatology* **34**, 395–403.

[27] Manns, M.P., McHutchison, J.G., Gordon, S.C., Rustgi, V.K., Shiffman, M., Reindollar, R., Goodman, Z.D., Koury, K., Ling, M.-H., Albrecht, J.K. and the International Hepatitis Interventional Therapy Group. (2001) Peginterferon alfa-2b plus ribavirin compared with interferon alfa-2b plus ribavirin for initial treatment of chronic hepatitis C: a randomised trial. *Lancet* **358**, 958–965.

[28] Russo, M.W. and Fried, M.W. (2003) Side effects of therapy for chronic hepatitis C. *Gastroenterology* **124**, 1711–1719.

Hepatology: A Practical Approach
B. Al Knawy, M.L. Shiffman, R.H. Wiesner (editors)

Chapter 4
Hepatitis D

Stephanos J. Hadziyannis[a], *Dimitrios Vassilopoulos*[b] *and George V. Papatheodoridis*[b]

[a]Department of Medicine and Hepatology, The Henry Dunant Hospital, 107 Messogion Avenue, 115 26 Athens, Greece

[b]2nd Academic Department of Medicine, Athens University School of Medicine, Hippokration General Hospital, 114 Vas Sofias Ave., 115 21 Athens, Greece

1. Introduction 101
  1.1 Disease definition 101
  1.2 Disease prevalence and incidence 101
2. Pathophysiology 102
3. Clinical Features 103
4. Diagnosis 104
5. Management 107
  5.1 Medical therapeutics 107
  5.2 Surgical procedures 107
  5.3 Prevention including family screening 108
6. Prognosis 108
References 108

1. INTRODUCTION

1.1 Disease definition

Hepatitis D is an infection caused by a satellite virus (or subviral agent) of hepatitis B virus (HBV), the hepatitis D virus (HDV) [1]. HDV infection occurs only in the presence of a concurrent or underlying chronic HBV infection. In the first setting, infection of the naïve host with both viruses (HBV and HDV) results in an acute hepatitis that is almost invariably self-limited (*co-infection*) [2]. Alternatively, an individual who is already chronically infected by HBV becomes infected with HDV leading either to an acute exacerbation of the underlying chronic liver disease or to a chronic HDV infection (*super-infection*) [2].

1.2 Disease prevalence and incidence

An estimated 5% of HBV-infected persons are considered to be HDV infected which accounts for 10–15 million HDV-infected individuals worldwide [3]. The distribution of HDV infection shows a significant geographical variation with areas of high, intermediate and low endemicity. Areas of high endemicity include parts of South America, certain South Pacific Islands, parts of West Africa and Northern India. The major determinant of HDV prevalence appears to be the route of transmission (parenteral vs. non-parenteral). High prevalence of HDV infection has been observed among intravenous drug users and their sexual partners, even in areas with low HBV endemicity such as most Western countries. Intrafamilial transmission is another well-established mode of HDV transmission in several parts of the world including the Mediterranean area.

Overall, during the last two decades a major decrease in the prevalence of HDV infection (acute and chronic) has been noted worldwide [3,4]. This epidemiological trend is mainly attributed to the significant decrease in the incidence of HBV infection as a result of widespread immunization programs and effective blood screening programs as well as to the general improvement of socioeconomic conditions including the use of disposable needles and syringes. This trend is best illustrated in countries such as Italy and Greece where the prevalence of HDV infection has significantly decreased [4,5]. For example, in Italy the number of HDV-infected individuals among HBV-infected persons has decreased from 23% in 1987 to 14% in 1992 and 8% in 1997 [4].

2. PATHOPHYSIOLOGY

HDV is a defective small single-stranded RNA virus that utilizes the envelope proteins of HBV for its assembly and infectivity [1]. The HDV particles are almost spherical with a diameter of approximately 38 nm and are comprised of a

- *ribonucleoprotein particle (RNP)* containing the HDV genomic RNA (~ 1.7 kb) complexed with approximately 70 copies of the hepatitis delta antigen (HDAg) and an
- *outer envelope* containing lipids and mixtures of the three HBV surface proteins (HBsAg, Pre-S1, Pre-S2).

The genome of HDV consists of a 1679-nucleotide (nt) negative stranded single-stranded circular RNA called δRNA, which represents the smallest genome known to cause human infection [1]. The HDV RNA is similar to that of plant viroids and virusoids RNAs and due to its significant intra-molecular base pairing (~ 70%) it is shaped in a rod-like structure. Replication of the *genomic RNA* proceeds through RNA-directed RNA transcription, probably utilizing the host RNA polymerase II. Two types of complementary RNAs called *antigenomic RNA* and *m-RNA* are produced during transcription in the nucleus of infected hepatocytes. The full-length positive stranded antigenomic RNA (~ 1.7 kb) serves as the template for the transcription back to the circular HDV genome while the m-RNA that is approximately 0.8 kb in size, is being translated into the small hepatitis delta antigen (HDAg-S). The HDAg-S (24 kDa) is 195 amino acids (aa) long and is necessary for HDV RNA replication.

During RNA replication, a small percentage (30–50%) of antigenomic transcripts undergo post-transcriptional RNA editing by an enzyme called double-stranded RNA adenosine deaminase (ADAR). This editing leads during translation to the addition of 19 aa downstream of the small HDAg, creating the large HDAg (HDAg-L, 214 aa, 27 kDa). The HDAg-L inhibits RNA replication but at the same time is necessary for virion formation.

The HDV enters hepatocytes through an unknown receptor on the surface of liver cells (most likely utilizing the same receptor as HBV). HDV then replicates in the nucleus of infected hepatocytes which is the only site where active HDV infection has been documented. The exact sequence of events that occur during HDV replication and give rise to the production of the different RNAs and HDV proteins have not been clarified. The most prevailing model of HDV replication is the double rolling-circle model proposed by Taylor [1].

So far, three different genotypes of HDV have been identified [6]. Genotype I is the predominant strain in North America and Europe whereas genotype II predominates in the East Asia and genotype III in South America and parts of Africa. A more severe course of HDV infection has been postulated for patients infected with genotypes I and III. This may be related to differences in virological characteristics between the different genotypes. In a recent study, genotype II HDV strains displayed a decreased efficiency of viral packaging and assembly compared to genotype I isolates, which may in part explain the less severe course of genotype II HDV infection [7]. However, adequate long-term longitudinal studies examining the role of the various genotypes in the natural course of acute or chronic HDV infection are lacking.

The mechanisms of HDV-induced liver disease have not been delineated but as is the case with other hepatotropic viruses (HBV, HCV) they are assumed to be predominantly immune mediated. Cellular immune responses (mainly CD4-mediated) are considered crucial in the control of HDV replication on the one hand and in the induction of liver inflammation on the other. In HIV-infected patients or in animals (woodchucks) receiving immunosuppressive therapy (cyclosporine), the levels of HDV viremia were higher indicating a role of T cell-mediated suppression of viral replication. Similarly, in patients with inactive chronic HDV infection, strong CD4 responses were observed suggesting a role of these cells in the control of HDV viremia [8].

3. CLINICAL FEATURES

The clinical features of HDV infection resemble those associated with other forms of viral hepatitis, but they may be generally more severe. Acute HDV infection results from acquisition of both HBV and HDV at the same time in individuals previously susceptible to both viruses (HDV co-infection) (Figure 1) or from acquisition of only HDV in patients already chronically infected with HBV (HDV super-infection) (Figure 2). The incubation period of HDV ranges from 3 to 7 weeks probably depending on the size of the viral inoculum. The acute hepatitis phase may run sub-clinically or present clinically as a typical acute viral hepatitis with preceding non-specific symptoms (fatigue, anorexia, nausea) followed by clay-colored stools, dark urine and jaundice. Acute HDV co-infection often presents with a biphasic pattern of serum aminotransferases values that corresponds to two distinct episodes of hepatitis 1–2 weeks apart, one related to HBV and one to HDV (Figure 1). The interval between and the sequence of these two episodes are probably associated with the relative size of the HBV and HDV inoculum [2].

Acute hepatitis D may become fulminant. It is estimated that the proportion of patients with severe or fulminant hepatitis is higher in acute hepatitis D than in other forms of acute viral hepatitis. Acute HDV super-infections are considered to run a more severe course than co-infections, but fulminant liver failure may develop in both cases. In Western countries, the risk for development of fulminant hepatitis is highest among intravenous drug users who develop acute HBV and HDV co-infections on pre-existing chronic HCV infections. Frequent development of severe or fulminant hepatitis D, even as epidemics, has been described in South America and has been associated with genotype III HDV strains that are prevalent in these areas.

Acute HDV infection may progress to chronicity. Acute HBV and HDV co-infection has a self-limited course in the vast majority of cases, while acute HDV super-infection usually progresses to chronic hepatitis D. The different outcomes between HDV co-infections and super-infections are mainly related to the duration of infection with the helper HBV. Acute hepatitis B runs a self-limited course in more than 95% of adult patients with or without HDV co-infection and thus HDV cannot outlive the episode of acute hepatitis. In contrast in super-infections, HDV is superimposed on already well-established chronic HBV infections, and thus HBV remains after the episode of acute hepatitis and favors the persistence of HDV (Figure 2) [2].

Chronic hepatitis D like all other forms of chronic viral hepatitis may be completely asymptomatic or present with non-specific symptoms, such as mild fatigue or vague right hypochondrial pain. The spectrum of biochemical abnormalities and disease severity is wide, ranging from sub-clinical and sub-biochemical chronic infections to cases with high

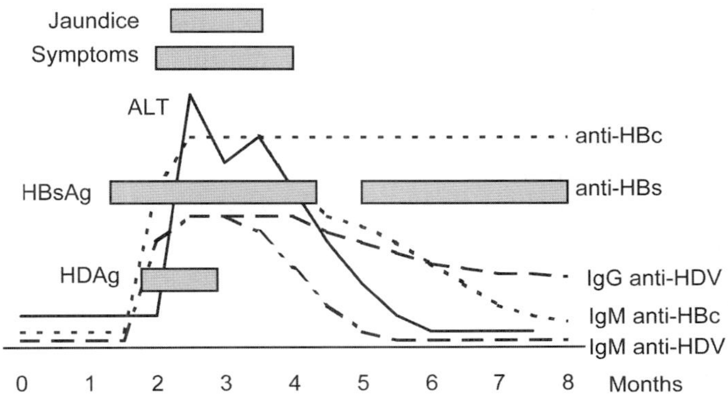

Figure 1. Typical course of acute HBV and HDV co-infection.

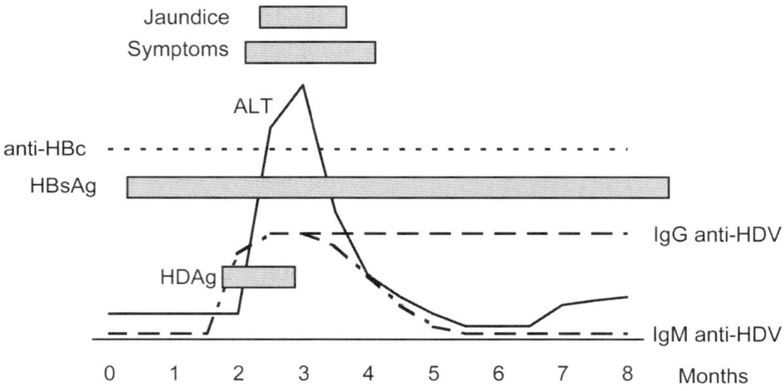

Figure 2. Typical course of acute HDV super-infection on chronic HBV infection.

disease activity and rapid progression to liver cirrhosis and decompensation. Chronic hepatitis D was initially associated with more severe liver disease and more frequent and/or more rapid development of cirrhosis compared to chronic hepatitis B or non-A, non-B/C. Subsequently, however, large population surveys in Greek communities and other parts of the world of high HDV endemicity showed that the clinically overt cases with rapid progression represent the tip of the clinical iceberg of chronic HDV infection and that the majority of chronically HDV-infected individuals remain asymptomatic and without biochemical abnormalities [2,3].

A pattern of latent HDV infection has been described in liver transplant patients. Latent HDV infections were considered as those with expression of HDV, but not HBV, in the liver and were associated with little or no liver injury. Sensitive polymerase chain reaction (PCR) assays, however, subsequently showed that these latent HDV infections of liver grafts do not represent autonomous HDV infections but low levels of HDV synthesis accompanied by very low levels of HBV expression. Although such latent HDV infections have not been detected in non-transplant patients, anti-HDV positive and HBsAg negative individuals with persistently normal liver enzymes might be similar cases [2].

Hepatocellular carcinoma may develop in patients with chronic HDV infection, but the role of HDV in the pathogenesis of hepatocellular carcinoma remains uncertain. Cirrhosis has almost universally been present in cases of hepatocellular carcinoma associated with HDV. Although it has been suggested that HDV infection may hasten the development of hepatocellular carcinoma in chronically HBV-infected patients, this may be related not directly to HDV itself but to the acceleration of the course of liver disease and rapid development of cirrhosis in patients with active chronic hepatitis D.

Several extrahepatic manifestations have been described to develop in association with both chronic hepatitis B and C, but not with chronic hepatitis D. However, several non-specific autoantibodies, such as antinuclear or smooth muscle antibodies, may be detected in patients with chronic hepatitis D perhaps more commonly than in patients with chronic hepatitis B or C. In addition, type III anti-liver–kidney microsomal antibodies (anti-LKM3) appear to be present relatively specifically in chronic hepatitis D. The autoantigen of anti-LKM3 has been recently specified to be UDP-glycuronyl-transferase, but their significance and exact pathogenetic role, if any, remain unclear.

4. DIAGNOSIS

The diagnosis of HDV infection can be based on the evaluation of the following markers: (a) antibodies against the HDV antigen (anti-HDV) in serum, (b) HDV antigen (HDAg) in serum and in liver, and (c) HDV RNA in serum and in liver (Table 1).

Detection of anti-HDV represents the hallmark of diagnosis of HDV infection. Both IgG and IgM class

Table 1. Serologic markers of HBV and HDV in the course of HDV infections.

Serologic marker	Acute HBV and HDV co-infection	Past HBV and HDV co-infection	Acute HDV super-infection	Chronic HDV infection
HBsAg	Positive	Negative	Positive	Positive
Anti-HBc	Positive	Positive	Positive	Positive
Anti-HBs	Negative	Positive	Negative	Negative
HBeAg	Positive/negative	Negative	Negative/positive	Negative
Anti-HBe	Negative/positive	Positive	Positive/negative	Positive
IgM anti-HBc	Positive	Negative	Negative	Negative
Serum HBV-DNA	Detectable for short period	Undetectable	Undetectable or in low levels	Undetectable or in low levels
IgG anti-HDV	Positive – late period	Positive – low titers	Positive – late period	Positive – high titers
IgM anti-HDV	Positive – high titers	Negative	Positive – high titers	Positive[a]
HDAg	Positive – early period	Negative	Positive – early period	Positive[b]
Serum HDV-RNA	Detectable for short period	Negative	Detectable	Detectable

[a]IgM anti-HDV titers may fluctuate with exacerbations of disease activity in chronic hepatitis D.
[b]HDAg may be intermittently detected in low titers by Western blot assays in chronic hepatitis D.

anti-HDV can be detected in serum by enzyme- or radio-immune assays. Detection of IgG class anti-HDV is mainly used in clinical practice, but IgM class anti-HDV may also be determined in certain laboratories. In acute HDV infections, serum IgG anti-HDV may be initially undetectable or present in very low titers. Therefore, testing of serial serum samples drawn during the late convalescence period and evaluation of their anti-HDV titers are required, if the diagnosis of a possible acute HDV infection should be based only on IgG anti-HDV determinations. In contrast, serum IgM anti-HDV in relatively high titers appears early in the course of acute HDV infections, but it tends to disappear within weeks if the infection resolves. Titers of IgG anti-HDV may also decrease several months after an acute HDV infection has resolved, but IgG anti-HDV remain detectable in low titers in the majority of such cases. Titers of IgG anti-HDV remain persistently high (greater than 1:10,000) in cases with progression to chronic HDV infection. IgM anti-HDV may also be detected in patients with chronic hepatitis D and its presence has been considered to represent a marker of HDV-induced liver damage. In particular, several data suggest that levels of IgM anti-HDV increase in response to HDV-induced liver damage and thus such high levels represent a surrogate marker of liver necroinflammation immunologically induced by HDV, while IgM anti-HDV levels decrease with the remission of HDV-related liver disease [9].

HDAg may be detected in serum by enzyme- or radio-immune assays or Western blot analysis, which has the best sensitivity for HDAg. Serum HDAg appears in high titers very early in the course of acute HDV infections, but it rapidly disappears if the acute infection resolves (Figures 1 and 2). Serum HDAg may also be detected in chronic HDV infections, but its titers tend to be lower and thus they are usually detectable only by Western blot analysis, which is not widely available. HDAg can also detected in liver tissue (in nuclei of hepatocytes) by immunohistochemistry. Liver HDAg represents a reliable marker of current HDV infection, which can be readily evaluated in cases with available liver biopsies [2].

HDV RNA can be detected in serum by hybridization or reverse transcription PCR (RT-PCR) assays and in liver tissue by *in situ* hybridization. The sensitivity for serum HDV RNA detection is certainly much better with RT-PCR than with hybridization assays. HDV RNA appears in serum very early in the course of acute HDV infections and remains persistently detectable only in cases who progress to chronicity. Serum HDV RNA (probably of fluctuating levels) remains always detectable by

RT-PCR during the course of chronic HDV infections. Currently, RT-PCR can detect HDV RNA from serum concentrations of 10–100 copies of HDV genome per milliliter and it is the most sensitive technique for the detection of current HDV infection. Thus, undetectable serum HDV RNA by RT-PCR and positive anti-HDV practically mean therapeutically or spontaneously eradication of HDV infection (past HDV infection). Since HDV genome contains very few highly conserved regions, particular attention is required for the choice of suitable primers for the amplification of HDV. It should be noted, however, that the reliability of RT-PCR for HDV RNA seems to be well established in experienced laboratories and its usefulness has been shown in the early diagnosis of acute HDV infection, estimation of infectivity as well and follow-up or evaluation of histologic severity of chronic HDV infection and monitoring of antiviral therapy in chronic hepatitis D [2].

Since HDV infection always requires the presence of HBV, serologic tests of HBV infection should also be considered. Acute HBV and HDV co-infection may be suspected in patients presenting with acute hepatitis, probably with a biphasic pattern of biochemical activity, and the diagnosis is confirmed by the detection of (a) IgM antibody to the core antigen of HBV (IgM anti-HBc) usually with positive HBsAg in serum (patients with early serum HBsAg clearance and thus negative HBsAg on hospital admission may also be observed) and (b) markers of acute HDV infection (Table 1). Markers of acute HDV infection are considered to be the seroconversion to IgG anti-HDV (IgG anti-HDV undetectable in the early phase and detectable in increasing titers later in the course of infection), the detection of serum IgM anti-HDV, or serum HDAg or serum HDV RNA. The last three markers may also be detected in cases with chronic ongoing HDV infection, but their detection in a patient with acute hepatitis and serologic evidence of acute HBV infection can be safely interpreted as acute HDV infection (Table 1).

Acute HDV super-infection should be suspected in previously known chronic HBV carriers presenting with acute hepatitis or in patients presenting with acute hepatitis and serologic evidence of chronic HBV infection. The diagnosis of acute HDV super-infection is confirmed by the detection of (a) serum HBsAg without IgM anti-HBc and (b) markers of acute HDV infection (Table 1). The most reliable HDV marker of acute HDV super-infection is the seroconversion to IgG anti-HDV.

The possible presence of chronic HDV infection should be evaluated in the initial diagnostic work-up of any patient with chronic HBV infection, since there is no clinical symptom or sign or laboratory finding that may differentiate patients with only chronic HBV than those with chronic HBV and HDV infections. The determination of serum IgG anti-HDV, which is the most widely available marker of HDV, can be safely used for the initial diagnosis or exclusion of chronic HDV infection (Figure 3). Whenever a new case of chronic HDV infection is made, the evaluation of the severity of chronic infection and the need for antiviral therapy should follow. Thus, liver function tests, full blood count and prothrombin time, serologic markers of activity of HDV infection (serum HDV RNA or IgM anti-HDV or HDAg by Western blot, if available) and the severity of liver histologic lesions are usually evaluated (Figure 3). If a liver biopsy is performed, the detection of HDAg in liver tissue may be used as

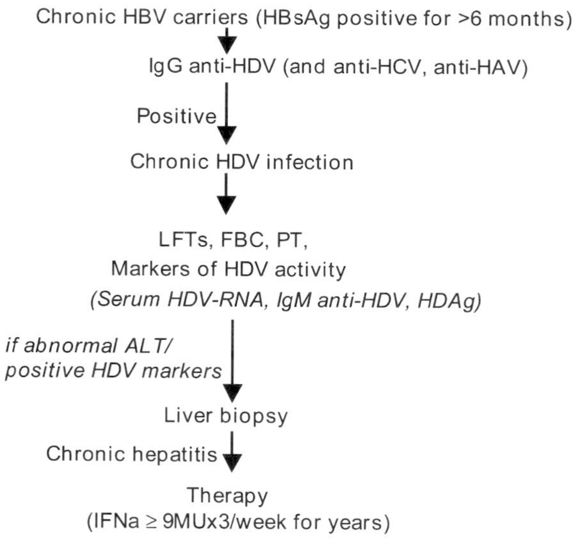

Figure 3. Management of patients with chronic HDV infection in clinical practice. LFTs, liver function tests; FBC, full blood count; PT, prothrombin time; IFN-α, interferon-α.

a reliable marker of HDV activity. In addition, the activity of HBV by determination of serum HBV DNA levels as well as the presence of current infection with hepatitis C virus (HCV) and of past infection with hepatitis A virus (HAV) by detection of the respective antibodies should also be examined.

5. MANAGEMENT

5.1 Medical therapeutics

Interferon-α (IFN-α) has been evaluated in all forms of chronic viral hepatitis, including hepatitis D. However, clinical trials of IFN-α therapy in chronic hepatitis D are rather small and thus no firm conclusion can be drawn. It seems that IFN-α in high dosage of at least 9 MU thrice weekly can achieve biochemical remission in the majority of treated patients, which is usually accompanied by decrease in levels or clearance of serum HDV RNA and significant histologic improvement in liver necroinflammatory activity. The efficacy of high IFN-α dosage is superior than achieved by the usual dosage of 3 MU thrice weekly. Unfortunately, most of responders relapse soon after discontinuation of 12-month courses even after treatment with high IFN-α doses. Since resolution of chronic hepatitis D has been described after several years of continuous IFN-α therapy [10], relatively high doses of IFN-α are usually given for very prolonged periods in patients with chronic hepatitis D. Sustained response after discontinuation of therapy should be expected only in patients who clear serum HBsAg during therapy.

Lamivudine is a nucleoside analogue that has been recently used in all subgroups of patients with chronic hepatitis B mainly because of its potent inhibition of HBV replication, oral administration, excellent tolerance, and absence of serious side effects. However, lamivudine monotherapy seems to be rather ineffective in the treatment of chronic hepatitis D. In a recent small study including five patients with chronic hepatitis D, a 12-month course of lamivudine, given at a dose of 100 mg daily, had a profound effect only on HBV viremia without any effect on HDV RNA levels, ALT activity, or histologic lesions [11]. Moreover, the combination of lamivudine with high dose of IFN-α was also not found to have any considerable effect in patients with chronic hepatitis D [12]. Recent *in vitro* data suggest that other anti-HDV approaches resulting from the better understanding of the life cycle of HDV might develop in the future, such as the ribozymes or antisense probes, which in combination with IFN-α have shown some promising initial results in the treatment of RNA viruses [13].

Summarizing the medical treatment of chronic hepatitis D in current clinical practice, we may conclude that IFN-α remains the only therapeutic option despite its limited efficacy. Given the well-known frequent side effects and contraindications of IFN-α, therapy should be considered only in patients with active (persistently increased ALT activity) and compensated chronic liver disease, while the presence of liver decompensation, hepatocellular carcinoma, or other extrahepatic conditions associated with shortened life span should be considered as contraindications to therapy. IFN-α should be given in high doses of at least 9 MU thrice weekly and the efficacy of therapy should be first evaluated after 6 months. Patients who maintain abnormal ALT activity should discontinue therapy, while IFN-α should continue for many years in those who show biochemical response. The best duration of therapy in patients with chronic hepatitis D responding to IFN-α remains undetermined and some researchers suggest that it may have to continue for life. IFN-α may be discontinued without high risk of relapse only in the patients who had cleared serum HBsAg during therapy.

5.2 Surgical procedures

Patients with HDV-related fulminant acute hepatitis or end-stage decompensated cirrhosis are candidates for orthotopic liver transplantation. In fact, HDV-related liver disease is a favorable indication for liver transplantation, at least compared to HBV-related liver disease, since HDV patients carry a much lower risk of graft reinfection [14]. HDV transplant patients should be treated with long-term therapy of hepatitis B immune globulin, which has been shown to significantly reduce further the relatively low risk of HBV and/or HDV post-transplant recurrence.

5.3 Prevention including family screening

Prevention of spread of HDV infection can be accomplished by the universal anti-HBV vaccination. However, successful anti-HBV vaccination will prevent the HBV and HDV co-infections in individuals previously susceptible to HBV, but it will have no effect on the incidence of HDV super-infections among chronic HBV carriers. Several attempts in experimental animals have been shown that it may be possible to prepare an anti-HDV vaccine of recombinant HDAg with or without HBsAg or more recently DNA-based immunization strategies in order to induce specific T-helper-1 immune responses against the HDAg [15–17]. Despite some promising initial experimental data, more research is clearly needed to confirm such findings and to evaluate the immunogenicity and protective efficacy of any potential anti-HDV vaccine in chronic HBV carriers.

The ongoing universal immunization against HBV is expected to lead to worldwide eradication of both HBV and HDV in the future. In the meantime, chronically infected HBV individuals, mainly parenteral drug users, should be advised to modify their behavior in an effort to reduce their exposure to other hepatitis viruses. Patients with chronic HDV infection should also be advised to reduce their exposure to risk factors for other hepatitis viruses and should be offered anti-HAV vaccination, in case they are susceptible to HAV. Moreover, patients with chronic HDV infection should be counseled to avoid factors that accelerate the progression of their liver disease, such as alcohol consumption. The family screening of an individual with HDV infection is the same with that of an individual for HBV infection. Thus, all first-degree relatives and sexual partners should be screened for serological markers of HBV and HDV infection.

6. PROGNOSIS

The prognosis of patients with HDV infection depends largely on their clinical presentation. Thus, the prognosis of cases with acute HBV and HDV co-infection is favorable, since most of them will resolve spontaneously. In contrast, acute HDV super-infections have a worse prognosis, since they are usually associated with more severe morbidity during the acute phase and almost always progress to chronic HDV infections. The prognosis is dismal for patients with HDV-associated acute fulminant hepatitis, who usually survive only if they undergo liver transplantation promptly. Among individuals with chronic HDV infections, those with persistently normal liver enzymes have a rather benign form of chronic HDV infection which has probably no effect on their survival. On the other hand, patients with active chronic hepatitis D expressed by abnormal aminotransferases levels and significant changes on liver biopsy have a worse prognosis compared not only to patients with inactive chronic HDV infection but also to patients with active chronic hepatitis B. The latter subgroup of patients with chronic HDV infection has been shown to progress frequently and rapidly to liver cirrhosis and to respond poorly to antiviral therapy. It has been estimated that approximately one-third of patients with HDV-related cirrhosis will die within 5 years, unless they undergo orthotopic liver transplantation.

REFERENCES

[1] Taylor, J.M. (1999) Hepatitis delta virus. *Intervirology* **42**, 173–178.

[2] Hadziyannis, S.J. (1999) Hepatitis D. *Clin. Liver Dis.* **3**, 309–325.

[3] Hadziyannis, S.J. (1997) Review: hepatitis delta. *J. Gastroenterol. Hepatol.* **12**, 289–298.

[4] Gaeta, G.B., Stroffolini, T., Chiaramonte, M., Ascione, T., Stornaiuolo, G., Lobello, S., Sagnelli, E., Brunetto, M.R. and Rizzetto, M. (2000) Chronic hepatitis D: a vanishing disease? An Italian multicenter study. *Hepatology* **32**, 824–827.

[5] Hadziyannis, S.J., Dourakis, S.P., Papaioannou, C., Alexopoulou, A., Hadziyannis, E.S. and Gioustozi, A. (1993) Changing epidemiology and spreading modalities of hepatitis delta virus infection in Greece. *Prog. Clin. Biol. Res.* **382**, 259–266.

[6] Casey, J.L., Brown, T.L., Colan, E.J., Wignall, F.S. and Gerin, J.L. (1993) A genotype of hepatitis D virus that occurs in northern South America. *Proc. Natl Acad. Sci. USA* **90**, 9016–9020.

[7] Hsu, S.C., Syu, W.J., Sheen, I.J., Liu, H.T., Jeng, K.S. and Wu, J.C. (2002) Varied assembly and RNA editing efficiencies between genotypes I and II hepatitis D virus and their implications. *Hepatology* **35**, 665–672.

[8] Nisini, R., Paroli, M., Accapezzato, D., Bonino, F., Rosina, F., Santantonio, T., Sallusto, F., Amoroso, A., Houghton, M. and Barnaba, V. (1997) Human CD4 + T-cell response to hepatitis delta virus: identification of multiple epitopes and characterization of T-helper cytokine profiles. *J. Virol.* **71**, 2241–2251.

[9] Borghesio, E., Rosina, F., Smedile, A., Lagget, M., Niro, M.G., Marinucci, G. and Rizzetto, M. (1998) Serum immunoglobulin M antibody to hepatitis D as a surrogate marker of hepatitis D in interferon-treated patients and in patients who underwent liver transplantation. *Hepatology* **27**, 873–876.

[10] Lau, D.T., Kleiner, D.E., Park, Y., Di Bisceglie, A.M. and Hoofnagle, J.H. (1999) Resolution of chronic delta hepatitis after 12 years of interferon alfa therapy. *Gastroenterology* **117**, 1229–1233.

[11] Lau, D.T., Doo, E., Park, Y., Kleiner, D.E., Schmid, P., Kuhns, M.C. and Hoofnagle, J.H. (1999) Lamivudine for chronic delta hepatitis. *Hepatology* **30**, 546–549.

[12] Wolters, L.M., van Nunen, A.B., Honkoop, P., Vossen, A.C., Niesters, H.G., Zondervan, P.E. and de Man, R.A. (2000) Lamivudine–high dose interferon combination therapy for chronic hepatitis B patients co-infected with the hepatitis D virus. *J. Viral Hepat.* **7**, 428–434.

[13] Madejon, A., Bartolome, J. and Carreno, V. (1998) In vitro inhibition of the hepatitis delta virus replication mediated by interferon and trans-ribozyme or anti-sense probes. *J. Hepatol.* **29**, 385–393.

[14] Samuel, D., Zignego, A.L., Reynes, M., Feray, C., Arulnaden, J.L., David, M.F., Gigou, M., Bismuth, A., Mathieu, D. and Gentilini, P. (1995) Long-term clinical and virological outcome after liver transplantation for cirrhosis caused by chronic delta hepatitis. *Hepatology* **21**, 333–339.

[15] Fiedler, M., Lu, M., Siegel, F., Whipple, J. and Roggendorf, M. (2001) Immunization of woodchucks (*Marmota monax*) with hepatitis delta virus DNA vaccine. *Vaccine* **19**, 4618–4626.

[16] Huang, Y.H., Wu, J.C., Tao, M.H., Syu, W.J., Hsu, S.C., Chi, W.K., Chang, F.Y. and Lee, S.D. (2000) DNA-based immunization produces Th1 immune responses to hepatitis delta virus in a mouse model. *Hepatology* **32**, 104–110.

[17] Mauch, C., Grimm, C., Meckel, S., Wands, J.R., Blum, H.E., Roggendorf, M. and Geissler, M. (2001) Induction of cytotoxic T lymphocyte responses against hepatitis delta virus antigens which protect against tumor formation in mice. *Vaccine* **20**, 170–180.

Hepatology: A Practical Approach
B. Al Knawy, M.L. Shiffman, R.H. Wiesner (editors)

Chapter 5
Hepatitis E

Mohammad Sultan Khuroo[a], *Saleem Kamili*[b], *Mehnaaz Sultan Khuroo*[c] *and Hamad Al Ashgar*[d]

[a]Consultant Transplant Hepatology (MBC 72), Department of Liver Transplantation, Hepato-biliary and Pancreatic Surgery, King Faisal Specialist Hospital and Research Centre, Post Box 3354, Riyadh 11211, Saudi Arabia

[b]Division of Viral Hepatitis, Centers for Disease Control and Prevention, Atlanta, GA, USA

[c]Department of Pathology, Shri-Ramachandra Medical College and Research Institute, Porur, Chennai, India

[d]Section of Gastroenterology (MBC 46), Department of Medicine, King Faisal Specialist Hospital and Research Centre, Post Box 3354, Riyadh 11211, Saudi Arabia

1. Introduction 111
2. Historical Background 111
3. Hepatitis E Virus 112
4. Epidemiology 112
   4.1 Disease prevalence 112
   4.2 Global distribution 114
   4.3 Modes of transmission 114
   4.4 Seroprevalence 116
5. Pathogenesis 116
6. Liver Histology 116
7. Clinical Profile 117
8. Diagnosis 119
9. Natural History and Prognosis 119
10. Control 119
Addendum 120
References 120

1. INTRODUCTION

Hepatitis E is an enterically transmitted, self-limiting acute viral hepatitis caused by well-characterized RNA virus, the hepatitis E virus (HEV). The disease is ecologically dependent and is a major health problem in regions of the world with unsafe water supplies and bad sewage disposal. The disease causes large-scale water-borne epidemics of viral hepatitis and is the most common cause of acute sporadic hepatitis and fulminant hepatic failure in such countries. Hepatitis E has been reported in the developed countries as an imported disease by travelers to endemic areas and recently, as a cause of a small percentage of sporadic and fulminant hepatic failure in persons without history of travel to endemic areas. Seroprevalence data reveal a global distribution of the infection. The infection is prevalent in a wide range of animal species and human infection may have a zoonotic origin. The disease has peculiar and as yet unexplained epidemiological characteristics including repeated waves of large-scale epidemics in the endemic zones, occurrence of disease in adult population, and high incidence and severity of disease in pregnant women. A recombinant vaccine for hepatitis E has passed through phase I study and phase II and III trials are underway.

2. HISTORICAL BACKGROUND

Hepatitis E was first recognized during an epidemic of hepatitis, which occurred in Kashmir valley in 1978 [1]. The epidemic involved an estimated 52,000 cases of icteric hepatitis with 1650 cases of fulminant hepatic failure and 1560 deaths. The disease had unique clinical and epidemiological features and sera lacked serological markers of acute hepatitis A and hepatitis B. Very soon after the description of the Kashmir epidemic, hepatitis E was retrospectively traced to an epidemic of acute viral hepatitis, which had occurred in Delhi, India in 1955–1956 [2]. In the late 1950s and 1960s, a number of epidemics of jaundice were reported in the literature. These epidemics had classical epidemiological features of hepatitis E. None of these has had serological confirmation of hepatitis E due to lack of availability of sera. Similar epidemics of jaundice had occurred in Europe and the United States in the 18th and 19th century. These data point to the fact that hepatitis E is an ancient disease discovered recently. It can be postulated that the disease existed in its epidemic form globally in the past and has only recently become restricted to certain geographical regions with unsafe water supplies and bad sewage disposal.

Balayan *et al.* [3] successfully transmitted the disease into himself by self-ingesting acute phase stool suspensions from a water-borne epidemic of non-A hepatitis in Central Asia. Reyes *et al.* [4] cloned and sequenced HEV. Yarbough *et al.* [5] developed the enzyme immunoassay (EIA) for detection of antibodies to HEV.

3. HEPATITIS E VIRUS

HEV particles are small, non-enveloped, 32–34 nm in diameter, with spikes and indentations on the surface (Figure 1). The viral genome is a single-stranded, positive-sense, polyadenylated RNA molecule of 7.5 kb and is organized into three overlapping open reading frames (ORF). ORF1 is 5079 base pairs and encodes a 1693 amino acid polyprotein consisting of non-structural proteins that are involved in genome replication and viral protein processing. ORF1 has sequences containing motifs characteristic of viral methyl transferase, papain-like cysteine protease, helicase and RNA-dependent RNA polymerase. In addition, ORF2 consists of 1980 base pairs and has three probable glycosylation sites and encodes a viral capsid protein. ORF3 is 369 base pairs and overlaps ORF1 and ORF2 by 1 and 328 base pairs, respectively [6]. ORF3 encodes a 123-amino acid protein (pORF3), which is expressed intracellularly. Recent studies of the biology of HEV replication have shown that pORF3 may be capable of associating with the liver cell cytoskeleton [6].

Genetic heterogeneity of HEV has become a matter of intense study [7]. A recent analysis has suggested that HEV isolates segregate into four major genotypes and at least nine different groups. Genotype 1 has very little genetic diversity with a single group (Group 1) and includes isolates from India, Burma, Pakistan and some regions of Africa, namely Chad and Algeria. Genotype II (Group 2) is represented by the Mexican isolate and several isolates from Nigeria. Genotype III has high level of diversity within it and includes five groups (Groups 3–7). Group 3 consists of two human US isolates (US1 and US2) and swine US isolate. Group 4 consists of the Italian isolate and the swine isolate from New Zealand. Group 5 consists of single isolate from Greece and two isolates from Spain and an isolate from swine sewage. Group 6 consists of second Greek isolate and Group 7 consists of the Argentine and the Austrian isolates. Genotype IV includes group 8 (isolate Ct1) and group 9 (isolate Cs15) from China. However, there is immunological cross-reactivity between structural proteins of all HEV isolates, suggesting that the virus has a single serotype. Hepatitis E virus bears structural similarity to caliciviruses; however, it lacks phylogenetic relatedness to caliciviruses and appears to produce different (putative) enzymes. These factors have led to the Calicivirus Study Group of the International Committee on Taxonomy of Viruses to propose that HEV be taken out of the family Caliciviridae and be given an "unassigned" status.

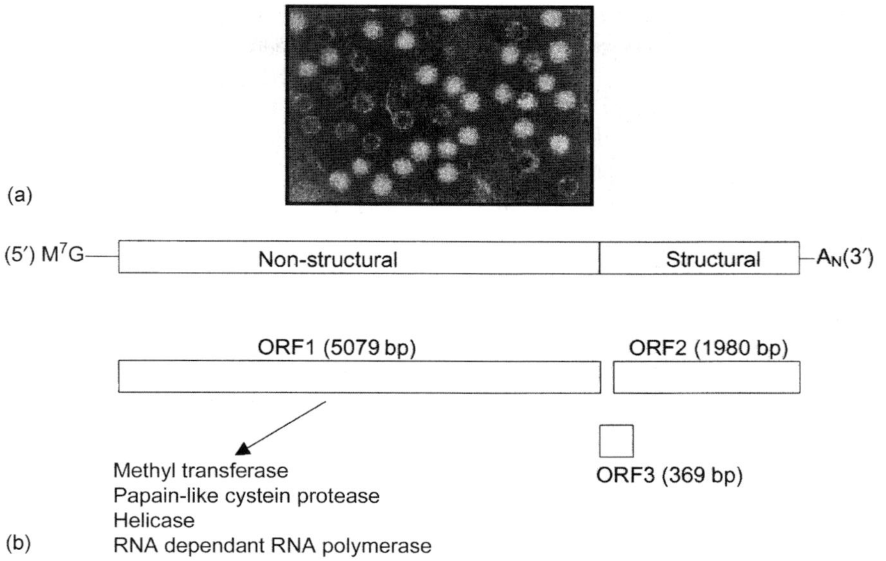

Figure 1. Hepatitis E virus. (a) Electron micrograph of 32-nm virus particle viewed by immune electron microscopy in infective inoculum (fecal sample) with convalescent phase serum from a patient as antibody source. (b) Genomic organization. ORF, open reading frame; bp, base pairs.

4. EPIDEMIOLOGY

4.1 Disease prevalence

Epidemiological features of hepatitis E have several peculiar characteristics, which remain unexplained. Hepatitis E presents as repeated large-scale water-borne epidemics of jaundice in high endemic areas occurring every 10–20 years. Hepatitis E is a disease of adult population. During epidemics, attack rate in adults is higher than in children. The sporadic disease is also common in adults in most endemic regions of the world. Hepatitis E epidemic and sporadic disease have been reported in children in few reports [8,9].

Hepatitis E has increased incidence and severity in pregnant women. In fact, the major cause of mortality in the epidemics is the high rate of fulminant hepatitis in pregnant women. Data collected from an outbreak of hepatitis E in Kashmir (1979) showed that the frequency of hepatitis was greater in pregnant (17.3%) than in non-pregnant (2.1%) women and in men (2.8%). The frequency of the disease in the first, second and third trimesters were 8.8, 19.4 and 18.6%, respectively. Severe disease in the form of fulminant hepatic failure developed more often in pregnant women (22.2%) than in non-pregnant women (none of whom had this complication) and in men (2.8%). Fulminant hepatitis developed exclusively in the third trimester. The nutritional status of women in the area affected by the outbreak or in those women who developed fulminant hepatic failure was assessed as good. The overall mortality in pregnant women was found to be 20% [10].

The epidemiology of sporadic acute viral hepatitis and its relationship with pregnancy have been recently studied. HEV was the most common cause of sporadic acute viral hepatitis in this endemic area. High proportion of pregnant women and increased severity of disease in pregnancy were limited to patients with hepatitis E. Sporadic acute hepatitis caused by other hepatitis viruses did not show any special predilection to or increased severity in pregnant women. Acute liver failure in pregnant women caused by HEV infection was an explosive disease with short pre-encephalopathy period, rapid development of cerebral edema and high occurrence of disseminated intravascular coagulation and may represent a severe manifestation of a Schwartzmann-like phenomenon [11]. The reason for increased incidence and severity of hepatitis E in pregnant women is not known.

The mechanism underlying the survival of hepatitis E in the endemic regions is a matter of continuing debate. During epidemics, disease spreads by gross water contamination. How does the agent continue to survive in the inter-epidemic period? Serial transmission of subclinical disease among susceptible individuals is a possibility. However, data point to the fact that person-to-person transmission does not occur. The environmental reservoirs of HEV are especially water supplies and sewage. Against this is the fact that HEV is a labile virus when exposed to high concentrations of salt, freeze thawing and pelleting. Recently, considerable interest has been generated by the data suggesting that HEV may be a zoonotic disease. If so, a wide variety of animals may be reservoirs of the virus and spread the diseases to humans under proper environmental situations [12].

4.2 Global distribution

Global distribution of hepatitis E is broadly divided into three zones (Figure 2) [8,9]. The disease has high endemicity in a broad region encompassing the Indian subcontinent, Southeast Asia, central Asia, eastern, northern, and western Africa and some parts of North America (Mexico). In a high endemic zone, hepatitis E presents as large-scale epidemics of jaundice and is the cause of around one half of the acute sporadic viral hepatitis and fulminant hepatic failure. The endemic zone of hepatitis E includes a number of countries in the Middle East and North Africa, namely Turkey, Saudi Arabia, Kuwait and Egypt, few countries from Southeast Asia and South America. In these countries hepatitis E causes over one quarter of cases of acute sporadic hepatitis and fulminant hepatic failure. However, large water-borne epidemics of jaundice have not been reported from these countries. In non-endemic zone, the disease accounts for less than 1% of reported cases of acute viral hepatitis. Such cases are associated with travel to the HEV-endemic regions. Recently, isolated cases of hepatitis E have been reported from Australia, New Zealand, the Western Europe and the United States among persons with no history of travel to the endemic regions of the disease. The origin of such cases has been of great interest as the virus in such patients is a novel HEV isolate and is closely related to HEV isolate naturally infecting swine. This has raised the issue of zoonotic origin of hepatitis E in such countries.

4.3 Modes of transmission

The fecal–oral route is the predominant mode of transmission [1,9]. There is convincing evidence that epidemics are related to consumption of fecally contaminated drinking water. All reported epidemics are limited to regional water supplies with a highly compressed epidemic curve of the disease suggesting a single common source of spread. Fecal contamination of drinking water source and time relation between contamination and occurrence of the disease have been elegantly shown in some epidemics. Increase in other water-borne diseases and lack of occurrence of disease in people from the epidemic using alternative water sources (especially well water) are other pointers to the water being as an incriminating source of transmission. Further, the genomic sequences of HEV have been detected in sewage water from endemic and non-endemic regions. Mechanism of water contamination differs from one region to other; however, it follows a uniform pattern in repeated epidemics of the same region. Contamination of the water has been documented in the following environmental settings: (1) heavy rains, (2) flooding and recession of flood waters after which rivers change their course, (3) contamination of open drinking water sources (rivers, streams, unprotected wells) with raw sewage. This information is important to know in order to control the epidemics.

Following epidemics secondary waves of hepatitis usually do not occur, suggesting that person-to-person contact transmission is not a major factor in the evolution of the outbreaks. During sporadic infections, secondary attack rates among household members are only 0.7–2.2%; in contrast, 50–75% of susceptible household contacts of hepatitis A are known to become infected. However, a significantly higher rate of spread by contact has been reported in some epidemics. These epidemics have been of protracted type and new cases of jaundice appeared for months after the main epidemic was over. The

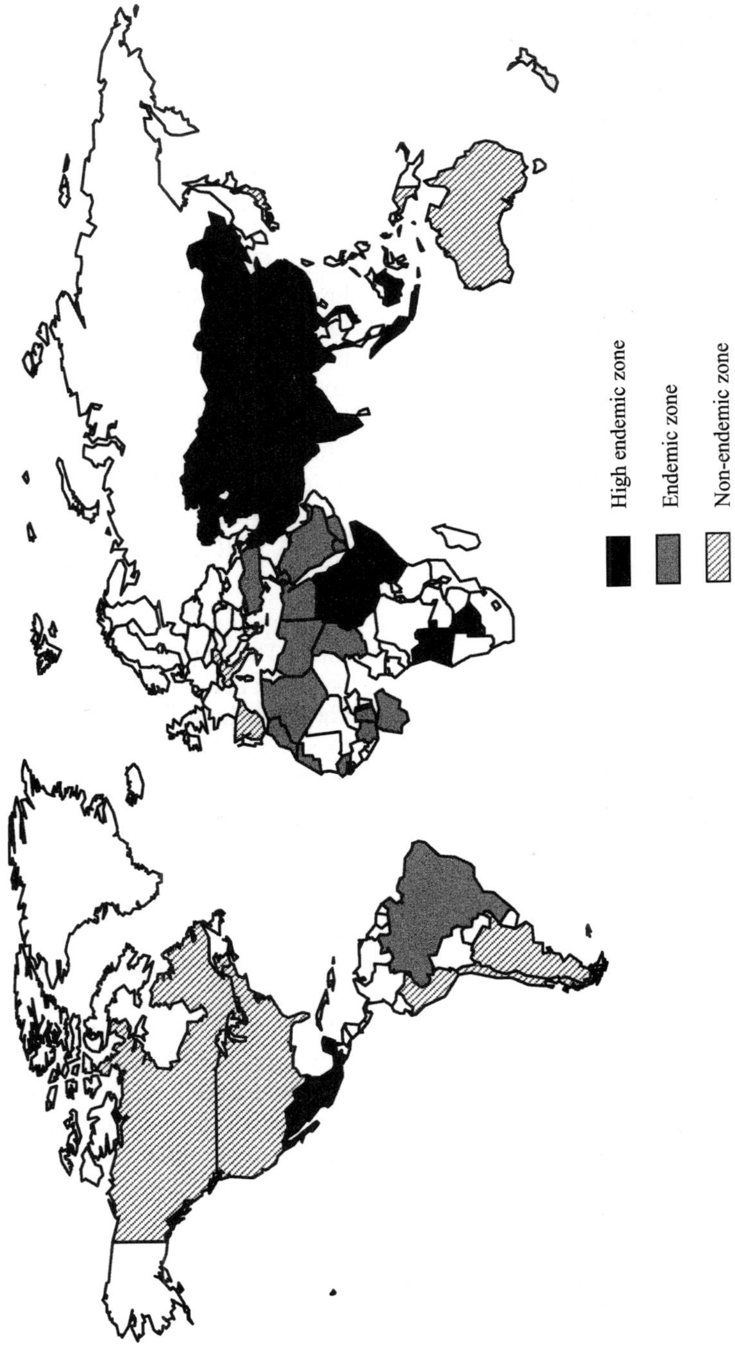

Figure 2. Global distribution of hepatitis E.

mode of transmission responsible for sporadic infections is unclear [1,9].

Vertical transmission of HEV infection from mother to infant is known to occur. In one study, six of eight babies born to mothers who had either acute uncomplicated hepatitis or fulminant hepatic failure from HEV infection in the third trimester of pregnancy were found to have evidence of HEV infection. Of these six babies, five had serological evidence of HEV infection acquired before birth [13].

The information regarding the parenteral transmission of HEV is scarce and only a few studies from endemic areas have been published. These studies have pointed to frequent occurrence of subclinical HEV infections in the endemic areas and transmission of HEV following transfusions from otherwise healthy viremic donors [9].

Recent data suggest that hepatitis E may be a zoonotic disease, particularly in the non-endemic zones. Antibodies to HEV have been detected in a wide range of animal species including swine, cattle, sheep and rodents from endemic and non-endemic areas. HEV RNA has been detected in feces of domestic swine in Nepal. Piglets and lambs have been shown to develop elevated liver enzymes, liver cell injury and fecal shedding of virus after experimental infection with human HEV. Moreover, human and swine HEV isolates in the United States are phylogenetically related and possess cross-species infectivity [12,14].

4.4 Seroprevalence

Seroprevalence data of HEV (IgG anti-HEV) have been studied globally and need explanation. The antibody prevalence in high endemic regions is around 4–20% and in endemic regions is around 4–16%. These prevalence rates are much lower than expected as hepatitis E causes repeated epidemics and is the most common cause of sporadic acute viral hepatitis in such areas. The antibody prevalence in non-endemic regions is around 1–5%. These prevalence rates are much higher than expected as hepatitis E causes less than 1% of sporadic viral hepatitis in such regions, mostly in persons who have recently visited endemic areas of hepatitis E. Only isolated cases of hepatitis E have been reported in such regions in persons who have not visited endemic areas [9].

Age-specific seroprevalence of HAV and HEV in endemic areas differs from each other. HAV is a highly pathogenic agent with strong person-to-person transmission. HAV exposure occurs very early in life and the majority of the population is exposed and protected by the end of their first decade. Against this, IgG anti-HEV prevalence in such countries is low, with maximum prevalence of around 30–40% in the third decade of life and onwards. This suggests that HEV is an agent with low pathogenicity, does not spread by person-to-person transmission and a large dose of the virus is needed for infection. This occurs through gross fecal contamination of water supplies [1,9].

5. PATHOGENESIS

The hepatitis E virus enters the body via the oral route. The site of primary replication is presumed to be in the intestinal canal. The virus reaches the liver via portal vein. The liver appears to be the sole target of infection and once established viral replication occurs, leading to viral shedding in bile. The pathogenesis of hepatitis E may be a combination of direct cytotoxicity and immunologic mechanisms [9].

Sequence of events has been well studied based on experimental infection in animals, self-ingestion in humans and natural acquired infection (Figure 3). The incubation period of the disease after oral exposure is 4–5 weeks. HEV is detected in stools approximately 1 week prior and as long as 2 weeks after onset of illness. Viremia is detected for at least 2 weeks after onset of illness. Most patients have monophasic enzyme elevation; however, biphasic enzyme elevation, prolonged fecal excretion and viremia can occur in around 10% of patients [9].

6. LIVER HISTOLOGY

Liver biopsies in patients with hepatitis E reveal portal triaditis, cholestasis, lobular inflammation and

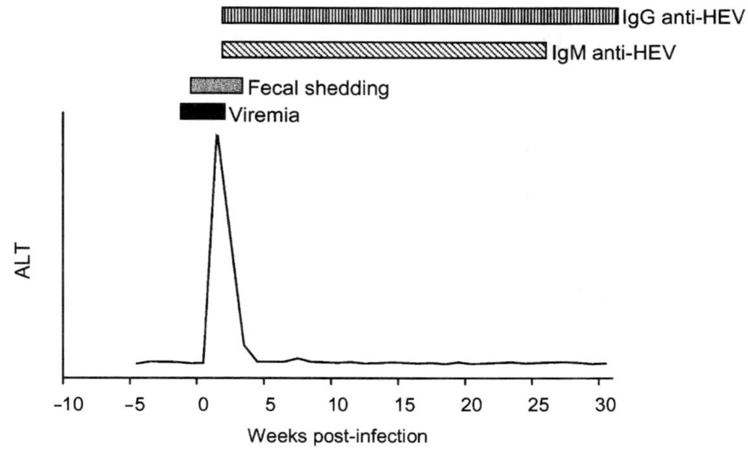

Figure 3. Sequence of events in hepatitis E virus infection. Note early appearance of IgG and IgM antibodies to HEV, short period of fecal shedding and viremia in early disease period and monophasic enzyme elevation.

degeneration of varying degrees, suggestive of acute viral hepatitis. However, nearly half of these patients have distinctive morphological changes designated as "cholestatic viral hepatitis". The changes include: absence of diffuse lobular degeneration and inflammation; predominance of focal necrosis; marked intrahepatocytic and intracanalicular cholestasis with characteristic bile plugs in the lobules, leading to pseudo-ductular formation around these; and portal triaditis with mono-nuclear cells infiltration with occasional polymorphonuclear leukocytes [1].

Liver histology in experimentally infected animals showed acidophilic types of hepatocytic degeneration and focal hepatic necrosis accompanied by accumulation of mononuclear macrophages and activated Kupffer cells; a less striking feature was the presence of lymphocytes in inflammatory infiltrates. The majority of these lymphocytes are positive for cytotoxic/suppressor phenotypes by immunostaining. The cholestatic hepatitis observed in human infection does not develop in experimental animals [9].

7. CLINICAL PROFILE

Hepatitis E is the cause of most epidemics of viral hepatitis in adults in endemic areas. It is the most common cause of acute sporadic hepatitis and fulminant hepatic failure in such areas (Figure 4). The disease can occur in a number of situations, which include intrauterine infections, neonatal hepatitis and hepatitis E superinfection on hepatitis B carriers and those with chronic liver disease. Hepatitis E can exist as unapparent infections in endemic areas and proportion of such infections to those of icteric disease is around 10:1. In addition hepatitis E infects western travelers to endemic areas. Isolated cases of hepatitis E occur in such countries in persons who have not traveled to endemic areas [9].

The clinical and biochemical picture of hepatitis E is similar to those of infection with other hepatitis viruses and encompasses a wide variety of symptoms. Incubation period varies from 15 to 45 days. Prodromal (preicteric) symptoms are generally more severe and can last for up to 10 days. These include fever with chills (44%), anorexia (79%), malaise (95%), epigastric pain (41%), nausea and vomiting (46%), arthralgia (75%) and urticaria (20%). The icteric phase begins abruptly, with the appearance of jaundice, dark urine, and clay-colored stools. Liver enzyme and serum bilirubin show a monophasic elevation with return to normal in 3–6 weeks. Prolonged intrahepatic cholestasis lasting from 3 to 6 months occurs in about 20% patients and simulates large bile duct obstruction. A small percentage of patients show a biphasic enzyme elevation, however, no chronic liver disease or chronic hepatitis is known to develop after hepatitis E. Generalized lymphadenopathy is known to occur

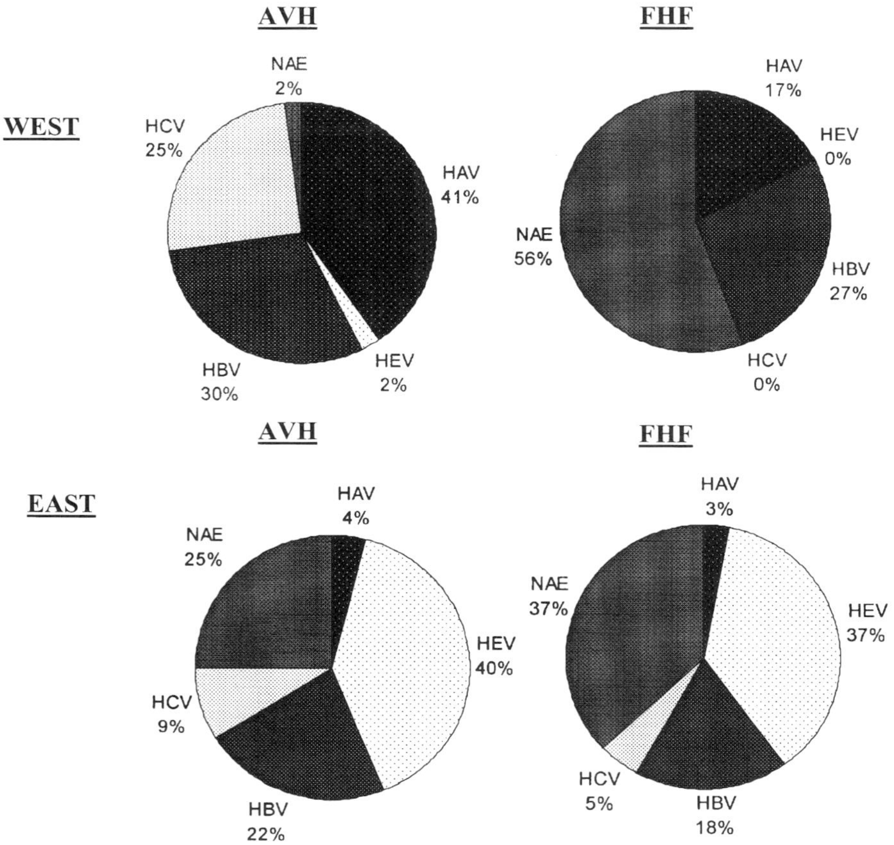

Figure 4. Etiology of acute sporadic viral hepatitis and fulminant hepatic failure in the West and the East [8,9].

during the course of illness and disease can present with spontaneous rupture of the spleen. HEV infection can cause severe intravascular hemolysis, unusually high levels of bilirubin and renal failure needing hemodialysis in patients with glucose-6-phosphatase dehydrogenase deficiency. Cryoglobinemia and other extrahepatic manifestations have not been reported with hepatitis E. HEV antibodies were found in 13% of patients who had autoimmune chronic hepatitis, raising the possibility that HEV may trigger this condition. However, this may be a epiphenomenon associated with hypergammaglobinemia of autoimmune hepatitis [15].

Fulminant hepatic failure caused by hepatitis E is common in pregnant women especially in the second and third trimester. The disease has shorter pre-encephalopathy period (days from onset of disease to encephalopathy), higher occurrence of cerebral edema and disseminated intravascular coagulation when compared to the disease caused by other hepatitis viruses and agents [16].

Intrauterine HEV infections transmitted transplacentally from the infected mother commonly cause fetal or neonatal deaths from massive hepatic necrosis and metabolic disturbances, namely hypoglycemia and hypothermia. Babies who survive may present with subclinical hepatitis or icteric acute hepatitis [13].

HEV commonly superinfects patients with chronic hepatitis B carriers. In endemic areas, 20–30% patients with HEV infections have underlying hepatitis B carrier state [15]. Such patients usually present with more serious symptoms of hepatitis, namely deep jaundice, ascites, and other signs of liver failure without the presence of encephalopathy.

Mortality in such patients is high and death occurs with sepsis and renal failure. HEV infection is also common in patients with chronic liver diseases in endemic areas. In one study eight (8.3%) of the 97 patients with chronic liver disease had acute HEV infection as against none of the 40 age- and sex-matched healthy subjects [15]. HEV superinfection in patients with chronic liver disease presents with severe hepatic decompensation leading to increased morbidity and mortality [17].

8. DIAGNOSIS

HEV infection should be looked for in a number of clinical situations in endemic areas. These include patients who contract disease during epidemics or outbreaks of jaundice, acute sporadic hepatitis, fulminant hepatic failure, liver disease in pregnancy, neonatal hepatitis and decompensation of otherwise stable chronic liver disease. In the developing countries evidence for such infections should be looked for in patients who have developed acute hepatitis, fulminant hepatic failure or elevated liver enzymes after recent travel to endemic areas. Rarely HEV infection may occur in patients who had never traveled to endemic areas. Because of these reports, hepatitis E testing should be done in patients with acute hepatitis of otherwise undetermined etiology [18].

ELISA for detection of IgM-anti-HEV is a reliable and sensitive marker of recent HEV infection. It is detected in over 95% of patients with HEV infection. The antibody can be detected as early as 4 days after the onset of symptoms and antibody titers are highest when the serum transaminases peak. IgM anti-HEV is undetectable by 4–5 months after acute infection [19].

IgG anti-HEV is detected in 90–100% of patients with acute infection. The antibody levels peak 30–40 days after the onset of the disease and the antibody may persist for up to 8–14 years. Thus, IgG anti-HEV is useful in seroprevalence studies of hepatitis E.

Hepatitis E virus RNA in serum, liver and stool using PCR techniques have been developed and employed by many laboratories for diagnosis of HEV infection [13]. However, yield of such tests is highest in samples taken within 7 days of the onset of the disease. Also such tests are not feasible for routine diagnosis especially in the developing countries [1].

Liver histology in HEV infection may be indistinguishable from that of acute hepatitis caused by other hepatitis viruses. However, a subgroup of patients with HEV infection has distinctive morphological changes and may give a clue to diagnosis in such cases [1].

9. NATURAL HISTORY AND PROGNOSIS

HEV infection is a self-limiting infection and chronic carrier state and chronic liver disease is not known to occur. The case fatality rate is 0.5–4.0%. Pregnant women especially in the second and third trimester have mortality ranging from 20 to 42%. In endemic areas hepatitis E is the commonest cause of acute liver failure. Acute liver failure occurs in a high proportion of pregnant women, mostly in the third trimester. Pregnant women with acute liver failure caused by hepatitis E have shorter duration of illness, shorter pre-encephalopathy period, lower serum bilirubin and more frequent development of cerebral edema than non-pregnant women with acute liver failure. A high proportion of pregnant women with acute liver failure develop disseminated intravascular coagulation. Early predictors of poor outcome of acute liver failure in endemic areas have been recently determined and include age >40 years, prothrombin time >30 s, grade of coma >2 and non-E etiology. Prognosis of acute liver failure caused by hepatitis E is better than acute liver failure caused by hepatitis B and hepatitis non-A to E. Pregnancy *per se* or duration of pregnancy does not influence the mortality from acute liver failure in endemic areas [16].

10. CONTROL

As hepatitis E is an ecologically determined disease, its control would depend upon improved sanitation, proper sewage disposal and supply of safe potable water. Mass education during and between outbreaks advising the public to follow proper hygienic precautions and to use boiled drinking water may be helpful. As the morbidity and mortality are seen mainly in pregnant women, special attention is needed in this population during epidemics [1,9].

Human immunoglobulins contain a low level of IgG anti-HEV and use of these has not been useful in disease or infection protection and as given conflicting results in clinical trials. However, sera containing high titer anti-HEV have been found to be protective in animals and humans and will be most useful in pregnant women during epidemics of hepatitis E.

Of great interest is the subject of vaccination against hepatitis E. Many different ORF2 antigens have shown to induce antibodies. However, in the majority of cases, it has not been shown that the resulting antibodies are neutralizing and could serve as vaccine candidates. Only three ORF2 antigens (TrpE-C2, Burma 62 kDa, and Pakistan 55 kDa) have been shown to induce antibodies that neutralize the virus. Thus far, only one vaccine has progressed to the stage of clinical trials. The 56-kDa recombinant vaccine developed at NIH, USA has been licensed to SmithKline Beecham and is currently being evaluated by the Walter Reed Army Institute of Research and in Nepal. In a phase 1 trial, the vaccine was found to be safe and immunogenic in 88 American volunteers. Based on these results a further phase 1 evaluation was performed in Nepal, where hepatitis E is endemic. Three doses of the vaccine (5 or 20 μg) were injected into 22 Nepalese volunteers at 0, 1 and 6 months. Serious adverse reactions were not observed and all the volunteers seroconverted. A phase II–III trial has been planned and its results will be seen with great interest. The approach of DNA vaccination, a novel vaccine technology, is also being explored against hepatitis E in the preclinical models. A candidate DNA vaccine encoding HEV ORF2 was shown to induce anti-HEV antibodies that recognized native HEV antigens. Further, DNA vaccine trials in non-human primates, immunized with an HEV ORF2 DNA cassette, conferred protection in the immunized animals [20].

A number of questions have to be sorted out for hepatitis E vaccination. These include: (a) the nature of immunity given by the vaccine in humans, (b) whether immunity is long term or not, (c) whether monovalent vaccine protects against all isolates of HEV, and (d) the neutralization epitopes of HEV and how broadly these are shared. Once a vaccine and/or HEV-Igs are available for human use, a number of potential situations can be exploited for use of either or both. These include: (a) pregnant women during epidemic to prevent fatalities – HEV-Igs with or without vaccine, (b) control of epidemic – vaccine, (c) western tourists and military traveling to endemic areas – vaccine, (d) pregnant women in high endemic and endemic regions to protect against epidemic and sporadic disease – vaccine, (e) universal vaccination in endemic areas to control the disease. This will depend upon the potency of the vaccine, its delivery route and cost. At present we can see the future of hepatitis E as progress towards a siege and final control [20].

ADDENDUM

Since the submission of the chapter some important information about hepatitis E has been published and needs to be added to the chapter.

Frequent transmission of HEV by blood transfusion was reported recently in a study in which post-transfusion HEV infection developed in 22 anti-HEV negative transfused patients; the infection was traced to their four respective donors who were asymptomatic but were viremic (Khuroo *et al.* (2004) *J. Gastroenterol. Hepatol.* **19**, 778–784). A direct evidence of zoonosis for HEV infection was reported from Japan; nucleotide sequences amplified from a left over portion of the deer meat were identical to those from patients who developed hepatitis E after consuming the meat. Patients' family members who ate none or very little of the deer meat remained uninfected (Suzuki *et al.* (2002) *N. Engl. J. Med.* **347**, 1456).

REFERENCES

[1] Khuroo, M.S. (1980) Study of an epidemic of non-A, non-B hepatitis: possibility of another human hepatitis virus distinct from post-transfusion non-A, non-B type. *Am. J. Med.* **68**, 818–823.

[2] Wong, D.C., Purcell, R.H., Sreenivasn, M.A., Prasad, S.R. and Pavri, K.M. (1980) Epidemic and endemic hepatitis in India: evidence for a non-A, non-B hepatitis etiology. *Lancet* **2**, 867–869.

[3] Balayan, M.S., Andzjaparidze, A.G., Savinskaya, S.S., Ketiladze, E.S., Braginiski, D.M., Savinov, A.P. and Poleschuk, F. (1983) Evidence of a virus in non-A, non-B hepatitis transmitted via the fecal–oral route. *Intervirology* **20**, 23–31.

[4] Reyes, G.R., Purdy, M.A., Kim, J., Luk, K.-C., Young, L.M., Fry, K.M. and Bradley, D.W. (1990) Isolation of a cDNA from the virus responsible for enterically transmitted non-A, non-B hepatitis. *Science* **247**, 1335–1339.

[5] Yarbough, P.O., Tam, A.W., Fry, K.E., Krawczynski, K., McCaustland, K.A., Bradley, D.W. and Reyes, G.R. (1991) Hepatitis E virus: identification of type-common epitopes. *J. Virol.* 5790–5797.

[6] Zafrullah, M., Ozdener, M.H., Panda, S.K. and Jameel, S. (1997) The ORF3 protein of hepatitis E virus is a phosphoprotein that associates with the cytoskeleton. *J. Virol.* **71**, 9045–9053.

[7] Schlauder, G.G. and Mushahwar, I.K. (2001) Genetic heterogeneity of hepatitis E virus. *J. Med. Virol.* **65**, 282–292.

[8] Krawczynski, K., Kamili, S. and Agarwal, R. (2001) Global epidemiology and medical aspects of hepatitis E. *Forum (Genova)* **11**, 166–179.

[9] Khuroo, M.S. (1996) Hepatitis E virus: another addition to the existing alphabet of human hepatitis viruses. *Ann. Saudi Med.* **16**, 308–319.

[10] Khuroo, M.S., Teli, M.R., Skidmore, S., Sofi, M.A. and Khuroo, M.I. (1981) Incidence and severity of viral hepatitis in pregnancy. *Am. J. Med.* **70**, 252–255.

[11] Khuroo, M.S. and Kamili, S. (2003) Etiology, clinical course and outcome of acute sporadic hepatitis in pregnancy. *J. Viral Hepat.* **10**, 61–69.

[12] Meng, X.J., Lehman, J.R., Webb, D.M., Tsareva, T.S., Haynes, J.S., Thacker, B.J., Halbur, P.G. and Emerson, S.U. (1997) A novel virus in swine is closely related to the human hepatitis E virus. *Proc. Natl Acad. Sci. USA* **94**, 9860–9865.

[13] Khuroo, M.S., Kamili, S. and Jameel, S. (1995) Vertical transmission of hepatitis E virus. *Lancet* **345**, 1025–1026.

[14] Meng, X.J., Halbur, P.G., Shapiro, M.S., Govindarajan, S., Bruna, J.D., Mushahwar, I.K., Purcell, R.H. and Emerson, S.U. (1998) Genetic and experimental evidence for cross-species infection by swine hepatitis E virus. *J. Virol.* **72**, 9714–9721.

[15] Khuroo, M.S., Rustgi, V.K., Dawson, G.J., Mushahwar, I.K., Yattoo, G.N., Kamili, S. and Khan, B.A. (1994) Spectrum of hepatitis E infection in India. *J. Med. Virol.* **43**, 281–286.

[16] Khuroo, M.S. and Kamili, S. (2003) Etiology and prognostic factors in acute liver failure in India. *J. Viral Hepat.* **10**, 224–231.

[17] Hamid, S., Atiq, M., Shehzad, F., Yasmeen, A., Nissa, T., Salam, A., Siddiqui, A. and Jafri, W. (2002) Hepatitis E virus superinfection in patients with chronic liver disease. *Hepatology* **36**, 474–478.

[18] Centers for Disease Control and Prevention (1993) Hepatitis E among US travelers, 1989–92. *MMWR Morb. Mortal. Wkly Rep.* **42**, 1–4.

[19] Dawson, G.J., Chau, K.H., Cabal, C.M., Yarbough, P.O., Reyes, G.R. and Mushawar, I.K. (1992) Solid-phase enzyme linked immunosorbent assay for hepatitis E virus IgG and IgM antibodies utilizing recombinant antigens and synthetic peptides. *J. Virol. Methods* **38**, 175–186.

[20] Kamili, S. (2002) Immunity to hepatitis E virus: new insights and future challenges. *Ind. J. Gastroenterol.* **21**, 136–138.

Hepatology: A Practical Approach
B. Al Knawy, M.L. Shiffman, R.H. Wiesner (editors)

Chapter 6
Other Hepatitis Viruses

Federico G. Villamil, Sonia M. Soria and Valeria I. Descalzi

Hepatology and Liver Transplantation Unit, Fundación Favaloro, Avenida Belgrano 1782, Piso 5, 1093 Capital Federal, Buenos Aires, Argentina

1. Introduction 123
2. Herpes Viruses 127
   2.1 Epstein–Barr virus infection 127
   2.2 CMV infection 129
   2.3 Herpes simplex virus infection 130
3. Flaviviruses 131
   3.1 HGV infection 131
4. Circoviruses 134
   4.1 TT virus infection 134
   4.2 SENV infection 135
5. Conclusions 136
References 137

1. INTRODUCTION

Whenever someone is found to have elevated aminotransferases, the first thought that comes to the mind of the physician is that the patient may have some type of hepatitis. Although the term hepatitis etymologically implies an inflammatory condition of the liver, it is well known that aminotransferases are frequently elevated in non-inflammatory liver disease such as steatosis, ischemia or toxic-induced hepatotoxicity, among others. The next step in the evaluation of this prototype patient at the time of the first visit is whether hepatitis is acute or chronic. Adults with acute hepatitis frequently develop jaundice or symptoms such as fatigue, short-lived fever, nausea or vomiting and abdominal discomfort due to hepatomegaly. The acute nature of the disease is strengthened by the finding of a markedly elevated AST and specially ALT. Acute hepatic failure is defined by coagulopathy and fulminant hepatic failure by the onset of encephalopathy in patients with acute liver failure. However, patients with acute hepatitis may be completely asymptomatic and, if studied late in the course of the disease, may have mild increase of liver enzymes. Conversely, reactivation of some types of chronic hepatitis may have a clinical presentation indistinguishable from that of acute hepatitis. Once a presumptive diagnosis of acute hepatitis is established, the next goal is to investigate the etiology, irrespective of the severity of the disease. Clinical parameters and liver tests are of little help in this regard. An exception could be, for example, a young patient with prolonged fever, pharyngitis, skin rash and palpable adenopathy where the diagnosis of infectious mononucleosis requires little confirmation. Similarly, drug-induced and acute alcoholic liver disease should be initially suspected at the time of completing the medical history. However, serological or virological testing is required in the vast majority of cases to search for an etiologic agent. Although the epidemiology of viral infections is quite variable in different geographic areas, initial testing for patients with a presumed diagnosis of acute viral hepatitis worldwide should include IgM anti-hepatitis A virus (HAV) antibody (anti-HAV), IgM anti-hepatitis B core antibody (anti-HBc), hepatitis B surface antigen (HBsAg) and anti-hepatitis C virus (HCV) antibody (anti-HCV). If these tests come back negative, the diagnosis of acute hepatitis A and B can be excluded. Acute hepatitis C is frequently anicteric and asymptomatic and therefore remains undiagnosed in the majority of cases. Because seroconversion to anti-HCV requires several weeks, the diagnosis of acute hepatitis C mostly relies on the detection of HCV RNA in serum by polymerase chain reaction (PCR). Virological markers for HCV infection should be part of the initial work-up in patients with a history of parenteral exposure 2–6 months before the onset of acute hepatitis. Patients with hepatitis delta virus (HDV) infection frequently present as acute hepatitis due to either coinfection with hepatitis B virus (HBV) or superinfection of chronic carriers of HBsAg. Therefore, serological and/or virological markers for HDV infection should be investigated only after the diagnosis of HBV infection is established. Hepatitis E virus (HEV) infection is endemic in Asian countries such as India and Pakistan, several regions of Africa and Mexico. Consequently, IgM anti-HEV should be part of the initial work-up for acute hepatitis only in these areas. In non-endemic regions, acute hepatitis E should be suspected in persons who traveled to areas where HEV infection is prevalent a few weeks before clinical onset. Types I and II autoimmune hepatitis may initially present as acute or fulminant hepatitis. Testing for autoantibodies and gamma-globulin in patients with acute hepatitis and negative markers for viral infections is essential to achieve a rapid diagnosis and for prompt initiation of therapy. Similarly, acute or even fulminant hepatitis may be the first clinical manifestation of Wilson's disease. The association of acute hepatitis with hemolytic anemia, neurological symptoms and acute renal failure, in the more severe forms of the disease, should raise the suspicion of this metabolic condition. Investigation of ceruloplasmin, urinary copper and Kayser–Fleischer rings is necessary to confirm the diagnosis of Wilson's disease. A substantial number of patients with acute or fulminant hepatitis have negative viral, immunologic and metabolic diagnostic markers and are thus classified as indeterminate, cryptogenic or non-A–E hepatitis. The term indeterminate hepatitis is preferable to non-A–E hepatitis because it does not necessarily imply a viral etiology. A number of hepatotropic or systemic viruses may produce acute hepatitis (Table 1). Testing for these infrequent viral infections is indicated after ruling out all common causes of acute viral hepatitis, unless clinical features present at the time of initial presentation strongly suggest a particular disease as mentioned above for infectious mononucleosis. The diagnostic algorithm for acute hepatitis is shown in Figure 1.

Chronic hepatitis is defined clinically as increased aminotransferases for at least 6 months. This minimal follow-up period has been proposed for the timing of liver biopsy in patients who do not normalize liver tests after a recognized episode of acute hepatitis. However, when clinical, biochemical or radiological evidences of chronic liver disease are present at the time of the initial consultation, it is unnecessary to postpone the diagnostic work-up and liver biopsy. The majority of patients with chronic hepatitis are asymptomatic. For this reason, incidental finding of chronic hepatitis, even in patients with established cirrhosis, is the rule rather than the exception. The most prevalent causes of chronic hepatitis can be suspected at the time of obtaining the medical history. Viral hepatitis appears as the most likely diagnosis in patients with parenteral risk factors whereas a history of extrahepatic autoimmune disorders and increased levels of gamma-globulin is highly suggestive of autoimmune hepatitis, particularly in females. Alpha-1-antitrypsin deficiency, hemochromatosis and Wilson's disease may occasionally present with chronic elevation of ALT. Therefore, metabolic causes of chronic hepatitis should be considered from the start in young patients with a family history of non-alcoholic cirrhosis or in those who present the typical extrahepatic manifestations of these hereditary diseases. As mentioned for the differential diagnosis of acute hepatitis, a good medical history is essential to rule out drug-induced chronic hepatitis. Initial testing to investigate the etiology of chronic hepatitis should include HBsAg, anti-HCV and anti-nuclear (ANA) and anti-smooth muscle (ASMA) antibodies. Whenever a patient with chronic hepatitis is found to be HBsAg-positive, investigation of hepatitis B e antigen (HBeAg), anti-HBe and HBV DNA is necessary to establish if the disease is due to replication of wild type or precore mutant HBVs or to superinfection of chronic non-replicative carriers with HDV or other viruses. Immunosuppressed patients, and to a much

Table 1. Serologic, virologic and other methods for the diagnosis of infection with herpesviruses, flaviviruses and circoviruses in patients who present with acute of chronic hepatitis of uncertain etiology.

Agent	Diagnostic tests		
	Serologic	Virologic	Other
Herpesviruses			
Epstein–Barr virus	Heterophile AB, IgM/IgG anti-VCA, anti-EA, anti-NA	EBV DNA	EBER-1 in tissues
Cytomegalovirus	IgM/IgG anti-CMV	CMV DNA CMV RNA	pp65 antigenemia Culture, biopsy
Herpes simplex virus	IgM/IgG anti-HSV 1 and 2	HSV DNA	Culture, biopsy
Flaviviruses			
Hepatitis G virus	Anti-E2	HGV RNA	
Circoviruses			
TT virus	Available but not validated	TTV DNA	
SEN virus	Not available	SENV DNA	

lesser degree immunocompetent patients, may have chronic HCV infection without detectable anti-HCV. In theses cases, investigation of HCV RNA in serum is necessary to confirm the diagnosis of hepatitis C. Type II autoimmune hepatitis is an infrequent but well described cause of chronic hepatitis, especially in children and young adults. Therefore, type 1 anti-liver–kidney–microsomal antibody (anti-LKM-1) should be requested in patients with chronic hepatitis of non-viral etiology and with negative ANA and ASMA. Alpha-1-antitrypsin deficiency, hemochromatosis or Wilson's disease may present as chronic hepatitis in the absence of any extrahepatic manifestations.

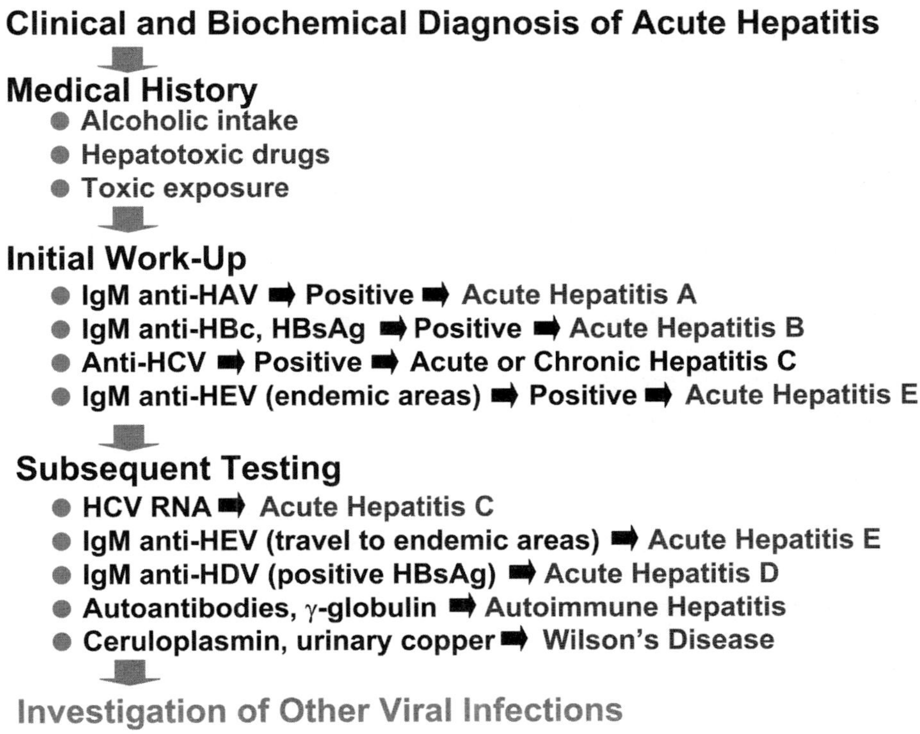

Figure 1. Diagnostic algorithm for acute hepatitis. (*For colored version, see Plate XV on page 570 at the end of the book.*)

Specific testing for metabolic etiologies is indicated in patients with chronic hepatitis of uncertain etiology. Patients with non-alcoholic steatosis or steatohepatitis frequently present with chronic elevation of ALT. The increased fat content of the liver may be detected on a routine abdominal ultrasound disclosing increased parenchymal echogenicity. The main goal of liver biopsy in patients with chronic hepatitis is to assess the severity of inflammation (grading) and fibrosis (staging). In addition, histological examination may be helpful to establish the etiology of the disease. Examples of these are the finding of steatosis or steatohepatitis not detected by ultrasound or unusual diseases such as giant-cell hepatitis. Not infrequently, liver biopsies obtained from patients with chronic elevation of ALT are normal or reveal minimal and non-specific inflammatory changes. Investigation of other viral infections is therefore indicated in patients with a confirmed diagnosis of cryptogenic chronic hepatitis after clinical, biochemical and histological evaluations. The diagnostic algorithm for chronic hepatitis is shown in Figure 2.

Viruses of the Herpesviridae family produce a systemic infection that frequently involves the liver, among other organs or tissues. The differential diagnosis with classic viral hepatitis is relatively simple in the majority of cases due to the presence of characteristic extrahepatic manifestations. However, some patients infected with herpes viruses may present with acute or even fulminant non-A–E hepatitis in the absence of systemic manifestations. Specific serological or virological testing is required to certify the diagnosis and thus to avoid misclassification of these cases as hepatitis of indeterminate etiology. Infection with herpes viruses is usually self-limited in immunocompetent hosts. Primary infection with these agents is followed by persistence of the virus in a latent form that can reactivate under the effects of immunosuppression. Therefore, infection with herpes viruses is frequently associated with severe or fatal hepatitis and lymphoproliferative diseases in patients with congenital immunodeficiencies, transplant recipients and carriers of the human immunodeficiency virus (HIV). In this chapter we will describe the prevalence, clinical features and

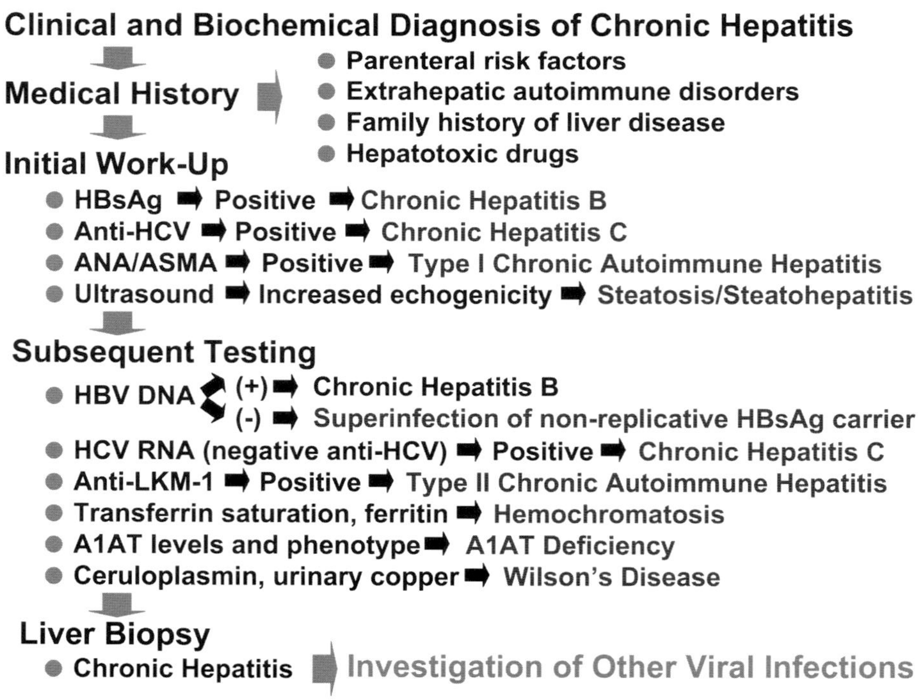

Figure 2. Diagnostic algorithm for chronic hepatitis. (*For colored version, see Plate XVI on page 571 at the end of the book.*)

diagnosis of acute infection by herpes viruses only among immunocompetent hosts.

After the discovery of HAV, HBV, HCV, HDV and HEV, it became clear that a substantial proportion of acute and chronic liver diseases may be due to infection with one or more unrecognized viruses. Around 10% of patients with posttransfusion hepatitis, 20% with community-acquired hepatitis, 30% with chronic liver disease, 40–50% with fulminant hepatic failure and the majority with hepatitis-associated aplastic anemia have negative serological and/or virological markers for all known hepatotropic viruses and are thus provisionally classified as non-A–E hepatitis. In the past, identification of a new pathogen mostly relied on the visualization or isolation of the agent or the demonstration of a specific antibody response. However, following cloning of HCV, molecular approaches such as representational difference analysis and host gene expression profiling have been utilized to search for new viruses. These viral discovery programs resulted in the identification of a number of agents such as hepatitis G virus (HGV) also known as GB virus C (GBV-C) and members of the so called superfamily of human circoviruses including the prototype TT virus (TTV), TTV variants such as SANBAN, YONBAN and TUSO1 and the SEN virus (SENV). Members of the Circoviridae family are small single-stranded, non-enveloped, circular DNA viruses that probably emerged from a common ancestor and were previously associated with diseases in animals. Despite being structurally similar, these agents have little sequence and amino acid homology. After extensive research and hundreds of publications, it is still unclear if any of these new viruses cause a particular liver disease. To prove causality, a newly discovered pathogen should fulfill the Koch's postulates which establish that the agent: (1) must be isolated, cultured and be present in every case of the disease, (2) is not found as an "innocent bystander" or in association with other diseases and (3) should reproduce the disease when inoculated into a susceptible animal. So far, a causal relationship has been very difficult to establish with these new viruses for a number of reasons. First, the prevalence of infection is relatively high in healthy individuals and is similar among patients with cryptogenic or with a well-defined etiology of acute and chronic liver diseases. Secondly, the majority of infected patients do not manifest significant clinical, biochemical and histological evidence of hepatitis. Finally, replication of these agents in hepatocytes has not been unequivocally proven.

2. HERPES VIRUSES

2.1 Epstein–Barr virus infection

Epstein–Barr virus (EBV) is a linear DNA virus that was initially identified in 1964 by electron microscopy of a cell culture obtained from a patient with Burkitt's lymphoma. Shortly after, EBV was found to be the causative agent of infectious mononucleosis. Two strains, denominated EBV-1 and EBV-2, have been recognized. Most infections in Europe and North America are due to the EBV-1 strain. EBV replicates in B-lymphocytes and epithelial cells. The major EBV envelope glycoprotein binds to the surface of lymphocytes through a specific receptor. Replication of EBV in B-lymphocytes produces latent infection with immortalization of the cells. These resting B-lymphocytes produce no detectable virus and represent the reservoir of EBV within the human body and therefore the source for reactivation. In contrast, replication of EBV in epithelial cells, predominantly of the oropharynx, is associated with active production of virions and cell lysis. Symptoms and signs of infectious mononucleosis are due to the heavy infiltration of infected organs and tissues by reactive T-cells originated in response to EBV [1]. Administration of acyclovir interrupts viral shedding but does not modify the clinical manifestations of the disease. EBV infection has a high prevalence worldwide. Antibodies against the virus are found in 90% or more of the adult population. The age of acquisition of EBV infection is lower in areas of low socioeconomic level. Transmission occurs mostly via saliva and oral secretions and requires close contact. For this reason, infectious mononucleosis is popularly known as "the kiss disease". EBV infection has an incubation period of 4–7 weeks. Clinical presentation is closely related to the age at infection. Primary EVB infection is largely asymptomatic in infants and children and is followed by lifelong immunity. Conversely, 50% of adolescents or young adults with primary EBV infection develop infectious mononucleosis characterized by the classic triad of fever, lymphadenopathy and exudative pharyngitis [1]. Hepatomegaly is found in 10–15% and splenomegaly in around 50% of patients with uncomplicated mononucleosis. Clinical jaundice is infrequent accounting for only 5% of cases [1–3]. Routine laboratory tests usually show relative and absolute lymphocytosis and atypical mononuclear cells which, although nonspecific, are useful to reinforce the suspicion of EBV infection in patients with typical clinical findings. Liver tests are abnormal in a large proportion of patients with symptomatic infectious mononucleosis. Mild increases in aminotransferases, alkaline phosphatase and bilirubin levels are found in 80%, 60% and 45% of patients, respectively [1–3]. A number of diagnostic assays are available to diagnose EBV infection [1–3] (Table 1). Heterophile antibodies with autoreactive specificities appear early in the course of infection and are regarded as a direct product of the activation and proliferation of B-cells induced by EBV. Reactivity of the Paul–Bunnel–Davidsohn and monospot tests is based on the property of heterophile antibodies to agglutinate or lyse sheep, goat, horse or bovine red blood cells. The monospot assay has a sensitivity of 80% and a specificity of 99% for the diagnosis of primary EBV infection. Negative results are encountered mostly in children or when the sample is obtained very early during the course of infection. In addition, preparations utilizing horse red blood cells have more false-negative results than those obtained from sheep or bovine. Testing for EBV-specific markers is indicated in patients with undetectable heterophile antibodies or when considered necessary due to the severity of the disease or the presence of atypical features. Serological assays are available to detect antibodies against the EBV viral capsid (anti-VCA), early (anti-EA) and nuclear (anti-NA) antigens. Traditional tests based on indirect immunofluorescence have been commercialized for more than 20 years. More recently, several ELISA assays and automatic systems for the simultaneous detection of IgG and IgM antibodies to EBV have been introduced. However, none of them have gained widespread acceptance. IgM anti-VCA appears shortly after primary infection followed, a few weeks later, by detection of anti-EA in 80% of cases. Titers of both antibodies rapidly decline during recovery and convalescence, at the time when anti-NA becomes detectable in conjunction with rising titers of IgG anti-VCA. The serologic profile of acute EBV infection is defined by the presence of IgM anti-VCA, with or without anti-EA, in the absence of anti-NA. However, it should be noted that most commercially available IgM kits lack specificity and have significant intra- and inter-assay variability. Cytomegalovirus virus (CMV) infection and rheumatoid factor may interfere with IgM anti-VCA. Importantly, false-positive results may also occur in patients with acute viral hepatitis of proven etiology and in chronic liver diseases. In addition, IgM may be persistently detected months after primary infection and may become positive again during reactivation. Qualitative and quantitative PCR assays allow the detection of EBV DNA in peripheral blood and tissues. Molecular testing is very useful for the diagnosis and monitoring of therapy in immunosuppressed patients with EBV-associated lymphoproliferative diseases but may also serve as a confirmation test for patients with atypical clinical presentations or whenever the results of serology are unclear or contradictory. EBV-induced lymphoproliferation is associated with the expression of several genes including nuclear antigens, latent membrane proteins and two short RNAs denominated EBER-1 and EBER-2, the first of which may be detected in infected tissues by *in situ* hybridization.

Occasionally, patients with acute EBV infection may present with icteric hepatitis and markedly elevated ALT, but without the usual clinical features of infectious mononucleosis [2–4]. Histologically acute EBV hepatitis is characterized by mixed and dense portal inflammatory infiltrates composed of small lymphocytes, large atypical lymphocytes, plasma cells, eosinophils and histiocytes. Variable degrees of bile duct damage have been described which may explain the frequent elevation of alkaline phosphatase in patients with infectious mononucleosis. Compared to classic acute hepatitis, EBV infection is associated with less hepatocyte necrosis and more sinusoidal inflammation which has been denominated "the mononucleosis pattern". EBV-related fulminant hepatitis has also been well described both in immunosuppressed and immunocompetent patients and is associated with a mortality rate of 80–90% [4]. X-linked lymphoproliferative disease is an inherited disease of males characterized by a defect of immune regulation that renders the patient unable to control EBV infection. Affected children develop fatal infectious mononucleosis, acquired agammaglobulinemia or malignant lymphoma during the first years of life. Fatal mononucleosis is primarily due to massive lymphoid infiltration of liver and bone marrow resulting in fulminant hepatitis and viral-associated hemophagocytic syndrome leading to pancytopenia, hemorrhage and infection [1–4]. Histological analysis of cases with fulminant hepatitis revealed massive or submassive necrosis, predominantly in zone 1 of the acinus, variable degrees of inflammation and expression of EBV DNA or EBV-antigens in liver tissue. It has been suggested that massive necrosis in primary EBV infection may result from an intense virus-induced host immune response involving both B- and T-cells, in analogy to what has been described for HBV infection. There is no conclusive evidence that EBV replicates in hepatocytes that, in addition, lack specific viral receptors. Therefore, direct cytopathic damage of EBV to hepatocytes is highly unlikely and appears not to be the mechanism for the development of massive hepatic necrosis [4,5].

In summary, mild and self-limited hepatitis is a frequent finding in infectious mononucleosis. A peripheral blood smear showing atypical lymphocytes combined with the detection of heterophile antibodies is sufficient to confirm the diagnosis of primary EBV infection in the vast majority of patients. Testing for specific antibodies and/or viral nuclear acids is indicated to confirm the diagnosis of EBV infection in patients who present with acute hepatitis in the absence of the typical clinical features of infectious mononucleosis. EBV is an unusual cause of fulminant hepatitis among immunocompetent patients. Congenital or acquired immune deficiencies should be suspected whenever primary EBV infection is confirmed in patients with fulminant hepatic failure.

2.2 CMV infection

Human CMV is a linear, double-stranded, enveloped DNA virus that was isolated in 1956 by three independent groups of investigators. However, the term "cytomegalia" was proposed in the 1920s to describe presence of the nuclear inclusion bodies in different infected cell types. Although several related strains of CMV have been identified the genetic differences do not allow classification into well-defined genotypes. Infection with multiple strains of CMV occurs both in immunocompetent and immunosuppressed individuals. Primary CMV infection is followed by persistence of the virus in a latent form, as described for EBV. Reactivation of CMV infection is a frequent event in immunocompromised hosts. Envelope glycoproteins are the major target for neutralizing antibodies whereas the cellular immune response is mostly directed to the pp65 tegument antigen. CMV replicates *in vivo* and *in vitro* in neutrophils, monocytes, B- and T-lymphocytes, endothelial cells and epithelial cells of the liver, salivary glands, lung and gastrointestinal tract among others. Latent infection occurs mostly in monocytes, macrophages and endothelial cells. CMV has a worldwide distribution and high penetration in the community where humans are the only reservoir for infection [6]. The prevalence of CMV infection ranges from 40% to 100% in adults from different geographic areas and is closely related to socio-economic conditions. Infection is acquired early in life in developing countries in contrast to developed countries where it occurs mostly in adolescents and young adults. Several modes of transmission have been demonstrated. CMV is the most common congenital and perinatal viral infection worldwide, accounting for approximately 1% of live births. Mother-to-baby transmission can occur intra-uterus, at birth by passage through a contaminated uterine cervix or postnatal through breastfeeding. Person-to-person transmission, via infected saliva, and sexual transmission are the most important routes for spread of CMV after puberty. Posttransfusion CMV infection occurs in only 5% of seronegative recipients of seropositive blood [6]. In contrast, seronegative transplant recipients grafted with a CMV-positive organ donor have a high risk of CMV infection and disease. CMV infection may be diagnosed in a number of ways [6,7] (Table 1). A viral lysate-based enzyme immunoassay has been available for many years to detect IgM and IgG antibodies to CMV envelope glycoproteins. More recently, new commercial tests were developed utilizing recombinant CMV antigens without significant increase in sensitivity or specificity. Detection of IgG anti-CMV indicates previous exposure to the virus and is not useful for the diagnosis of primary infection, unless seroconversion is demonstrated. Serologic diagnosis of acute CMV infection is not reliable due to a relatively high frequency of false-positive results of IgM anti-CMV observed in several diseases including acute and chronic hepatitis. The rate of interference with IgM-based assays varies according to the antigen preparation used. In addition, IgM anti-CMV is frequently positive in patients with reactivation of CMV infection. Isolation of the virus in culture was, until recently, the only method to confirm CMV infection. Unfortunately, isolation of CMV from cultured human fibroblasts may require as much as 1 month, rendering this method unsuitable for a timely diagnosis and instrumentation of therapy. These difficulties have been overcome by the development of new sensitive and reliable diagnostic methods. The shell vial assay is a rapid culture method that may identify CMV only 24–48 hours after inoculation with blood or other clinical specimens. Detection of pp65 antigen in leukocytes by immunofluorescence is another sensitive technique for the diagnosis of CMV infection. In addition, antigenemia has a rapid turnover time and is semiquantitative. At present, the most sensitive diagnostic test for CMV infection is the detection and quantification of CMV nucleic acids by molecular methods. Several commercial assays are available to detect CMV DNA or CMV RNA such as PCR, signal amplification, hybrid capture and nucleic acid sequence-based amplification (NASBA). Viral load directly reflect the magnitude of CMV replication. Consequently, the finding of high serum levels of CMV DNA increases the likelihood of disease. Lastly, histological examination of liver, kidney, lung, gastrointestinal and other tissues may reveal the characteristic "owl's eye" nuclear inclusions which are almost diagnostic of CMV infection. When inclusions are not present or when the etiology of inclusion bodies is not clear, detection of specific antigens or nucleic acids in infected cells by immunohistochemistry or *in situ* hybridization is useful to confirm the diagnosis of CMV infection.

Primary CMV infection rarely causes clinical disease in immunocompetent individuals. Symptomatic patients usually present with a mononucleosis-like illness with pharyngitis, lymphadenopathy, splenomegaly and atypical lymphocytosis being less common than in classic EBV-infectious mononucleosis. CMV-mononucleosis is more frequent among patients who acquired the infection through blood transfusions. Mild and self-limited hepatitis is a frequent finding in acute CMV infection. However, some patients present with icteric hepatitis without the extrahepatic clinical manifestations of primary CMV infection [8]. Liver biopsy, which is rarely indicated, often reveals portal and lobular inflammation with mild hepatocyte necrosis. CMV also causes granulomatous hepatitis. CMV inclusions may be found in hepatocytes, biliary epithelium, Kupffer cells and endothelial cells. However, inclusion bodies are absent in the vast majority of immunocompetent patients with CMV infection. There are very few well-documented cases of CMV-induced fulminant hepatitis in non-immunosuppressed patients. In the majority of reports, diagnosis of acute CMV infection was based on serology, which lacks specificity. Recent publications suggest that CMV is a hepatotropic agent and that liver cells support the complete cycle of viral replication [8].

In summary, CMV rarely causes disease in immunocompetent persons. Mild and self-limited elevation of aminotransferases is common in CMV-mononucleosis. Modern diagnostic methods such as shell vial culture, antigenemia or molecular tests are required to confirm CMV infection in patients with primary CMV infection presenting as acute hepatitis. CMV is an extremely unusual cause of fulminant hepatic failure.

2.3 Herpes simplex virus infection

Herpes simplex virus (HSV) is a double-stranded enveloped DNA virus. Similar to the other members of the Herpesviridae family, HSV induces latent infection that may reactivate in persons with underlying conditions that impair host defense mechanisms. Two well-defined serotypes were identified in 1968 and named HSV 1 (HSV-1) and 2 (HSV-2). Both variants are biologically and epidemiologically different. HSV-1 infects primarily non-genital sites and is spread by close personal contact. The oral mucosa is the most frequent portal of entry. In contrast, HSV-2 usually infects the genitalia and is transmitted by sexual contact.

Vaginitis or infection of the uterine cervix or endometrium are the most frequent entry sites. HSV infects almost 100% of individuals at some time during their lives. Genital herpes is one of the most common sexually transmitted diseases. Sensitive and specific serologic assays have been developed to detect IgM and IgG antibodies to type-specific envelope glycoproteins of both HSV-1 and HSV-2 by enzyme immunoassay, radioimmunoassay or Western blot. Viral culture was, for many years, the gold standard for the diagnosis of HSV infection. At present, detection of HSV DNA by PCR in serum or other specimens is considered the most sensitive diagnostic method (Table 1). The vast majority of HSV infections in healthy persons are asymptomatic or result in localized disease such as herpes stomatitis. However, disseminated primary or reactivated HSV infection may occur in neonates, malnourished children, immunocompromised hosts, pregnant women and rarely in healthy adults. Genital herpes is more common in pregnant than in non-pregnant women and is frequently reactivated during gestation. In addition, it has been suggested that pregnancy is an immunocompromised state with a deficient cell-mediated immune response. Disseminated HSV infection carries a high fatality rate and is characterized by severe necrotic visceral lesions preferentially involving the liver, adrenal glands and brain. Patients with herpetic hepatitis typically present with malaise, fever, hepatomegaly and mucocutaneous lesions [9,10]. However, oral or genital herpetic lesions may be absent in around 30% of cases. The combination of markedly elevated aminotransferases with slight or no increase in bilirubin and leukopenia with lymphopenia provides an important clue to differentiate this disease from other causes of acute hepatitis. Computed tomography scan often reveals scattered low-density areas in the liver parenchyma that do not enhance with intravenous contrast. The majority of patients go on to develop fulminant hepatic failure and disseminated intravascular coagulation. Liver biopsy provides the most rapid and reliable diagnosis. The transjugular method is often required due to the severe coagulopathy. Histologically, herpetic hepatitis is characterized by well-demarcated areas of focal or confluent hemorrhagic necrosis with little or no inflammation. Viable hepatocytes located at the periphery of the necrotic tissue contain the typical Cowdry type A nuclear inclusion bodies that allow a prompt diagnosis of HSV infection [9,10]. When the etiology of inclusion bodies needs further confirmation, immunohistochemistry with specific antibodies may be utilized to detect specific HSV antigens in the nuclei, cytoplasm or cell membrane of infected hepatocytes. Early diagnosis and prompt initiation of therapy with intravenous acyclovir are essential to improve the chances of survival and to avoid the need for liver transplantation.

In summary, herpetic hepatitis is a severe and well recognized but rare disease in adult patients with no immunologic deficiencies. The combination of fever, anicteric hepatitis and leukopenia is useful to differentiate this condition from other etiologies of acute liver failure at the time of clinical presentation. Liver biopsy may allow a prompt diagnosis by revealing the typical histological features of herpetic hepatitis. Lack of awareness is the major contributing factor to the high fatality rate of disseminated HSV infection.

3. FLAVIVIRUSES

3.1 HGV infection

A hepatitis agent isolated in 1967 from a surgeon with acute hepatitis was designated GBV. The infectivity of GBV was confirmed by serial propagation in tamarins. Gene amplification of serum samples obtained after multiple passages in primates allowed the identification in 1995 of three flavivirus-like genomes that were denominated GBV-A, GBV-B and GBV-C. It was later found that only GBV-C produced human infection. Almost simultaneously, molecular amplification and cloning of serum samples from monkeys inoculated with serum from a patient with community-acquired non-A–C hepatitis led to the discovery of HGV in 1996 by an independent group of investigators. Subsequent studies showed that GBV-C and HGV were almost identical with 86% nucleotide homology and 100% amino acid identity. It was then concluded that they were two isolates of the same virus [11]. To facilitate reading, the term HGV will be used in this chapter for both agents. HGV genome is a single-stranded, positive sense RNA of 9392 nucleotides in length. It contains a long open reading frame encoding a single polypeptide of 2783 amino acids. HGV has only 25% homology with HCV and other flaviviruses and has been classified as a member of the new *Hepacivirus* genus within the Flaviviridae family. Four different variants or genotypes of HGV have been described according to their geographic origin. HGV has less genetic heterogeneity than HCV and lacks a hypervariable region in the E2 domain. The rate of mutations is low and remains constant over time. Diagnosis of HGV infection requires the detection of HGV RNA in serum by qualitative or quantitative PCR (Table 1). The most sensitive assays utilize primers from the 5′UTR region of the genome. Eighteen French laboratories with expertise in molecular biology received a common panel containing positive and negative samples for HGV. The mean sensitivity of the PCR assays to detect HGV RNA among different laboratories was only 75% (38–100%) with an overall specificity of 98% (71–100%) [12]. This may partially explain the marked reported variations of HGV prevalence in both low- and high-risk groups worldwide. Investigation of serum HGV RNA by quantitative PCR or branched-DNA assays is of little clinical utility. An ELISA assay to detect HGV antibodies has been developed utilizing recombinant proteins from the E2 region (anti-E2). Interestingly, anti-E2 was found mostly in individuals who were not viremic. In contrast to anti-HCV, anti-E2 appear to be neutralizing and to confer protective immunity. Several studies showed that the prevalence of HGV infection was much higher utilizing anti-E2 than PCR for HGV RNA. This suggests that spontaneous recovery appears to be more frequent in HGV infection than in HCV infection. The prevalence of HGV infection worldwide exceeds that of HCV and was found to be higher than initially expected. Transmission of HGV may occur via transfusions of blood or blood products, percutaneous exposure to infected blood and through non-parenteral routes. Posttransfusion HGV infection has been well documented. In the NIH study, 10% of patients who received blood transfusions developed new HGV infection compared to only 0.6% of non-transfused controls [11] (Table 2). Patients with transfusion-associated HGV infection were non-viremic at baseline and became HGV RNA-positive a few weeks after being transfused. In addition, retrospective testing showed that all patients who developed transfusion-associated HGV infection received blood from viremic donors. Only one-third of patients with new HGV infection cleared the virus within 3 years of follow-up. Therefore, the majority of HGV RNA-positive patients in this and other studies developed persistent viremia. A high prevalence of HGV infection has been reported among patients with thalassemia or hemophilia (20–38%), intravenous drug abusers (24–75%) and patients on chronic hemodialysis (4–57%). Percutaneous exposure was found to be a significantly more frequent risk factor for HGV infection than a history of blood transfusions in many of the reported series. The existence of non-parenteral modes of HGV transmission may explain the high frequency of infection among healthy individuals (1–10%) and blood donors (0.5–12%). Studies utilizing anti-E2 have shown that as much as 20% of the general population may be infected with HGV. The prevalence of HGV infection among blood donors was 1.3–1.7% in the United States, 0.5–9.7% in European countries, 0.5–1.7% in Japan, 10% in Brazil, 4% in India and 12%

Table 2. Incidence of HGV, TTV and SENV infections after blood transfusions and prevalence of infection with these agents in transfusion-associated hepatitis non-A–E and hepatitis C in the National Institute of Health trials.

Author	Agent	Incidence of infection		Prevalence of infection	
		Transfused patients	Non-transfused controls	Non-A–E hepatitis	Hepatitis C
Alter [11]	HGV	35/357 (9.8%)	1/157 (0.6%)	3/13 (23%)	6/63 (9.5%)
Matsumoto [15]	TTV	48/182 (26%)	6/127 (4.7%)	3/13 (23%)	18/45 (40%)
Umemura [21]	SENV	86/286 (30%)	3/97 (3%)	11/12 (92%)	20/49 (41%)

in Egypt. The rates of infection are much higher in commercial compared to volunteer blood donors. Sexual transmission of HGV appears likely based on the high reported rates of HGV infection among commercial sex workers (13–25%), men who have sex with men (10–13%), sexual partners of index cases (22%) and HIV-positive patients with high risk sexual behavior but no parenteral risk factors (16%). Small concentrations of HGV have been found in semen. However, the most conclusive available data to suggest sexual transmission was the documentation at the molecular level of identical viral sequences of HGV RNA between spouses. Similarly, infection with the same strain of HGV has been found in mother–infant pairs. Vertical transmission of HGV appears to be higher than with HCV. Follow-up of infected infants showed that infection persisted in 91% at 1 year and 57% at 2 years. A relatively high prevalence of HGV infection has been reported in many liver diseases with well-defined etiologies such as acute hepatitis, fulminant hepatitis and chronic viral hepatitis with or without cirrhosis or hepatocellular carcinoma (HCC) [13]. However, the impact of coexisting HGV infection in the pathogenicity of diseases with an identified cause and the primary etiologic role of HGV in patients with acute or chronic cryptogenic hepatitis is far from being proven. A weak association between HGV infection and posttransfusion non-A–E hepatitis was reported by the NIH group and later confirmed by other groups. HGV RNA was detectable in only 23% of cases with non-A–E hepatitis and in 10% of those with HCV infection [11] (Table 2). Among patients with HCV infection, ALT levels paralleled HCV RNA levels. However, in patients infected with HGV alone, the increase in ALT was modest and was temporally unrelated to the fluctuations of HGV RNA. The prevalence of HGV infection in a study of community-acquired hepatitis in the United States was 25% in hepatitis A, 32% in hepatitis B, 20% in hepatitis C and only 9% in non-A–E hepatitis [14]. Although persistent viremia was documented in 75% of cases, none of the individuals infected with HGV alone developed chronic hepatitis or significant liver damage. A large multicenter study from Japan showed HGV infection in 10% of 3043 patients with chronic hepatitis C, 6% of 778 patients with chronic hepatitis B and only 5% among those with non-A, non-C chronic liver diseases [13]. It has been clearly shown that clinical, biochemical or histological parameters of liver damage, levels of serum HCV RNA or response to interferon therapy did not differ in patients with hepatitis C with or without HGV infection. Coexisting HGV infection occurs in patients with all HCV genotypes. There is also no evidence to suggest that HGV is a risk factor for the development of HCC. HGV infection has been found in 10%–22% and 41%–67% of patients before and after liver transplantation, respectively. These high rates of infection are thought to be related to the frequent need for transfusions of blood or blood products in the transplant setting. Both *de novo* and recurrent HGV infection have been described in as much as 86% of transplant recipients. However, the vast majority of patients with posttransplant HGV infection do not develop graft injury. Initial reports suggested that a more virulent strain of HGV was associated with fulminant hepatitis. It was later found that these mutations were also present in patients with chronic hepatitis and healthy persons. In addition, the reported rates of HGV infection (16–50%) are similar in patients with fulminant hepatic failure of indeterminate cause and in those with an established etiology. Finally, intravenous inoculation of chimpanzees with HGV resulted in infection but not in liver damage. This is another strong argument against the pathogenicity of HGV. Controversy exists regarding whether HGV is able to replicate in hepatocytes [11]. Attempts to detect a negative-stranded RNA intermediate of HGV in liver tissue have been mostly negative. Interestingly, antigenomic viral RNA has been found in lymphocytes, bone marrow and spleen suggesting that HGV may be a primarily lymphotropic agent.

In conclusion, HGV is a novel flavivirus that can produce both acute and chronic infection in humans. The majority of infected patients carry the virus for years in the absence of significant liver damage. At present, no conclusive evidence exists to regard HGV as a hepatitis virus. HGV infection is benign, is not associated with poor outcomes and may account for a minority of cases with unexplained acute or chronic liver diseases.

4. CIRCOVIRUSES

4.1 TT virus infection

TTV was first identified in 1997 in a Japanese patient with non-A–G transfusion-associated hepatitis and was named after the initials of the index case. The TTV genome is a circular, negative sense, single-stranded DNA of 3852 base pairs in length. The coding region of the virus is variable whereas the non-coding region is well preserved. TTV has a high degree of genomic variability. At least 16 major genotypes have been identified which differ from one another by more than 30% of the DNA sequence. Mixed infections are common. Up to five different genotypes have been isolated in a serum sample obtained from a single patient. Diagnosis of TTV infection is based on the detection of serum TTV DNA by PCR (Table 1). The genomic areas selected for designing the primers markedly influence the rate of detection of TTV DNA. Primers from the non-coding regions allow the detection of all TTV genotypes, whereas those obtained from the coding region detect primarily four genotypes. Although serological assays for both IgM and IgG class anti-TTV antibodies have been developed, they have not yet been validated in large series of patients with acute or chronic liver diseases. TTV infection has a worldwide distribution and broad penetration in the community. The wide range in the reported prevalence of TTV infection may be due to true geographic differences or to the primers selected for the detection of TTV DNA by PCR. TTV is unequivocally transmitted by blood transfusions. In the NIH study, acute TTV infection was diagnosed in 26.4% of transfused patients compared to only 4.7% in non-transfused controls [15] (Table 2). In addition, a strong association was found between the transfusion volume and the rate of TTV infection. The high prevalence observed among hemodialysis patients and patients with a history of intravenous drug abuse suggests that TTV may also be transmitted by the percutaneous route. However, many studies found no difference in the frequency of TTV infection among high- and low-risk groups. In addition, the elevated prevalence of infection among blood donors and healthy subjects suggest that TTV may be spread by non-parenteral modes including fecal–oral, horizontal, sexual and vertical transmission [15–19]. TTV has been isolated from bile, feces, tears and saliva. Rates of TTV infection higher than 80% have been reported in healthy persons from rural areas of developing countries living under poor hygienic conditions. These findings suggest direct fecal–oral transmission of TTV or horizontal transmission due to infectious saliva. Sexual transmission has been suggested based on the elevated reported rates of TTV infection among commercial sex workers and men who have sex with men and particularly because of the progressive increase in prevalence of infection with the number of lifetime sex partners. Mother-to-infant transmission of TTV may also occur. The virus has been detected in maternal blood, cord blood, amniotic fluid and breast milk. The existence of vertical transmission of TTV is strengthened by studies in which genetic relatedness was documented in mother–infant pairs. Interestingly, TTV-like sequences have been detected in 20%–30% domestic animals such as chickens, pigs and sheep, which may constitute a reservoir for human infection. TTV produces both acute and chronic infection. Among 21 viremic patients of the NIH study, clearance of serum TTV DNA occurred in 38% at 1 year and 67% at 5 years of follow-up [15]. The remaining patients developed persistent viremia for up to 22 years. Initial reports from Japan showed that TTV DNA was present in around 50% of patients with cryptogenic fulminant and chronic hepatitis. It was then suggested that TTV was the causative agent of non-A–E liver diseases. These initial observations were supported by the finding of higher rates of TTV infection in patients with acute or chronic liver diseases of unknown origin compared to blood donors. However, when more sensitive PCR assays became available, TTV DNA was detected in a large proportion of healthy adults and children, blood donors and patients with fulminant or chronic hepatitis of different etiologies [16–19]. The reported prevalence of TTV infection in blood donors was 30–90% in Japan, 14–28% in other Asian countries, 2–14% in Europe, 7.5–10% in the United states and 62% in Brazil. In addition, many studies showed that TTV infection was present in a similar proportion of patients with well-identified causes of liver disease and in those classified as cryptogenic [16–19]. The finding of TTV DNA and replicative intermediates in liver tissue suggest that TTV may be a hepatotropic agent. However, a number of pieces of evidences strongly suggest that TTV may not cause liver damage. The first argument against pathogenicity of TTV is the overwhelming prevalence of infection in entirely healthy persons and blood donors. Secondly, in the majority of reported studies, no association was found between TTV DNA and ALT levels. Third, inoculation of chimpanzees with TTV resulted in acute infection with identical viral sequences to the human inocula but without any biochemical or histological evidence of liver damage. Lastly, the rate of TTV infection in the NIH study was almost identical among patients with non-A–E hepatitis (23%) and patients who received blood transfusions but did not develop hepatitis (22%) [15]. Absence of pathogenicity has also been demonstrated among patients with liver diseases of well-identified etiology coinfected or superinfected with TTV. New TTV infection did not influence the severity or persistence of acute HCV infection, as demonstrated in the NIH study. Similarly, many studies showed that the clinical, biochemical, virological and histological abnormalities were similar among patients with chronic hepatitis B or C with or without TTV infection [16–19]. The finding of similar rates of TTV infection in patients with HBV- and HCV-cirrhosis with or without HCC suggests that TTV does not influence the development of malignancy [17,18]. In conclusion, TTV infection is not the causative agent of non-A–E hepatitis, does not play a significant role in the pathogenesis of chronic liver disease of other etiologies and is not a risk factor for the development of HCC.

4.2 SENV infection

In 1999, a small single-stranded, circular DNA virus of approximately 3800 nucleotides was discovered in the serum of an intravenous drug abuser with HIV infection and was named SENV after the initials of the patient. Although SENV is structurally similar to the prototype TTV, less than 55% nucleotide homology and less than 37% amino acid homology exist between both agents [20]. Phylogenetic analysis revealed eight different variants. Genotypes D (SENV-D) and H (SENV-H) have been the most extensively studied because they were found to be more prevalent in patients with posttransfusion hepatitis than in the general population. No assays are available to detect antibodies or to assess immune response to SENV. Therefore, diagnosis relies on the detection of serum SENV DNA by PCR (Table 1). SENV produces both acute and chronic infection. In the NIH study, 55% of patients with new SENV infection cleared the virus within 6 months and 74% after 5 years of follow-up [21]. Infection for more than 1 year was observed in 45% and up to 12 years in 13% of patients. Mutations of SENV are much higher than in other DNA viruses being similar to the rates observed in RNA viruses. This may allow the virus to evade the host immune response and produce persistent infection as described for HCV. SENV is unequivocally transmitted by blood transfusions. One-third of transfused patients of the NIH series developed new SENV infection compared to only 3% of non-transfused controls [21] (Table 2). The prevalence of infection increased linearly with the volume of transfusions, being 45% in patients who received 13 or more units of blood. More importantly, molecular linkage was demonstrated in donor–recipient pairs. A study performed in Taiwan showed SENV infection in 54% of patients with intravenous drug abusers, 68% in hemophiliacs and hemodialysis patients and in 90% of thalassemic patients. This suggests the existence of other parenteral routes of transmission. The reported prevalence of SENV infection in blood donors is around 2% in the United States, with similar rates before and after screening for HCV, 2% in Italy, and 10% in Japan. A recent report from Japan showed SENV infection in 56% of the inhabitants of a highly endemic area for HCV and 61% in another region of low endemicity where no association was found between SENV infection and blood transfusions, surgical history or folk medical practices. Previous reports from Japan showed that the prevalence of HCV infection in endemic areas is low in people aged less than 40 years followed by a sharp increase after age 50. In contrast, the prevalence of SENV infection remained relatively constant from ages 18 to 70. This suggests that SENV infection may be endemic in certain regions of Japan and that the virus may be transmitted by non-parenteral routes. The reported prevalence of SENV infection in healthy adults was much lower in the United States (2%–3%) and Taiwan (15%). A strong association between acute SENV infection and the development of transfusion-associated non-A–E hepatitis was reported by investigators of the NIH [21]. SENV DNA was detected in 11 of 12 (92%) patients with non-A–E posttransfusion hepatitis and in 55 of 225 (24%) patients who received transfusions but did not develop hepatitis (Table 2). In this study viremia was detected before or at the same time of the ALT elevation. In addition, the levels of serum SENV DNA tended to parallel the levels of aminotransferases. A SENV RNA replicative intermediate was recovered from liver tissue in two patients. This suggests that SENV may be a hepatotropic agent although these observations need further confirmation. The prevalence of SENV infection in patients with hepatitis C ranged from 21% to 67% in different series [22–24]. However, SENV infection had no effects on the persistence or severity of HCV infection. Serum HCV RNA levels were similar in patients with hepatitis C with or without SENV infection suggesting that this virus does not interfere with HCV replication as has been described for HAV and HBV [23,24]. SENV infection has been reported in around one-third of patients with fulminant hepatitis of indeterminate etiology from Japan and Taiwan. However, in the Japanese series SENV DNA was also detectable in 33% of patients with fulminant hepatitis of well-identified causes. A study from Taiwan showed SENV infection in 41% of patients with chronic hepatitis B, 54% with HBV-positive HCC, 67% with chronic hepatitis C and 76% with HCV-positive HCC. These preliminary results suggest that SENV is not an important risk factor for HCC among patients with chronic viral hepatitis. Based on the reported experience it appears that SENV can cause hepatitis in some patients. However, the majority (83%) of patients of the NIH study with posttransfusion SENV infection did not develop hepatitis [21]. Therefore, the strong association between SENV infection and non-A–E hepatitis does not prove causality. The effects of α-interferon therapy in patients with HCV-SENV co-infection were recently analyzed [23,24]. In one report from Japan the rate of HCV sustained virological response did not differ between patients with and without SENV co-infection. After interferon therapy SENV DNA disappeared from serum in 69% of patients suggesting that this agent is highly sensitive to antiviral therapy, although spontaneous viral clearance may have occurred in a substantial number of individuals. Interestingly, all patients with a sustained clearance of serum HCV RNA had normal ALT despite the presence of SENV DNA in serum. Conversely, lack of response to interferon with persistence of HCV viremia was associated with elevated ALT despite clearance of SENV. This reinforces the concept that patients infected with SENV alone have mild or no hepatitis. Opposite results were found in a study from the United States utilizing combination therapy with α-interferon and ribavirin. A sustained virological response was obtained in 53% of patients with HCV alone and in only 17% of those infected with HCV and SENV suggesting that co-infection might adversely affect the outcome of treatment. Larger trials are required to clarify these controversial observations.

Among the newly discovered human circoviruses, SENV appears as the only member of this family that may have a causative role in non-A–E posttransfusion hepatitis and perhaps in some cases of fulminant hepatitis and cryptogenic chronic liver diseases.

5. CONCLUSIONS

After isolation and cloning of HCV, viral discovery programs utilizing sophisticated techniques allowed the identification of several transmissible agents in less than a decade. These new viruses are now well characterized and sensitive molecular diagnostic assays have been developed. However, these notable advances in virological research have not translated into major practical benefits for the physician dealing with patients with acute or chronic liver diseases of uncertain etiology.

Primary infection with herpesviruses accounts for a minority of cases of acute or fulminant non-A–E hepatitis. Today, the identification of such cases is relatively simple. Modern and sensitive diagnostic assays for EBV, CMV and HSV are easily available in most clinical laboratories as they are routinely used in immunosuppressed hosts such as transplant recipients or HIV-positive patients.

HGV, TTV and SENV are transmitted by parenteral and non-parenteral routes. However, none of them unequivocally produces liver disease or is regarded as the proven causative agent of non-A–E hepatitis.

Therefore, it is highly unlikely that diagnostic assays for these new agents will become widely available. It is even unclear whether testing for HGV or TTV is indicated for patients with cryptogenic liver disease in clinical practice. Further studies are required to clarify the role of SENV in acute and less likely chronic non-A–E hepatitis. According to the trend observed in recent years, it is highly probable that new viruses will be identified in the near future. In the meanwhile, a large number of patients with acute hepatitis, fulminant hepatic failure and chronic liver disease will remain in the cryptogenic category.

REFERENCES

[1] Cohen, J.I. (2000) Epstein–Barr virus infection. *N. Engl. J. Med.* **343**, 481–492.

[2] Markin, R.S., Linder, J., Zuerlein, K., Mroczek, E., Grierson, H.L., Brichacek, B. and Purtilo, D.T. (1987) Hepatitis in fatal mononucleosis. *Gastroenterology* **93**, 1210–1217.

[3] White, N.J. and Juel-Jensen, B.E. (1984) Infectious mononucleosis hepatitis. *Semin. Liver Dis.* **4**, 301–306.

[4] Feranchak, A.P., Tyson, R.W., Narkewicz, W.R., Karrer, F.M. and Sokol, J.S. (1998) Fulminant Epstein–Barr hepatitis: orthotopic liver transplantation and review of the literature. *Liver Transplant. Surg.* **4**, 469–476.

[5] Mason, A., Sallie, R., Perrillo, R., Rayner, R., Xu, L., Dohner, D.E., Dehner, M., Naoumov, N., Gelb, L., Saha, B., O'Grady, J. and Williams, R. (1996) Prevalence of herpesviridae and hepatitis B virus DNA in the liver of patients with non-A, non-B fulminant hepatic failure. *Hepatology* **24**, 1361–1365.

[6] De Jong, M.D., Boucher, C.A.B., Danner, S.A., Gazzard, B., Griffiths, P.D., Katlama, C., Lange, J.M., Richman, D.D. and Vella, S. (1998) Summary of the international consensus symposium on management of HIV, CMV and hepatitis virus infections. *Antiviral Res.* **37**, 1–16.

[7] Weber, B., Berger, A. and Rabenau, H. (2001) Human cytomegalovirus infection: diagnostic potential of recombinant antigens for cytomegalovirus antibody detection. *J. Virol. Methods* **96**, 157–170.

[8] Sinzger, C., Bissinger, A.L., Viebahn, R., Oettle, H., Radke, C., Schmidt, C.A. and Jahn, G. (1999) Hepatocytes are permissive for human cytomegalovirus infection in human liver cell culture and *in vivo*. *J. Infect. Dis.* **180**, 976–986.

[9] Klein, N.A., Mabie, W.C., Shaver, D., Latham, P.S., Adamec, T.A., Pinstein, M.L. and Riely, C.A. (1991) Herpes simplex virus hepatitis in pregnancy. Two patients successfully treated with acyclovir. *Gastroenterology* **100**, 239–244.

[10] Aboguddah, A., Stein, H.B., Phillips, P., Amar, J. and English, R. (1991) Herpes simplex hepatitis in a patient with psoriatic arthritis taking prednisone and methotrexate. Report and review of the literature. *J. Rheumatol.* **18**, 1406–1412.

[11] Alter, H.J., Nakatsuji, Y., Melpolder, J., Wages, J., Wesley, R., Shih, J.W. and Kim, J.P. (1997) The incidence of transfusion-associated hepatitis G virus infection and its relation to liver disease. *N. Engl. J. Med.* **336**, 747–754.

[12] Lefrere, J.-J., Lerable, J., Mariotti, M., Bogard, M., Thibault, V., Frangeul, L., Loiseau, P., Bouchardeau, F., Laperche, S., Pawlotsky, J.M., Cantaloube, J.F., Biagini, P., de Lamballerie, X., Izopet, J., Defer, C., Lepot, I., Poveda, J.D., Dussaix, E., Gerolami, V., Halfon, P., Buffet-Janvresse, C., Ferec, C., Mercier, B., Marcellin, P., Martinot-Peignoux, M. and Gassain, M. (2000) Lessons from a multicentre study of the detectability of viral genomes based on a two-round quality control of GB virus C/hepatitis G virus polymerase chain reaction assay. *J. Virol. Methods* **85**, 117–124.

[13] Iino, S., Sato, S.-I., Kumada, H., Toda, G., Ishii, H., Miyake, K., Hino, K., Ichida, T., Akahane, Y., Kiyosawa, K., Kobayashi, K.-I., Hayashi, N., Kuroki, T., Tsuji, T., Sata, M., Sakai, T. and Yano, M. (1999) Involvement of GBV-C/HGV in liver diseases in Japan. *Hepatol. Res.* **13**, 153–159.

[14] Alter, M.J., Gallaher, M., Morris, T.T., Moyer, L.A., Meeks, E.L., Krawczynski, K., Kim, J.P. and Margolis, H.S. (1997) Acute non-A–E hepatitis in the United States and the role of hepatitis G virus infection. *N. Engl. J. Med.* **336**, 741–746.

[15] Matsumoto, A., Yeo, A.E.T., Shih, J.W.K., Tanaka, E., Kiyosawa, K. and Alter, H.J. (1999) Transfusion-associated TT virus and its relation to liver disease. *Hepatology* **30**, 283–288.

[16] Gimenez-Barcons, M., Forns, X., Ampurdanes, S., Guilera, M., Soler, M., Soguero, C., Sanchez-Fueyo, A., Mas, A., Bruix, J., Sanchez-Tapias, J.M., Rodes, J. and Saiz, J.C. (1999) Infection with a novel human DNA virus (TTV) has no pathogenic significance in patients with liver diseases. *J. Hepatol.* **30**, 1028–1034.

[17] Kato, T., Mizokami, M., Orito, E., Nakano, T., Tanaka, Y., Ueda, R., Hirashima, N., Iijima, Y., Kato, T., Sugauchi, F., Mukaide, M., Shimamatsu, K., Kage, M. and Kojiro, M. (1999) High prevalence of TT virus infection in Japanese patients with liver diseases and in blood donors. *J. Hepatol.* **31**, 221–227.

[18] Tagger, A., Donato, F., Ribero, M.L., Binelli, G., Gelatti, U., Portera, G., Albertini, A., Fasola, M., Chiesa, R. and Nardi, G. (1999) A case-control study on a novel DNA virus (TT virus) infection and hepatocellular carcinoma. *Hepatology* **30**, 294–299.

[19] Tuveri, R., Jaffredo, F., Lunel, F., Nalpa, B., Pol, S., Feray, C., Marcellin, P., Thibault, V., Delagneau, J.F., Opiolon, P., Scarpa, B., Brechot, C. and Theirs, V. (2000) Impact of TT virus infection in acute and chronic, viral- and non-viral-related liver diseases. *J. Hepatol.* **33**, 121–127.

[20] Tanaka, Y., Primi, D., Wang, R.Y.H., Umemura, T., Yeo, A.E., Mizokami, M., Alter, H.J. and Shih, J.W. (2001) Genomic and molecular evolutionary analysis of a newly identified infectious agent (SEN virus) and its relationship to the TT virus family. *J. Infect. Dis.* **183**, 359–367.

[21] Umemura, T., Yeo, A.E., Sottini, A., Moratto, D., Tanaka, Y., Wang, R.Y., Shih, J.W., Donahue, P., Primi, D. and Alter, H.J. (2001) SEN virus infection and its relationship to transfusion-associated hepatitis. *Hepatology* **33**, 1303–1311.

[22] Umemura, T., Alter, H.J., Tanaka, E., Yeo, A.E., Shih, J.W., Orii, K., Matsumoto, A., Yoshizawa, K. and Kiyosawa, K. (2001) Association between SEN virus infection and hepatitis C in Japan. *J. Infect. Dis.* **184**, 1246–1251.

[23] Umemura, T., Alter, H.J., Tanaka, E., Orii, K., Yeo, A.E., Shih, J.W., Matsumoto, A., Yoshizawa, K. and Kiyosawa, K. (2002) SEN virus: response to interferon alfa and influence on the severity and treatment response of coexistent hepatitis C. *Hepatology* **35**, 953–959.

[24] Rigas, B., Hasan, I., Rehman, R., Donahue, P., Wittkowski, K.M. and Lebovics, E. (2002) Effect on treatment outcome of coinfection with SEN viruses in patients with hepatitis C. *Lancet* **358**, 1961–1962.

Hepatology: A Practical Approach
B. Al Knawy, M.L. Shiffman, R.H. Wiesner (editors)

Chapter 7

Liver Disease in AIDS

J.C. Servoss, K.E. Sherman and R.T. Chung

Gastrointestinal Unit GRJ724, Massachusetts General Hospital, Fruit Street, Boston, MA 02114, USA

1. Introduction 139
2. Causes of Liver Disease in Patients with HIV 140
   2.1 Viral 140
      2.1.1 Hepatitis A 140
      2.1.2 Hepatitis B 142
      2.1.3 Hepatitis C 144
   2.2 Non-hepatotropic viruses 145
      2.2.1 CMV 145
      2.2.2 HSV and other viruses 145
   2.3 Fungal liver disease 145
      2.3.1 Candida, histoplasmosis and aspergillus 145
      2.3.2 Parasites 146
3. Other Infectious Etiologies of Liver Disease in AIDS 146
4. Neoplasms of the Liver 147
   4.1 Kaposi's sarcoma and non-Hodgkin's lymphoma 147
   4.2 Hepatocellular carcinoma 147
5. Hepatotoxicity of HAART 148
6. Hepatotoxicity in Coinfected Patients with HBV or HCV 148
7. Alcoholic Liver Disease in Patients with AIDS 150
8. Metabolic Liver Disease – Hepatic Steatosis 150
9. AIDS Lipodystrophy and Liver Dysfunction 150
10. Orthotopic Liver Transplantation in HIV-Infected Patients 151
References 151

1. INTRODUCTION

Diseases of the liver are increasingly important causes of morbidity and mortality in patients infected with HIV. The advent of highly active antiretroviral therapy (HAART) has seen extended survival and a substantial decrease in the frequency of traditional opportunistic infections. However, successful immune reconstitution has opened the door for more chronic opportunists such as the hepatotropic viruses and other forms of chronic liver disease (Table 1). In fact, mortality attributable to end-stage liver disease has increased steadily since 1996, and in some populations, is now the leading cause of death in HIV patients [1]. Other important complications include both the direct and indirect effects of these medications on the liver. All classes of antiretroviral therapy (ART) can directly cause hepatotoxicity. In addition, they can lead to metabolic alterations that secondarily affect the liver. Thus, identification, evaluation, and management of liver disease are cardinal components of the care of patients with HIV infection (Algorithms 1 and 2).

Table 1. Diseases of the liver.

Viral hepatitis
Hepatotropic viruses
Hepatitis A
Hepatitis B
Hepatitis C
Hepatitis D
Non-hepatotropic viruses
Cytomegalovirus (CMV)
Herpes simplex
Epstein–Barr virus
Varicella-zoster virus
Fungi
Candida albicans
Histoplasma capsulatum
Aspergillus spp.
Parasites
Pneumocystis carinii
Microsporidia spp.
Cryptosporidia spp.
Toxoplasma gondii
Leishmania donovani
Bacteria
Bartonella henselae
Granulomatous
Mycobacterium tuberculosis
Mycobacterium avium complex (MAC)
Toxic–metabolic
Nucleoside reverse transcriptase inhibitors (NRTIs)
Non-nucleoside reverse transcriptase inhibitors (NNRTIs)
Protease inhibitors (PIs)
Fatty liver
Non-alcoholic steatohepatitis (NASH)
AIDS lipodystrophy
Alcohol
Other medications
Neoplasia
Kaposi's sarcoma
Non-Hodgkin's lymphoma
Hepatocellular carcinoma
AIDS cholangiopathy
Cryptosporidium
Microsporidium
CMV
MAC

Adapted from Chung, R.T. and Sherman, K.E. (2003) Hepatic and hepatobiliary diseases, in *AIDS Therapy*, eds. Dolin, R., Masur, H. and Saag, M.S., 2nd edition, (Churchill Livingstone, Philadelphia) pp. 902–920, with permission.

2. CAUSES OF LIVER DISEASE IN PATIENTS WITH HIV

2.1 Viral

2.1.1. Hepatitis A

Hepatitis A virus (HAV) is an enterovirus that is transmitted almost exclusively via the fecal–oral route. Epidemiologic studies have shown that there is an increased prevalence of hepatitis A among HIV-infected individuals. Risk groups include homosexual men and injection drug users [2]. A recent analysis of HIV(+) versus HIV(−) controls infected with HAV has shown that HIV(+) individuals, despite having lower aminotransferase elevations, had a higher HAV load and longer period of viremia. Indeed, some of the patients had completely asymptomatic viremia, which may explain the higher rates of transmission among these risk groups [3]. Despite this increased duration of viremia, the typical self-limited course of hepatitis A is usually not altered in patients with HIV. Persons harboring chronic hepatitis C virus may be at increased risk for hepatic complications when acutely infected with hepatitis A virus. These patients have been found to have an increased incidence of fatal acute hepatitis A [4]. Thus, those persons coinfected with HCV and HIV can be assumed to be at high risk for severe hepatitis A. For this reason, the Centers for Disease Control (CDC) now recommends that all HIV-infected patients at risk for HAV, as well as those patients with chronic hepatitis B and C, should be vaccinated against HAV.

The diagnosis of acute hepatitis A is made by serologic testing for IgM antibodies against HAV. There are no data regarding risk of false negative reactions related to HIV-associated immunosuppression. Many laboratories will also test for the IgG antibody, a hallmark of previously cleared infection or of immunization. Treatment of acute HAV in the HIV(+) patient remains supportive until symptoms have resolved.

2.1.2. Hepatitis B

Because of shared epidemiologic risks and routes of transmission, there is an increased prevalence of

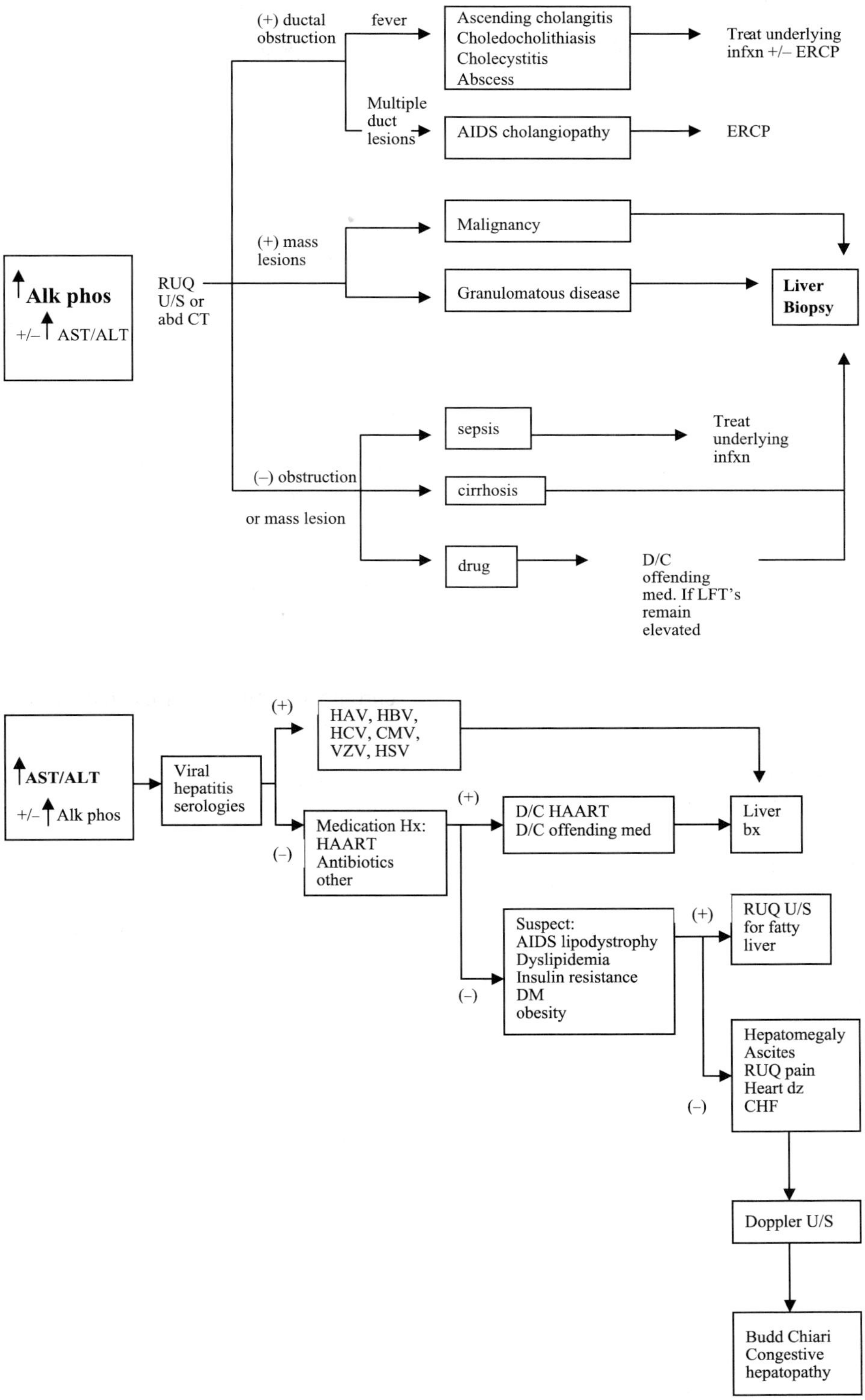
Alk phos
+/– AST/ALT
RUQ U/S or abd CT
(+) ductal obstruction
fever
Ascending cholangitis
Choledocholithiasis
Cholecystitis
Abscess
Treat underlying infxn +/– ERCP
Multiple duct lesions
AIDS cholangiopathy
ERCP
(+) mass lesions
Malignancy
Granulomatous disease
Liver Biopsy
sepsis
Treat underlying infxn
(–) obstruction or mass lesion
cirrhosis
drug
D/C offending med. If LFT's remain elevated
AST/ALT
+/– Alk phos
Viral hepatitis serologies
(+)
HAV, HBV, HCV, CMV, VZV, HSV
(–)
Medication Hx: HAART Antibiotics other
(+)
D/C HAART
D/C offending med
Liver bx
(–)
Suspect: AIDS lipodystrophy Dyslipidemia Insulin resistance DM obesity
(+)
RUQ U/S for fatty liver
(–)
Hepatomegaly Ascites RUQ pain Heart dz CHF
Doppler U/S
Budd Chiari Congestive hepatopathy

Algorithm 1.

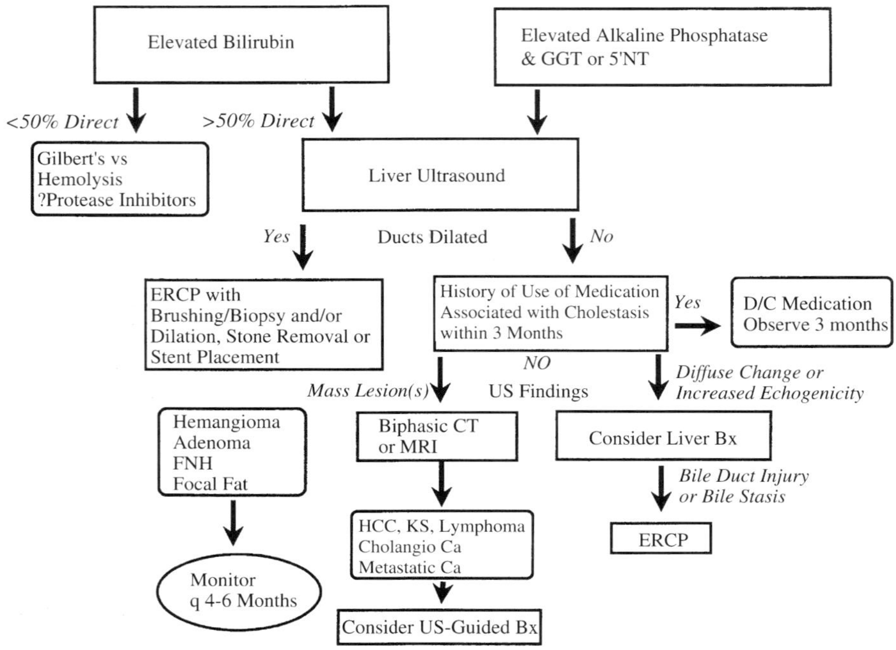

Algorithm 2.

hepatitis B virus (HBV) patients infected with HIV. Up to 95% of persons with AIDS in some cohorts have serologic markers of prior HBV infection (anti-HBs or anti-HBc+) and 10–15% are chronic carriers (HBsAg+) [2]. In the vast majority of acute infections in immunocompetent persons, the cytotoxic T lymphocyte (CTL) response that recognizes and eliminates virus-infected hepatocytes is sufficient to clear the virus. However, with the functional impairment of the cellular immune response accompanying HIV infection, HBV clearance rates are diminished and an increased frequency of both chronic infection and replication are observed. Markers of persistent HBV replication, HBeAg and HBV DNA, are found in increased frequency in patients with HIV, along with a lower alanine aminotransferase activity, and in the short term, likely less immunopathogenic liver injury [5].

However, over the long term, unchecked viral replication is likely to have adverse impact on the natural history of chronic HBV disease. With regard to the effect of HIV on the progression of HBV liver disease, one retrospective study of HIV/HBV coinfected patients compared to HBV mono-infected patients showed a higher histological activity index in HIV(+) patients. There was also a higher mortality rate in coinfected individuals [6]. A major limitation of this study was the majority of the patients were also infected with hepatitis delta virus (HDV), which could also account for the histologic progression of liver disease. More recently, however, two studies of homosexual men, excluding patients coinfected with HCV or HDV, also found progressive disease on liver biopsies [7], and an increase in liver-attributable mortality [8], reinforcing the concept that HIV hastens the progression of HBV-associated liver disease. Successful immune recovery in persons coinfected with HIV and HBV has been associated with well-described flares of hepatitis B, occasionally with hepatic decompensation [9]. This is likely a result of the cellular recognition of hepatocytes infected with high levels of virus replicating under unchecked conditions. Thus, serologic assessment for HBV in all patients with HIV becomes paramount.

The diagnosis of acute hepatitis B (HBV) infection in HIV(+) patients is also made serologically. Hallmarks of acute infection include the presence of hepatitis B surface antigen (HBsAg) and/or IgM antibody to the virus core antigen (anti-HB core). Presence of anti-HBc IgM suggests acute infection in the "window period". Anti-HB core IgG is a sign of more remote infection or chronic infection with HBV. For those patients with chronic infection, markers of viral replication should also be assessed, including hepatitis B e antigen (HBeAg), and a quantitative HBV DNA level (traditionally by hybridization or branched chain techniques, though more sensitive PCR-based methods are becoming popular), which will also detect active viremia. It is important to note that in some cases, HIV(+) patients may have ongoing viral replication in the face of negative tests for HBsAg and HBeAg [10]. In these situations, a quantitative HBV DNA will allow the clinician to discern the presence of viremia. These patients will often harbor only anti-HB core IgG as a marker of infection. The clinical significance of this finding is still under active investigation.

Currently, there are three FDA-approved treatment regimens for actively replicating chronic HBV infection. These include interferon-α (IFN) and lamivudine (3TC), and adefovir dipivoxil. IFN is administered as a daily dose of 5 million units (MU) subcutaneously (SQ) daily or 10 MU SQ three times a week (TIW) for 16 weeks. Loss of HBV DNA or seroconversion from HBeAg(+) to anti-HBe occurs in approximately 40% of adult Caucasian patients along with a decrease in inflammation on liver biopsy. However, clearance of HBV DNA can be preceded by a flare of hepatitis (increased transaminases) thought secondary to immune-mediated hepatocyte necrosis. These flares occur in approximately 63% of responders and 27% of non-responders [11]. IFN is associated with numerous side effects such as depression and bone marrow suppression. These adverse effects as well as lower efficacy have limited its use in HIV–HBV coinfection.

Lamivudine is a nucleoside analogue which competes with dCTP for incorporation into the growing DNA chain. Clinical trials in monoinfected patients have shown that lamivudine 100 mg po qd for 12 months results in a normalization of ALT in 50–70% and loss of HBeAg in 30%. However, seroconversion to anti-HBe only occurs in 15–20% of patients [12]. Given this low rate of seroconversion, chronic suppressive treatment has been employed, particularly for those with more advanced disease on liver biopsy, i.e., fibrosis. Lamivudine has activity against both the HIV reverse transcriptase and the HBV DNA polymerase making it particularly useful in treating HIV persons coinfected with HBV.

Widespread use of lamivudine has resulted in the emergence of lamivudine-resistant strains of HBV. The most common is the YMDD (tyrosine–methionine–aspartate–aspartate) mutant. Mutations in the YMDD active site motif of the DNA polymerase confers resistance to lamivudine in 15–30% after 1 year of treatment, 60% after 3 years of treatment. These mutations result in bulky side chains which sterically hinder the binding of lamivudine to the nucleotide binding site. Lamivudine-resistant patients will flare HBV DNA and ALT levels on therapy, but levels of these markers are typically lower than pre-treatment values. This is likely the result of the impaired replicative ability of the YMDD mutant. As a result, when compared to placebo, continued medical treatment with lamivudine is associated with continued suppression of wild-type HBV DNA and histologic improvement. Flares of hepatitis can occur in up to 40% of patients with HBeAg(+) infection. These flares occur in the setting of emergence of YMDD mutant, HBeAg seroconversion, clearance of mutant virus, or transient hepatic decompensation [13]. In HIV persons coinfected with HBV who are on lamivudine as part of their HAART regimen, the emergence of the YMDD mutant is almost universal (90% at 4 years). The emergence of the mutant is heralded by a new rise in HBV DNA or a rise in aminotransferase levels. YMDD breakthrough or lamivudine withdrawal may result in serious hepatic injury and death [14]. In this situation, lamivudine should be continued and alternative nucleotide analogues, such as adefovir or tenofovir might be considered.

Adefovir and tenofovir are nucleotide reverse transcriptase inhibitors that have activity against HIV reverse transcriptase and HBV DNA polymerase. In a recent study, 550 HIV infected patients were randomized to tenofovir 300 mg po qd versus placebo for 24 weeks. Of these patients, 14 (12 treatments, 2 placebos) were coinfected with HBV. All of these patients had received lamivudine, and seven had YMDD mutations. There was a mean decrease in HBV DNA $-4.63 \log_{10}$ in the tenofovir group, and $+1.23 \log_{10}$ in the placebo group ($p = 0.04$) at 24 weeks. Of note, tenofovir was not associated with any new HBV mutations and was well tolerated [15]. This agent has not been prospectively evaluated in randomized clinical trials to date, though such studies are underway.

Adefovir dipivoxil is another nucleotide reverse transcriptase inhibitor that has been recently approved for use in HBV monoinfected patients. Like tenofovir, adefovir has activity against both the HIV reverse transcriptase and HBV DNA polymerase and has not been associated with new HBV mutations. A French study [16] reported interim data from a 96-week study of adefovir 10 mg po daily on 35 persons coinfected with HIV/HBV. Subjects had well-controlled HIV on ART including lamivudine, detectable HBV DNA, and documented lamivudine (YMDD mutant) resistance. Adefovir yielded a mean decrease in HBV DNA was $-3.4 \log_{10}$ copies/ml at week 24, $-4.07 \log_{10}$ copies/ml at week 48, and $-4.77 \log_{10}$ copies/ml at week 72. Nine subjects had undetectable HBV DNA (<1000 copies/ml) at week 72 and 9% of subjects seroconverted from HBeAg(+) to HBeAg(−). In the 14 subjects with paired liver biopsies performed at 1 year, median inflammatory and fibrosis scores decreased, as did ALT. Adefovir was well tolerated and was not associated with the development of adefovir resistance mutations in the HIV reverse transcriptase.

2.1.3. Hepatitis C

In a manner analogous to HBV, the common routes of transmission for HIV and hepatitis C virus (HCV) have been associated with an increase in prevalence of HCV among HIV(+) individuals. The prevalence of HCV among HIV(+) patients may range from 5 to 85%, depending on risk factors for acquisition in isolated cohorts. Among injection drug users, the prevalence is anywhere from 52 to 92%, and from 4 to 14% among homosexual men [5]. An analysis of the heterogenous, US ACTG cohort revealed an overall prevalence of 16.1% among HIV-infected patients [17]. Like HBV, hepatitis C (HCV) is cleared and controlled by the action of host CTLs. In the setting of immune suppression by HIV, HCV replication is increased. HIV infection has been clearly associated with an accelerated natural history of HCV. The most informative data have come from hemophilia cohorts, in whom the timing of HIV and HCV infection can be more precisely ascertained. The Multicenter Hemophilia Cohort Study prospectively examined 223 patients with hemophilia. Of those coinfected with HIV and HCV, there was a liver failure rate of 8.8% when HCV had been present for >10 years [18]. More recently, in a retrospective cohort study of injection drug users, HIV coinfection was associated with higher HCV RNA levels, worsening liver disease on liver biopsy as well as a decreased response to interferon [19]. Conversely, HCV has also been suggested in some studies to accelerate the progression of HIV. In particular, in one study of injecting drug users, HCV was associated with a more rapid progression to AIDS and death, compared to non-genotype 1 HCV patients [20]. The same study suggested that HCV infection can blunt the immune recovery induced by HAART [20]. However, controversy still exists, as HAART-related immune recovery in the short term does not appear to be adversely affected by HCV coinfection [2]. Because of high coinfection rates, all persons with HIV should be screened for HCV.

The diagnosis of chronic HCV infection can be made through the detection of HCV antibodies via an ELISA assay. Higher false negative rates are seen in patients with advanced immunodeficiency (CD4 <100). However, in general, low false negative rates have been observed in HIV cohorts entering clinical trials [17]. For those patients who test (+) for anti-HCV, detection of HCV RNA by PCR will help to differentiate those persons with active viremia from those who have cleared infection remotely. High false positive and false negative rates of detection mandate that two HCV RNA assays be performed to confirm or deny infection in those with negative serologic assays.

Current therapy for HCV monoinfection is combination therapy with pegylated-interferon-α-2b (PEG-IFN) and ribavirin (RBV). PEG-IFN is longer acting than IFN and permits for once weekly dosing. PEG-IFN and RBV therapy for 48 weeks results in a 54% sustained virologic response (SVR), defined as HCV RNA clearance 6 months following completion of therapy [21]. SVR is associated with an arrest in fibrosis progression and even regression over the long term. However, as with IFN, PEG-IFN is associated with side effects such as depression, fatigue and anemia that are especially problematic in coinfected persons. In HIV(+) persons coinfected with HCV, up to 29% of patients prematurely discontinue IFN/RBV combination treatment [22]. In addition, RBV antagonizes the phosphorylation of thymidine analogues such as AZT or d4T in *in vitro* systems. To date, there is little evidence of clinically relevant antagonism *in vivo*. This competitive competition may also increase serum/tissue levels of concomitantly administered ddI, which may lead to mitochondrial injury characterized by lactic acidosis and even liver failure [23].

A trial of IFN/RBV versus PEG-IFN/RBV in HIV–HCV coinfected persons is being conducted through the US Adult AIDS Clinical Trial Group. The 24-week interim analysis revealed a virologic response rate of 15% in the IFN/RBV group versus 44% in the PEG-IFN/RBV group ($p = 0.0003$). In those patients who failed to achieve a virologic response at week 24, there was improvement in histology in both the IFN/RBV (40%) and the PEG-IFN/RBV (26%) arms [24]. An upcoming trial will specifically examine the effect of suppressive therapy with PEG-IFN on inflammation and fibrosis progression in those coinfected patients who fail to achieve virologic clearance.

2.2 Non-hepatotropic viruses

2.2.1. CMV

Cytomegalovirus (CMV) is the most common infectious pathogen in patients with AIDS. There is a wide range of clinical manifestations of CMV from asymptomatic seropositivity to esophagitis, diarrhea, GI bleeding, hepatitis with or without biliary involvement, and fulminant multiorgan disease. CMV in the liver causes a hepatitis-like picture with elevations of aminotransferases. CMV may also elicit a granulomatous response in the liver in which case the alkaline phosphatase can also be elevated. Since many patients with HIV/AIDS are seropositive for CMV, the diagnosis of active hepatic CMV infection is made by liver biopsy. Histologic findings of CMV include characteristic viral inclusions, which can be seen in Kupffer cells, hepatocytes, and in association with granulomas. Monoclonal antibody staining or *in situ* hybridization can confirm the presence of the virus in the liver [25]. The treatment for CMV hepatitis includes intravenous ganciclovir.

2.2.2. HSV and other viruses

In patients with HIV who present with disseminated herpes simplex virus (HSV) infection, liver involvement can be significant. HSV causes a severe, acute hepatitis with marked aminotransferase elevations. Diagnosis can be made using HSV DNA PCR assays, which may reveal high levels of viremia, or by liver biopsy which disclose intranuclear inclusions typical for HSV. In order to distinguish CMV from HSV, immunohistochemical staining should be performed. Treatment for disseminated HSV infection or HSV hepatitis includes prompt administration of intravenous acyclovir [2].

Other herpetic viruses implicated in liver disease in HIV patients include varicella-zoster (VZV) and Epstein–Barr virus. Liver involvement in VZV infection occurs with disseminated disease. Diagnosis is typically made with identification of the classic dermatomal rash associated with VZV. Treatment includes intravenous acyclovir [2].

2.3 Fungal liver disease

2.3.1. Candida, histoplasmosis and aspergillus

Candidal infection of the liver is rare with the exception of disseminated candidal infection. In the setting of neutropenia and/or severe immunocompromise, candidal infection of the liver can result in hepatic micro- or macro-abscesses which can be diagnosed by radiologic studies (ultrasound or abdominal CT scan) and subsequent liver biopsy [25]. Liver biopsy will reveal yeast forms characteristic of candida. Abscesses in the liver will also result in an elevated alkaline phosphatase with or without cholestasis. The treatment for disseminated candidiasis is intravenous amphotericin.

Similar to candida, hepatic infection with *Histoplasma capsulatum* typically occurs in HIV patients with advanced immunocompromise and disseminated histoplasmosis. The manifestation of histoplasmosis in the liver includes the formation of caseating granulomas resulting in alkaline phosphatase as well as aminotransferase elevations. If hepatic histoplasmosis is suspected, liver or bone marrow biopsy can be performed. In the former, fungal organisms can be seen within the granulomas. In bone marrow biopsies, which have been shown to have a higher diagnostic yield than liver biopsies, stainable yeast can also be seen [26]. Since it is difficult to grow the organism in culture, serologic testing for complement fixing antibodies is a useful adjunct in the diagnosis of histoplasma infection [2]. Similar to disseminated candidal infection, intravenous amphotericin is the treatment of choice for disseminated histoplasmosis.

Aspergillus species can also infect the liver of HIV patients with advanced immunocompromise and disseminated infection. *Aspergillus* spp. typically form caseating granulomas in the liver, cholestasis and abscess formation. Alkaline phosphatase elevations usually predominate. Further diagnosis by liver biopsy can reveal the fungal forms in the granulomas or abscess, and the treatment is intravenous amphotericin.

2.3.2. Parasites

Although hepatic involvement with *Pneumocystis carinii* (PCP) is rare, cases of individuals, who inhaled pentamidine for prophylaxis against PCP pneumonia, have been described. Inhaled pentamidine does not protect extrapulmonary sites, such as liver and spleen, from infection [27]. Diagnosis of PCP in the liver is done by liver biopsy, which shows discrete areas of granular necrosis with minimal inflammation as well as a foamy eosinophilic exudate [2]. Treatment for extrapulmonary PCP includes intravenous bactrim or pentamidine.

In addition to PCP, other parasites such as *Microsporidium*, *Toxoplasma gondii*, and *Cryptosporidium* can also infect the liver. Hepatic involvement with *Microsporidium* has been described in isolated case reports. *T. gondii* in the liver is seen with disseminated infection and presents with elevated alkaline phosphatase. *Cryptosporidium* has been implicated in cases of acalculous cholecystitis, biliary tract obstruction, and secondary sclerosing cholangitis [28].

Visceral leishmaniasis is caused by *Leishmania donovani*, which is endemic in the Mediterranean, central Asia, Russia, the Middle East, China, India, Pakistan, Bangladesh, Africa, Central America, and South America [29]. The primary vector for leishmaniasis is the sandfly. Once amastigotes are ingested by the sandfly, they become flagellated promastigotes. Once the promastigotes enter the human reservoir, they are taken up by macrophages in the reticuloendothelial system of the liver and spleen where replication occurs. The clinical presentation of visceral leishmaniasis includes an ulcerated or papular skin lesion at the site of the sandfly bite. After a 2–6-month incubation period, patients may develop intermittent fevers, diarrhoea, weight loss and painful hepatosplenomegaly. Biochemical tests may reveal elevated liver function tests (LFTs), a polyclonal hypergammaglobulinemia as well as pancytopenia. On physical exam, there may be lymphadenopathy, impressive hepatosplenomegaly and evidence of ascites or jaundice. The cutaneous gray hyperpigmentation that gave rise to the name "kala-azar", or "black fever" is usually only seen in India. On histopathologic examination of the liver, amastigotes can be found in Kupffer cells or within non-caseating granulomas. Infection with leishmaniasis can lead to hepatocyte necrosis and fibrosis. Although the liver may appear cirrhotic on radiographic examination, complications of end-stage liver disease are rarely seen. The diagnosis of visceral leishmaniasis can be made using serologic tests such as ELISA, immunofluorescence, or direct agglutination. More definitive diagnosis occurs with visualization of amastigotes in hepatic, splenic, or lymph node tissue, or bone marrow aspiration. Treatment includes at least 4 weeks of pentavalent antimonial compounds such as Pentostam which is available through the Centers for Disease Control and Prevention. Alternative agents include amphotericin B and aminosidine [30].

3. OTHER INFECTIOUS ETIOLOGIES OF LIVER DISEASE IN AIDS

Along with their immunocompetent counterparts, patients with HIV are susceptible to the same wide range of infectious agents that affect the liver (Table 1). However, there are particular organisms highlighted here that are seen primarily or more commonly in patients with AIDS.

Bacterial infection. Bacillary angiomatosis is a bacterial infection seen primarily in patients with HIV/AIDS, or other immunocompromised states. The disease is most commonly caused by *Bartonella henselae*, and is associated with an exposure to cats infected with the bacteria. The bacilli can infect the liver, lymph nodes, pleura, bronchi, bones, brain, bone marrow and spleen. The most common clinical presentation is that of blood-red papular skin lesions, and possibly fever and sepsis. However, infection can occur without the skin manifestations. Markers of infection in the liver include elevated aminotransferases as well as the presence of peliosis hepatis, or blood-filled cysts in the liver. On liver biopsy, clusters of bacteria are surrounded by these blood-filled cysts [31]. The diagnosis of *Bartonella* infection is done by polymerase chain reaction-based methods on serum [32]. First-line treatment for *Bartonella* is erythromycin 2 g daily for 6 weeks, or doxycycline may be used.

Granulomatous liver disease. A myriad of pathogens can cause granulomatous liver disease in patients with HIV. The most common of these agents is *Mycobacterium avium* complex (MAC). MAC can be found in the livers of up to 80% of patients who die because of AIDS. Similar to *M. tuberculosis*, the clinical presentation of MAC disease in the liver includes low grade fever, night sweats, fatigue, and malaise. The typical biochemical feature of liver infestation is an elevated alkaline phosphatase, a reflection of the space-occupying granulomas in the liver. The treatment of MAC infection in the liver is a 3–4-drug regimen for 3 months. Most commonly, a macrolide (erythromycin, azithromycin) is combined with two or three of the following: ethambutol, rifampin, or ciprofloxacin [33,2].

AIDS cholangiopathy. AIDS cholangiopathy is a disorder of the biliary tree characterized by (1) isolated papillary stenosis or (2) intrahepatic strictures akin to sclerosing cholangitis, or a combination of the two. Extrahepatic bile duct strictures can also be seen. The syndrome is thought to be caused by infectious agents such as *Cryptosporidium*, *Microsporidium*, *CMV*, and *MAC*. The presenting symptoms include those of ascending cholangitis: fever, right upper quadrant pain, and jaundice. On occasion, patients may also have hepatomegaly. Biochemical tests typically reveal a predominantly obstructive picture with an alkaline phosphatase elevation out of proportion to the transaminases. AIDS cholangiopathy can be diagnosed by ERCP. MRCP has also been utilized with some success. Ultrasound or CT may demonstrate intrahepatic segmental dilation, but fail to clearly permit diagnosis of this condition. Treatment of the causative organisms does not change the course of the disease. Only papillotomy or stenting of dominant strictures is employed as treatment strategies for papillary stenosis and intra- or extrahepatic strictures, respectively. Neither of these measures will necessarily affect the elevation of alkaline phosphatase, nor halt progression of disease. There are no prospective studies that describe the effect of HAART-associated immune reconstitution on disease progression.

4. NEOPLASMS OF THE LIVER

4.1 Kaposi's sarcoma and non-Hodgkin's lymphoma

In the setting of progressive immunosuppression from AIDS, persons with HIV are at higher risk for two malignancies of the liver, Kaposi's sarcoma and non-Hodgkin lymphomas. While Kaposi's more commonly presents with skin manifestations, it can also be seen in the luminal gastrointestinal tract as well as in the liver. Non-Hodgkin's lymphomas (NHL) are usually of the B-cell subtype. Kaposi's and NHL liver lesions typically present as infiltrative lesions with an elevated alkaline phosphatase out of proportion to transaminases. The lesions can be visualized by ultrasound or abdominal CT and diagnosis should be confirmed by liver biopsy [2].

4.2 Hepatocellular carcinoma

With the increasing prevalence of HBV and HCV coinfection and subsequent end-stage liver disease in the HIV population, hepatocellular carcinoma will become a more common source of morbidity and mortality. As with monoinfected patients, HCC should be suspected in any person with chronic viral hepatitis or cirrhosis who experiences worsening of their LFTs or other sign of hepatic decompensation. Screening α-fetoprotein serum tests and ultrasonography should be performed semiannually in those patients with HBV- or HCV-related cirrhosis. When the index of suspicion is high, abdominal CT and MRI with contrast are more sensitive tests than ultrasonography to detect small HCC. Treatments for HCC currently include resection (in well-compensated hosts), radiofrequency ablation and chemoembolization, though liver transplantation for small intrahepatic HCCs is the only proven long-term cure in HIV(−) patients, as it removes the underlying pre-malignant substrate tissue [2]. Ongoing trials examine the effectiveness of liver transplant for ESLD in HIV(+) recipients.

5. HEPATOTOXICITY OF HAART

Since the introduction of HAART, AIDS-related morbidity and mortality has declined. However, a significant impediment to the initiation or continuation of HAART is treatment-related hepatotoxicity (Table 2). In 6–30% of patients, HAART has been associated with significant elevations of liver enzymes [34]. In fact, Clark *et al.* [35] recently reported six cases of acute liver failure (ALF) secondary to HAART therapy, five of which were fatal. The median duration of therapy was 12.5 months, but the ALF was neither related to duration of HAART, nor the specific type of therapy.

Nucleoside reverse transcriptase inhibitors (NRTIs), such as AZT, d4T, ddI and ddC, competitively inhibit the viral reverse transcriptase of HIV, resulting in premature viral chain termination. NRTIs have been associated with mitochondrial toxicity which manifests clinically as lactic acidosis and microvesicular fatty liver. The incidence of grade 3 or 4 hepatotoxicity (ALT > 5× ULN) is approximately 5% for patients on dual nucleoside therapy [2].

Protease inhibitors (PIs), such as indinavir, ritonavir, saquinavir, and nelfinavir, prevent new virion particles from being released from infected CD4 cells. Although all PIs inhibit the HIV protease, they each produce their own unique hepatotoxicity. The incidence of indinavir hepatotoxicity is approximately 6%. Indinavir's effect on the liver has been described as a hypersensitivity reaction presenting as a severe elevation of ALT and AST [36]. Saquinavir and nelfinavir have similar rates of hepatotoxicity and appear to have a direct toxic effect on hepatocytes. Ritonavir at higher doses has been associated in one study with the highest risk of hepatotoxicity, 27–32%. In this same study, risk factors for developing hepatotoxicity on HAART included use of ritonavir and a CD4 count increase of $0.05 \times 10^9\ l^{-1}$ [37]. However, ritonavir, a potent P450 inhibitor, is now used at considerably lower doses to boost levels of other concomitantly administered PIs, and the incidence of severe hepatotoxicity with these regimens is not yet established.

Non-nucleoside reverse transcriptase inhibitors (NNRTIs), such as nevirapine and efavirenz can also be associated with significant hepatotoxicity. In a recent prospective study of 568 patients on an NNRTI containing regimen, grade 3 or 4 hepatotoxicity was seen in 15.6 and 8% of patients on nevirapine or efavirenz containing regimens, respectively. Remarkably, more half of these grade 3 or 4 elevations occurred after the first 12 weeks of therapy suggesting that hepatotoxicity is not always an early event [34]. These findings are supportive by a retrospective study of the US Adult AIDS Clinical Trial Group (ACTG). Over 9000 patients enrolled in 21 ACTG studies were followed for HAART-related hepatotoxicity. There was a high rate of severe ART hepatotoxicity irrespective of class at 9%. Among the NNRTIs, nevirapine had the highest rate of grade 3/4 hepatotoxicity at 10.4%, followed by efavirenz at 9.8%. Most of the treatment discontinuation occurred after 24 weeks of therapy, emphasizing the concept that NNRTI-related hepatotoxicity can occur at any time during treatment [38].

6. HEPATOTOXICITY IN COINFECTED PATIENTS WITH HBV OR HCV

The preponderance of studies show that coinfection with viral hepatitis predisposes patients to hepatotoxicity. Two studies by Johns Hopkins have shown

Table 2. Hepatotoxicity of drugs commonly used in patients with HIV.

Type of drug	Pattern of injury		Cholestatic	Granulomas	Mixed
	Hepatocellular	Microvesicular steatosis			
Analgesics	Acetaminophen Ibuprofen Indomethacin Salicylates		Propoxyphene		Naproxen Piroxicam Sulindac
Anticonvulsants	Phenytoin	Valproate	Phenytoin	Phenytoin	Carbamazepine Phenobarbital
Antimicrobials	Acyclovir Ampho B Ethionamide Isoniazid Ketoconazole Metronidazole Penicillins Pentamidine Pyrazinamide Quinacrine Rifampin Sulfonamides Dapsone Tetracycline TMP-SMX 5-Flucytosine	Tetracycline (IV)	Albendazole Azithromycin Erythromycin Ketoconazole Rifampin Thiabendazole TMP-SMX	TMP-SMX	TMP-SMX
Antiretrovirals					
NRTI		ddC d4T ddI AZT			
NNRTI	Nevirapine Efavirenz				
PI	Indinavir Saquinavir Nelfinavir Ritonavir (Inhib. P450)				
Miscellaneous	Disulfiram Vitamin A Prochlorperazine			Anabolic steroids Chlorpromazine Contraceptive steroids Prochlorperazine	Chlordiazepoxide Diazepam

From Chung, R.T. and Sherman, K.E. (2003) Hepatic and hepatobiliary diseases, in *AIDS Therapy*, 2nd edition, eds. Dolin, R., Masur, H. and Saag M.S. (Churchill Livingstone, Philadelphia) pp. 902–920, with permission.

that coinfection with HBV or HCV has conferred an increased risk of hepatotoxicity. In the first study, HBV- or HCV-infected patients on non-ritonavir regimens had a 3.7-fold increased risk of severe hepatotoxicity [37], although it should be noted that the majority of coinfected patients (88%) did not develop any hepatotoxicity [37]. In the second study, the authors demonstrated that any grade of hepatotoxicity was seen in at least 70% of HCV patients and that there was a 2-fold increased risk of severe hepatotoxicity in patients coinfected with HCV or HBV [34]. A recent small study from

Madrid examined the role of specific HCV genotype in the development of HAART-related hepatotoxicity [39]. HIV/HCV-infected patients were followed for 9 months during which 17% developed severe hepatotoxicity. The incidence of severe hepatotoxicity was highest in the genotype 3 group (33%), compared to genotypes 1, 2, and 4. Multivariate analysis identified genotype 3 HCV as an independent risk factor for the development of hepatotoxicity.

7. ALCOHOLIC LIVER DISEASE IN PATIENTS WITH AIDS

The most recent study examining the effect of alcohol on liver disease progression on patients with HIV was a cohort study of 244 patients from France [40]. This study compared 122 HIV +/HCV + coinfected patients with 122 HIV −/HCV + patients and examined the fibrosis rate. They also analyzed risk factors for the development of fibrosis. They found that progression to fibrosis was more rapid in patients coinfected with HIV and HCV versus HCV alone. Their multivariate analysis also demonstrated that alcohol consumption of >50 g/day, CD4 count <200 cells/mm^3, and age at HCV infection >25 years old were also independent risk factors for more rapid fibrosis progression. The same independent risk factors were observed in coinfected patients. It can therefore be concluded that alcohol also compresses the natural history of fibrosis progression in patients coinfected with HIV and HCV. Thus, patients with HIV–HCV coinfection should be strongly advised to abstain from alcohol consumption.

8. METABOLIC LIVER DISEASE – HEPATIC STEATOSIS

The most common histologic finding on liver biopsies of patients with HIV is macrovesicular fatty infiltration. It can be associated with several metabolic abnormalities including obesity, weight loss or weight gain, diabetes, hyperlipidemia, hyperalimentation, and alcohol use. The typical finding on liver biopsy is macrovesicular steatosis randomly distributed throughout the liver lobule. Usually there is little concomitant inflammation. Of note, a substantial subset of patients with steatosis will also have fibrosis on liver biopsy and will be at increased risk for the development of cirrhosis. In patients with HIV infection, steatosis has been associated with antiretroviral medications including AZT, d4T, ddC, ddI, as well as protease inhibitors (Table 2). With regard to diagnosis, macrovesicular steatosis can result in elevations of transaminases and alkaline phosphatase. Physical exam may reveal hepatomegaly. Fatty liver may be suggested by radiologic studies, such as ultrasound or abdominal CT scan, which show increased echogenicity of the liver. However, the reliability of these findings in a setting where fibrosis is present has not been established. Therapy for macrovesicular steatosis is treatment of the underlying disease. For patients on antiretrovirals, withholding medications are recommended when grade 3 LFT elevations occur. If the LFT elevations are persistent, liver biopsy is generally recommended to evaluate whether fat or other injury is present [2].

9. AIDS LIPODYSTROPHY AND LIVER DYSFUNCTION

AIDS lipodystrophy is syndrome of metabolic and fat distribution changes that have been described in the HIV population. The changes manifest in combinations as lipoatrophy or lipohypertrophy and are frequently associated with dyslipidemia, insulin resistance, and fatty liver disease [41]. Initial reports linked AIDS lipodystrophy with PI-containing regimens, but now lipodystrophy can be seen irrespective of ART class. Carr *et al.* [42] has described a syndrome of lipoatrophy, lactic acidosis and liver dysfunction associated with ART therapy. In this case-control study NRTIs were associated with a partially reversible syndrome of fatigue, nausea, hepatomegaly, lactic acidosis and abnormal LFTs ($\leq 4\times$ upper limit of normal). The abnormal LFTs occurred over 3–6 months prior to diagnosis of the syndrome. Most cases discontinued therapy secondary to fatigue or lactic acidosis. Four cases maintained NRTI therapy and had stable LFTs over 1–3 months of follow-up. The diagnosis should be entertained when characteristic physical changes of fat redistribution are accompanied by LFT elevations.

10. ORTHOTOPIC LIVER TRANSPLANTATION IN HIV-INFECTED PATIENTS

In the pre-HAART era, HIV infection was considered an absolute contraindication to orthotopic liver transplantation (OLT) because of poor patient survival due to complications from immunosuppressive therapy. As a consequence, from 1987 to 1991, there were only 14 OLT cases reported among four different centers (Pittsburgh, Massachusetts General Hospital, Deaconess Hospital (MA), Cambridge, and Omaha) [43]. Of these 14 cases, five were secondary to viral hepatitis; the other etiologies of liver failure were unknown. Seven of 14 had an AIDS-defining illness at the time. Only four patients were alive 9 months post-OLT, 10/14 died. In the post-HAART era, the outcomes have been variable. Nowak *et al.* [44] reported four cases of OLT, three of whom were coinfected with HCV. Three subjects were alive after 9, 14, and 36 months. One patient died after 3 months. Prachalias *et al.* [43] from King's College reported five cases of OLT in HIV-infected patients. Three patients were coinfected with HCV, and two had ALF, one from HBV and the other from non-A, non-B, non-C hepatitis. No patients had AIDS-defining illnesses. All three HCV coinfected patients died from recurrent HCV. The other two patients transplanted for ALF were alive, 4 and 34 months after transplantation with no HIV-related complications.

A more recent, multicenter experience of OLT in HIV-infected patients has shown more promising results. Ragni *et al.* [45] reported 23 cases of OLT in HIV-infected patients. Fourteen patients were HCV coinfected. Survival at 12, 24, and 36 months after OLT was 90.9, 75.9 and 75.9% which was comparable to age- and race-matched HIV-negative controls from the United Network for Organ Sharing (UNOS), $p = 0.643$. Maintenance of HIV control post-OLT with HAART was uniformly successful in those patients who tolerated HAART. Predictors of poor survival included coinfection with HCV ($p = 0.037$), post-OLT antiretroviral intolerance ($p = 0.007$), post-OLT CD4 < 200 cells/ul ($p = 0.005$), and post-OLT HIV viral load > 400 copies/ml ($p = 0.016$). Type of antiretroviral or immunosuppressive therapy did not affect survival. This study demonstrates that HIV infection should no longer be a contraindication to OLT. However, diligent assessment of HIV status and antiretroviral tolerance will be critical to the evaluation of potential OLT candidates.

REFERENCES

[1] Bica, I., McGovern, B., Dhar, R., Stone, D., McGowan, K., Scheib, R. and Snydman, D.R. (2001) Increasing mortality due to end-stage liver disease in patients with human immunodeficiency virus infection. *Clin. Infect. Dis.* **32**, 492–497.

[2] Chung, R.T. and Sherman, K.E. (2003) Hepatic and hepatobiliary diseases, in *AIDS Therapy*, eds. Dolin, R., Masur, H. and Saag, M.S., 2nd edition (Churchill Livingstone, Philadelphia, PA) pp. 902–920.

[3] Ida, S., Tachikawa, N., Nakajima, A., Daikoku, M., Yano, M., Kikuchi Yasuoka, A., Kimura, S. and Oka, S. (2002) Influence of human immunodeficiency virus type 1 infection on acute hepatitis A virus infection. *Clin. Infect. Dis.* **34**(3), 379–385.

[4] Vento, S., Garofano, T., Renizini, C., Caincilli, F., Casali, F., Ghironzi, G., Ferraro, T. and Concia, E. (1998) Fulminant hepatitis associated with hepatitis A virus superinfection in patients with chronic hepatitis C. *NEJM* **338**, 286–290.

[5] Kim, A.Y., Chung, R.T. and Polsky, B. (2000) Human immunodeficiency virus and hepatitis B and C coinfection: pathogenic interactions natural history, and therapy. *AIDS Clin. Rev.*, 263–306.

[6] Houset, C., Pol, S., Carnot, F., Dubois, F., Nalpas, B., Housset, B., Berthelot, P. and Brechot, C. (1992) Interaction between human immunodeficiency virus type 1 infection, hepatitis delta virus and hepatitis B virus infections in 260 chronic carriers of hepatitis B virus. *Hepatology* **15**, 578–583.

[7] Colin, J.F., Cazals-Hatem, D., Loriot, M.A., Martinot-Peignoux, M., Pham, B.N., Auperin, A., Degott, C., Benhamou, J.P., Erlihger, S., Valla, D. and Marcellin, P. (1999) Influence of human immunodeficiency virus infection on chronic hepatitis B in homosexual men. *Hepatology* **29**, 1306–1310.

[8] Thio, C.L. *et al.* (2002) Liver disease mortality in HIV–HBV coinfected persons, *9th Conference on Retroviruses and Opportunistic Infections*. Abstract 656.

[9] Carr, A., Samaras, K., Chisholm, D.J. and Cooper, D.A. (1998) Pathogenesis of HIV-protease inhibitor-associated peripheral lipodystrophy, hyperlipidaemia and insulin resistance. *Lancet* **351**, 1881–1883.

[10] Hofer, M., Joller-Jemelka, H.I., Grob, P.J., Luthy, R. and Opravil, M. (1998) Frequent chronic hepatitis B virus infection in HIV-infected patients positive for antibody to hepatitis B core antigen only. Swiss HIV cohort study. *Eur. J. Clin. Microbiol. Infect. Dis.* **17**, 6–13.

[11] Feldman, M., Scharschmidt, B.F. and Sleisinger, M.H. (editors) (1998) *Sleisenger and Fordtran's Gastrointestinal and Liver Disease* (Saunders, Philadelphia), 6th edition.

[12] Lok, A.S. *et al.* (2002) *UptoDate Online*.

[13] Lok, A.S., Heathcote, E.J. and Hoofnagle, J.H. (2001) Management of hepatitis B: 2000 – summary of a workshop. *Gastroenterology* **120**, 1828–1853.

[14] Bessesen, M., Aaranda-Michel, J., Condreay, L., Lawrence, S. and Sherman, K.E. (1999) Chronic active hepatitis B exacerbations in HIV-infected patients treated with lamivudine. *Clin. Infect. Dis.* **28**, 1032–1036.

[15] Cooper, D. (2002) *9th Conference on Retroviruses and Opportunistic Infections*. Abstract 124.

[16] Benhamou, Y., Bochet, M., Thibault, V. *et al.* (2002) Adefovir dipivoxil 10 mg suppresses HBV viral replication in HIV–HBV coinfected patients with lamivudine resistant HBV, *9th Conference on Retroviruses and Opportunistic Infections*. Abstract 123.

[17] Sherman, K.E., Rouster, S.D., Chung, R.T. and Rajicic, N. (2002) Hepatitis C virus prevalence among patients infected with human immunodeficiency virus: a cross-sectional analysis of the US adult AIDS Clinical Trials Group. *Clin. Infect. Dis.* **34**(6), 831–837.

[18] Eyster, M.W., Diamondstone, L.D., Lien, J.M., Ehmann, W.C., Quan, S., Goedert, J.J. and for the Multicenter Hemophilia Cohort Study, (1993) Natural history of hepatitis C virus infection in multitransfused hemophiliacs: effect of coinfection with human immunodeficiency virus. *J. Acquir. Immune Defic. Syndr.* **6**, 602–610.

[19] Di Martino, V., Rufat, P., Boyer, N., Renard, P., Degos, F., Martinot-Peignoux, M., Matheron, S., Le Moing, V., Vachon, F., Degott, C., Valla, D. and Marcellin, P. (2001) The influence of human immunodeficiency virus coinfection on chronic hepatitis C in injection drug users: a long-term retrospective cohort study. *Hepatology* **34**, 1193–1199.

[20] Greub, G., Ledergerber, B., Battegay, M., Grob, P., Perrin, L., Furrer, H., Burgisser, P., Erb, P., Boggian, K., Piffaretti, J.C., Hirschel, B., Janin, P., Francioli, P., Flepp, M. and Telenti, A. (2000) Clinical progression, survival, and immune recovery during antiretroviral therapy in patients with HIV-1 and hepatitis C virus co-infection: the Swiss HIV cohort study. *Lancet* **356**, 1800–1805.

[21] Manns, M.P., McHutchison, J.G., Gordon, S.C., Rustgi, V.K., Shiffman, M., Reindollar, R., Goodman, Z.D., Koury, K., Ling, M., Albrecht, J.K. and the International Hepatitis Interventional Therapy Group, (2001) Peginterferon alfa-2b plus ribavirin compared with interferon alfa-2b plus ribavirin for initial treatment of chronic hepatitis C: a randomized trial. *Lancet* **358**, 958–965.

[22] Landau, A., Batisse, D., Piketty, C., Duong Van Huyen, J.P., Bloch, F., Belec, L., Bruneval, P., Weiss, L., Jian, R. and Kazatchkine, M.D. (2001) Long-term efficacy of combination therapy with interferon-alpha 2b and ribavirin for severe chronic hepatitis C in HIV-infected patients. *AIDS* **15**(16), 2149–2155.

[23] Lafeuillage, A., Hittinger, G. and Chadapaud, S. (2001) Increased mitochondrial toxicity with ribavirin in HIV/HCV coinfection. *Lancet* **357**(9252), 280–281.

[24] Chung, R.T. *et al.* (2002) *9th CROI*, LB-15.

[25] Feldman, M., Friedman, L.S. and Sleisenger, M. (2002) *Sleisenger and Fordtran's Gastrointestinal and Liver Disease: Pathophysiology, Diagnosis and Management* (Saunders, Philadelphia), vol. 1, 7th edition, p. 500.

[26] Cappell, M.S. (1991) Hepatobiliary manifestations of acquired immune deficiency syndrome. *Am. J. Gastroenterol.* **86**, 1–15.

[27] Rockley, P.F., Wilcox, C.M., Moynihan, M., Hewan-Lowe, K. and Schwartz, D. A. (1994) Splenic infection simulating lymphoma: an unusual presentation of disseminated *Pneumocystis carinii* infection. *South. Med. J.* **87**, 530.

[28] Schneiderman, D.J. (1988) Hepatobiliary abnormalities of AIDS. *Gastroenterol. Clin. N. Am.* **17**(3), 615–630.

[29] Smith, D.H. (1984) Visceral leishmaniasis: human aspects, in *Recent Advances in Tropical Medicine*, ed. Gilles, H.M. (Churchill Livingstone, Edinburgh) pp. 79–87.

[30] Feldman, M., Friedman, L.S. and Sleisenger, M. (2002). *Sleisenger and Fordtran's Gastrointestinal*

and Liver Disease: Pathophysiology, Diagnosis and Management, vol. 2, 7th edition, pp. 1352–1353.

[31] Feldman, M., Scharschmidt, B.F. and Sleisenger, M. (1998). *Sleisenger and Fordtran's Gastrointestinal and Liver Disease: Pathophysiology, Diagnosis and Management* (Saunders, Philadelphia), vol. 2, 6th edition, p. 1186.

[32] Gasquet, S., Maurin, M., Brouqui, P., Lepidi, H. and Raoult, D. (1998) Bacillary angiomatosis in immunocompromised patients. *AIDS* **12**, 1793–1803.

[33] Horsburgh, C.R., Metchock, B., Gordon, S.M., Havlik, J.A., McGowan, J.E. and Thompson, S.E. (1994) Predictors of survival in patients with AIDS and disseminated *Mycobacterium avium* complex disease. *J. Infect. Dis.* **170**, 573–577.

[34] Sulkowski, M.S., Thomas, D.L., Mehta, S.H., Chaisson, R.E. and Moore, R.D. (2002) Hepatotoxicity associated with nevirapine or efavirenz-containing antiretroviral therapy: role of hepatitis C and B infections. *Hepatology* **35**, 182–189.

[35] Clark, S.J., Creigton, S., Portman, B., Taylor, C., Wendon, J.A. and Cramp, M.E. (2002) Acute liver failure associated with antiretroviral treatment for HIV: a report of six cases. *J. Hepatol.* **36**(2), 295–301.

[36] Baru, N., Leaf, H.L., Wieczorek, R.L. and Margolis, D.M. (1997) Severe hepatitis in three AIDS patients treated with indinavir. *Lancet* **349**, 924–925.

[37] Sulkowski, M.S., Thomas, D.L., Chaisson, R.E. and Moore, R.D. (2000) Hepatotoxicity associated with antiretroviral therapy in adults infected with human immunodeficiency virus and the role of hepatitis C or B infection. *JAMA* **283**, 74–80.

[38] Servoss, J.C., Sherman, K.E., Robbins, G., Liou, S., Reisler, R., Polsky, B., Murphy, R., Theodore, D., Miskovsky, E., Peters, M. and Chung, R.T (2001) Hepatotoxicity in the US Adult AIDS Clinical Trial Group, *DDW*. Abstract 102394.

[39] Nunez, M., Rios, P., Martin-Carbonbero, L., Perez-Olmeda, M., Gonzalez-Lahoz, J. and Soriano, V. (2002) Brief report: role of hepatitis C virus genotype in the development of severe transaminase elevation after the introduction of antiretroviral therapy. *J. Acquir. Immune Defic. Syndr.* **30**, 65–68.

[40] Benhamou, Y., Bochet, M., Di Martino, V., Charlotte, F., Azria, F., Coutellier, A., Vidaud, M., Bricaire, F., Opolon, P., Katlama,, Poynard, T. and for the MULTIVIRC Group, (1999) Liver fibrosis progression in human immunodeficiency virus and hepatitis C virus coinfected patients. *Hepatology* **30**, 1054–1058.

[41] Shevitz, A., Wanke, C.A., Falutz, J. and Kotler, D.P. (2001) Clinical perspectives on HIV-associated lipodystrophy syndrome: an update. *AIDS* **15**, 1917–1930.

[42] Carr, A., Miller, J., Law, M. and Cooper, D.A. (2000) A syndrome of lipoatrophy, lactic acidaemia and liver dysfunction associated with HIV nucleoside analogue therapy: contribution to protease inhibitor-related lipodystrophy syndrome. *AIDS* **14**, F25–F32.

[43] Prachalias, A.A., Pozniak, A., Taylor, C., Srinivasan, P., Muiesan, P., Wendon, J., Cramp, M., Williams, R., O'Grady, J., Rela, M. and Heaton, N.D. (2001) Liver transplantation in adults coinfected with HIV. *Transplantation* **72**(10), 1684–1688.

[44] Nowak, P., Schvarcz, R., Ericzon, B.G., Flamholc, L. and Sonnerborg, A. (2003) Follow-up of antiretroviral treatment in liver transplant recipients with primary and chronic HIV type 1 infection. *AIDS Res. Hum. Retroviruses* **19**(1), 13–19.

[45] Ragni, M., Belle, S., Im, K., Neff, G., Roland, M., Stock, P., Heaton, N., Humar, A. and Fung, J (2003) Survival in HIV-infected liver transplant recipients, *10th Conference on Retroviruses and Opportunistic Infections*. Oral Abstract 155.

Hepatology: A Practical Approach
B. Al Knawy, M.L. Shiffman, R.H. Wiesner (editors)

Chapter 8
Non-Viral Infections of the Liver

Mohammad Sultan Khuroo

Consultant Transplant Hepatology (MBC 72), Department of Liver Transplantation, Hepato-biliary and Pancreatic Surgery, King Faisal Specialist Hospital and Research Centre, Post Box 3354, Riyadh 11211, Saudi Arabia

1. Non-Viral Infections Involving the Liver as a Primary Target Organ 156
1.1 Pyogenic liver abscess 156
1.1.1 Etiology 156
1.1.2 Clinical features 158
1.1.3 Diagnosis 158
1.1.4 Treatment 159
1.1.5 Prognosis 159
1.2 Amebic liver abscess 159
1.2.1 Life cycle 160
1.2.2 Clinical features 160
1.2.3 Diagnosis 160
1.2.4 Treatment 161
1.2.5 Prognosis 161
1.3 Hepatic hydatid disease 161
1.3.1 Epidemiology 161
1.3.2 Life cycle 162
1.3.3 Pathology 162
1.3.4 Clinical features 162
1.3.5 Diagnosis 163
1.3.6 Treatment 164
1.4 Hepatobiliary and pancreatic ascariasis 165
1.4.1 Epidemiology 165
1.4.2 Life cycle 166
1.4.3 Clinical features 166
1.4.4 Diagnosis 168
1.4.5 Treatment 168
1.4.6 Control 168
1.5 Hepatic schistosomiasis 168
1.5.1 Epidemiology 168
1.5.2 Life cycle 169
1.5.3 Pathology 170
1.5.4 Clinical features 170
1.5.5. Diagnosis 170
1.5.6 Treatment 171
1.6 Liver flukes: fascioliasis 171
1.6.1 Life cycle 171
1.6.2 Clinical features 171
1.6.3 Diagnosis 171
1.6.4 Treatment 171

1.7 Liver flukes: clonorchiasis and opisthorchiasis 171
1.7.1 Life cycle 172
1.7.2 Clinical features 172
1.7.3 Diagnosis 172
1.7.4 Treatment 172
2. Non-viral Infections, which Involve the Liver as a Part of Multiorgan Infection 172
2.1 Hepatobiliary tuberculosis 172
References 174

The liver serves as the initial site of filtration of absorbed luminal contents and it is particularly susceptible to contact with microbes of all varieties. Both the portal venous circulation and biliary tract provide convenient routes of invasion of such infections from the gastrointestinal tract. Furthermore, the rich vascular supply of the liver renders it susceptible to secondary infection as a consequence of several systemic infections.

1. NON-VIRAL INFECTIONS INVOLVING THE LIVER AS A PRIMARY TARGET ORGAN

The liver is commonly affected by a group of unrelated hepatotrophic viruses causing the clinical syndrome of viral hepatitis. Other than hepatitis viruses, the liver can be affected by a large group of infectious agents involving the liver as a primary target organ (Table 1). Many of such infections are endemic in tropical countries. However, more and more of these infections are seen in Western countries because of the increasing number of immigrants from the developing countries and occurrence of these infections in patients of AIDS and organ transplant patients.

1.1 Pyogenic liver abscess

Pyogenic liver abscess is responsible for 8–20 cases per 100,000 hospital admissions. Pyogenic abscesses most often occur in patients over 40 years of age, with a peak incidence in the sixth decade. No significant sex, ethnic, or geographic differences exist in disease frequency. About one half of patients have solitary abscess. Abscesses involve right lobe in 75%, left lobe in 20%, and caudate lobe in 5% of cases [1].

1.1.1 Etiology

Suppurative cholangitis as a result of bile duct stones, benign and malignant biliary strictures, and endoscopic, radiologic, and operative biliary interventions are the major identifiable causes of pyogenic liver abscess. In endemic areas, *Ascaris lumbricoides* and *Clonorchis sinesis* can invade biliary tree, cause cholangitis and commonly predispose to liver abscesses [2]. Abscesses secondary to biliary disease are usually multiple. Pylephlebitis from diverticulitis, pancreatitis, omphalitis, inflammatory bowel disease, or postoperative infection can result in liver abscess. In the preantibiotic era, pyogenic liver abscess commonly occurred in the setting of appendicitis with associated pylephlebitis [3]. Patients with overwhelming sepsis frequently have multiple microabscesses of liver. Liver abscess can be caused by *Salmonella typhi*, *Mycobacterium tuberculosis* and *Brucella* spp. *Yersinia enterocolitica* infection has a special predilection for patients with hemochromatosis [4]. Secondary infection of an amebic liver abscess, hydatid cyst, liver hematoma, or liver metastases can also occur. Liver abscess after embolization of hepatic tumors has also been described. Lastly, cryptogenic liver abscess constitutes 20–60% of cases in various studies [1].

Most pyogenic liver abscesses are polymicrobial. The frequently isolated organisms include *Escherichia coli*, *Klebsiella pneumoniae*, *Streptococci viridans*, and *Enterococcus faecalis*. Infections with anaerobic organisms are increasingly recognized. The common anaerobes isolated include *Bacteroides* spp., *Fusobacterium* spp., anaerobic streptococci, *Actinomyces*

Table 1. Non-viral infections, which involve the liver as a primary target organ.

Disease	Agents	Endemic areas	Manifestations	Diagnosis	Treatment
Pyogenic liver abscess	*E. coli*, *K. pneumoniae*, Enterococci, anaerobes	Worldwide	Insidious onset, fever, RUQ pain and tenderness	US or CECT and aspiration	IV antibiotic plus image-guided drainage
Amebic liver abscess	*Entamoeba histolytica*	Tropical and subtropical areas	Acute onset, fever, RUQ pain and tenderness	US or CECT plus serology	Metronidazole plus diloxanide furoate
Hepatic hydatid disease	*Echinococcus granulosis*	Sheep and cattle raising areas	Incidental, mass lesion, infection, rupture	US or CECT plus serology	Surgery or PAIR and albendazole
Hepatobiliary and pancreatic ascariasis (HPA)	*Ascaris lumbricoides*	Developing countries	Biliary colic, cholangitis, cholecystitis, pancreatitis, liver abscess	US and ERCP	Anthelminthic therapy and worm extraction
Hepatic schistosomiasis	*S. mansoni*, *S. japonicum*, *S. intercalatum*, *S. makongi*	Asia, Africa, South America, Caribbean	Portal hypertension	Serology, hepatic imaging, ova in stool/rectal or liver biopsy	Praziquantel therapy and treat portal hypertension
Fascioliasis	*Fasciola hepatica*	Cattle and sheep raising areas	Cholangitis, cholestasis	Eggs in feces/bile ERCP	Bithionol, extraction at ERCP
Clonorchiasis/ opisthorchiasis	*C. sinesis*, *O. viverrini*, *O. felineus*	Southeast Asia	Cholangitis, cholestasis, cholangiocarcinoma	Ova in stool, ERCP	Praziquantel therapy and therapeutic ERCP

spp., and rarely *Clostridia* spp. Some authors consider the microaerophilic streptococci to be among the most common causes of liver abscess. *Staphylococcus aureus* infections are most common in children with monomicrobial abscesses [1].

1.1.2 Clinical features

In the past, patients typically presented with acute onset abdominal pain (89%), high fever with rigors and chills (67%), and right upper quadrant tenderness (70%). Since the introduction of antibiotics, the presentation of pyogenic liver abscess has become less acute, often insidious and characterized by malaise, low-grade fever, and dull abdominal pain. Symptoms may be present for 1 month or more before a diagnosis is made. Jaundice is a late finding, unless the abscess occurs as a result of biliary obstruction. Accordingly, a high index of suspicion is required to make a timely diagnosis of pyogenic liver abscess [3].

1.1.3 Diagnosis

Laboratory findings include anemia, leukocytosis, an elevated erythrocyte sedimentation rate, and abnormal liver function tests, especially an elevated serum alkaline phosphatase. Blood cultures may be positive in 50–90% of cases depending on culture technique and specimen handling.

Diagnostic imaging studies are essential in making the diagnosis of pyogenic liver abscess. Sonography has high sensitivity (94%) and reveals hypoechoic lesions with enhanced through-sound transmission (fluid), high internal echoes (debris), and high intensity linear echoes with reverberation artifacts (gas). It is the imaging method of choice in patients

(a)

(b)

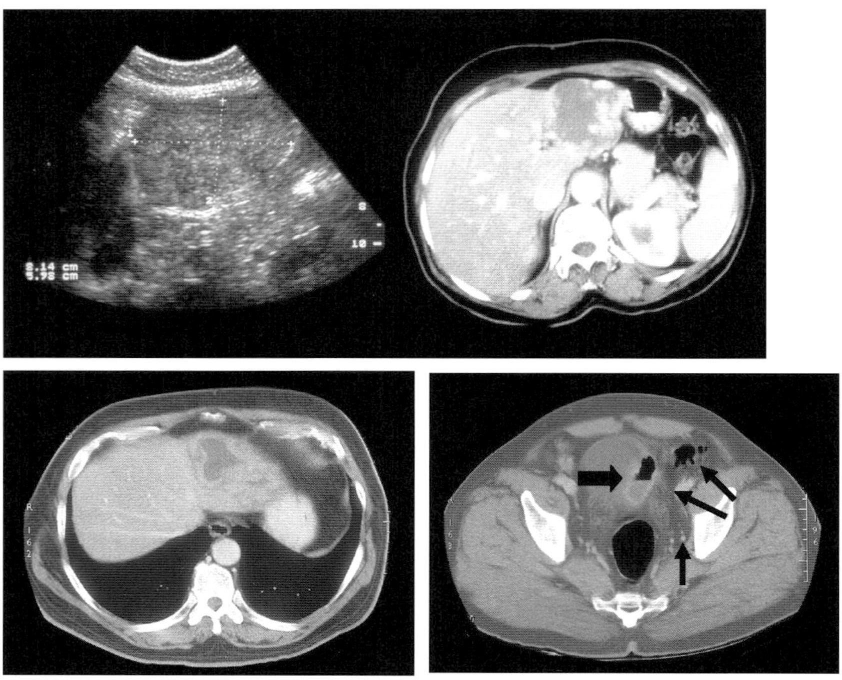

Figure 1. (a) Liver abscess caused by brucellosis. A 30-year-old woman who presented with fever, arthralgia, hepatomegly, and elevated serum alkaline phosphatase. Left panel: A transverse sonogram of the left lobe of liver shows an 8 × 6 cm mass with heterogenous echogenicity. Right panel: contrast-enhanced CT scan image of liver shows hypodense mass in the left lobe with thick ring enhancement of the margins. (b) Liver abscess secondary to sigmoid diverticulitis. A 70-year-old male who presented with fever, pain in left lower quadrant and mass in the left iliac fossa. Left lobe liver was enlarged and tender. Contrast enhanced CT scan. Left panel: CT scan image of the liver shows a hypodense lesion in the left lobe liver with thick enhancing margins. Right panel: CT scan image of the pelvis shows hypodense lesion around the sigmoid colon and an air filled cavity involving the left bladder wall.

with suspected biliary disease, and in children, pregnant women, and patients with contraindication to intravenous contrast. Contrast enhanced computed tomography (CECT) has high sensitivity (100%), and visualizes the abscesses better because contrast enhancement highlights the unaffected liver. On CECT, pyogenic liver abscesses are highly complex hypoechoic lesions with internal septation and irregular margins with a "rim" of contrast enhancement in 20% of cases and gas inside the lesion in 19–28% of cases. CECT is the procedure of choice when the precise location of an abscess and its relationship with adjacent structures is needed and in postoperative patients with open wounds and surgical drains (Figure 1). MR imaging of the liver is a sensitive technique for detecting and characterizing hepatic lesions. An MR scan of the liver abscess typically shows a homogenous hypointense signal with well-defined margins on a T1-weighted image. On a T2-weighted image, the abscess has a hyperintense signal that can appear heterogeneous depending on the fluidity and debris of the necrotic exudates. Technetium sulfur colloid scanning of the liver has a sensitivity of 70–80% in pyogenic liver abscess. However, this modality of imaging is rarely performed now for this purpose.

Diagnostic aspiration of the abscess cavity can be performed at sonography or CT and aspirated material should be cultured for aerobic, anaerobic, and microaerophilic organisms [1].

1.1.4 Treatment

Treatment of pyogenic liver abscess requires antibiotic therapy and image-guided drainage of the abscess and such regimen is successful in 85–90% of patients. Percutaneous aspiration with catheter drainage has been employed in the past. Recent data have shown that aspiration of cavity contents without catheter placement gives equal results. Antibiotic therapy alone is an option for small liver abscesses not amenable to drainage or in those in whom drainage presents with unacceptable risk. Surgical drainage is reserved in the following situations: (i) percutaneous drainage is unsuccessful, (ii) there is coexisting intraabdominal disease requiring surgery, and (iii) abscess is complicated by rupture or extension into adjacent structures. Antibiotics should be started as soon as the diagnosis of pyogenic liver abscess is suspected. Earlier, combination antibiotic therapy consisting of ampicillin and aminoglycoside has been the most frequently employed regimen. However, the prevalence of resistant strains of enterobacteriaceae has resulted in the use of β-lactam/β-lactamase inhibitor antibiotic combination (i.e., ampicillin/sulbactam, ticarcillin/clavulinic acid, piperacillin/tozabactam) in place of ampicillin and an aminoglycoside for initial empiric therapy. Addition of metronidazole or clindamycin is recommended to cover anaerobic organisms. Antibiotic therapy should be optimized when culture and antibiotic sensitivity are available. In most situations, patients require a prolonged course of antibiotics, consisting of an initial 2 weeks course of intravenous antibiotics, followed by six additional weeks of suitable oral antibiotic [1].

1.1.5 Prognosis

The mortality without treatment approaches 100%. The mortality rate for patients treated with antibiotics and percutaneous drainage is 16%. Bad prognostic indicators are: (i) delay in making a diagnosis, (ii) multiple organisms cultured from blood, (iii) jaundice, (iv) hypoalbuminemia, (v) a pleural effusion, and (vi) associated co-morbid illnesses [1,3].

1.2 Amebic liver abscess

Amebic liver abscess is the most common extraintestinal manifestation of *Entamoeba histolytica* infection. Amebiasis occurs worldwide, but is most common in tropical and subtropical regions. *E. histolytica* infected 40–50 million people worldwide, resulting in 40,000–100,000 deaths per year. Amebic liver abscess occurs in approximately 8.5% of all patients with amebic infection. Amebiasis occurs with equal frequency in men and women; however, amebic liver abscess occurs 3–10 times more often in men. Infections occurring in developed countries are confined to certain high risk groups, including travelers, immigrants, and homosexual males [5].

1.2.1 Life cycle

During its life cycle, *E. histolytica* exists as trophozoite and cyst forms. Amebic infection is acquired by ingestion of cyst through contaminated food or water. In the small intestine the cyst wall undergoes digestion allowing the amebae to develop into invasive trophozoites. The trophozoites travel to colon and cause invasive colonic disease. In some cases the invasive trophozoites are carried via the portal circulation to the liver resulting in the formation of an abscess. The abscess fluid is typically "anchovy sauce" in appearance resulting from the lysis of liver cells, red blood cells, and connective tissue. Leukocytes are usually absent, unless the abscess is secondarily infected. Amebae are found in the cyst wall, invading normal liver tissue. Amebic abscesses are characteristically located in the right lobe under the dome of the diaphragm. Majority (>80%) of patients have a solitary lesion.

1.2.2 Clinical features

Amebic liver abscess most often occurs in the age group 20–45 years. Most patients present with an acute illness and duration of symptoms is usually less than 2 weeks. Clinical symptoms and signs include low-grade fever and chills; right upper quadrant pain and tenderness, and hepatomegaly. Pleuritic chest pain and radiation of the pain to the right shoulder are common in abscesses involving diaphragmatic surface of the liver. Left lobe abscess presents with toxemia; epigastric pain, tenderness, and guarding; and a large epigastric mass. During the course of illness one-third of patients develop jaundice. Jaundice develops in patients with a large abscess, or multiple abscesses, or an abscess situated at the porta hepatis. Multiple liver abscesses usually present with high fever, toxemia, jaundice, and encephalopathy [5,6].

Complications of amebic liver abscess include secondary bacterial infection of the abscess, rupture of the abscess into adjacent viscera, and compression of the bile ducts, portal vein, or hepatic outflow tract by expanding abscess. Secondary bacterial infection occurs in 20% of patients and present with toxemia, high fever and features of hepatic encephalopathy. *E. coli* and *Klebsiella pneumonae* are usual organisms infecting amebic abscess. Abscess can rupture into pleura causing empyema; into lung causing hepatobronchial fistula; into pericardium causing pericarditis or pericardial effusion; and peritoneum causing amebic peritonitis. Left lobe abscess has a greater propensity to rupture into peritoneum or pericardium [7].

1.2.3 Diagnosis

High index of suspicion is required in patients living in or migrated from endemic areas or in those who have traveled to such areas in the recent past. Most patients exhibit mild anemia, leukocytosis, and elevated serum alkaline phosphatase. Serum bilirubin is elevated in patients with large or multiple abscesses. Diagnosis is made on hepatic imaging and amebic serology. Chest radiographs are abnormal in 50% of patients and reveal elevation of the right hemidiaphragm, pleural effusion, or evidence of atelectasis with diminished excursion of the right hemidiaphragm. Ultrasound and CECT are useful in delineating and localizing the abscess as well as to monitor the response to treatment. The appearances of amebic liver abscess are similar to that of pyogenic liver abscess. Aspiration of amebic liver abscess is now rarely necessary for establishing the diagnosis due to high sensitivity of serologic tests. Many serologic tests can be used in the diagnosis of invasive amebiasis. Indirect hemagglutinin test has been widely used in the past and is approximately 90% sensitive for detecting amebiasis. In contrast, enzyme immunoassay has a sensitivity of 99% and specificity greater than 90% in patients with amebic liver abscess. The serologic test becomes positive early in the disease course and stays positive up to 20 years after infection. Thus a positive test in an endemic area should be read with caution as it can represent either a previous exposure or a current infection.

Amebic liver abscess needs to be differentiated from pyogenic liver abscess in endemic areas and it is important in view of different treatment regimen employed in the two entities and different response to therapy (Table 2).

1.2.4 Treatment

Metronidazole, 800 mg three times per day orally for 10 days is curative in over 90% of patients with amebic liver abscess. Clinical improvement is usually seen within 3–5 days. After clinical cure, abscess cavity disappears in 6–9 months. Alternative

Table 2. Differentiating features of pyogenic and amebic liver abscess.

Feature	Pyogenic liver abscess	Amebic liver abscess
Distribution of disease	Worldwide	Tropical and subtropical regions
Age of occurrence	Above 40 years	20–45 years
Sex distribution	Equal	3–10 times more in males than females
Number	Often multiple (50%)	Often single (80%)
Location	Either lobe	Often right lobe under dome of diaphragm
Duration of illness	Usually > 1 month	Often < 2 weeks
Symptoms	Low grade fever, RUQ pain and tenderness	Same
Jaundice	Mild unless associated with biliary disease	Moderate in large and multiple abscesses
Blood culture	Positive (50–90%)	Negative
Hepatic imaging	Mass lesion with fluid component	Same
Amebic serology	Negative	Positive
Treatment	IV antibiotics plus drainage	Metronidazole plus diloxanide furoate
Mortality	16%	2–18%
High risk groups	Jaundice, low albumin, co-morbid disease	Multiple abscesses, left lobe abscess, high bilirubin, encephalopathy, low albumin

agents include secnidazole 500 mg orally three times per day, tinidazole 600 mg orally twice per day for 7 days, or chloroquine 600 mg orally as a single dose per day for 2 days followed by 300 mg orally given as a single dose per day for 14–21 days. A luminal amebicide, diloxinide furoate 500 mg three times per day for 10 days is often used to eradicate intestinal carriage of the organism. Unlike pyogenic liver abscess, needle aspiration or abscess drainage offers no additional therapeutic benefit. Aspiration is indicated in patients with persistent symptoms after 5 days of medical therapy and in those with: (i) very large abscess, (ii) abscess involving the left lobe, (iii) abscess which shows signs of imminent rupture, (iv) abscess with secondary bacterial infection. Open surgical drainage is indicated in abscess, which has ruptured into peritoneum or adjacent viscera.

1.2.5 Prognosis

Amebic liver abscess has an overall mortality of 2–18%. Predictors of poor prognosis include: hyperbilirubinemia, encephalopathy, hypoalbuminemia, left lobe abscess and multiple abscesses [7].

1.3 Hepatic hydatid disease

Hydatid disease, also known as echinococcosis or hydatidosis, is a zoonotic infection caused by larval forms (metacestodes) of the tapeworms of the genus *Echinococcus* and is characterized by development of expanding cysts in the liver and other body organs. Within the genus *Echinococcus*, four species are recognized. *E. granulosus* causes cystic hydatid disease, *E. alveolaris* causes alveolar hydatid disease, *E. vogeli* and *E. oligarthrus* cause polycystic hydatid disease. The most clinically relevant form is cystic echinococcosis caused by *Echinococcus granulosus* [8].

1.3.1 Epidemiology

E. granulosus is a cosmopolitan parasite. Endemic regions include southern South America (Uruguay and Argentina), the Mediterranean region, Middle East, many parts of Africa (especially Kenya), southern and central Russia, Central Asia and many regions in China (especially Xinjiang province). Majority of patients reported in Austria, Germany, and Switzerland are immigrants from the Mediterranean region. The disease has been eradicated in Iceland and disease load significantly diminished in New Zealand, Tasmania, and Cyprus by control measures. In the United States, most infections are seen in immigrants from endemic areas, but autochthonous transmission is currently recognized in Alaska, California, Utah, Arizona, and New Mexico. The annual incidence of human infection in endemic areas varies widely (<1 to 220 per 100,000 per annum) from region to region [8].

1.3.2 Life cycle

E. granulosis requires two hosts for completion of the life cycle. Adult tapeworms, which measure 3–4 mm in length, inhabit the small intestines of the dog, the definitive host. Sheep and cattle are the intermediate hosts. Dogs infected with the tapeworm pass eggs in their feces. When ingested by a suitable intermediate host, the oncospheres hatch in the small intestines, become activated, penetrate the epithelial layer and migrate via blood or lymphatic vessels to the viscera. In the viscera the oncosphere undergoes a series of reorganization events involving degeneration, cell proliferation, differentiation, and vesiculation resulting in the formation of primary vesicle (metacestode). Metacestode develops into hydatid cyst by a process unique for each species of *Echinococcus*. Scoleces are formed within the cysts which when ingested by the definitive host (eating offal of intermediate host) develop into adult tapeworms. Metacestodes develop in the liver and other viscera of intermediate hosts and under natural conditions host assemblages are linked together in predator–prey relationship. Human beings become incidental intermediate hosts and do not complete the life cycle of the parasite.

1.3.3 Pathology

E. granulosus cysts following primary infection may inhabit any anatomic site. The two most common organs involved are liver (65%) and lungs (25%). Cysts of the sylvan strain predominantly localize in the lungs. Other less common sites affected by cysts include the muscles (5%), spleen (1%), bones (3%), kidneys (2%), heart (1%), pancreas (1%), and central nervous system (1%). Majority of patients have single organ involvement (87%) and harbor a solitary cyst (72%). Secondary infection follows cyst rupture and scoleces can grow in peritoneum, pleura, bronchial tree, and bile ducts or be carried via blood stream to distant organs. Cyst size ranges from 1 to 15 cm and cyst growth varies from 1 to 30 mm/yr.

Hydatid cyst wall consists of inner germinal layer and outer laminated membrane. Surrounding is the pericyst, which has outer zone of compressed liver cells, middle zone of heavy lymphoplasmocytic infiltrate, and inner tough zone formed of collagen (Figure 2). The cyst fluid is crystal clear with a specific gravity of 1012 and contains salts, enzymes, proteins, and toxic substances, and is antigenic. The germinal layer forms small cellular masses projecting into the cyst cavity, which vesiculate to form brood capsules. In each brood capsule multiple protoscolices (head of the future worm) develop on the inner surface of their walls by asexual budding. Brood capsules and protoscolices may be released into the cyst fluid to form hydatid sand. Protoscolices have a potential to develop into adult tapeworm within the gut of the definitive host, differentiate into secondary cysts when released following cyst rupture (ectogenic vesiculation) and form daughter cysts within the mother cyst by endogenic vesiculation. Each daughter cyst is a true replica of the mother cyst and has a germinal layer and laminated membrane and contains brood capsules and protoscolices. Daughter cysts may be packed together in the mother cyst (multivesicular cyst) or float freely in the mother cyst cavity. In older cysts the contents degenerate forming a gelatinous amber-colored structure called the matrix. Matrix gives pseudo-tumor appearance on imaging tools and can be confused with pus by the surgeon. Calcification can occur in the pericyst, mother cyst, and daughter cyst. Calcification of endocyst indicates that the cyst is non-viable. However, calcification of pericyst is found in one-third of cysts and occurs in all stages of cyst development [8].

1.3.4 Clinical features

Infections are usually acquired during childhood, however, most cases of cystic hydatid disease present in adults in third to fifth decades of life, with equal sex distribution. The clinical features depend upon the organ involved, site of organ involvement, and stage of cyst development and viability of the cyst contents. Majority of the cysts produce no symptoms and are detected as incidental findings on routine imaging or at autopsy. Symptoms of the disease are related to expanding mass, pressure on adjacent structures, infection and rupture of cyst contents into surrounding body cavities. Uncomplicated liver cysts usually present with dull ache in the right upper quadrant or

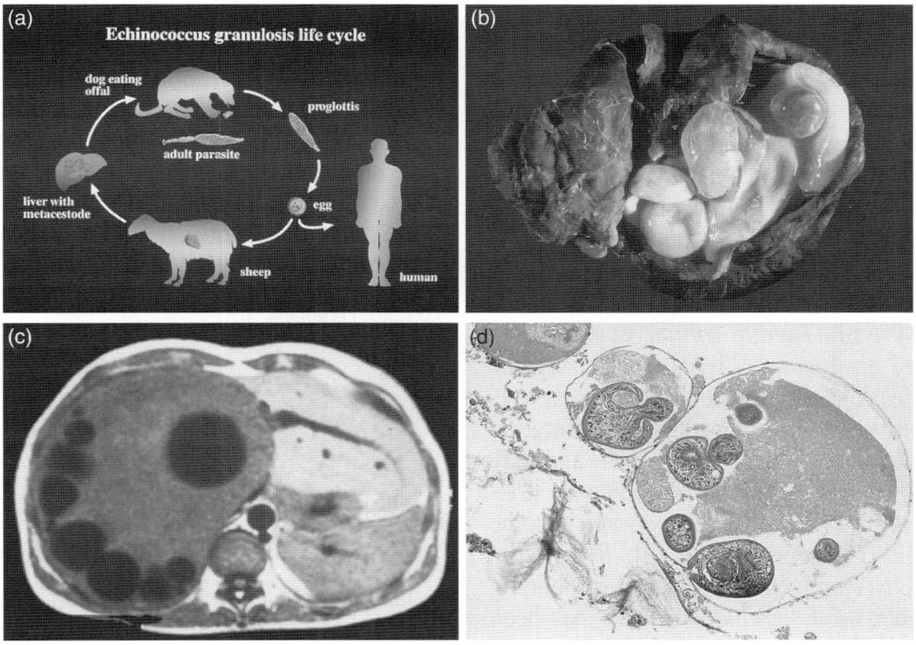

Figure 2. (a) Life cycle of *Echinococcus granulosus*. The parasite completes the life cycle between dog, the definitive host and sheep, the intermediate host. Human beings become incidental intermediate hosts and do not complete the life cycle of the parasite. (*Source:* Khuroo, M.S. (2002) Hydatid disease: current status and recent advances. *Ann. Saudi Med.* **22**, 56–64) (b) Resected hydatid cyst liver with peripheral coating (pericyst), ivory white laminated membranes, and glistening rounded daughter cysts. (c) Hydatid cyst liver. An axial T_1-weighted MR image shows a large rounded lesion occupying the whole right lobe of the liver. The lesion reveals multiple rounded low signal lesions (daughter cysts). The remainder of the contents reveal high signal (matrix). (d) Histology of the hydatid cyst. Multiple protoscolices (both eviginated and invaginated) are seen attached to the endocyst. (*For colored version, see Plate XVII on page 572 at the end of the book.*)

a feeling of abdominal swelling or distension. Clinical examination is unremarkable except for enlarged liver with a rounded mass felt on its surface. A hydatid thrill may be elicited on a large mass pointing to its fluid content. Rarely the mass is calcified giving it a hard consistency and needs to be differentiated from a primary or secondary liver tumor. A large cyst in the hilar region can compress the common hepatic duct causing cholestasis. Hepatic vein or inferior vena cava compression can cause Budd–Chiari syndrome. Cyst rupture into the biliary tree causes obstruction of the ducts by daughter cysts and laminated membranes and presents as biliary colic, cholangitis, and progressive cholestasis. Cyst contents may block the ampullary orifice causing acute pancreatitis. Cyst rupture into the peritoneum causes immediate life threatening anaphylaxis and if the person survives, the scoleces implant on the peritoneal surface resulting in extensive peritoneal hydatidosis. Cyst can rupture into the pleural cavity or lung and can establish cysto-bronchial fistula. Rarely cyst can grow on to the skin along a sinus tract following surgery or percutaneous drainage of the cyst. Infection of the cyst follows tear in the laminated membrane and soilage of the cyst with bile or blood. Infected hydatid cyst has clinical features of a liver abscess [8,9].

1.3.5 Diagnosis

Routine hematological and biochemical tests do not help in diagnosis of cystic hydatid disease. Serology and imaging tools establish diagnosis.

Serology detects specific serum antibodies or circulating antigen by a variety of immunodiagnostic methods. Of these, the enzyme immunosorbent assay (ELISA) employing hydatid fluid antigen for detection of echinococcal antibodies (IgG) in the serum is most widely used. This test has a sensitivity of 80–100% and specificity of 88–96% in hepatic cysts. However, the sensitivity of this test is around 50–56% in pulmonary cysts and cysts involving other organs. False positive test can occur in normal persons from endemic areas and in those with other parasitic infections. Positive test results need confirmation by the arc-5 immunoelectrophoretic (IEP) test, which detects antibodies against immunodominant and specific antigen (antigen 5) of the cestode. This test does not cross-react with non-cestode parasites. Cross-reaction with *Taenia solium* cysticercosis does occur and need to be differentiated in regions where both infections are prevalent. Serological tests have limitations in monitoring patients after surgery, percutaneous drainage, or drug therapy. The antibody titers rise following surgery and percutaneous drainage. The titers start falling at 3 months and become negative in 12–24 month period [9]. PCR using recombinant DNA antigens is valuable in defining particular species of *E. granulosus*. This has been effectively applied for control of the disease and development of an animal vaccine.

Abdominal cysts particularly in the liver and cysts in soft tissues are well visualized by ultrasound. Cysts may appear univesicular, rounded with well-defined margins containing pure fluid or multivesicular (daughter cysts) with pure fluid collection in each vesicle. Cysts may have hyperechoic solid pattern (pseudotumor appearance) or may have reflective wall suggestive of calcification. Rupture of liver cysts into the bile ducts can be suspected on ultrasound. Ultrasound appearances in such cases include dilated bile ducts, non-shadowing echogenic structures within the ducts, and loss of continuity of the cyst wall adjacent to the bile duct representing site of communication. However, ERCP is the recommended tool and reveals filling defects of varying shape and size in the dilated bile ducts and leakage of contrast medium into the cyst cavity.

Computed tomography is the method of choice to detect lung, brain, and bone cysts. It has advantage over ultrasound for cysts at other sites for better documentation of site, size, and structure of cyst and for monitoring of lesions during chemotherapy and following surgery. Magnetic resonance imaging may show a characteristic intense rim. Angiography and scintigraphy have no major advantage over above imaging tools and are rarely employed in this setting.

Diagnostic puncture of cysts is only justified when imaging and serological tests do not permit discrimination between hydatid cyst and neoplasm. It carries risk of anaphylaxis and spillage of cyst contents with secondary echinococcosis [9].

1.3.6 Treatment

Treatment options for cystic hydatid disease are surgery, drug therapy, and percutaneous drainage [10,11].

Surgery has the potential to remove cysts and lead to complete cure. Surgical procedure of choice is cystectomy with removal of the germinal and laminated layers and preservation of pericyst. Cavity is either drained or closed, or tightly packed with omentum (omentoplasty). Occasionally, cyst is removed by total pericystectomy, partial hepatectomy, or segmentectomy. Surgery is treatment of choice in large hepatic cysts with multiple daughter cysts, subcapsular or pedenculated liver cysts, infected liver cysts, cysts communicating with bile ducts, and cysts in the lungs, brain, kidney, bones, and other organs. Surgery is contraindicated in patients at extremes of age, pregnant women, patients with co-morbid diseases and in those with multiple cysts and cysts, which are difficult to access. Operative mortality varies from 0.5 to 4.0% in centers with adequate medical and surgical facilities. Cyst fluid spillage can occur during surgery resulting in anaphylaxis and/or secondary echinococcosis (2–25% of cases).

Two benzimidazoles (mebendazole and albendazole) and praziquantel, an isoquinolone derivative have scolicidal activity and have been used in over 1000 well-documented patients with cystic hydatid disease. Mebedazole is poorly absorbed and scolicidal drug levels are achieved with a daily dose of 40–50 mg/kg administered orally in divided doses. Albendazole is better absorbed and the usual daily dose is 10–15 mg/kg. Drug dosing with a fat-rich meal improves intestinal absorption. Cyclic treatment (three 1-month courses with intervals of 14 days) has been widely used. Recent data show that uninterrupted drug therapy for 3–6 months has better efficacy with no increase in adverse effects. Praziquantel is administered at a dose of 40 mg/kg once a week concomitantly with benzimidazoles and has been shown to increase the scolicidal activity of the imidazoles. Chemotherapy achieves a cyst disappearance of 30%, partial response in another 30%, and no response in 40%. It is effective in small cysts (<4 cm diameter), cysts with thin walls and in younger patients. It is indicated in patients who are at high risks for surgery, in patients with multiple peritoneal cysts, to prevent secondary echinococcosis after spillage during surgery and as a concomitant therapy with percutaneous drainage. Imidazoles are hepatotoxic, can cause neutropenia, thrombocytopenia, alopecia and are potentially embryotoxic and teratogenic.

Recently percutaneous drainage of hepatic hydatid cysts, popularly known in Europe as the PAIR (Puncture, Aspiration, Installation of scolicidal agent and Respiration) technique has gained acceptance. The procedure is minimally invasive, cost effective, involves reduced hospital stay and has less morbidity and mortality than surgery. It is the treatment of choice in patients with hepatic hydatid cysts who either refuse surgery or have significant co-morbid diseases. The procedure is highly effective in intact univesicular and multivesicular cysts with few large daughter cysts, cysts with diameters of over 5 cm, and multiple cysts in different liver segments. Cysts relapsing after surgery or failed to regress following chemotherapy are amenable to percutaneous drainage. The procedure cannot be done in superficial or pedenculated cysts, small volume cysts, cysts with honeycomb appearance (multiple small daughter cysts), cysts with dominant solid component, and those with infection or communicating with bile ducts. Procedure is associated with possible complications of liver puncture (bleeding, bile peritonitis), anaphylaxis, allergic reactions, and biliary communications. Inadvertent installation of sclerosing agent into a cyst with biliary communication can cause sclerosing cholangitis. Long-term follow-up has shown that secondary echinococcosis does not occur following percutaneous drainage.

Endoscopic therapy has been used in a small number of patients with hepatic cysts, which have ruptured into bile ducts. At ERCP, endoscopic sphincterotomy is performed; laminated membranes and daughter cysts are extracted and a nasobiliary drain is placed in the bile duct. The cyst regresses and disappears over the next 4–6 weeks. Laparoscopic removal of hepatic cysts has been reported and liver transplant has been performed in extensive hepatic hydatidosis not amenable to surgical resection. None of these modalities have been evaluated in controlled trials.

1.4 Hepatobiliary and pancreatic ascariasis

Ascariasis is a helminthic infection of humans caused by the nematode *A. lumbricoides*. Hepatobiliary and pancreatic ascariasis (HPA) is one of the most common and well-described entities caused by ascaris. Ascarides in the duodenum enter the ampullary orifice and can block it; they can advance further to the bile duct and hepatic ducts. While in the common duct, the cystic duct can be blocked by worms entering its orifice. Less often, worms can reach the gallbladder or enter the pancreatic duct [2].

1.4.1 Epidemiology

Ascariasis has a global distribution. It has been estimated that more than 1.4 billion throughout the world are infected with *A. lumbricoides*. Ascariasis is highly endemic in China and Southeast Asia, with prevalence rates of 41–92%. In the Indian subcontinent, ascariasis is highly endemic in Kashmir (70%), Bangladesh (82%), and Central and Southwest India (20–49%). In Africa, the overall prevalence of the infection varies from 15 to 27%. The prevalence is high in Latin America and has not changed over the years. The prevalence in Japan dropped considerably after the end of World War II: 70–80% up to 1955, 13% in 1962, and 0.04% in 1992. In Europe, the prevalence is low in large cities but may be high in rural areas and can reach up to 52% in some rural areas. In the United States, ascariasis is the third most common helminth infection (exceeded only by hookworm and *Trichuris trichuria* infections). Of the 4 million people infected in the United States, a large percentage are immigrants from developing countries with infection rates of 20–60%.

The magnitude of the problem of HPA in an endemic area was often underestimated in the past as worms move actively in and out of the bile duct from the duodenum and usually are not present in the ducts at the time of imaging or surgery. In prospective studies and with the use of ultrasonography and endoscopic retrograde cholangiopancreatography (ERCP) early in the disease, HPA is as common as gallstones as the cause of biliary and pancreatic disease in endemic areas.

HPA is more common in women than men (female-to-male ratio of 3:1) with a mean age of occurrence being 35.0 years (range 4–70 years). Children do suffer from HPA but less often than adults. This is possibly due to the smaller size of the bile ductal system making it difficult for the worms to enter. Pregnant women are particularly prone to HPA, and worms reach the gallbladder more often than in non-pregnant women. The majority of patients with HPA have had previous surgery on the biliary tree, including cholecystectomy, choledocholithotomy, or sphincteroplasty, performed for gallstones. Endoscopic sphincterotomy predisposes patients to HPA in endemic areas in view of the widened ampullary orifice and easier passage of worms into the bile ducts.

1.4.2 Life cycle

The normal habitat for the adult worm is the jejunum in humans. Ascaris eggs are passed in the feces. The fertilized eggs require 10–15 days in the soil for embryonation before they are infective. *A. lumbricoides* is a soil-transmitted helminth and requires moist, shady soil for embryonation of the eggs. The eggs in the soil remain viable and capable of infection for a period up to 10 years. The infection occurs by ingestion of the embryonated eggs. After ingestion, the shell of the embryonated egg is dissolved by gastric juice, and the embryo emerges in the duodenum as the rhabdoid larva 200–300 μm long and 13–15 μm thick. The larvae penetrate the surface epithelium of the intestinal mucosa, enter the veins of the portal system and are carried to the liver. In the liver, larvae move freely in the sinusoids. Some may subsequently pass via hepatic veins to the heart and lungs. The larvae break through the capillary wall and enter the alveolar space and the bronchial tree. During this passage, larvae molt twice and grow considerably in length and width. They ascend the tracheobronchial tree and larynx to the hypopharynx, where they are swallowed. On reaching the small intestines, the larvae attain sexual maturity in 2–3 months. In the upper gastrointestinal tract, they molt again before becoming mature worms (Figure 3). The time from the larval infection to maturation is usually 4 months.

1.4.3 Clinical features

HPA can cause five distinct clinical presentations [2].

1. *Biliary colic*. Biliary colic presents as sudden right hypochondrial pain associated with nausea and vomiting usually lasting just a few days. The pain may be recurrent in nature or severely prolonged demanding large doses of narcotic analgesics. The usual features of cholangitis, such as fever and jaundice, are absent. In most patients, worms are invading the ampullary orifice of the duodenum (Figure 3). Removal of the worms from the ampullary orifice and their extraction by mouth leads to rapid relief of symptoms in those patients.
2. *Acalculous cholecystitis*. The patients present with pain in the right hypochondrium, referred across to the back and lower angle of the scapula and to the right shoulder associated with vomiting and low-grade fever (37.2–37.8°C). Most of the patients have tenderness and guarding in the right hypochondrium, and a mass is palpable in the right hypochondrium. As judged by ultrasonography, the gallbladder is distended (>4 cm transverse diameter), and there is increased thickness of the gallbladder wall (4 mm) and sludge in the gallbladder. Most of the patients respond to treatment without complications.
3. *Acute cholangitis*. The patients present with hypochondrial pain and high-grade fever (38.3–40°C); jaundice; a tender enlarged liver; pronounced leukocytosis, and raised serum bilirubin, serum alkaline phosphatase, and serum alanine aminotransferase. In patients with pyogenic cholangitis, pus is seen exuding out of the papilla at duodenoscopic examination or recovered on bile aspiration at ERCP. These patients are critically ill with hypotension and metabolic acidosis (endotoxic shock). Treatment includes

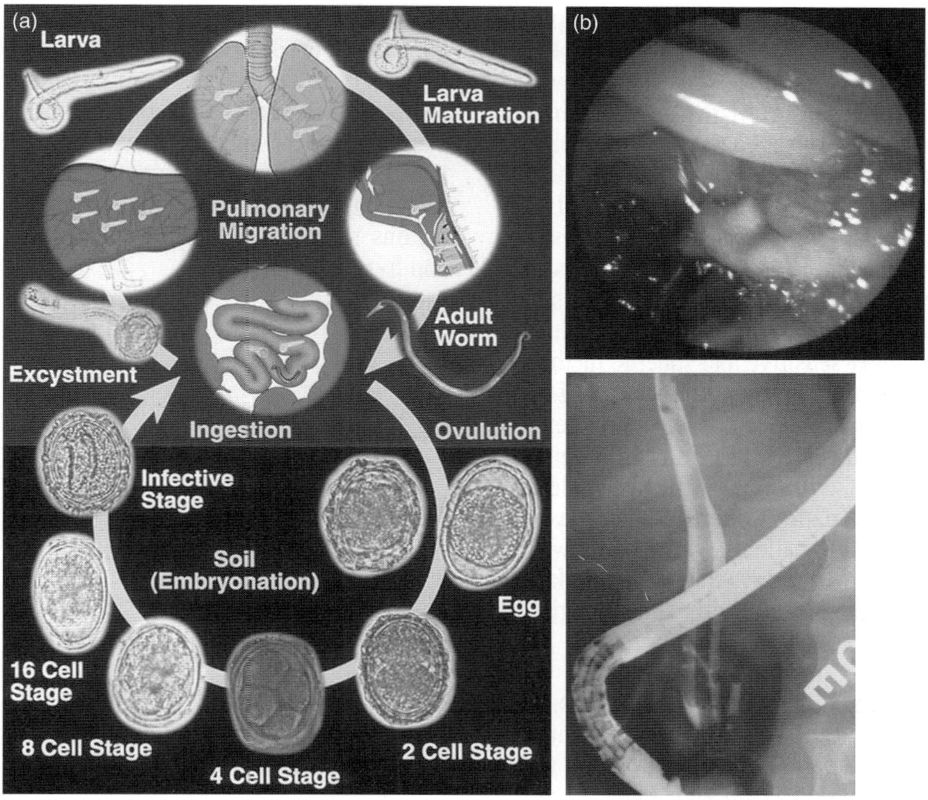

Figure 3. (a) Life cycle of *Ascaris lumbricoides*. (*Source*: Khuroo, M.S. (1996) Ascariasis. *Gastroenterol. Clin. N. Am.* **25**, 553–577.) (b) Endoscopic retrograde cholangiogram of a 30-year-old woman who presented with recurrent episodes of biliary colic of 7 days duration. Top panel. Duodenoscopic view of the papilla showing an Ascaride in the ampullary orifice with its tail in the duodenal lumen. Bottom panel. Cholangiogram. A long linear smooth filling defect in the common bile duct and across the papilla representing the portion of the Ascaride that had entered the bile duct. (*Source*: Khuroo *et al.* (1993) *Gastrointest. Endosc.* **39**, 680–685, Fig. 1, p. 682.) (*For colored version, see Plate XVIII on page 573 at the end of the book.*)

broad-spectrum antibiotics followed by specific antibiotic treatment when bile culture and sensitivity results are known. The patients with pyogenic cholangitis also need urgent surgical or endoscopic biliary decompression and drainage.

4. *Acute pancreatitis*. The patients present with epigastric pain referred to the back, vomiting, and raised serum amylase and alkaline phosphatase. Ninety percent of patients had mild pancreatitis and 10% had severe pancreatitis. Ultrasonography reveals an enlarged echo poor pancreas or pseudocyst. A small group of patients with massive ascaris invasion and hemorrhagic pancreatitis die. All other patients recover rapidly with palliative treatment or extraction by mouth of worms invading the ampullary orifice of the duodenum [12].
5. *Hepatic abscess*. The patients present with right upper quadrant pain, high fever, tender enlarged liver with intercostal tenderness, and edema of the right chest wall. Ultrasonography reveals an echo-poor lesion in the right lobe or left lobe (or both), and ultrasound-guided aspiration reveals pus, which yields ova of *A. lumbricoides*.

1.4.4 Diagnosis

Laboratory tests do not help in the diagnosis of HPA. Identification of ascaris eggs in the stool has little diagnostic value in endemic areas.

Diagnosis of HPA can be made by ultrasonography and ERCP [2]. The characteristic sonographic findings of worms in the ducts have been well described. The bile ducts are dilated and contain a thick, long, linear or curved, non-shadowing echogenic strip containing a central, longitudinal anechoic tube, probably representing the alimentary canal of the worm. These structures show characteristic writhing movement within the ducts. The worms in the gallbladder have much more characteristic appearances and can be identified with ease. Ultrasonography is a highly sensitive and specific method for detection of worms in the biliary tree. This investigation is non-invasive, can be used in patients with symptoms, and repeated frequently to monitor movement of worms in the ducts. Because ultrasonography cannot visualize duodenal ascariasis, more than half of the patients with HPA with worms in the duodenum and invading the ampullary orifice cannot be diagnosed with this imaging modality.

ERCP has an advantage as a diagnostic tool in that it permits identification of the worms in the duodenum and those across the papilla. On cholangiogram, the worms in the ducts appear as smooth, linear filling defects (Figure 3). ERCP, in addition, has therapeutic potential, allowing removal of worms from the ducts or the duodenum.

1.4.5 Treatment

The rational treatment for biliary ascariasis is to treat cholangitis by conservative means and affect the paralysis of worms in the intestines by oral administration of anthelmintic agents, from where they are expelled by effective peristaltic activity of the intestines [2]. Several drugs are available and effective for treatment of ascariasis. Pyrantel pamoate, mebendazole, and albendazole, however, are drugs of first choice against ascariasis. The administration of an anthelmintic agent into the biliary tree at cholangiography cannot be advocated as treatment for biliary ascariasis because it impedes the migration of live worms out of ducts into the duodenum.

Endoscopic intervention is performed when patients do not respond to energetic symptomatic treatment within the first few days of hospitalization or when worms have not moved out of the ducts into the duodenum at 3 weeks [13]. Worm extraction is successful in all patients from the ampullary orifice and in more than 90% of patients from the bile or pancreatic duct. After worm extraction, patients with biliary disease or acute pancreatitis have rapid relief of symptoms. Few (6%) patients developed complications related to endoscopy, including cholangitis and hypotension.

1.4.6 Control

Theoretically, there should be no difficulty in controlling ascariasis in the community. There are excellent drugs such as pyrantel pamoate and mebendazole for treating individual patients and for mass chemotherapy, and, if they are combined with health education and improved sanitation, infection rates can be greatly reduced. However, cultural practices, inadequate financial resources, and the enormous biotic potential of the worms prevent any serious attempt at control in endemic areas.

1.5 Hepatic schistosomiasis

Schistosomiasis is a disease caused by certain species of the genus *Schistosoma*. Hepatic schistosomiasis is caused by *S. mansoni*, *S. japonicum*, *S. intercalatum*, and *S. makongi*. *S. haematobium* causes urinary schistosomiasis. Hepatic schistosomiasis is characterized by granuloma formation in the liver with hepatic fibrosis leading to portal hypertension [14].

1.5.1 Epidemiology

Schistosomiasis is endemic in 75 countries in tropical and subtropical areas of Africa, Asia, South America, and the Caribbean. It has been estimated that over 200 million people worldwide harbor schistosomial infection. The endemicity of the disease depends upon the prevalence of the intermediate host snail species, patterns of water exposure, and other sociocultural factors. Mass movement of populations during conflicts or famine and water development projects (e.g., irrigation, dams, and fish farming) alters water usage practices and lead to an increased risk of exposure of non-immune populations to schistosomes through contact with contaminated fresh water.

Infection with schistosomiasis begins in childhood, as early as 6 months of age, with peak incidence usually between 10 and 14 years of age in areas with high disease prevalence, and in late adolescence in less intensely infected populations. The incidence of the disease in adults gradually decreases [14].

1.5.2 Life cycle

Schistosomiasis requires two hosts for completion of its life cycle: a sexual stage in humans and an asexual stage in the intermediate host, the snail. Adult worms of *S. mansoni* and *S. intercalatum* reside in the inferior mesenteric veins; while adult worms of *S. japonicum* and *S. mekongi* reside in the superior mesenteric vein of the infected humans (Figure 4). Eggs either migrate through the vascular wall into the intestinal submucosa, or are carried by the portal circulation into the liver. Eggs in the submucosa find their way into the intestinal lumen and are excreted in the feces into static or slow moving fresh water bodies, and hatch at temperatures in the 20–30°C range. After hatching, the released ciliated miracidia penetrate the intermediate host, the snail and lose the cilia and develop into a primary sporocyst. Asexual stage of development in the snail takes 3–5 weeks, resulting in the release of hundreds of cercariae. These fork-tailed, larval forms of the parasite actively swim in the search of a human host. The cercaria attaches to the epidermis by an oral sucker and penetrates intact skin. The cercaria shed their forked tails and the resulting schistomosula migrate through the venous circulation to the heart and then the lungs, where they reside and continue to mature for 2–3 weeks. The developing worms eventually reach the left side of heart and are carried to the portal circulation. The female and male worms reach maturity and mating occurs with the male occupying the gynecophoric

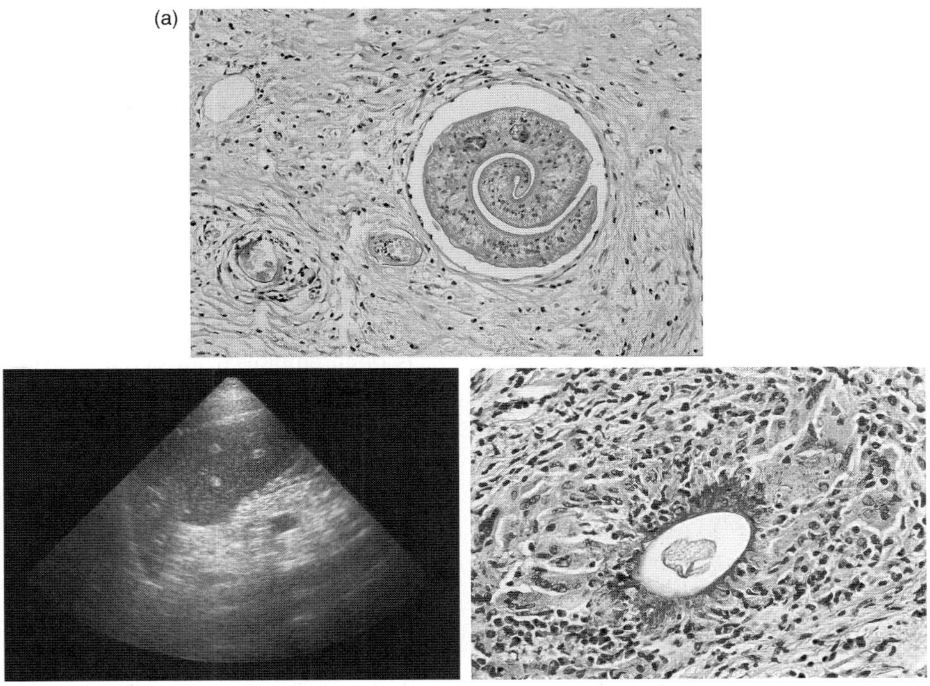

Figure 4. (a) Microscopic examination of a mesenteric mass in a 40-year-old male who had laparotomy for intestinal obstruction. A mesenteric mass with adhesions to the bowel loops was seen at surgery. Histology of the mass shows an adult worm of *Schistosoma mansoni* curved up in the mesenteric vein. Two eggs, oval in shape and with lateral spines (*Schistosoma mansoni* eggs) are placed nearby. (b) A 30-year-old male who presented with variceal bleed secondary to hepatic schistosomiasis. Left panel: A transverse sonogram through hilum of the liver shows an echogenic mass surrounding the portal vein. Right panel: Liver biopsy shows an *S. mansoni* egg with a lateral spine. Eosinophilic fibrinoid material is surrounding the egg, the Hoeppli–Splendore reaction. (*For colored version, see Plate XIX on page 574 at the end of the book.*)

canal of the female. The adult worms remain in a state of continuous copulation within the vessels, eventually migrating against the portal blood flow to the mesenteric venous plexus. Adult worms survive an average of 3–5 years [14].

1.5.3 Pathology

Schistosome eggs in the intestinal submucosa elicit an intense granulamatous response that can lead to inflammatory or ulcerative lesions in the intestinal wall. Eggs in the liver lodge in the small portal vein tributaries and lead to granuloma formation causing pyelophlebitis, peripyelophlebitis, and periportal fibrosis. The granulomas are rich in eosinophils, lymphocytes, macrophages, and plasma cells. Grossly the liver is enlarged but may be normal or even small in the later stages. The surface is often irregular and left lobe may be disproportionately enlarged. The characteristic lesion of hepatic schistosomiasis is "clay pipestem" lesion. This is described as wide bands of fibrosis around portal veins. The parenchyma between the areas of fibrosis is usually well preserved and the disease does not cause cirrhosis [15].

1.5.4 Clinical features

Disease syndromes associated with schistosomiasis include cercarial dermatitis, larval pneumonitis, acute schistosomiasis (Katayama fever), and chronic schistosomiasis. Chronic schistosomiasis presents as two polar forms – intestinal and hepatic syndromes. Hepatic disease causes portal hypertension manifesting by splenomegaly, esophageal varices, and portosystemic collateral shunts at other sites. Liver is enlarged particularly at the left lobe. The disease may stay asymptomatic for a number of years. Bleeding from esophageal varices is a major complication. Variceal bleed in hepatic schistosomiasis is better tolerated than variceal bleeding in posthepatitic or alcoholic cirrhosis and encephalopathy is not usually precipitated following bleed. Hypersplenism may present with anemia, leucopenia, and thrombocytopenia. Synthetic functions of the liver namely serum bilirubin, serum albumin, and prothrombin time are well within normal limits. In the late stages of disease, patient presents with features of hepatic decompensation namely ascites, encephalopathy, and muscle wasting. Liver is shrunken and serum albumin is low and prothrombin time is elevated. However, stigmata of cirrhosis namely jaundice, spider naevi, palmer erythema, testicular atrophy, and gynecomastia are not seen. Patients with hepatic schistosomiasis may be co-infected with hepatitis B or hepatitis C. Co-infections with HBV or HCV cause rapid deterioration of liver functions in patients with hepatic schistosomiasis with development of severe, irreversible periportal fibrosis and end stage liver disease [14].

1.5.5 Diagnosis

Diagnosis needs a high suspicion and residence or travel to endemic area may give a clue in patients who are asymptomatic with splenomegaly, hypersplenism, or heme-positive stools. The demonstration of parasite eggs in stool specimens remains the gold standard for diagnosis of schistosomiasis. Biopsy of rectal mucosa is more sensitive than fecal egg detection for the diagnosis. Crush technique for detection of eggs in the mucosal biopsies is particularly valuable. Serologic tests have been developed to detect specific antibodies against *S. mansoni* adult worm antigens. The detection of antischistosomial antibodies is a useful tool to diagnose the infection in persons who have visited endemic areas. However, a positive test in patients from endemic areas should be read with caution, as the test cannot differentiate past and recent infection. Abdominal imaging is often employed for defining liver size, periportal fibrosis, splenomegaly, and portosystemic shunts. Ultrasonography with Doppler is non-invasive, inexpensive, and sensitive tool to stage the severity of disease and monitor the response to therapy (Figure 4). Liver biopsy is helpful in excluding other causes of liver disease. The presence of schistosome eggs in the biopsy is seen as often as positive findings on stool examination or rectal biopsy [16].

1.5.6 Treatment

Hepatic schistosomiasis is managed by antischistosomial chemotherapy and measures to treat portal hypertension and its complications and hepatic failure on standard guidelines. Drug therapy eradicates the infection, prevents progression of disease, and interrupts egg excretion and disease dissemination. The effective drugs in current use are praziquantel and oxamniquine. Praziquantel is the drug of choice for all schistosomes. In *S. mansoni* and *S. intercalatum*, praziquantel 20 mg/kg per oral in two doses is administered on 1 day. In *S. japonicum* and *S. mekogi*, praziqantel 20 mg/kg in three doses is administered orally over 1 day. Cure rates of up to 90% have been reported with these regimens. Oxamniquine is an alternative drug for *S. mansoni* infection [14].

1.6 Liver flukes: fascioliasis

Fascioliasis is caused by the sheep liver fluke *Fasciola hepatica*. Mature flukes reside in the biliary tree and cause chronic obstructive biliary symptoms. Fascioliais is endemic in parts of Europe and Latin America, North Africa, Asia, the Western Pacific, and some parts of the United States.

1.6.1 Life cycle

Eggs are passed in the feces of the infected mammals into fresh water and hatch into miracidia. Miracidia penetrate the snail *Lymnaea truncu!ata*. Asexual stage of development in the snail takes 3–5 weeks, resulting in the release of hundreds of cercariae. Cercariae attach to aquatic plants such as watercress. Hosts become infected when they consume plants containing encysted metacercariae. The larvae bore into intestinal wall, enter the abdominal cavity, penetrate the hepatic capsule, and eventually settle in the bile ducts, where they attain maturity.

1.6.2 Clinical features

Three clinical syndromes are recognized: acute or invasive, chronic latent, and chronic obstructive. The acute phase corresponds to migration of young flukes through the liver and is marked by fever, pain right upper quadrant, urticaria, hepatomegaly, and eosinophilia. Liver tests reveal mild abnormalities. The latent phase corresponds to the settling of the flukes into the bile ducts and can last for months to years. Affected patients may experience vague gastrointestinal symptoms. Eosinophilia persists and fever can continue. The chronic obstructive phase is a consequence of intrahepatic and extrahepatic bile duct inflammation and hyperplasia evoked by the flukes. Recurrent biliary colic, cholangitis, cholelithiasis, and cholestasis may result. Liver tests reveal features of biliary obstruction. Long-term infection can lead to biliary cirrhosis and secondary sclerosing cholangitis.

1.6.3 Diagnosis

Diagnosis of acute infection is done by detection of antibodies by counter immuno-electrophoresis or enzyme immuno-electrophoresis (ELISA). Chronic infection can be diagnosed by detection of eggs in feces, duodenal aspirate, or bile. Hepatic imaging by ultrasonography or CECT is useful to define biliary dilatation and secondary hepatic changes due to cholestasis. ERCP will demonstrate adult flukes in the biliary tree and can be used to extract the parasites from the ducts [17].

1.6.4 Treatment

Bithionol is the drug of choice and is administered in a dose of 50 mg/kg/day for 10 days. Bacterial cholangitis needs aggressive treatment with intravenous antibiotics and bile duct strictures need appropriate management.

1.7 Liver flukes: clonorchiasis and opisthorchiasis

C. sinesis, *Opisthorchis viverrini*, and *Opisthorchis felineus* are trematodes of the family Opisthorchioidae. *C. sinesis* and *O. viverrini* are widespread in East and Southeast Asia and linked to lower socioeconomic status. *O. felineus* infects humans and domestic animals in eastern Europe.

1.7.1 Life cycle

All three parasites have similar life cycle. The adult flukes live in the bile ducts of the host and release eggs in the feces into fresh water. Eggs are consumed by snails, and hatch as free-swimming cercariae, which seek and penetrate fish or crayfish, encysting in skin or muscle as metacercariae. The mammalian host is infected on consumption of raw or undercooked fish.

The metacercariae excyst in the small bowel and migrate into the ampulla of Vater and into the bile ducts, where they mature into adult flukes. Infection can be maintained for two decades or longer.

1.7.2 Clinical features

Clinical manifestations are caused by the presence of adult flukes in the bile duct, which release eggs that cause severe inflammation and fibrosis. Fever, pain right hypochondrium, tender hepatomegaly, and eosinophilia are initial symptoms. Later features of chronic biliary obstruction occur. Patients develop cholelithiasis, cholecystitis, and recurrent pyogenic cholangitis. Liver tests reveal elevated serum bilirubin and alkaline phosphatase. Long-term infection leads to exuberant inflammation, marked biliary epithelial hyperplasia, and dysplasia, and a substantially increased risk of cholangiocarcinoma [18].

1.7.3 Diagnosis

Diagnosis is made by detection of characteristic fluke eggs in the stool except late in the disease. Cholangiography, at ERCP or PTC, reveals slender, uniform filling defects within intrahepatic ducts. Bile ducts reveal strictures, dilation, and sacculation mimicking sclerosing cholangitis.

1.7.4 Treatment

Praziquantel is the drug of choice and is administered in a dose of 75 mg/kg in three divided doses over 1 day. The response to therapy is suboptimal and recurrences are common. Dead flukes from the bile ducts need endoscopic or surgical therapy.

2. NON-VIRAL INFECTIONS, WHICH INVOLVE THE LIVER AS A PART OF MULTIORGAN INFECTION

A number of non-viral infections, which primarily involve other organ(s), do affect the liver occasionally and cause hepatic manifestations. These include invasive candidiasis, malaria, typhoid fever, tuberculosis, and leptospirosis. The etiological agents, endemic zones, high risk groups, organs involved and hepatic manifestation of these infections are shown in Table 3.

2.1 Hepatobiliary tuberculosis

Tuberculosis remains one of the major health problems in the world. WHO estimates that each year 8 million new cases of tuberculosis occur and approximately 3 million die from the disease. Tuberculosis is a disease of developing countries, however, its incidence is increasing in developed countries mainly in the immigrant population and in patients with AIDS.

Hepatobiliary tuberculosis is seen in number of situations [19]:

1. *Incidental.* Liver involvement is seen at autopsy in 25–50% of patients dying from active pulmonary tuberculosis. An autopsy study from West Africa found that 50% adults dying of AIDS have active tuberculosis and in 85% of them liver is involved.
2. *Miliary form.* This occurs due to hematogenous spread of the tubercle bacilli. Liver is involved by multiple granulomas. Miliary tuberculosis presents with fever, night sweats, anorexia, weakness and weight loss. Physical signs include hepatomegaly, splenomegaly, and lymphadenopathy. Elevation of serum alkaline phosphatase and other abnormal values in liver function tests are detected in patients with severe hepatic involvement. Liver biopsy revealed granulomas in high percentage of patients and usually gives clue to diagnosis.
3. *Granulomatous hepatitis.* Patients present with unexplained fever, jaundice, hepatomegaly, elevated alkaline phosphatase, and abnormality of other liver function tests. Imaging of the liver may be normal or reveal non-specific abnormalities. Laparoscopy is useful and shows cheesy white irregular nodules on the liver surface. Biopsy from such lesions reveals caseating granulomas. Granulomatous hepatitis with multiple granulomas in the liver may also be seen following vaccination with bacilli calmette-Guerin, especially in persons with impaired immune response.
4. *Nodular disease.* In this entity single or multiple focal masses develop in the liver and are seen as

Table 3. Non-viral infections which involve the liver as a part of multiorgan infection.

Disease (agent)	Endemic areas (high risk groups)	Organ involved	Hepatic manifestations
Invasive candidiasis (*Candida* spp.)	Worldwide (acute leukemia on immunosuppression)	Skin, lungs, GI tract, kidneys, liver, spleen	Chronic debilitating illness; high fever, RUQ pain, weight loss, hepatomegaly, elevated ALP; US or CECT reveals several hepatic hypoechoic lesions; treat with amphotericin or fluconazole, response 80%
Malaria (*Plasmodium* spp.)	Asia, Africa, South America	Red blood cells	Malarial hepatitis occurs in 11–25 infections, presents as jaundice, tender hepatomegaly, elevated liver enzymes, liver biopsy no inflammation; hepatic failure occurs in patients with severe *P. falciparum* infections; tropical splenomegaly syndrome presents as massive splenomegaly, elevated antimalarial antibodies and high serum IgM levels, liver biopsy reveals hepatic sinusoidal lymphocytosis (B lymphocytes), responds to long-term antimalarial therapy
Typhoid fever (*Salmonella* spp.)	Indian subcontinent, travel South/Central America	Peyer's patches, spleen, blood	Typhoid hepatitis occurs in 1–26% of patients, presents as jaundice, RUQ pain, elevated ALT; fulminant hepatic failure is rare; liver abscess can rarely occur
Leptospirosis (*Leptospira* spp.)	Tropical countries (sewage workers)	Blood, meninges, kidneys, liver	Liver is involved in second week, histology reveals mild lobular hepatitis and extensive cholestasis; hepatic disease presents with RUQ pain, severe jaundice, and minimal elevation of ALT; death due liver failure is rare
Tuberculosis (*Mycobactrium* spp.)	Developing countries (AIDS)	Lungs, intestines, other organs	The most common is diffuse parenchymal involvement, is characterized by formation of granulomas, occurs in patients with military tuberculosis; rarely tuberculous abscess or tuberculoma (focal lesion) can occur, these patients present with fever, weight loss, hepatomegaly, and raised serum alkaline phosphatase
Strongyloidosis (*S. stercoralis*)	Tropics and subtropics (AIDS, organ transplant)	Jejunum	Liver is affected in hyperinfection syndrome in immunosuppressed patients, patients present with jaundice and elevated liver enzymes, liver biopsy reveals eosinophilic granulomatous hepatitis with larvae in canaliculi and portal vein branches, larva can be detected in stool, Albendazole is the drug of choice

low-density non-enhancing lesions with or without peripheral rim enhancement. Such appearances need to be differentiated from lymphoma, fungal infection, and metastasis. Diagnosis is confirmed by image guided fine needle aspiration biopsy of the lesion.

5. *Tuberculous liver abscess*. Tuberculous abscesses in liver are extremely rare. Clinical picture and imaging resembles pyogenic or amebic liver abscess. Culture of the aspirated material clinches the diagnosis by growth of tubercle bacilli.
6. *Tubular disease*. These patients present with obstructive jaundice due to involvement of bile ducts. Bile ducts may be involved by enlarged tuberculous lymph node compressing the bile duct or diffuse involvement of the intrahepatic ducts by tubercle bacilli. ERCP reveals multiple intrahepatic biliary strictures, areas of dilatation, beading and ectasia, resembling sclerosing cholangitis or cholangiocarcinoma. Biliary stricture may occur at hilar region or distal common bile duct with dilatation of the intrahepatic ducts.

REFERENCES

[1] Johannsen, E.C., Sifri, C.D. and Madoff, L.C. (2000) Pyogenic liver abscesses. *Infect. Dis. Clin. N. Am.* **14**(3), 547–564.

[2] Khuroo, M.S., Zargar, S.A. and Mahajan, R. (1990) Hepatobiliary and pancreatic ascariasis in India. *Lancet* **335**, 1503–1506.

[3] Huang, C., Pitt, H.A., Lipsett, P.A., Osterman, F.A., Jr., Lillemoe, K.D., Cameron, J.L., and Zuidema, G.D. (1996) Pyogenic hepatic abscess. Changing trends over 42 years. *Ann. Surg.* **223**, 600–607.

[4] Vadillo, M., Corbella, X., Pac, V., Fernandez-Viladrich, P., and Pujol, R. (1994) Multiple liver abscesses due to *Yersinia enterocolitica* discloses primary hemochromatosis: three case reports and review. *Clin. Infect. Dis.* **18**, 938–941.

[5] Petri, Jr., W.A. and Singh, U. (1999) Diagnosis and management of amebiasis. *Clin. Infect. Dis.* **29**, 1117–1125.

[6] Akgun, Y., Tacyildiz, I.H. and Celik, Y. (1999) Amebic liver abscess: changing trends over 20 years. *World J. Surg.* **23**, 102–106.

[7] Sharma, M.P., Dasarathy, S., Verma, N., Saksena, S., and Shukla, D.K. (1996) Prognostic markers in amebic liver abscess: a prospective study. *Am. J. Gastroenterol.* **91**, 2584–2588.

[8] Ammann, R.W. and Eckert, J. (1996) Cestodes: echinococcosis. *Gastroenterol. Clin. N. Am.* **25**, 655–689.

[9] Lewall, D.B. (1998) Hydatid disease: biology, imaging and classification. *Clin. Radiol.* **53**, 863–874.

[10] Gil-Grande, L.A., Rodriguez-Caabeiro, F., Prieto, J.G., Sanchez-Ruano, J.J., Brasa, C., Aguilar, L., Garcia-Hoz, F., Casado, N., Barcena, R., and Alvarez, A.I. (1993) Randomized controlled trial of efficacy of albendazole in intra-abdominal hydatid disease. *Lancet* **342**, 1269–1272.

[11] Khuroo, M.S., Wani, N.A., Javid, G., Khan, B.A., Yattoo, G.N., Shah, A.H., and Jeelani, S.G. (1997) Percutaneous drainage compared with surgery for hepatic hydatid cysts. *N. Engl. J. Med.* **337**, 881–887.

[12] Khuroo, M.S., Zargar, S.A., Yattoo, G.N., Koul, P., Khan, B.A., Dar, M.Y., and Alai, M.S. (1992) Ascaris-induced acute pancreatitis. *Br. J. Surg.* **79**, 1335–1338.

[13] Khuroo, M.S., Zargar, S.A., Yattoo, G.N., Javid, G., Dar, M.Y., Boda, M.I., and Khan, B.A. (1993) Worm extraction and biliary drainage in hepatobiliary and pancreatic ascariasis. *Gastrointest. Endosc.* **39**, 680–685.

[14] DaSilva, L.C. and Carrilho, F.J. (1992) Hepatosplenic schistosomiasis. *Gastroenterol. Clin. N. Am.* **21**, 163.

[15] Helal, T.E.A., Danial, M.F. and Ahmed, H.F. (1998) The relationship between hepatitis C virus and schistosomiasis: histopathologic evaluation of liver biopsy specimens. *Hum. Pathol.* **29**, 743.

[16] Pereira, L.M.M.B., Domingues, A.L.C., Spinelli, V. and McFarlane, I.G. (1998) Ultrasonography of the liver and spleen in Brazilian patients with hepatosplenic schistosomiasis and cirrhosis. *Trans. R. Soc. Trop. Med. Hyg.* **92**, 639–642.

[17] Beers, B., Pringot, J., Geubel, A., Trigaux, J.P., Bigaignon and Dooms, G. (1990) Hepatobiliary fascioliasis: noninvasive imaging findings. *Radiology* **174**, 809–810.

[18] Dennis, M.J.S., Dennison, A.R. and Morris, D.L. (1989) Parasitic causes of obstructive jaundice. *Ann. Trop. Med. Parasitol.* **83**, 159.

[19] Alvarez, S.Z. (1998) Hepatobiliary tuberculosis. *J. Gastroenterol. Hepatol.* **13**, 833–839.

Hepatology: A Practical Approach
B. Al Knawy, M.L. Shiffman, R.H. Wiesner (editors)

Chapter 9
Nonalcoholic Fatty Liver Disease

Shiobhan R. Weston[a] *and Kris V. Kowdley*[b]

[a]University of California, San Francisco, CA, USA

[b]University of Washington, P.O. Box 356174, Seattle, WA 98195, USA

1. Introduction 176
2. NAFLD in Children 176
  2.1 Disease definition 177
    2.1.1 NAFLD and Syndrome X 177
  2.2 Prevalence and incidence 178
    2.2.1 NAFLD and hepatitis C 179
    2.2.2 NAFLD and diabetes secondary to advanced cirrhosis 179
  2.3 General demographics 179
  2.4 Pathophysiology 179
  2.5 The role of family history and familial metabolic factors 180
3. Evaluation of Suspected NAFLD 180
  3.1 Clinical history 180
  3.2 Clinical features 181
  3.3 Risk factors for NAFLD 181
    3.3.1 Risk factors for the progression of NASH 182
  3.4 Diagnosis 182
    3.4.1 Blood tests 182
    3.4.2 Other laboratory tests 182
    3.4.3 Imaging studies 183
    3.4.4 Pathological studies 183
    3.4.5 Other noninvasive tests 183
  3.5 Management 183
    3.5.1 Medical therapeutics 183
      3.5.1.1 Nonpharmacologic therapies 184
      3.5.1.2 Pharmacologic treatments 185
      3.5.1.3 Future pharmacotherapeutic directions 186
    3.5.2 Surgery 186
      3.5.2.1 Bariatric surgery 186
      3.5.2.2 Liver transplantation 186
    3.5.3 Prevention and family screening 186
4. Morbidity and mortality 186
5. Conclusion 187
References 187

Nonalcoholic fatty liver disease (NAFLD) has superseded hepatitis C as the liver disease epidemic of the new millennium. NAFLD has been described in all age groups. This "umbrella term" encompasses a broad histologic spectrum of fatty liver disease, which ranges from simple steatosis to diffuse inflammation (steatohepatitis), fibrosis, and cirrhosis. Central (visceral) obesity, noninsulin dependent diabetes mellitus, also known as "adult onset" or "type II diabetes", and dyslipidemia are the most commonly implicated risk factors for the development of NAFLD. All three risk factors share in common an association with insulin resistance. NAFLD is now recognized as a hepatic manifestation of insulin resistance syndrome. While steatosis is considered relatively benign, nonalcoholic steatohepatitis (NASH) may progress to cirrhosis and end-stage liver disease ultimately requiring liver transplantation. Weight loss, exercise, improved diabetic, and lipid control are recommended in those with identifiable risk factors. Although antioxidants and ursodeoxycholic acid are commonly prescribed, no pharmacologic treatments of proven efficacy are currently FDA approved for the treatment of NASH.

While the impact of the current global epidemic of obesity, diabetes, and hyperlipidemia as well as the recent increase in the prevalence of obesity and emergence of type II diabetes in children and adolescents on NAFLD is unknown, these epidemiological trends may have far reaching consequences unless active steps are taken to address the central issues of weight control, exercise, diet, and lifestyle. A NASH Clinical Research Network funded by the NIH comprising eight centers was established earlier this year in the US to expand our current understanding of the pathogenesis of NASH, to better define its natural history, and develop safe and effective individualized treatments.

1. INTRODUCTION

NAFLD is now regarded as the most common cause of chronic liver disease in the United States. It is estimated that as many as one-quarter of the American population probably have NAFLD [1]. The emergence of fatty liver disease has paralleled worldwide upward trends in the prevalence of obesity, diabetes, and dyslipidemia, all considered risk factors for disease development. The more severe histologic lesion within the NAFLD spectrum, NASH, has emerged as an important cause of liver-related morbidity and mortality. NAFLD has now been reported in Japan, Australia, Britain, Italy, Spain, and France as well as other parts of Europe and the Middle East, reflecting its worldwide distribution.

In the United States, the prevalence of obesity, defined as a body mass index (BMI) of $>30\ kg/m^2$, continues to increase dramatically (see Table 1). Estimates from the 1999–2000 National Health and Examination Survey (NHANES) carried out in 4115 adult men and women revealed an age-adjusted prevalence of obesity of 30.5% compared with 22.9% from NHANES III survey data (1988–1994). Corresponding rates for overweight, now defined as a BMI $\geq$ 25 are 64.5% up from 55.9% during this same period [2]. Hepatic steatosis is present in over 65% of obese patients, with figures exceeding 90% in those who are morbidly obese. Type II diabetes and dyslipidemia have followed similar upward trends worldwide. Based on US census figures as many as 30.1 million obese adults may have steatosis and 8.6 million may have steatohepatitis [3].

2. NAFLD IN CHILDREN

Age-adjusted rates for overweight and obesity in children in the US based on NHANES 1999–2000 survey data revealed a prevalence of overweight of 15.3% among 6–11 year olds and 15.5% among children aged 12–19 [4]. Based on ultrasonography and laboratory parameters [5], the projected prevalence of NAFLD in Japanese children is 2.6%, with prevalence rates of over 50% in the obese Italian pediatric population [6]. Prevalence figures for childhood NAFLD within North America are not known, as only a few published series exist.

Table 1. Classification of obesity.

Weight	Body mass index (BMI) (kg/m^2)
Underweight	<18.5
Normal weight	18.5–24.9
Overweight	25.0–29.9
Class I obesity	30.0–34.9
Class II obesity	35.0–39.9
Class III obesity	>40.0

NIH: Obesity Research 1998.

The largest of these, a Canadian series, describes 36 children with NAFLD between the ages of 4 and 16. Of 24 children who underwent a liver biopsy as part of their evaluation, 88% had histologic changes consistent with NASH and 71% had fibrosis [7]. This series is representative of the severity of the histologic lesion described in the majority of children and adolescents with available histology to date. As the prevalence and severity of obesity, type II diabetes and dyslipidemia continue to escalate, the disease burden from NAFLD will be more fully realized as it continues to gain international recognition as a significant public health issue.

2.1 Disease definition

The term nonalcoholic steatohepatitis (NASH) was initially coined by Jurgen Ludwig, a pathologist at the Mayo Clinic in 1980 [8]. Ludwig and colleagues described the syndrome of the typical histologic lesion of alcoholic hepatitis occurring in obese, diabetic women without excessive alcohol intake. NASH is considered only part of a histopathologic spectrum of liver injury now described collectively as NAFLD. The distinction between steatosis and NASH is important clinically. At the most benign end of this spectrum is simple steatosis in which fatty infiltration of the liver is the sole finding. As an isolated finding, steatosis may persist or even regress over time and is considered to be a largely benign condition which does not portend a poor prognosis [9]. In contrast, NASH is characterized by diffuse inflammation with necroinflammatory changes on liver histology that may progress to advanced fibrosis, cirrhosis, and hepatocellular carcinoma. Current data suggest that only the most severe form of fatty liver disease, NASH, is associated with significantly progressive cirrhosis and liver-related death. The etiology of NAFLD cannot be established on histologic grounds alone. A number of other causes including excess alcohol consumption, commonly used pharmaceutical agents, and disorders of lipid metabolism may potentiate hepatocellular injury. It is important to remember that NASH is a clinicopathologic diagnosis. As its name implies, NAFLD requires a careful history to confirm minimal or no alcohol ingestion; however it must be emphasized that there is no universal consensus as to what constitutes "minimal" alcohol intake. There is also no consensus as to the histologic grading of NAFLD. The two most widely quoted pathologic scoring systems are those of Brunt [10] and Matteoni [11] (see Figure 1). The histologic features most generally agreed upon include: (i) macrovesicular steatosis, (ii) centrilobular inflammation with a mixed cellular infiltrate, (iii) hepatocellular ballooning degeneration and necrosis, predominantly within zone 3, with or without Mallory's hyaline, and (iv) zone 3 perivenular or perisinusoidal fibrosis. In children, portal-based inflammation and fibrosis are more prominent. In contrast, the portal tracts in adults are relatively spared, unless co-existent liver pathology such as HCV is present. A second feature on liver pathology unique to children is the absence of Mallory's hyaline. The underlying reasons for these histologic differences are currently unknown. There remains controversy as to the role of hepatic iron deposition and HFE mutations in the pathogenesis of NASH. Most previous studies have been limited by small sample size or referral or selection bias [12].

2.1.1. NAFLD and Syndrome X

NAFLD shares many overlapping features with the insulin resistance syndrome, also known as "Syndrome X". These include (i) central obesity (ii) type II diabetes, and (iii) dyslipidemia [13]. Irrespective of the presence or absence of obesity, an association with insulin resistance is characteristic of the majority of cases described [14] (see Figure 2). In an Australian series which characterized 66 patients with NASH, 98% demonstrated insulin resistance and 87% fulfilled minimal WHO criteria for insulin resistance syndrome, lending additional support to the concept of NASH as the hepatic manifestation of this syndrome [15]. The role of insulin resistance in NASH versus other liver diseases with comparable histology has also been examined by this group in which 36 patients with less severe histologic NASH were compared with age- and sex-matched controls with HCV with comparable fibrosis. The prevalence of insulin resistance was found to be significantly higher in those with NASH (75%) versus 8.3% of those with Hepatitis C.

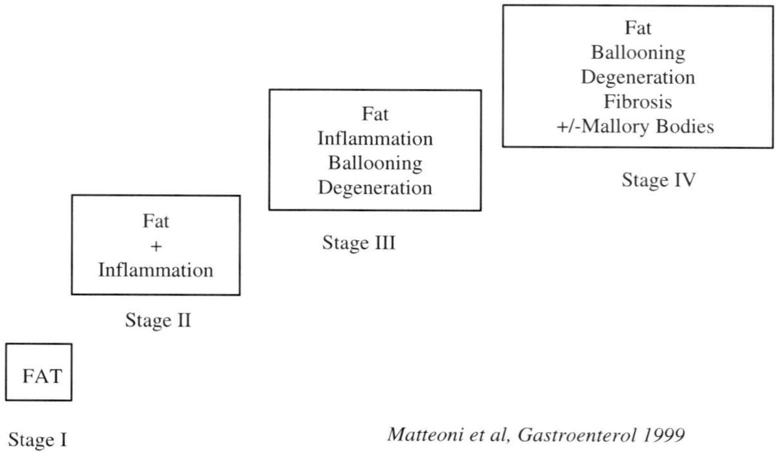

Figure 1. Proposed histologic spectrum NAFLD.

2.2 Prevalence and incidence

The true prevalence of NAFLD is difficult to evaluate, in large part because of the retrospective nature of most studies and the small number of patients who have undergone liver biopsy. Based on a large Canadian autopsy series, the overall prevalence of NASH is estimated to be 18.5% in obese and 2.7% in nonobese adults with bridging fibrosis or cirrhosis in 13.8% compared with 6.6%, respectively [16]. In this series a 2.6-fold increase in NASH was found in those with type II diabetes. Similar estimates based on autopsy data as well as from general population screening with ultrasound estimate the prevalence of NAFLD and NASH may be as high as 20 and 2–3%, respectively, in the general population [17].

NASH has also been recently appreciated as a probable cause of cirrhosis in patients with previously diagnosed cryptogenic cirrhosis, which now constitutes the third most common indication for liver transplantation. Over the course of this disease, NASH may lose its defining histologic feature of macrovesicular fat and may appear as a nonspecific hepatitis or bland cirrhosis. The similarities between the phenotypic and metabolic features of NASH and cryptogenic cirrhosis suggest that a substantial proportion of cases of cryptogenic cirrhosis may have evolved from advanced NASH. Over two-thirds of patients with cryptogenic cirrhosis have one or more risk factors for NASH [18]. Furthermore, post-transplant NAFLD develops in approximately one-third of patients transplanted for cryptogenic cirrhosis, lending further support to the concept that NASH accounts for cirrhosis in a number of patients originally thought to have cryptogenic disease [19].

Further prevalence data have been acquired from morbidly obese patients undergoing weight reduction surgery as well as from the evaluation of potential organ donors for living-related transplantation in whom 20–25% have been observed to have NAFLD [20]. Predominantly encountered in the

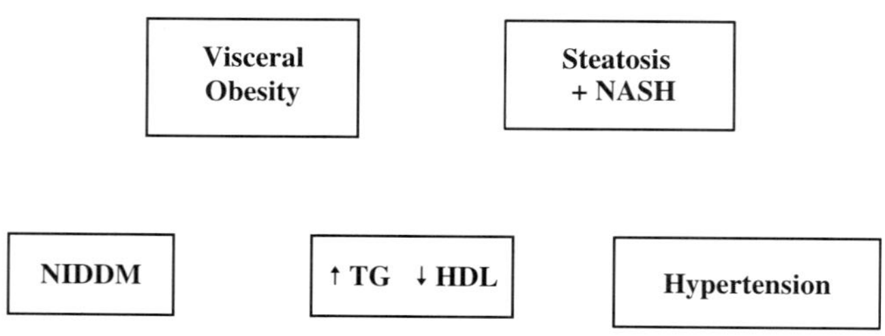

Figure 2. Metabolic X syndrome "syndrome of insulin resistance".

middle-aged population, advanced NAFLD is now becoming increasingly recognized in children and adolescents, commonly in association with morbid obesity, with documentation of cirrhosis at the time of index or follow-up biopsy [21]. Coincident with this, there has also been a dramatic increase in the prevalence of type II diabetes occurring in adolescents under the age of 18. Type II DM now accounts for approximately one-third of newly diagnosed diabetes among those in the pediatric age group [22].

2.2.1. NAFLD and hepatitis C

Steatosis may act synergistically to promote more rapid disease progression in those with HCV-related disease. Fatty changes are present in as many as 70% of HCV-infected patients. Whether steatosis is predominantly a histologic manifestation of Hepatitis C, or whether it occurs coincident with hepatitis C is a topic of active debate. Current evidence suggests that steatosis occurs as part of the disease process in hepatitis associated with HCV genotype 3 disease [23]. HCV genotype 3a has been found to be a stronger determinant of NAFLD than BMI. Interestingly, this group is among those most likely to respond to therapy [24]. In contrast, hepatic steatosis is thought to correlate with visceral obesity in patients with HCV genotype 1 infection and to correlate with more rapidly progressive fibrosis.

2.2.2. NAFLD and diabetes secondary to advanced cirrhosis

With diminishing synthetic function, as is typical of advanced fibrosis and cirrhosis, the liver's capacity to metabolize insulin is reduced, resulting in a state of hyperinsulinemia and insulin resistance. Therefore, insulin resistance may be a feature of advanced liver disease from any cause.

2.3 General demographics

NASH has been classically regarded as a disease of obese females with diabetes and dyslipidemia. However, NASH has now been reported in all age groups and is appreciated to be much more common in men than initially thought. In one study, a sizable number of patients with NASH were male, and 42% were nonobese with normal lipid and glucose profiles [25]. Although these findings were initially thought to reflect selection or referral bias, they were the first data to suggest that the clinical profile for NASH patients required further characterization. Subsequently, NAFLD has been reported an increasing number of men and also in children, some as young as 4 years of age [7]. Among children, NAFLD appears closely associated with visceral obesity. Studies to date show an increased predilection for NAFLD in boys. These gender differences in the prevalence of fatty liver in childhood might in part be explained by differences in fat distribution, as accumulation of visceral fat is more common in males irrespective of total body fat, especially in early childhood [26].

2.4 Pathophysiology

While the pathogenesis of NASH remains unclear, insulin resistance and derangements in lipid metabolism are thought to play a key role. A "two-hit" paradigm best describes the basic principles involved in pathogenesis (Figure 3). The first "hit" represents the accumulation of macrovesicular fat termed "steatosis" within the liver parenchyma. This occurs in the setting of insulin resistance characteristic of patients with obesity, type II diabetes, and dyslipidemia. The second "hit" is presumed to represent any number of processes that contribute to oxidative injury in the liver, possibly by disruption and interplay of the normal pathways of fatty acid transport and lipid metabolism alteration in mitochondrial uncoupling proteins (UCP-2), cytochrome p450 2E1, excess iron, activation of pro-inflammatory cytokines such as TNF-α, NF-kβ, IL-1, and other cascade pathways [27]. Other evidence points to a disorder involving mitochondrial fatty

"First hit" – Excess fat accumulation

↓

"Second hit" – Intrahepatic oxidative stress
Lipid peroxidation
TNF-alpha, cytokine cascade

Figure 3. Pathogenesis "2 Hit" paradigm.

acid β-oxidation linked with insulin resistance and increased visceral adiposity. Visceral fat is more insulin resistant and more susceptible to lipolysis than subcutaneous fat. Excess free fatty acids also decrease the effective utilization of glucose by muscle and contribute to peripheral insulin resistance, which acts to further promote the peripheral release of free fatty acids. Within the liver, free fatty acid accumulation leads to increased β-oxidation and lipid peroxidation. The common endpoint is an increase in oxidative stress within the liver with the subsequent formation of toxic free radical oxygen species and depletion of glutathione and vitamin E, resulting in loss of local antioxidant defenses. Triglycerides, which are synthesized from free fatty acids and exported as VLDL from the liver, produce an inhibitory effect upon peripheral insulin receptors resulting in glucose intolerance, hyperlipidemia, and steatosis. When the capacity of the liver to export VLDL is exceeded, free fatty acids accumulate within the liver.

The anti-obesity hormone leptin, derived from adipocytes may also play a role in the pathogenesis of NAFLD. Indirect evidence supporting a role for leptin comes from previous work in animal models where it has been shown to regulate triglyceride accumulation as well as fibrosis. Chitturi *et al.* have recently shown leptin levels to be independently associated with degree of steatosis, but not inflammation or fibrosis in patients with NAFLD. The authors speculate that peripheral leptin resistance may play a role in disease pathogenesis. However, serum leptin levels were not associated with BMI, the presence or absence of diabetes, or dyslipidemia [28].

2.5 The role of family history and familial metabolic factors

Unexplained familial cirrhosis associated with steatosis and risk factors for insulin resistance syndrome was first described in 1979 [29]. The evaluation of family members of three siblings with steatosis and idiopathic familial cirrhosis revealed five of nine additional family members with liver blood test abnormalities. Four of five were found to have steatosis on subsequent liver biopsy. Obesity and diabetes were associated features in this pedigree. More recently NASH-related cirrhosis and cryptogenic cirrhosis have been reported within families and in identical twins, lending further support for a genetic association [30]. While differentiation of inherited risks from that of shared common environmental exposure and chance occurrences is difficult, the coexistence of NASH and cryptogenic cirrhosis within these families suggests a common pathogenesis. Clinical features of insulin resistance syndrome (syndrome X) have also been described in kindreds with NASH, suggesting a role for familial metabolic factors [31]. The observation that some normal weight patients with insulin resistance have 1st-degree relatives with type II DM or hyperlipidemia suggests a role for genetic susceptibility and family history as potentially important contributing factors in etiopathogenesis. Previous work that led to the concept of "metabolic obesity in normal weight individuals", also lends additional support to insulin resistance as a plausible explanation for a common shared etiopathogenesis in lean and obese patients with fatty liver disease [32].

3. EVALUATION OF SUSPECTED NAFLD

3.1 Clinical history

A detailed weight history should be obtained in all patients suspected to have fatty liver disease including a history of obesity during childhood, adolescence, and adult life, as well as details of intentional rapid weight fluxes, commonly referred to as weight cycling. Past medical history should include special attention to exercise and dietary history with specific enquiry as to eating disorders such as anorexia and bulimia, in addition to factors specifically known to be associated with NAFLD: glucose intolerance, gestational or type II diabetes, hypertriglyceridemia, low HDL, and other disorders of lipid metabolism. A family history of liver disease as well as features specific to metabolic X syndrome (glucose intolerance, hypertriglyceridemia, hypertension, coronary heart disease) in 1st-degree blood relatives should also be specifically sought.

Exclusion of other diseases: By definition, NAFLD requires the careful exclusion of alcohol with corroboration of alcohol history. The exact amount of alcohol required to potentiate steatosis and amounts of alcohol ingestion considered safe in a person with fatty liver varies and is, in part, genetically determined. A daily intake of alcohol as little as 20 g (two drinks) in males and 10 g (one drink) in females is sufficient to produce alcohol injury in a genetically susceptible individual. Medication history should also include enquiry as to the use of specific potential hepatotoxic medications known to cause steatosis, as well as over-the-counter medications, natural supplements, and herbal products. As NAFLD is a disease of exclusion, risk factors for alcoholic, viral, autoimmune, and inherited liver disease (hemochromatosis and Wilson's disease) as well as systemic diseases such as celiac sprue, inflammatory bowel disease, and other endocrinopathies should be excluded. Finally, primary steatohepatitis associated with insulin resistance syndrome needs to be distinguished from secondary causes of steatohepatitis such as jejuno-ileal bypass, TPN, and other genetic or metabolic derangements (see Table 2).

3.2 Clinical features

Patients with steatosis or steatohepatitis are often initially discovered to have abnormal liver blood tests on routine medical screening, or at the time of application for medical or life insurance. The majority of patients with fatty liver disease "NAFLD" remain asymptomatic (75%). In those who do exhibit symptoms, fatigue, malaise, right upper quadrant fullness or discomfort associated with hepatic capsular distention are not infrequent complaints. Nonspecific abdominal pain is the most common reported symptom in childhood. Clinical features on physical examination, which may suggest the diagnosis, include truncal obesity, waist circumference of 37 cm in men and 32 cm in women. Hepatomegaly is found in up to 90% of patients. In children the most notable feature of insulin resistance that may lead to a diagnosis of NAFLD is the presence of obesity, as evidenced by a BMI ≥ the 85th percentile. Additionally acanthosis nigricans, a marker of insulin resistance, may be present in one-third of children and adolescents [7] and should be carefully looked for. Patients may not come to medical attention until they show evidence of hepatic decompensation as manifest by complications of portal hypertension: new-onset ascites, subacute bacterial peritonitis, variceal hemorrhage, or hepatocellular carcinoma. These later presentations are more typical of patients with "burnt-out NASH" or cryptogenic cirrhosis who have risk factors for NAFLD, but in whom disease has been previously clinically silent.

Table 2. Conditions associated with NAFLD.

Primary (associated with insulin resistance syndrome)
Obesity
Noninsulin dependant diabetes mellitus (NIDDM)
Dyslipidemia: hypertriglyceridemia, low HDL cholesterol
Secondary
Drugs amiodarone, methotrexate, corticosteroids, estrogens (tamoxifen, toremifine) calcium channel blockers (nifedipine, diltiazem), perhexiline, chloroquine, valproate, zidovudine
Surgical: jejuno-ileal bypass, gastroplexy, extensive small bowel resection, short bowel syndrome bilio-pancreatic diversion
Nutritional: total parenteral nutrition (TPN) protein-calorie malnutrition, B12 deficiency, starvation, and rapid weight loss, eating disorders (anorexia and bulimia)
Small bowel disease: jejunal diverticulosis with bacterial overgrowth, inflammatory bowel disease
Metabolic or genetic: dysbetaproteinemia, metabolic X syndrome, lipodystrophy, Prader–Willi syndrome Weber–Christian disease, Wolman's disease, cholesterol ester storage disorders galactosemia, fructose intolerance, acute fatty liver of pregnancy

3.3 Risk factors for NAFLD

Co-existing medical conditions such as obesity, type II diabetes, and disorders of lipid metabolism (hypertriglyceridemia and low HDL) are the most commonly associated risk factors for the development of NAFLD. However, not all patients have readily identifiable risk factors for the development of NAFLD. While the typical phenotypic profile may be absent, features to suggest underlying insulin resistance such as increased visceral adiposity or a family history of diabetes or hypertriglyceridemia in a 1st-degree relative also represent increased risk in this subset of patients. A family history of steatohepatitis or cryptogenic cirrhosis is also implicated as a risk factor. Thus, familial metabolic factors may also play a role in disease development. The exact interplay of a Western diet, lifestyle, and potential underlying genetic factors remains to be defined. The PPAR-γ receptor is linked to control of insulin sensitivity, glucose homeostasis, and blood pressure. Recently, two heterozygous germ-line mutations in humans have been reported in the ligand-binding domain of human PPAR-γ, providing indirect evidence for a genetic association.

3.3.1. Risk factors for the progression of NASH

Four risk factors are associated with more advanced NAFLD. These include (i) Age ≥ 45, (ii) Obesity (BMI ≥ 30), (iii) type II diabetes, and (iv) AST/ALT ratio <1.0 [33]. NASH superimposed on Hepatitis C has also recently been shown to be an independent risk factor for advanced fibrosis [19]. The effect of coexistent NAFLD and other liver diseases such as hemochromatosis is currently an area of active study.

Natural history studies show that there is only a 3–4% risk of progression to fibrosis in patients with simple or "bland" steatosis over a 10-year period [9]. It has been reported that 15% of individuals with simple steatosis progress to NASH; among patients who have biopsy-proven NASH, progression to fibrosis and cirrhosis during the first 10 years of follow-up is estimated to be as high as 40% [34]. Moreover, at the time of initial liver biopsy, advanced fibrosis may be present in up to 25% [35]. In some patients, NASH may remain undiagnosed and follow a clinically indolent course until steatosis disappears and "cryptogenic" cirrhosis is eventually diagnosed.

3.4 Diagnosis

NAFLD is a diagnosis of exclusion and relies on compatible liver histology along with a clinical history of "insignificant" alcohol intake, a term of highly variable definition. An approach to initial evaluation is shown in Figure 4.

3.4.1. Blood tests

Both steatosis and steatohepatitis are typically characterized by mild-to-moderate elevation of serum liver enzymes, with a two- to five-fold elevation in serum aspartate aminotransferase (AST) and alanine aminotransferase (ALT). A two- to three-fold elevation of serum gamma-glutamyl transferase and serum alkaline phosphatase occurs in <50% of cases [17]. Serum bilirubin levels are rarely elevated in the absence of advanced cirrhosis. The AST/ALT ratio in patients with simple steatosis or mild steatohepatitis is <1 in 65–90% of patients. This is in direct contrast to alcoholic hepatitis in which the AST/ALT ratio is often >1.5–2.0, and may be useful in distinguishing alcoholic from NAFLD when the alcohol history is uncertain. With advanced histologic disease, the AST/ALT ratio may be reduced or reversed. Thrombocytopenia should raise the index of suspicion for hypersplenism due to portal hypertension and prompt radiological imaging studies including duplex imaging of the portal and hepatic vasculature. Prolongation of prothrombin time, an increase in INR and decrease in serum albumin may develop with advanced hepatic cirrhosis.

3.4.2. Other laboratory tests

Fasting serum glucose and triglycerides are often elevated and HDL cholesterol may be low. A 2-h glucose test is also recommended in those with one of more signs of insulin resistance syndrome (hypertension, hyperlipidemia, acanthosis nigricans, or polycystic ovarian syndrome). An oral glucose tolerance test and fasting insulin level are not routinely performed in the evaluation of NAFLD in adults. When measured, a formal oral glucose tolerance test is considered to be more accurate than a fasting insulin but may be normal in metabolic X syndrome. Increased serum ferritin, an acute phase protein, may be present in up to 50% of patients and increased serum transferrin-iron saturation in approximately 10%, although hepatic iron is not typically increased. The heterozygous MZ phenotype of α-1-antitrypsin is present in 16.7% of patients with NASH, compared with a background prevalence of less than 3.6% in the general population [36]. Antinuclear antibody (ANA) and anti-smooth muscle antibody (ASM-AB) may be present in low titer, in the absence of accompanying autoimmune disease. Serum level of C-reactive protein may also be elevated, although it is relatively nonspecific.

1. Exclusion of Other Causes Of Liver Disease

HCV-Ab, HBsAg, HBcAb, AMA, ANA, anti-SMA
serum ferritin, transferrin iron saturation
ceruloplasmin, alpha-1 antitrypsin phenotype and serum level

Quantification of alcohol consumption + hepatotoxic medications

2. Radiologic Imaging

Ultrasound, CT, or MRI

3. Repeat LFT's 3 months after complete cessation of alcohcl and all hepatotoxic drugs

Figure 4. Initial work-up of patients with suspected NAFD.

3.4.3. Imaging studies

In evaluating a patient with abnormal liver enzymes, an abdominal ultrasound should be the initial radiologic screening modality to exclude other hepatobiliary disease. The prevalence of hepatomegaly on ultrasonography in patients with NAFLD may be as high as 90% [37]. The liver typically appears diffusely hyperechoic in relation to the spleen and is often referred to as "bright liver". While computerized tomography (CT) may offer improved accuracy over that of ultrasound, focal fat may appear similar to hepatoma, and may appear as a suspicious solitary hepatic lesion on either of these imaging modalities. Magnetic resonance imaging (MRI) offers an advantage over CT in this regard in that it can demonstrate fat as increased attenuation on T1-weighted signaling images, thereby allowing distinction of isolated suspicious hepatic lesions from focal fatty infiltration, as well as regions of focal fatty sparing [38]. Unfortunately, none of the above imaging modalities enable distinction of simple steatosis from NASH with or without necroinflammation and bridging fibrosis unless clear features of cirrhosis are present [39].

3.4.4. Pathological studies

Current noninvasive radiological imaging modalities cannot readily distinguish simple fatty liver from steatohepatitis and cirrhosis. Therefore, liver biopsy remains the most sensitive and specific tool by which to differentiate simple steatosis from steatohepatitis with or without fibrosis. This has important implications for staging of disease and prognosis and will have increasingly significant implications for medical management, as effective treatments become available.

3.4.5. Other noninvasive tests

Markers of liver fibrosis are currently being evaluated in patients with hepatitis C as a noninvasive means of assessing liver fibrosis. While the sensitivity and specificity of these blood tests remains to be evaluated in NAFLD, they may prove potentially useful in the initial evaluation of those patients most likely to benefit from a liver biopsy. Furthermore, they may provide a safe and inexpensive means of following disease over time, obviating the need for serial biopsies. Another promising candidate is MR spectroscopy. This technology can be used to detect triglyceride within hepatocytes, allowing for quantitative assessment of fatty infiltration [40]. MR spectroscopy may additionally provide a useful adjunct in the initial screening of patients for advanced NASH.

3.5 Management

3.5.1. Medical therapeutics

When present, associated co-morbid conditions in those with overlapping phenotypic features of syndrome X require a multidisciplinary team approach. If possible, therapeutic intervention should be directed towards the underlying etiology. All potentially implicated drugs should be discontinued if possible, with follow-up serial liver blood tests performed at 4–6 weeks and again as clinically indicated by the degree and pattern of enzyme elevation. A proposed algorithm for management of probable and definite NASH is shown in Figure 5.

3.5.1.1. Nonpharmacologic therapies. The cornerstone of any intervention plan should include dietary counseling, preferably with the help of a nutritionist and initiation of a regular exercise program.

3.5.1.1.1. Weight loss. A number of studies support the beneficial effects of gradual weight reduction on serum aminotransferases and steatosis, as detected by noninvasive imaging studies as well as liver histology. In those who are overweight, a target weight loss of 10% of initial body weight over a 6-month period is reasonable. A common error in the management of obese patients with NAFLD is the recommendation of rapid weight reduction. While weight reduction may successfully reduce fatty infiltration in patients with fatty liver, extreme weight loss over short periods of time, as occurs with weight reduction surgery or severe dieting, may be associated with progression to advanced disease. The proposed mechanism involves increased free fatty acid delivery to the liver resulting in increased lipid peroxidation, formation of reactive oxygen species, and a cascade of other cytokine and other inflammatory events leading to stellate cell activation, fibroblast formation, and acceleration of hepatic fibrosis. In theory, this mechanism may also operate in persons with rapid weight fluctuation as occurs with "weight cycling", representing multiple "second hits". In those who are overweight, a gradual weight reduction program is recommended, aiming for an average weight loss of 500 g per week in children [6] and 1600 g per week in adults [3]. Gradual and sustained weight loss may result in normalization of aminotransferases and reduction in liver volume, resulting in improvement in abdominal discomfort or pain.

3.5.1.1.2. Dietary modification. The American Heart Association guidelines recommend a 1200–1500 kcal/day diet in which 20–30% of calories are supplied as fat. In women, a 1000–1200 kcal/day diet and in men, a 1200–1500 kcal/day diet ultimately resulting in weight loss of 1–2 lb a week. Daily caloric intake can also be calculated by multiplying the patients current weight by 10 to establish the daily requirements needed to maintain current weight and then subtracting 500 or 100 kcal necessary to achieve a 1 or 2 lb weight loss per week, respectively.

3.5.1.1.3. Exercise program. Development of an exercise or physical activity program is essential to the facilitation and maintenance of weight loss. Increased aerobic activity improves peripheral

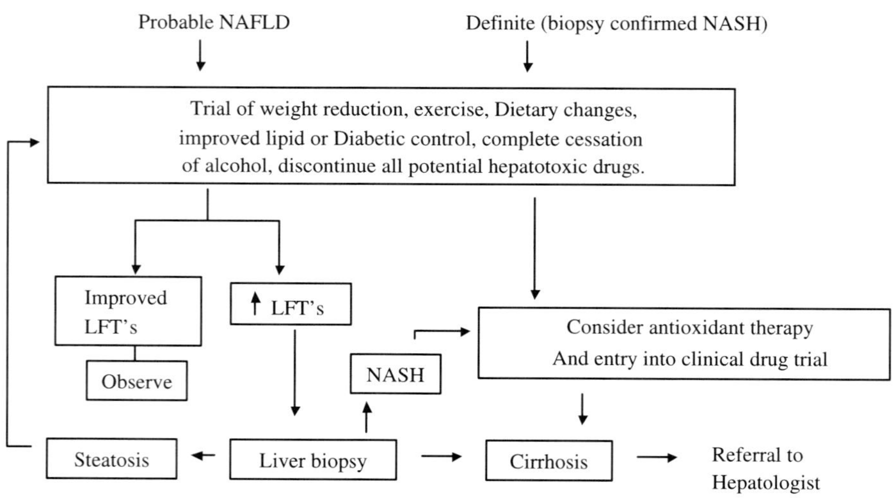

Figure 5. Management algorithm.

insulin resistance by stimulating insulin-independent uptake of glucose by skeletal muscle. Exercise has been shown to improve insulin sensitivity and reduces the risk of type II diabetes by 56% in the Finnish. US diabetic intervention studies also provide similar convincing evidence for this rationale. Thirty minutes or more of moderate-intensity aerobic physical activity for 3 or more days in a week is a reasonable target. For those who are unable to engage in more vigorous physical activity, walking for 30 min or as tolerated should be advocated.

3.5.1.1.4. Behavior modification. Lifestyle changes are instrumental in reducing risk factors for fatty liver disease and other components of metabolic X syndrome. While not all patients with NAFLD are overweight, obese children under age 10 are more likely to develop components of metabolic syndrome in adulthood and parental obesity is known to more than double the risk of adult obesity among both obese and nonobese children under the age of 10 [41]. Modification of lifestyle activity and eating habits are instrumental to management and optimization of risk factor control. The incorporation of behavioral biofeedback therapy under the guidance of a behavioral psychologist may assist with long-term goals, especially in those with compulsive eating and other eating disorders, namely bulimia and anorexia.

3.5.1.2. Pharmacologic treatments. While a number of promising agents have been studied in pilot phase I studies, there are currently no FDA approved medications for the primary treatment of NAFLD. Pharmacologic intervention should be directed towards management of co-morbid conditions.

3.5.1.2.1. Obesity. Pharmacotherapy should be reserved for individuals with a BMI >30 or >27 and one or more co-morbidities related to obesity who have failed other methods. There are currently three FDA approved therapies for use as adjuvant therapy for management of obesity. Phentermine, a norepinephrine-releasing agent is approved for short-term use for up to 3 months as an appetite suppressant. Two agents are currently approved for longer term use. The first of these, silbutramine, is a serotonin and norepinephrine reuptake inhibitor. Its side-effect profile is more favorable than phentermine and weight loss with this agent slows 6 months after initiation of therapy. Orlistat, a lipase inhibitor, inhibits both pancreatic and gastric lipase, decreasing intestinal fat absorption by 30%. This latter agent may prove a useful adjunct therapy in weight maintenance after reaching initial target loss.

3.5.1.2.2. Type II diabetes. Pharmacotherapy for diabetes should be considered in patients whose euglycemic control is unlikely to be attained or does not occur with nonpharmacotherapeutic intervention. Metformin is a logical treatment choice for obese patients with NIDDM. In addition to improvement in hepatic insulin sensitivity, the appetite suppressant properties of this agent provide additional therapeutic advantage.

In a recent study, treatment of NASH in nondiabetic patients with metformin for 4 months resulted in reduction in serum aminotransferases and liver volume, supporting an earlier report, which demonstrated a beneficial effect of metformin on insulin resistance in insulin-resistant *ob/ob* positive mice. However, it should be remembered that lactic acidosis has been previously reported in the setting of liver disease, and careful monitoring of patients, preferably in the context of clinical trials may be preferred. Other insulin sensitizing agents such as thiazolidinediones, which reduce circulating free fatty acids, triglycerides and circulating insulin levels, may also improve serum aminotransferases. Troglitazone, a thiazolidinedione and peroxisome proliferator-activated receptor gamma (PPARγ) ligand, introduced in the late 1990s for treatment of diabetes, was the first drug in this class studied in patients with NAFLD. However, this agent is not currently available because of hepatotoxicity. Rosiglitazone, another member of this drug class has been occasionally reported to have similar side effects. Therefore, the use of thiazolidinediones in nondiabetics outside the context of clinical trials cannot be recommended as primary treatment for NAFLD at this time.

3.5.1.2.3. Hyperlipidemia. Gemfibrozil given at a dose of 600 mg/day improves serum aminotransferases, independent of effects on weight. Clofibrate, which showed initial promise in decreasing hepatic triglycerides in animal studies, has not proved effective in pilot studies. Atorvastatin or other lipid-lowering agents belonging to the statin family may represent the pharmacotherapeutic agents with most promise. Because hepatotoxic effects may be a side effect of statin therapy, baseline and 2–3 monthly liver blood tests are recommended while on therapy.

3.5.1.3. Future pharmacotherapeutic directions. The development of rational pharmacotherapeutic intervention strategies with clinically relevant end-points will require a better understanding of the etiopathogenesis and natural history of NAFLD. Currently, there are no known treatment modalities of proven efficacy. While a number of treatments have been used in pilot studies, few studies have follow-up liver histology, limiting quantitative objective measurement of treatment response. Treatments with potential promise include: (i) agents directed against lipid peroxidation and oxidative stress such as vitamin E, ursodeoxycholic acid, silymarin, and *N*-acetylcysteine, *S*-adenosyl-methionine (SAMe), or betaine (ii) insulin-sensitizing agents such as metformin or thiazolidinediones, and (iii) lipid-lowering agents. Future potential therapeutic agents on the horizon include proinflammatory cytokine inhibitors such as neutralizing anti-TNF antibodies and pentoxyphylline, probiotics, iron depletion, modulators of mitochondrial function, and antifibrotic agents.

3.5.2. Surgery

3.5.2.1. Bariatric surgery. Open and laparoscopic bariatric surgery are medically approved as indicated treatment for patients with a BMI ≥ 40 or ≥ 35 with the presence of obesity-related co-morbidities. Steatosis and steatohepatitis are commonly seen in this patient population, often at the time of surgery. The effects of rapid weight loss on patients with pre-existing steatosis or steatohepatitis on liver histology and long-term effects of current day bariatric surgery techniques are largely unknown and are the focus of ongoing prospective evaluation at several North American centers.

3.5.2.2. Liver transplantation. Orthotopic liver transplantation or living-related organ donation for end-stage liver disease secondary to NAFLD and cryptogenic cirrhosis offers a potential, but not definitive therapeutic alternative. As with viral hepatitis and cholestatic liver disease, NAFLD may recur following transplantation and may also develop following transplantation for cryptogenic cirrhosis. The effect of weight gain, diabetes, and hyperlipidemia in the post-transplant period are common with the use of immunosuppressive agents. With the recent addition of sirolimus to the therapeutic armamentarium of current transplant pharmacologic regimens, NAFLD may assume increasing importance in future organ transplantation because of its hyperlipidemic effect.

3.5.3. Prevention and family screening

At present there are no formal guidelines for screening of family members with NAFLD. Nonetheless, most patients with NAFLD, independent of weight, have co-morbidities, which overlap with metabolic X syndrome including insulin resistance, dyslipidemia, systemic hypertension, and coronary heart disease. Specific public policy guidelines and recommendations will need to be developed and targeted at those at increased risk for obesity, diabetes, and dyslipidemia in both children and adults. Implementation of primary and secondary preventive measures involving lifestyle modification such as integration of daily exercise, changes in diet and eating habits will be required to curb the potential ramifications of obesity and obesity-related consequences for future generations.

4. MORBIDITY AND MORTALITY

According to Matteoni *et al.*, liver disease is now the second leading cause of death in patients with NAFLD with rates equaling those from coronary heart disease. The liver-related death rate was estimated to be 11% in those patients with advanced NAFLD compared with a crude adjusted death rate of 9.5 per 100,000 for the general US population [11]. The outcome of cirrhosis and liver-related death is not uniform across the spectrum of NAFLD. Most liver-related deaths occur in those with histologically advanced disease. At the time of initial diagnosis, severe fibrosis is recognized in one-third of patients. While in general there is minimal morbidity and need for transplantation during the long-term follow-up of patients with

NASH, as many as 20% of patients may have a progressive course, resulting in cirrhosis. Cirrhosis and liver-related deaths occur in 25 and 8% of patients over a 10-year period, respectively. Moreover, hepatocellular carcinoma (HCC) is now increasingly realized in patients with cryptogenic cirrhosis, and features suggestive of NAFLD are more frequently observed in this patient population compared with age- and sex-matched HCC patients with underlying viral- or ethanol-related disease [42].

Although not listed by United Network for Organ Sharing (UNOS) as a separate indication for liver transplantation, 2.9% of liver transplants were performed for NASH at The Mayo Clinic between 1993 and 1999. Grade II steatosis was present in 60% of patients transplanted for NASH, compared with 15% transplanted for alcoholic liver disease and hepatitis C. NASH recurred in one-third of transplant recipients, in some as early as 6 weeks, with progression to cirrhosis in 12.5% after 2 years. One- and 3-year patient survival rates were 93 and 81.2%, respectively [36]. Overall survival rates after liver transplantation for NASH at the Mayo Clinic were 72 and 58% at 1 and 5 years, respectively.

5. CONCLUSION

After more than 20 years, NAFLD has finally come to the forefront of hepatology, and is now recognized as possibly the most common cause of liver disease in the Western world. Its importance as a public health problem lies in its prevalence and proclivity to progress to cirrhosis. The prevalence of fatty liver disease will likely continue to rise coincident with current global trends in obesity, diabetes, and dyslipidemia. Although the vast majority of affected persons have simple steatosis, the disease burden of advanced NASH will likely become increasingly significant in children and adults. Targeted primary and secondary preventative measures will continue to play a significant role as first line management in the foreseeable future. The long-term effects of these intervention strategies, particularly behavior modification, will likely assume the greatest clinical importance in children. Finally, the importance of liver biopsy will play an increasing role in staging of disease in both the pediatric and adult population as obesity trends continue and new effective pharmacologic treatments become available.

REFERENCES

[1] Kim, W.R., Brown, Jr., R.S., Terrault, N.A. and El Serag, H. (2002) Burden of liver disease in the United States: summary of a workshop. *Hepatology* **36**(1), 227–242.

[2] Flegal, K.M., Carroll, M.D., Ogden, C.L. and Johnson, C.L. (2002) Prevalence and trends in obesity among US adults, 1999–2000. *J. Am. Med. Assoc.* **288**(14), 1723–1727.

[3] Angulo, P. (2002) Nonalcoholic fatty liver disease. *N. Engl. J. Med.* **346**(16), 1221–1231.

[4] Ogden, C.L., Flegal, K.M., Carroll, M.D. and Johnson, C.L. (2002) Prevalence and trends in overweight among US children and adolescents, 1999–2000. *J. Am. Med. Assoc.* **288**(14), 1728–1732.

[5] Tominaga, K., Kurata, J.H., Chen, Y.K., Fujimoto, E., Miyagawa, S., Abe, I. and Kusano, Y. (1995) Prevalence of fatty liver in Japanese children and relationship to obesity. An epidemiological ultrasonographic survey. *Dig. Dis. Sci.* **40**(9), 2002–2009.

[6] Franzese, A., Vajro, P., Argenziano, A., Puzziello, A., Iannucci, M.P., Saviano, M.C., Brunetti, F. and Rubino, A. (1997) Liver involvement in obese children. Ultrasonography and liver enzyme levels at diagnosis and during follow-up in an Italian population. *Dig. Dis. Sci.* **42**(7), 1428–1432.

[7] Rashid, M. and Roberts, E.A. (2000) Nonalcoholic steatohepatitis in children. *J. Pediatr. Gastroenterol. Nutr.* **30**(1), 48–53.

[8] Ludwig, J., Viggiano, T.R., McGill, D.B. and Oh, B.J. (1980) Nonalcoholic steatohepatitis: Mayo Clinic experiences with a hitherto unnamed disease. *Mayo Clin. Proc.* **55**(7), 434–438.

[9] Teli, M.R., James, O.F., Burt, A.D., Bennett, M.K. and Day, C.P. (1995) The natural history of nonalcoholic fatty liver: a follow-up study. *Hepatology* **22**(6), 1714–1719.

[10] Brunt, E.M., Janney, C.G., Di Bisceglie, A.M., Neuschwander-Tetri, B.A. and Bacon, B.R. (1999) Nonalcoholic steatohepatitis: a proposal for grading and staging the histological lesions. *Am. J. Gastroenterol.* **94**(9), 2467–2474.

[11] Matteoni, C.A., Younossi, Z.M., Gramlich, T., Boparai, N., Liu, Y.C. and McCullough, A.J. (1999) Nonalcoholic fatty liver disease: a spectrum of clinical

and pathological severity. *Gastroenterology* **116**(6), 1413–1419.

[12] Chitturi, S., Weltman, M., Farrell, G.C., McDonald, D., Liddle, C., Samarasinghe, D., Lin, R., Abeygunasekera, S. and George, J. (2002) FE mutations, hepatic iron, and fibrosis: ethnic-specific association of NASH with C282Y but not with fibrotic severity. *Hepatology* **36**:1 142–149.

[13] Reaven, G.M. (1998) Insulin resistance and human disease: a short history. *J. Basic Clin. Physiol. Pharmacol.* **9**(2–4), 387–406.

[14] Marchesini, G., Brizi, M., Morselli-Labate, A.M., Bianchi, G., Bugianesi, E., McCullough, A.J., Forlani, G. and Melchionda, N. (1999) Association of nonalcoholic fatty liver disease with insulin resistance. *Am. J. Med.* **107**:5 450–455.

[15] Chitturi, S., Abeygunasekera, S., Farrell, G.C., Holmes-Walker, J., Hui, J.M., Fung, C., Karim, R., Lin, R., Samarasinghe, D., Liddle, C., Weltman, M. and George, J. (2002) NASH and insulin resistance: insulin hypersecretion and specific association with the insulin resistance syndrome. *Hepatology* **35**:2 373–379.

[16] Wanless, I.R. and Lentz, J.S. (1990) Fatty liver hepatitis (steatohepatitis) and obesity: an autopsy study with analysis of risk factors. *Hepatology* **12**(5), 1106–1110.

[17] Falck-Ytter, Y., Younossi, Z.M., Marchesini, G. and McCullough, A.J. (2001) Clinical features and natural history of nonalcoholic steatosis syndromes. *Semin. Liver Dis.* **21**(1), 17–26.

[18] Caldwell, S.H., Oelsner, D.H., Iezzoni, J.C., Hespenheide, E.E., Battle, E.H. and Driscoll, C.J. (1999) Cryptogenic cirrhosis: clinical characterization and risk factors for underlying disease. *Hepatology* **29**(3), 664–669.

[19] Ong, J.P., Younossi, Z.M., Speer, C., Olano, A., Gramlich, T. and Boparai, N. (2001) Chronic hepatitis C and superimposed nonalcoholic fatty liver disease. *Liver* **21**(4), 266–271.

[20] Dixon, J.B., Bhathal, P.S. and O'Brien, P.E. (2001) Nonalcoholic fatty liver disease: predictors of nonalcoholic steatohepatitis and liver fibrosis in the severely obese. *Gastroenterology* **121**(1), 91–100.

[21] Molleston, J.P., White, F., Teckman, J. and Fitzgerald, J.F. (2002) Obese children with steatohepatitis can develop cirrhosis in childhood. *Am. J. Gastroenterol.* **97**(9), 2460–2462.

[22] Fagot-Campagna, A. (2000) Emergence of type 2 diabetes mellitus in children: epidemiological evidence. *J. Pediatr. Endocrinol. Metab.* **13**(Suppl. 6), 1395–1402.

[23] Monto, A., Alonzo, J., Watson, J.J., Grunfeld, C. and Wright, T.L. (2002) Steatosis in chronic hepatitis C: relative contributions of obesity, diabetes mellitus, and alcohol. *Hepatology* **36**(3), 729–736.

[24] Rubbia-Brandt, L., Leandro, G., Spahr, L., Giostra, E., Quadri, R., Male, P.J. and Negro, F. (2001) Liver steatosis in chronic hepatitis C: a morphological sign suggesting infection with HCV genotype 3. *Histopathology* **39**(2), 119–124.

[25] Bacon, B.R., Farahvash, M.J., Janney, C.G. and Neuschwander-Tetri, B.A. (1994) Nonalcoholic steatohepatitis: an expanded clinical entity. *Gastroenterology* **107**(4), 1103–1109.

[26] Kral, J.G., Schaffner, F., Pierson, Jr., R.N. and Wang, J. (1993) Body fat topography as an independent predictor of fatty liver. *Metabolism* **42**(5), 548–551.

[27] Tilg, H. and Diehl, A.M. (2000) Cytokines in alcoholic and nonalcoholic steatohepatitis. *N. Engl. J. Med.* **343**(20), 1467–1476.

[28] Chitturi, S., Farrell, G., Frost, L., Kriketos, A., Lin, R., Liddle, C., Samarasinghe, D. and George, J. (2002) Serum leptin in NASH correlates with hepatic steatosis but not fibrosis: a manifestation of lipotoxicity?. *Hepatology* **36**:2 403–409.

[29] Altman, A.R., Gottfried, E.B., Paronetto, F. and Lieber, C.S. (1979) Idiopathic familial cirrhosis and steatosis in adults. *Gastroenterology* **77**(6), 1211–1216.

[30] Willner, I.R., Waters, B., Patil, S.R., Reuben, A., Morelli, J. and Riely, C.A. (2001) Ninety patients with nonalcoholic steatohepatitis: insulin resistance, familial tendency, and severity of disease. *Am. J. Gastroenterol.* **96**(10), 2957–2961.

[31] Struben, V.M., Hespenheide, E.E. and Caldwell, S.H. (2000) Nonalcoholic steatohepatitis and cryptogenic cirrhosis within kindreds. *Am. J. Med.* **108**(1), 9–13.

[32] Ruderman, N.B., Schneider, S.H. and Berchtold, P. (1981) The "metabolically-obese," normal-weight individual. *Am. J. Clin. Nutr.* **34**(8), 1617–1621.

[33] Angulo, P., Keach, J.C., Batts, K.P. and Lindor, K.D. (1999) Independent predictors of liver fibrosis in patients with nonalcoholic steatohepatitis. *Hepatology* **30**(6), 1356–1362.

[34] Neuschwander-Tetri, B.A. (2000) Nonalcoholic steatohepatitis: an evolving diagnosis. *Can. J. Gastroenterol.* **14**(4), 321–326.

[35] Diehl, A.M., Goodman, Z. and Ishak, K.G. (1988) Alcohol like liver disease in nonalcoholics. A clinical and histologic comparison with alcohol-induced liver injury. *Gastroenterology* **95**(4), 1056–1062.

[36] Charlton, M., Kasparova, P., Weston, S., Lindor, K., Maor-Kendler, Y., Wiesner, R.H., Rosen, C.B. and Batts, K.P. (2001) Frequency of nonalcoholic

steatohepatitis as a cause of advanced liver disease. *Liver Transpl.* **7**(7), 608–614.

[37] Powell, E.E., Cooksley, W.G., Hanson, R., Searle, J., Halliday, J.W. and Powell, L.W. (1990) The natural history of nonalcoholic steatohepatitis: a follow-up study of forty-two patients for up to 21 years. *Hepatology* **11**(1), 74–80.

[38] Mitchell, D.G., Palazzo, J., Hann, H.W., Park, C.H., Tempany, C., Chako, A. and Rubin, R. (1992) Mass-like hepatic hypertrophy: MRI findings with histologic correlation. *Magn. Reson. Imaging* **10**(4), 541–547.

[39] Saadeh, S., Younossi, Z.M., Remer, E.M., Gramlich, T., Ong, J.P., Hurley, M., Mullen, K.D., Cooper, J.N. and Sheridan, M.J. (2002) The utility of radiological imaging in nonalcoholic fatty liver disease. *Gastroenterology* **123**:3 745–750.

[40] Ricci, C., Longo, R., Gioulis, E., Bosco, M., Pollesello, P., Masutti, F., Croce, L., Paoletti, S., de Bernard, B., Tiribelli, C. and Dalla Palma, L. (1997) Noninvasive in vivo quantitative assessment of fat content in human liver. *J. Hepatol.* **27**:1 108–113.

[41] Whitaker, R.C., Wright, J.A., Pepe, M.S., Seidel, K.D. and Dietz, W.H. (1997) Predicting obesity in young adulthood from childhood and parental obesity. *N. Engl. J. Med.* **337**(13), 869–873.

[42] Bugianesi, E., Leone, N., Vanni, E., Marchesini, G., Brunello, F., Carucci, P., Musso, A., De Paolis, P., Capussotti, L., Salizzoni, M. and Rizzetto, M. (2002) Expanding the natural history of nonalcoholic steatohepatitis: from cryptogenic cirrhosis to hepatocellular carcinoma. *Gastroenterology* **123**:1 134–140.

Hepatology: A Practical Approach
B. Al Knawy, M.L. Shiffman, R.H. Wiesner (editors)

Chapter 10

Alcohol-Induced Liver Disease

W. Carey

The Cleveland Clinic Foundation, 9500 Euclid Avenue, Cleveland, OH 44195, USA

1. Introduction 191
   1.1 Definition 191
   1.2 Disease prevalence 191
   1.3 General demographics 192
2. Pathophysiology 192
3. Clinical Features 194
   3.1 History 194
   3.2 Steatosis (fatty liver) 194
   3.3 Acute alcoholic steatohepatitis 194
   3.4 Cirrhosis 194
4. Diagnosis 194
   4.1 Blood tests 194
   4.2 Imaging studies 195
   4.3 Pathology 195
5. Management 196
   5.1 Medical therapeutics 196
      5.1.1 Acute alcoholic steatohepatitis 196
   5.2 Surgical procedures 198
   5.3 Prevention 198
6. Prognosis and Natural History 198
References 198

1. INTRODUCTION

1.1 Definition

Alcohol (ethanol) is consumed throughout the secular world. Even when taken in small amounts, histologic changes in the liver (steatosis – macrovesicular fat within hepatocytes) may be observed. Such changes are without deleterious consequences. In most, ingestion of large amounts of alcohol for a long time produces no additional liver damage. In about 20%, however, serious injury, most importantly acute alcoholic steatohepatitis, fibrosis, or cirrhosis will develop. Hepatoma may be a late consequence in alcoholic cirrhosis but will not be considered further in this chapter. Since the spectrum of liver injury caused by alcohol is great it should not be surprising that clinical features will vary accordingly. This chapter will principally describe the clinical and pathological spectrum of alcoholic steatosis, steato-hepatitis, and cirrhosis.

1.2 Disease prevalence

The prevalence of alcohol-induced liver disease parallels cultural attitudes towards alcohol consump-tion. In devout Muslim countries, alcohol-related liver disease is relatively uncommon. In many

Western countries (US, France, United Kingdom), alcohol-induced liver disease is a health problem of major proportions. There is a clear relationship between *per capita* alcohol consumption and alcohol-related cirrhosis [1]. Nearly one-half of all cirrhotic deaths in the US are from alcoholic liver disease, and over US$ 1.6 billion are spent annually caring for such patients [2,3]. Many reports of the impact of alcohol on the liver are confounded by the frequent simultaneous presence of multiple liver insults, especially hepatitis C.

1.3 General demographics

As mentioned *per capita* alcohol consumption correlates well with the prevalence of liver disease. Decreased alcohol-related liver disease is observed when alcohol becomes unavailable because of war, legal prohibition, or for other reasons. Women are more susceptible to development of progressive alcoholic liver disease. They are more likely to develop acute alcoholic steatohepatitis and cirrhosis, and require less alcohol to do so [4].

Women who drink as few as seven drinks (one "drink" is either one 12 oz bottle of beer, a 4 oz glass of wine, or 1 oz of "spirits") per week may develop significant liver disease [5]. The reason for women's increased susceptibility for liver disease is poorly understood. It may lie in differences in absorption (more gastric absorption), or may be due to changes in the way alcohol is metabolized, or to gender-related difference in the induction of the numerous pathophysiologic perturbations described below.

Social and genetic differences appear to play a role in the likelihood that uncontrolled alcohol use will occur. But since none of the metabolites of alcohol degradation is sufficient to cause progressive liver disease, the role of genetic differences in producing liver damage remains to be elucidated.

2. PATHOPHYSIOLOGY

A small amount of alcohol is absorbed by the stomach. Most is absorbed by the small bowel. Its metabolism is almost exclusively hepatic. Multiple enzymatic pathways are involved including alcohol dehydrogenase and catalases. Most, however, is metabolized by the mitochondrial ethanol oxidizing system (MEOS). Cytochrome P450 enzymes, particularly isoenzyme 2E1 is responsible for a major portion of metabolism and this is an inducible enzyme. Figure 1 shows the relative contribution made to alcohol metabolism by the enzyme systems in non-drinkers and in chronic drinkers. This change occurs because of the induction of the cytochrome P450 system by alcohol. Polymorphism in alcohol

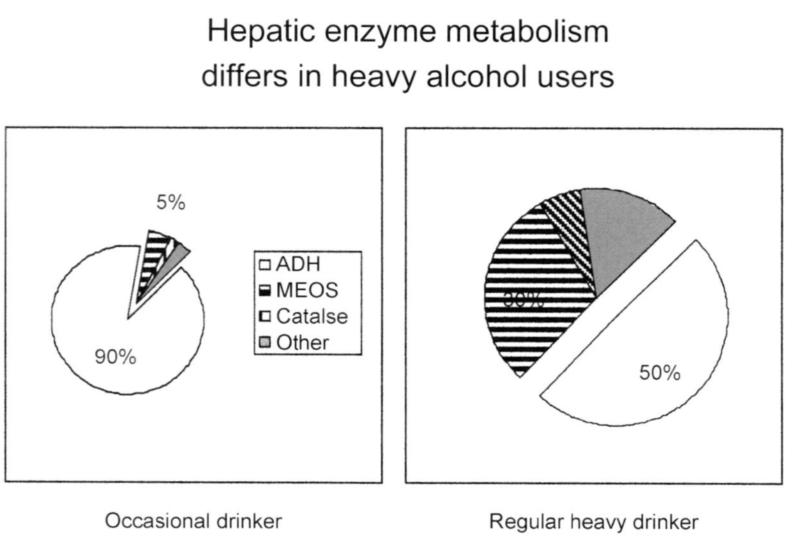

Figure 1. Chronic alcohol ingestion alters the pathways of alcohol metabolism by induction of the cytochrome P450 enzyme system.

metabolizing enzymes has been offered as an explanation for the variable susceptibility of alcoholics to progressive liver injury [6]. Despite polymorphism, alcohol metabolism by all individuals produces the same metabolites (acetaldehyde and acetate), neither of which produces steatohepatitis, fibrosis, or cirrhosis. Therefore, factors other than direct hepatotoxicity of alcohol and its metabolites must be responsible for development of progressive alcoholic liver injury.

The gut may play a role in the development of progressive liver disease in some alcoholics. It has recently been shown in alcohol-fed rats that induction of a "leaky gut" allows endotoxins to reach the portal circulation and a heightened susceptibility of the liver induction of changes of acute alcoholic hepatitis [7]. Humans with alcoholic chronic liver disease also have increased intestinal permeability [8]. Activation of Kupffer cells by endotoxin appears to be an important step in eliciting a polymorphonuclear response in alcoholic liver injury [9].

Alternate mechanisms of response to the presence of free radicals generated during alcohol metabolism may play a role [10]. The role of oxidative stress, endotoxins, and cytokines all appear to have a role in the induction of steatohepatitis, fibrosis, and cirrhosis. Higher levels of endotoxin, lipid peroxidation, nuclear factor kappa B, chemokines, monocyte chemotactic protein 1, macrophage inflammatory protein 2, tumor necrosis factor alpha, and cyclo-oxygenases are all elevated in a rat model of acute alcohol liver injury [11]. Intercellular adhesion molecule (ICAM)-1 may mediate early leukocyte infiltration of the liver, and ICAM-1 may be responsible for eliciting TNF-1 response [12]. Figure 2 summarizes many possible factors in the production of steatohepatitis and beyond, as well as demonstrating the reversibility of steatosis, and the lesser reversibility of steatohepatitis.

Finally, multiple hepatic injuries may explain why some who abuse alcohol are more likely than others to develop fibrosis and cirrhosis. Many with alcoholic liver injury are also infected with hepatitis C virus, for example [13]. Among alcoholics, hepatitis C is more prevalent with more advanced disease, especially cirrhosis [14]. The combination of alcohol and hepatitis C appears to result in more rapid development of fibrosis and cirhosis than either insult

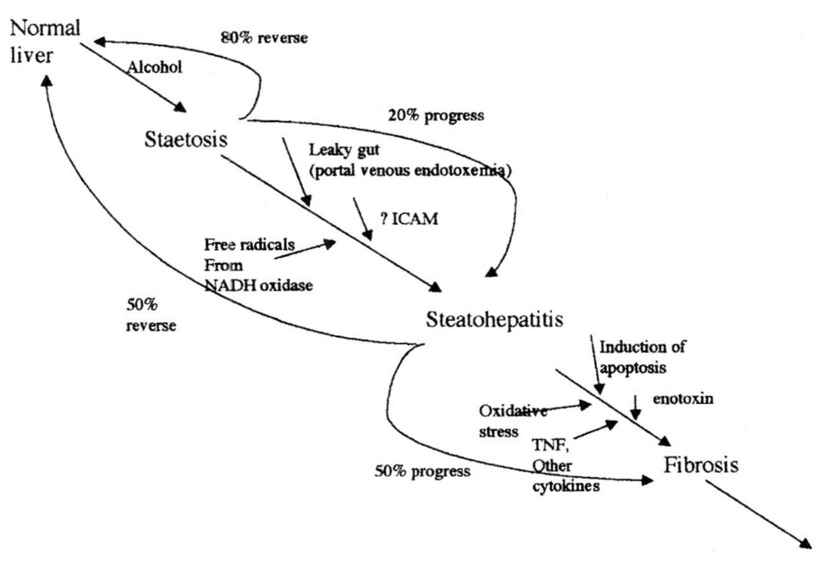

Figure 2. Alcohol produces liver injury in stages. Steatosis is 100% reversible. Only 20% of alcoholics pass from steatosis to steatohepatitis. Steatohepatitis is 50% reversible. Cirrhosis is irreversible.

alone. Iron may also serve as a co-factor for alcoholic liver injury.

3. CLINICAL FEATURES

3.1 History

It is axiomatic that alcohol-induced liver disease requires a history of moderate to heavy alcohol ingestion over many years. However, those most at risk for alcohol-induced liver disease are most likely to minimize or even deny heavy alcohol ingestion. Consideration of liver disease caused by alcohol, therefore, begins with a history, but must never end with history.

Approximately 60 g alcohol per day for women, and 80 g for men taken over 10–12 years are required to produce progressive alcoholic liver disease [15]. A brief period of heavy alcohol intake is generally insufficient to cause serious alcohol-induced liver disease. Other causes of hepatic dysfunction must be sought in those whose alcohol intake is modest or of short duration.

3.2 Steatosis (fatty liver)

Nearly all who consume even modest amounts of alcohol develop fat in the liver. This early benign and reversible phase of liver injury produces no symptoms or signs. Typical (but not diagnostic) laboratory abnormalities are discussed below.

3.3 Acute alcoholic steatohepatitis

The individual with acute alcoholic steatohepatitis may feel entirely well, and have a normal physical exam. Early symptomatic acute alcoholic hepatitis usually presents with fatigue, loss of appetite, and sometimes vomiting. Low-grade temperature elevations may be present. The physical examination at this stage may show typical features of the alcoholic: spider telangiectasias, parotid gland enlargement, and hepatomegaly. As the illness becomes more severe, the patient becomes quite ill with nausea, jaundice, and often stigmata suggesting cirrhosis, such as ascites. Decreased muscle mass may also be present.

3.4 Cirrhosis

The individual with alcohol-induced cirrhosis may be indistinguishable from others with cirrhosis, but frequently have some or all of the features noted above. The development of ascites, variceal hemorrhage, or hepatic encephalopathy often makes the diagnosis of cirrhosis obvious. In others, only laboratory parameters suggest, and a liver biopsy confirms, the presence of cirrhosis.

4. DIAGNOSIS

4.1 Blood tests

The cardinal laboratory finding in acute alcoholic liver injury is a modest elevation of the aspartate transaminase (AST), formerly referred to as serum glutamic-oxaloacetic transaminase (SGOT). With simple alcoholic steatosis, the alanine aminotransferase (ALT) formerly referred to as serum glutamate-pyruvic transaminase (SGPT) may be also mildly elevated. The gamma glutamyl transpeptidase (GGTPP) is usually elevated, but this test is not particularly useful [16]. When only steatosis is present, the other liver enzymes are usually normal. In cases of acute alcoholic steatohepatitis the AST remains elevated, but not markedly so. The ALT is usually either normal or just slightly elevated. Regardless of the severity of the disease, the AST rarely goes as high as 400 u/dl. The ratio of AST:ALT is usually >2.

Severe alcoholic hepatitis results in impairment of liver synthetic function. Abnormalities in the prothrombin time and serum albumin reflect this. Serum bilirubin elevation also parallels the severity of the alcoholic steatohepatitis. Severe disease is most often defined by a high value of the discriminant function formula:

$$\textit{Discriminant function} = 4.6\,[\text{prothrombin time (in seconds)}] + [\text{serum bilirubin (mg/dl)}] \geq 32$$

Values of 32 or higher correlate with a 50–80% short-term mortality. For this reason those with a high discriminant function are most often considered for special additional treatment (see below).

Leukocytosis is frequently seen in acute alcoholic steatohepatitis; indeed "leukemoid" reactions are described. An elevated white blood cell count in this setting does not mandate the use of antibiotics, although a search for possible infection by chest X-ray, and appropriate cultures should be undertaken. Severe dietary deficiencies are frequent in the individual who has been drinking heavily and laboratory tests may reflect this. Transient hemolysis (Zieve's syndrome) may be present when an acute alcoholic patient is first seen. This usually remits after a few days of adequate nutrition. When cirrhosis is present, laboratory findings typical for that condition may also be seen.

4.2 Imaging studies

Imaging studies in cases of alcohol-induced liver injury primarily identify two attributes: fat and (when present) cirrhotic changes (irregular liver surface, splenomegaly, ascites, varices, etc.). Imaging studies are not required as part of the investigation of otherwise typical alcohol-induced liver disease, and no imaging feature is pathognomonic of alcohol as the cause of liver disease. On the other hand, many cases of alcoholic steatosis, and steatohepatitis, first come to light because an imaging study was done for some other purpose. Ultrasonography, computerized tomography, and magnetic resonance imaging will be considered here (Table 1).

A recent report directly compares all three imaging techniques done prospectively in 25 consecutive patients with fatty liver (steatosis, steatohepatitis, fibrosis, cirrhosis). These patients, in fact, had non-alcoholic fatty liver disease, but the spectrum of histology was precisely that seen in alcoholic liver disease. None of the three imaging tests was able to distinguish steatosis alone from the more aggressive steatohepatitis. Signal changes consistent with fatty liver were not uniformly present until more than 33% of hepatocytes (as judged by biopsy) contained fat. Intraobserver error was at least moderate for all

Table 1. Imaging characteristics of fatty liver with or without steatohepatitis.

Ultrasonography	Computerized tomography	Magnetic resonance imaging
Signal features		
Increase in fine echoes	Decreased signal in liver(compared, for example, to spleen)	Decreased signal in in-phase images, compared to opposed-phase images
Patterns		
Diffuse hyperechoic nodules	Diffuse focal sparing	Diffuse focal sparing

tests (least discordance for MRI, and most for computerized tomography) [17]. In summary, imaging studies are of limited utility in the diagnosis of steatosis, and not helpful in identifying those with more aggressive disease. Considerable fat may be present within the liver even when scanning studies are normal. Ultrasonography performs about as well as more expensive testing.

4.3 Pathology

The histologic abnormality that is direct and dose related is steatosis – fat accumulation in the hepatocyte cytoplasm. Macrovesicular fat typically displaces the cell nucleus to the cell periphery. Steatosis occurs within hours of alcohol ingestion and is completely reversible. Even on a chronic basis, steatosis is well tolerated, does not usually elicit a fibrotic response, and is not likely to result in cirrhosis. Most of the finding characteristic for alcohol-induced liver injury may also been seen in the non-alcoholic. Care must be taken to avoid assuming that because certain histologic features are present, the etiology of the liver disease must be from alcohol. An excellent review of the pathology of alcoholic hepatitis is available [18]. Figure 3a–c shows the typical histologic findings of steatohepatitis and alcoholic cirrhosis. Certain features are shared by alcoholic and non-alcoholic fatty liver disease, as indicated in Table 2.

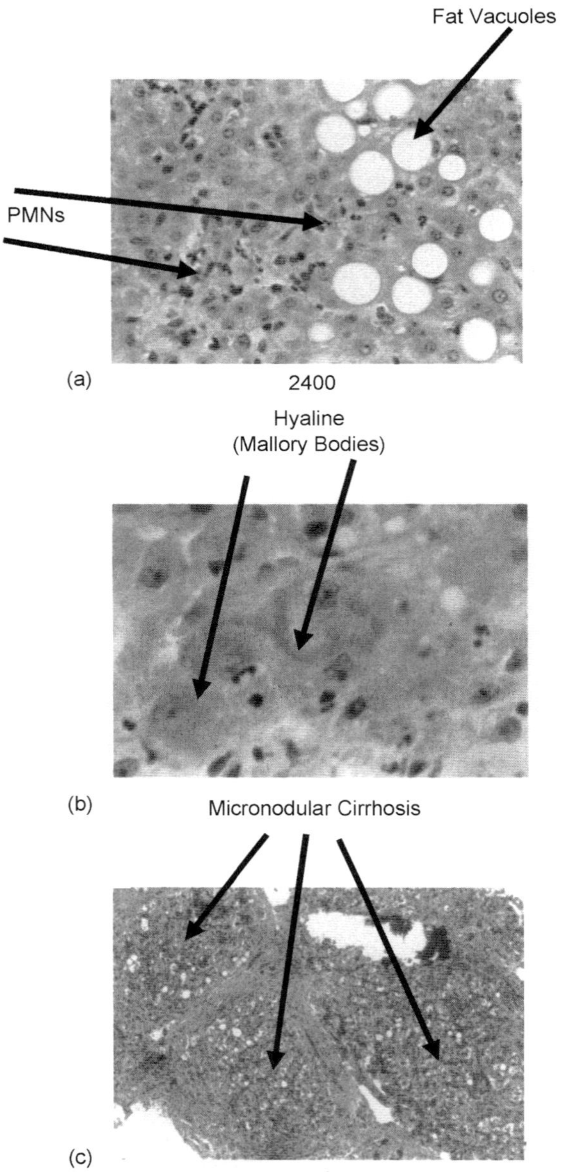

Figure 3. (a) Liver biopsy showing infiltration by polymorphonuclear cells (PMNs). Many hepatocytes contain fat vacuoles. Note the displacement of the cell nucleus to the periphery of the hepatocytes. These changes are typical for acute alcoholic hepatitis. (b) High-power view of hepatocytes. In the cytoplasm is a ropy material, variously called hyaline, Mallory bodies, and sometimes alcoholic hyaline. Mallory bodies are seen in non-alcoholic steatohepatitis as well. (c) Well-developed cirrhosis due to alcohol. Trichrome stain reveals broad fibrous septa (blue), and small nodules (2–4 mm) of regenerating hepatocytes. Although some fat vacuoles are seen, most other features of active alcoholic liver disease are absent.

Liver biopsy is helpful, but not essential in establishing the diagnosis of alcohol-induced liver disease. Liver biopsy may be relatively contraindicated in sicker patients with acute alcoholic steatohepatitis due to coagulation defects and ascites. Even in the sickest patients, liver biopsy employing the transvenous route may be done if the information to be obtained is deemed to be sufficiently important. In many cases, it is reasonable to proceed to develop a therapeutic plan without a biopsy. In most cases, a biopsy should be considered once the acute episode is over so that the amount of structural liver damage can be assessed.

5. MANAGEMENT

5.1 Medical therapeutics

A clinical practice guideline on the management of alcoholic liver disease has recently been published [19].

Fatty liver. This may require no treatment, since fatty liver from modest alcohol intake has not been shown to represent a progressive process. The serendipitous finding of a fatty liver by ultrasound, with normal or slightly abnormal liver tests should initiate discovery of the individual's drinking pattern. Other risk factors for fatty liver should also be elucidated (obesity, diabetes, lipid abnormalities, etc.), and, where appropriate, treated. The patient should be counseled about the deleterious health consequences of excess alcohol intake. Referral to a chemical dependence specialist should be considered in selected cases. Fatty liver from alcohol is reversible within a few weeks of alcohol abstinence.

5.1.1 Acute alcoholic steatohepatitis

Milder cases may be treated on an outpatient basis. Of paramount importance is cessation of alcohol. Most individuals with this condition have lost control over their drinking and should be referred to a health professional with expertise in the field of alcohol and chemical dependency. Nutrition, often

Table 2. Histologic features of alcohol induced, and non-alcoholic fatty liver disease, demonstrating considerable overlap.

	Non-alcoholic fatty liver disease	Alcoholic fatty liver disease
Reversible liver lesions		
Steatosis	++++	++++
Ballooned hepatocytes	++++	++++
Hepatocyte necrosis	++++	++++
Progressive liver lesions		
Lobular polymorphonuclear inflammation	+++	++++
Mallory hyaline	+++	++++
Megamitochondria	++++	++++
Fibrosis	++++	++++
Sclerosing hyaline necrosis	+	+++
Cholestasis	0	++
Microvesicular steatosis "foamy degeneration"	+ (Reye's syndrome, drugs, acute fatty liver of pregnancy)	++
Cirrhosis	++	++

+ indicates relative frequency of finding.

neglected, is important. Those with more severe disease, especially when the discriminant function is >32 (see above) should initially be admitted to hospital. This step underscores to patient and family the seriousness of the condition and allows for certain discontinuation of alcohol and institution of needed nutritional and pharmacological treatment. Attention should be directed not only to the liver disease, but to possible other end-organ damage, including brain and heart. During the first 72 h vigilance to possible emergence of alcohol withdrawal syndrome is necessary, and should be treated aggressively when present.

Sicker patients with alcoholic hepatitis often have marked anorexia. The role of nutrition in the management of this condition is underscored by studies which show that an aggressive nutritional approach by use of enteral feedings results in improved survival when compared to merely encouraging the patient to eat [20,21]. Special protein diets (low in aromatic amino acids, rich in branched chain amino acids) are costly and not worth the expense.

Pharmacotherapy for alcoholic hepatitis should be considered for sicker patients with acute alcoholic hepatitis. Most often considered are corticosteroids. Some, but not all, studies indicate the value of corticosteroids [22]. Metaanalysis of published studies provides reasonably clear guidelines for the use of corticosteroids (e.g. 30–40 mg prednisone daily for 1 month) for severe disease [23].

When first seen, some patients with severe alcoholic hepatitis appear septic even when they are not. A search for infection should be undertaken. Finding none, the use of corticosteroids should not be unreasonably withheld. When corticosteroids cannot be used, alternative therapies may be considered. Anabolic steroids, propylthiouracil, insulin, and glucagon and antifibrotics are all subjects of a few favorable reports, but on balance appear to be of limited value in the management of severe acute alcoholic hepatitis.

Pentoxifylline, a tumor necrosis factor inhibitor, has recently been reported to be of benefit. Given in a dosage of 400 mg orally three times daily for a month, patients developed hepatorenal syndrome less often, and had improved survival compared to those given placebo [24]. This study is promising, but needs confirmation. Studies comparing the effect of corticosteroids and pentoxifylline in the management of acute alcoholic hepatitis are also needed. Etanercept binds and neutralizes unbound serum tumor necrosis factor (TNF). There is reason to consider this agent in therapy for acute alcoholic hepatitis. Despite encouraging pilot study data [25], a randomized prospective double blind study of etanercept together with prednisolone unexpectedly showed increased mortality after 2 months [26] in those who received etanercept. This agent should not be used in the treatment of acute alcoholic hepatitis outside of research trials.

Chronic therapy of the patient with severe alcoholic liver disease has been attempted. Colchicine does not appear to be helpful. One study suggests a role for propylthiouracil (PTU), especially for those who continue to drink a modest amount of alcohol. A 50% reduction (from 25% seen in placebo-treated patients, to 13% in PTU-treated patients) in 2-year mortality was seen in patients who received PTU 150 mg twice daily [27]. This approach has not been widely embraced, in part because there are no supporting studies demonstrating its value. It is also difficult to select patients who might benefit, especially since the amount of alcohol an individual consumes may vary from time to time, and in any event, may not be reliably reported to the physician.

5.2 Surgical procedures

The patient with advanced alcoholic liver disease has a high mortality risk. Liver transplantation is an option for the failing liver. Prior to transplantation, alcohol abstinence is generally required. This requirement, plus the short supply of donor organs, makes liver transplantation for severe alcoholic steatohepatitis inappropriate. However, the patient with alcoholic cirrhosis who has undergone rehabilitation and has had a significant period of alcohol abstinence is a good candidate for liver transplantation. Disease recurrence is a frequent occurrence for most diseases for which liver transplantation is done, and recurrent alcoholic liver disease is no exception. Although up to one-third of previous alcoholics will return to some form of drinking within 4 years after transplantation, often alcohol intake is insufficient to re-create liver disease. Recurrent alcoholic liver disease is uncommon, and outcomes quite good [28]. Patients with end-stage alcoholic cirrhosis should be considered for liver transplantation services.

5.3 Prevention

Prevention of alcohol-related liver disease is conceptually simple – avoidance of alcohol excess. However, in most parts of the world alcohol is deeply ingrained in the social, cultural, and religious fabric of life. Prevention of excessive use of alcohol requires a thorough understanding of its contextual basis. An excellent review of this topic is available [29].

6. PROGNOSIS AND NATURAL HISTORY

The prognosis of alcoholic liver disease is highly dependent on severity. Those with simple steatosis have an excellent prognosis, with or without continued drinking. Cessation of drinking will result in disappearance of steatosis within weeks. The lesion of alcoholic steatohepatitis may remit with alcohol cessation, but in about 50% of cases severe fibrosis or cirrhosis will result [30]. The prognosis for those with alcoholic steatohepatitis depends both on the severity of the disease, and upon the ability of the patient to abstain from alcohol. Several indices are available to predict survival in the setting of acute alcoholic hepatitis. The discriminant function is discussed above. Those with a discriminant score of 32 or higher have a 50% short-term mortality rate. A scoring system with even better ability to predict short-term survival in patients with alcoholic steatohepatitis is the Composite Clinical Laboratory Index. This Index requires information about hepatomegaly, splenomegaly, ascites, encephalopathy, clinical bleeding, spider telangiectasias, palmar erythema, peripheral edema, anorexia, weakness, and laboratory values for ALT, alkaline phosphatase, albumin, prothrombin time, and bilirubin. A CCLI of 6 correlates with a short-term mortality of 20%, whereas a CCLI of 21 predicts 100% short-term mortality [31]. Its complexity precludes its widespread use as a clinical tool despite its power to predict outcome. For short-term predictions of outcomes from acute alcoholic hepatitis, the discriminant function is the most practical; for predicting survival in those with alcoholic cirrhosis, the Child's Pugh score is most appropriate.

REFERENCES

[1] Dufor, M., Stinson, F.S. and FeCaces, M. (1993) Trends in cirrhosis morbidity and mortality: United States 1979–1988. *Semin. Liver Dis.* **13**, 109–116.

[2] Orholm, M., Sorenson, T.I., Bentsen, K., Hoyboye, G., Eghoje, K. and Christofferson, P. (1985) Mortality of alcohol-abusing men prospectively assessed in relation to history of abuse and degree of liver injury. *Liver* **5**, 253–260.

[3] Grant, B.F., DeBakey, S. and Zobeck, T.S. (1991) *Surveillance Report No. 18 – Liver Cirrhosis Mortality in the United States, 1973–1988* (National Institutes of Alcohol Abuse and Alcoholism, Rockville, MD).

[4] Norton, R., Batey, R. and Dwyer, T. (1987) Alcohol consumption and the risk of alcohol-related cirrhosis in women. *Br. Med. J.* **295**, 80–82.

[5] Becker, U., Deis, A., Sorensen, T.I.A., Gronbaek, M.N., Borch-Johnsen, K., Muller, C.F., Schnohr, P. and Jensen, G. (1996) Prediction of risk of liver disease by alcohol intake, sex, and age: a prospective population study. *Hepatology* **23**, 1025–1029.

[6] Frenzer, A., Butler, W.J., Norton, I.D., Wilson, J.S., Apte, M.V., Pirola, R.C., Ryan, P. and Roberts-Thompson, I.C. (2002) Polymorphism in alcohol-metabolizing enzymes, glutathione *S*-transferase and apolipoprotein E and susceptibility to alcohol-induced cirrhosis. *J. Gastroenterol. Hepatol.* **17**, 177–182.

[7] Mathurin, P., Deng, Q.G., Keshavarzian, A., Choudhary, S., Holmes, E.W. and Tsukamoto, H. (2000) Exacerbation of alcohol liver injury by enteral endotoxin in rats. *Hepatology* **32**, 1008–1017.

[8] Keshavarzian, A., Holmes, E.W., Patel, M., Iber, F., Fields, J.Z. and Pethkar, S. (1999) Leaky gut in alcoholic cirrhosis: a possible mechanism for alcohol-induced liver damage. *Am. J. Gastroenterol.* **94**, 200–207.

[9] Thurman, R.G. (1998) Alcoholic liver injury involves activation of Kupffer cells by endotoxin. *Am. J. Physiol.* **275**, G605–G611.

[10] Cardin, R., D'Errico, A., Fiorentino, M., Cecchetto, A., Naccarato, R. and Farinati, F. (2002) Hepatocyte proliferation and apoptosis in relation to oxidative damage in alcohol related liver disease. *Alcohol Alcohol.* **37**, 43–48.

[11] Nanji, A.A., Jokelainen, K., Fotouhinia, M., Rahemtulla, A., Thomas, P., Tipoe, G.L., Su, G.L. and Dannenberg, A.J. (2001) Increased severity of alcoholic liver injury in female rats: role of oxidative stress, endotoxin, and chemokines. *Am. J. Physiol. Liver Physiol.* **28**, G1348–G1356.

[12] Kono, H., Uesugi, T., Froh, M., Rusyn, I., Bradford, B.U. and Thurman, R.G. (2001) ICAM-1 is involved in the mechanism of alcohol-induced liver injury: studies with knock-out mice. *Am. J. Gastrointest. Liver Physiol.* **280**, G1289–G1295.

[13] Oshita, M., Hayashi, N., Kasahara, A., Hagiwara, H., Mita, E., Naito, M., Katayama, K., Kasahara, K., Fusamoto, H. and Kamada, T. (1994) Increased serum hepatitis C RNA levels among alcoholic patients with chronic hepatitis C. *Hepatology* **20**, 1115–1120.

[14] Pares, A., Barrera, J.M., Caballeria, J., Ercilla, G., Bruguera, M., Caballeria, L., Castillo, R. and Rodes, J. (1990) Hepatitis C virus antibodies in chronic alcoholic patients: associations with severity of liver injury. *Hepatology* **12**, 1295–1299.

[15] Grant, B.F., Dufour, M.C. and Harford, T.C. (1988) Epidemiology of alcoholic liver disease. *Semin. Liver Dis.* **8**, 12–25.

[16] Carey, W.D. (2000) How should a patient with an isolated GGT elevation be evaluated? *Cleve. Clin. J. Med.* **67**, 315–316.

[17] Saadeh, S., Younossi, Z.M., Remer, E.M., Gramlich, T., Ong, J.P., Hurley, M., Mullen, K.D., Cooper, J.N. and Sheridan, M.J. (2002) The utility of radiologic imaging in non-alcoholic fatty liver disease. *Gastroenterology* **123**(3), 745–750.

[18] Brunt, E. (2002) Alcoholic and non-alcoholic steatohepatitis. *Clin. Liver Dis.* **6**, 399–420.

[19] McCullough, A.J. and O'Connor, J.F.B. (1998) Alcoholic liver disease: proposed recommendations for the American College of Gastroenterology. *Am. J. Gastroenterol.* **93**, 2022–2036.

[20] Cabre, E., Gonzale-Huix, F., Abad-LaCruz, A., Esteve, M., Acero, D., Fernandez-Banares, F., Xiol, X. and Gassull, M.A. (1990) Effect of enteral nutrition on the short-term outcome of severely malnourished cirrhotics. *Gastroenterology* **98**, 715–720.

[21] Kearns, P.J., Young, H., Garcia, G., Blaschke, T., O'Hanlon, G., Rinki, M., Sucher, K. and Gregory, P. (1999) Accelerated improvement in alcohol liver disease with enteral nutrition. *Gastroenterology* **102**, 200–205.

[22] Ramond, M.J., Poynard, T., Rueff, B., Mathurin, P., Theodore, C., Chaput, J.C. and Benhamou, J.P. (1992) A randomized trial of prednisolone in patients with severe alcoholic hepatitis. *N. Engl. J. Med.* **326**, 507–510.

[23] Imperiale, T.F. and McCullough, A.J. (1990) Do corticosteroids reduce mortality from alcoholic hepatitis? A metaanalysis of the randomized trials. *Ann. Intern. Med.* **113**, 299–303.

[24] Akriviadis, E., Botla, R. and Briggs, W. (2000) Pentoxifylline improves short term survival in severe acute alcoholic hepatitis: a double-blind placebo-controlled trial. *Gastroenterology* **119**, 1637–1648.

[25] Menon, K.V.N., Stadheim, L., Kamath, P.S., Wiesner, R.H., Gores, G.J., Peine, C.J., and Shah, V. (2004)

A pilot study of the safety and tolerability of etanercept in patients with alcoholic hepatitis. *Am. J. Gastroenterol.* **99**, 225–260.

[26] Naveau, S., Chollet-Martin, S., Dharancy, S., Mathurin, P., Jouet, P., Piquet, M.-A., Davion, T.D., Oberti, F., Broet, P. and Emilie, D. (2004) A double-blind randomized controlled trial of Infliximab associated with prednisolone in acute alcoholic hepatitis. *Hepatology* **39**, 1390–1397.

[27] Orrego, H., Blake, J.E., Blendis, L.M., Compton, K.V. and Israel, Y.(1987) Long term treatment of alcoholic liver disease with propylthiouracil. *N. Engl. J. Med.* **317**, 1421–1427.

[28] Weisner, R.H., Lombardero, M., Lake, J.R., Everheat, J. and Detre, K.M. (1997) Liver transplantation for end-stage alcoholic liver disease: an assessment of outcomes. *Liver Transpl. Surg.* **3**, 231–239.

[29] Georgi, J.M. (2001) Transplantation in patients with alcoholic liver disease, in *Medical Care of the Liver Transplant Patient*, eds. Killenberg, P. and Clavien, P.-A., 2nd edition (Blackwell Science, Oxford).

[30] Pares, A., Caballeria, J. and Bruguera, M. (1986) Histologic course of alcoholic hepatitis: influence of abstinence, sex, and extent of hepatic damage. *J. Hepatol.* **2**, 33–42.

[31] Orego, H., Israel, Y., Blake, J.E. and Medline, A. (1983) Assessment of prognostic factors in alcoholic liver disease: towards a global quantitative expression of severity. *Hepatology* **3**, 896–905.

Hepatology: A Practical Approach
B. Al Knawy, M.L. Shiffman, R.H. Wiesner (editors)

Chapter 11
Alpha 1-Antitrypsin Deficiency

Suzanne Herten-Wittig[a], *James K. Stoller*[b] *and Zobair M. Younossi*[a]

[a]Center for Liver Diseases, Inova Fairfax Hospital, Falls Church, VA, USA

[b]Department of Pulmonary/Critical Care Medicine, The Cleveland Clinic Foundation, Cleveland, OH, USA

1. Introduction 201
2. Pathophysiology 202
3. Clinical Features 203
4. Diagnosis 204
5. Management 205
6. Prognosis 207
7. Conclusions 207
References 208

1. INTRODUCTION

Alpha 1-antitrypsin deficiency is a relatively common inherited disorder that can present in different ways, depending on which organ systems are affected. The primary organ systems involved are the liver and the lungs, with the end results being cirrhosis and emphysema, respectively. The mechanisms of disease differ in emphysema and cirrhosis, despite the fact that the predisposition involves the same genetic mutation. Although this disease is due to a single gene mutation, the clinical manifestations vary substantially, as there is allelic variability as well as differing degrees of cellular end organ injury. Recent advances in molecular biology have shed light on the pathophysiology of this disease. However, many unanswered questions remain, including optimal and effective therapeutic strategies. This chapter will review key aspects of alpha 1-antitrypsin (AAT) deficiency, focusing on liver disease. We present the genetics, pathophysiology, and clinical features of AAT deficiency. Finally, we discuss management and prognosis.

Alpha 1-antitrypsin deficiency was first identified in 1963 when individuals with a deficient alpha band on a serum protein electrophoresis were found to have early-onset COPD and a family history of emphysema [1]. Alpha 1-antitrypsin is a member of the family of serine protease inhibitors (also known as the serpins) which control vital intra- and extracellular pathways [2]. In the lung, alpha 1-antitrypsin protects connective tissue from destruction by neutrophil elastase, which is released by leukocytes. Affected patients with severe AAT deficiency are predisposed to panlobular basal emphysema, asthma, bronchiectasis, and, in some patients, vasculitis [3]. Many patients first develop these pulmonary symptoms and experience shortened survival and, as such, the prevalence of associated liver disease may be underestimated.

The gene that encodes alpha 1-antitrypsin is located on the long arm of chromosome 14 (14q32.1). Each individual inherits one allele from each parent and the two alleles are co-dominantly expressed. To date, over 100 allelic variants have been described. Most variants are due to point mutations (i.e., one base substitution or deletion). These variants can be classified into four groups: normal, deficient, null, and dysfunctional [4].

The normal phenotype (the so-called PI*MM, where PI stands for "protease inhibitor") characterizes 95% of Caucasian Americans and almost all non-Caucasians. Individuals with this phenotype have normal levels of fully functioning alpha 1-antitrypsin.

Patients with a deficient allele have an alpha 1-antitrypsin mutation that causes decreased levels of this protease inhibitor. Ten percent of people of European descent carry one of the two most common deficient alleles: the S mutation and the Z mutation. The S mutation, in which a valine substitutes for a glutamic acid residue at position 264 (i.e., summarized as Glu264Val), occurs more commonly than the Z allele. Patients who are homozygous for the S mutation (PI*SS) experience a 40% decrease in the serum concentration of alpha 1-antitrypsin. However, this minor decrease by itself does not pose a significant threat to health because their serum levels exceed a protective threshold (see below); individuals with the PI*SS phenotype are not at risk for emphysema or liver disease [5].

The Z allele (Glu342Lys), which occurs in 3% of the US population, causes an 85% decrease in plasma alpha 1-antitrypsin concentration [5]. Because each allele is expressed co-dominantly, ZZ homozygotes do not produce sufficient levels of alpha 1-antitrypsin to ensure protection of the lungs from proteolysis by neutrophil elastase. The 85% reduction in serum levels of AAT associated with the PI*ZZ phenotype produces serum levels below a so-called “protective threshold” value, which is felt to be the minimal level needed to confer lung protection against neutrophil elastase. Individuals with the Z allele are also at risk for liver disease, though the pathogenesis of liver disease relates to polymerization of Z-type protein within the hepatocytes rather than to unopposed proteolysis. Approximately 10% of PI*SZ individuals have serum levels below the protective threshold.

Patients with null and dysfunctional alleles are rare. Patients in the null group have a defect in transcription or translation and thus do not produce any alpha 1-antitrypsin. The absence of AAT in serum predisposes to severe emphysema, though null alleles are not associated with liver disease because null-type AAT does not accumulate within hepatocytes.

Finally, the rare patient with dysfunctional alpha 1-antitrypsin alleles produces alpha 1-antitrypsin with aberrant function. For example, patients with the Pittsburgh variant of alpha 1-antitrypsin present with a bleeding diathesis, because the dysfunctional alpha 1-antitrypsin acts as a thrombin inhibitor [5].

2. PATHOPHYSIOLOGY

As a member of the serine protease inhibitor (serpin) family, AAT is vulnerable to misfolding. A conformational change in AAT impairs its ability to bind to and neutralize neutrophil elastase function, and its ability to be secreted from the hepatocyte. As such, alpha 1-antitrypsin deficiency is an example of a “conformational disease”, which is primarily due to the polymerization of aberrant forms of the protein, most notably the Z-type protein [5].

Severe alpha 1-antitrypsin deficiency predisposes to emphysema, but also to the development of cirrhosis. A key pathophysiologic understanding of AAT deficiency is that the liver disease is not due to a deficiency of protease inhibition, but rather to polymerization of the variant protein within the hepatocytes, where the protein is mainly synthesized. The result is impaired secretion of alpha 1-antitrypsin from hepatocytes and accumulation of polymers of alpha 1-antitrypsin within liver cells that can be seen by light microscopy on liver biopsy. These polymers stain as PAS-positive inclusions in the rough endoplasmic reticulum of hepatocytes, and are a pathologic hallmark of AAT deficiency [6].

Because of this polymerization process, PI*ZZ type alpha 1-antitrypsin deficiency has also been called “inclusion body hepatocellular disease” [7]. Specifically, the single amino acid substitution (lysine for glutamic acid at position 342) that characterizes the Z protein causes abnormal protein folding, which predisposes to intrahepatocytic polymerization in a mechanism dubbed “loop sheet polymerization” [8]. Liver damage is found only in patients with the allelic variants of alpha 1-antitrypsin that aggregate and accumulate within hepatocytes, namely the Z, Mmalton, and Mduarte variants. The null phenotype does not predispose to cirrhosis because no protein is synthesized.

Though the precise mechanism of liver damage is incompletely understood, it appears that liver disease results from the net effect of intrahepatocyte polymerization and impaired cellular mechanisms to clear intrahepatocyte protein.

Molecular and biologic studies have shown that an intense inflammatory response, with production of interleukins (i.e., endotoxin, IL-6 and TNF), leads to increased production of alpha 1-antitrypsin. The elevated rate of synthesis is temperature-dependent; therefore, fever and inflammation should be aggressively treated in these patients to slow the production of abnormal proteins. The increased synthesis of the variant forms of alpha 1-antitrypsin can cause worsening transaminitis with faster progression to cirrhosis and end-stage liver disease [6].

3. CLINICAL FEATURES

The liver disease associated with alpha 1-antitrypsin deficiency characteristically affects two distinct age groups: newborns through first few years of life and adults over the age of 50. Children who present with alpha 1-antitrypsin deficiency classically present with acute hepatitis and jaundice. These symptoms follow and should be distinguished from the physiologic jaundice of the newborn. Alpha 1-antitrypsin deficiency should be suspected if a newborn has an elevated conjugated bilirubin during the first 4 months of life. Almost all of these newborns will have hepatomegaly and approximately half of them will have associated splenomegaly.

The largest study of the natural history of alpha 1-antitrypsin deficiency involved screening 200,000 Swedish newborns. The prevalence of the PI*ZZ phenotype was 1:1575 infants. Of those with this phenotype, 11% developed hepatocellular damage – starting as neonatal hepatitis and cholestasis between 4 days and 4 months after birth and persisting for up to 1 year. Other children manifested hepatomegaly with elevated transaminases but without evidence of hepatic decompensation. Of 14 children with neonatal hepatitis, 21% progressed to cirrhosis by age 7. The remainder remained healthy at age 8 with intermittent elevations of AST and ALT [9].

In the subset of newborns (10–15%) with neonatal hepatitis, 5% remained jaundiced, with cirrhosis and death resulting at 1 year. The remaining infants displayed one of the four clinical patterns (about 25% each):

1. resolution of hepatitis by age 3–10 years without hepatosplenomegaly;
2. development of cirrhosis with end-stage liver disease or death between 6 months and 17 years of age;
3. evidence of cirrhosis by histology but without symptoms for more than 10 years;
4. persistence of elevated transaminases without cirrhosis [10].

Adults with the PI*ZZ phenotype often present with pulmonary manifestations before liver dysfunction. As stated previously, AAT deficiency is under-recognized in adults. In reality, alpha 1-antitrypsin deficiency (PI*ZZ phenotype) may be one of the most common hereditary causes of chronic liver disease. Still some patients may not exhibit clinical manifestations despite severe deficiency of AAT. Other patients with liver disease may have more common risk factors or environmental exposures (e.g., alcohol, hepatitis B, or hepatitis C) which may preclude the physician's recognizing associated alpha 1-antitrypsin deficiency. In fact, retrospective studies have shown that there is an average delay of 7.2 years between the onset of symptoms and the confirmatory diagnosis of alpha 1-antitrypsin deficiency. In one study, over 40% of patients saw at least three physicians and 12% saw 6–10 physicians before the diagnosis was first made [11]. These observations underscore the need to heighten physicians' awareness of this disease. Notably, 2–3% of patients with chronic obstructive pulmonary disease have severe deficiency of alpha 1-antitrypsin, yet fewer than 10,000 of the expected 100,000 severely AAT-deficient Americans have been diagnosed [12].

Individuals with at-risk alleles may develop adult-onset cirrhosis or hepatoma, often without antecedent liver disease in childhood. Interestingly, hepatoma may occur in the absence of cirrhosis and thus patients identified as deficient in alpha 1-antitrypsin should be monitored accordingly. The risk of hepatoma is greater in males than in females. In an early study of 246 PI*ZZ homozygotes, cirrhosis occurred in 11.8% and hepatoma in 3.3% [13].

Patients with pulmonary manifestations of alpha 1-antitrypsin deficiency typically develop panacinar emphysema [1,14]. Afflicted patients may be non-smokers and are younger than would be expected to develop COPD (i.e., <50 years old). The pathogenesis of AAT-deficient emphysema is an imbalance between elastase (secreted from neutrophils in the lungs) and alpha 1-antitrypsin, which is the major elastase inhibitor in the lung interstitium. Neutrophil elastase destroys elastin, a component of the intra-alveolar matrix, and ultimately leads to emphysema [15,16]. Individuals with severe deficiency of AAT may also develop bronchiectasis or asthma, both of which lead to obstructive airway disease. Most patients with pulmonary symptoms are PI*ZZ homozygotes, and have a serum alpha 1-antitrypsin level below the threshold necessary to protect the lung from damage. The normal range of plasma alpha 1-antitrypsin levels is between 20 and 53 umol/l (150–350 mg/dl). PI*ZZ homozygotes often have levels as low as 5–6 umol/l (30–40 mg/dl). Pooled data suggest that a level of 11 umol/l (80 mg/dl) is the so-called "protective threshold" below which patients are susceptible to lung damage [3].

Not all patients who are severely deficient in alpha 1-antitrypsin will develop emphysema. Several risk factors predispose to the development of pulmonary disease in these patients. Other genetic modifiers of COPD risk are suspected but currently incompletely understood. These known risk factors include smoking, a parental history of COPD [17], and some occupational exposures. Smoking is very strongly associated with the development of fixed airway obstruction in these patients and actually can accelerate the onset of symptoms by as much as 19 years [18]. Non-smokers with the PI*SZ phenotype rarely develop COPD [19].

Individuals with COPD associated with alpha 1-antitrypsin deficiency share many features with the "typical", AAT-replete COPD patient, but also have distinctive clinical features. Like patients with AAT-replete COPD, the initial symptom is usually dyspnea on exertion, which is progressive in nature. Eventually, many will develop a chronic cough, sputum production, and wheezing. Unlike "typical", AAT-replete COPD patients, AAT-deficient patients will exhibit bullous changes that are more prominent, or at least as prominent, in the bases as in the apices on chest X-ray. In one large series, the mean age of onset of emphysema in alpha 1-antitrypsin-deficient patients was 46 years (± 11 years) versus 60–70 years in AAT-replete COPD patients [20].

Aside from the common manifestations of alpha 1-antitrypsin deficiency discussed above, other organs may be affected by AAT deficiency. Specifically, skin involvement may present as panniculitis, due to unopposed proteolysis in the skin. This mechanism is similar to that which causes proteolytic damage in the lung. Affected patients may present with inflammatory skin lesions. Another well-established association is Wegener's granulomatosis. Specifically, the frequency of deficient AAT alleles among individuals with Wegener's granulomatosis is higher than for the overall population, raising the possibility that deficient AAT phenotypes predispose to vasculitis. Current views suggest that AAT can bind proteinase 3, the antigen implicated in C-ANCA-positive vasculitis, and that AAT deficiency allows greater antigenicity. Other conditions speculated to be associated with AAT deficiency include vascular disease, such as fibromuscular dysplasia or aneurysms, inflammatory bowel disease, glomerulonephritis, IgA deficiency, and rheumatoid arthritis. Membranoproliferative glomerulonephritis has rarely been associated with the PI*ZZ phenotype; all affected patients have also had cirrhosis, raising the possibility that the membranoproliferative glomerulonephritis develops because of liver disease. Finally, the mechanism by which IgA nephropathy develops is felt to be related to Kupffer cell impairment, with resultant inability to remove IgA-containing complexes from the circulation and IgA deposition in the kidney [13].

4. DIAGNOSIS

Testing for alpha 1-antitrypsin deficiency should be considered (especially) in patients of Northern European descent with clinical, biochemical, or histological evidence of liver disease. Minor elevations in transaminases (AST or ALT <1.5 times the upper limit of normal) may be the only clue to underlying hepatic disease. In the context that AAT deficiency is under-recognized by clinicians, alpha 1-antitrypsin deficiency should be suspected and tested for in the following clinical circumstances: men >50 years old with chronic hepatitis, portal hypertension, cirrhosis or hepatocellular carcinoma [6]; a history of neonatal hepatitis; a personal or family history of "unexplained" liver disease or COPD, a personal history of COPD, especially in a non-smoker or with onset at an earlier than expected age (e.g., <50 years), or in an individual with a chest X-ray showing basilar hyperlucency. It is important to remember that in many instances, liver and lung disease may not coexist in the same patient.

The initial diagnostic test to perform in a patient suspected of having alpha 1-antitrypsin deficiency is a quantitative serum level of alpha 1-antitrypsin, usually performed by nephelometry. Because some available commercial standards may overestimate alpha 1-antitrypsin levels by 35–40%, high quality standards in testing are essential [4]. Cirrhosis should not lower serum levels and acute inflammation or infection can raise serum levels because AAT is an acute phase reactant, at least in heterozygotes [6] (Table 1).

Individuals with borderline or low alpha 1-antitrypsin concentrations should also undergo phenotypic analysis. Protease inhibitor (PI) phenotyping is performed by isoelectric focusing within a narrow pH gradient (pH 4–5) in a gel. Bands migrate according to their isoelectric points. The position of migration between the cathode and the anode determines the letter assigned to the variant, with

Table 1. Risk of pulmonary disease by serum level of alpha 1-antitrypsin.

Phenotype	AAT commercial level (mg/dl)	AAT true level (μmol/l)	Risk of pulmonary disease
Null–null	0	0	Extremely high risk
ZZ	20–45	2.5–7	High risk
SZ	75–120	8–19	Mild increased risk
SS	100–140	15–33	No increase
MZ	90–210	12–35	No increase
MM	150–350	20–48	No increase

The risk of pulmonary disease increases in individuals whose serum levels of AAT fall before the protective threshold value of 11 μmol (or ~ 80%).

the normal allele, M, migrating in the middle and the Z allele migrating most slowly [6]. Null alleles, for instance, do not produce any circulating protein and thus, have no isoelectric focusing bands. Very unusual variants may also require DNA/gene analysis. In addition to serum testing to establish the diagnosis of AAT deficiency, individuals with established alpha 1-antitrypsin deficiency should undergo a baseline chest X-ray, pulmonary function testing (especially with spirometry and diffusion capacity measurements), an assessment of oxygenation, and liver function tests [4].

Though not an essential part of management, liver biopsy can help to stage liver disease, rule out alternate etiologies for liver disease, and identify the alpha 1-antitrypsin polymers within hepatocytes. Neonates will often have one of the three classic histologic patterns:

1. hepatocellular damage with normal bile ducts and minimal inflammation;
2. varying degrees of portal fibrosis with ductal proliferation (often confused with biliary atresia);
3. hypoplasia of intrahepatic ducts [6].

A suggestive finding on light microscopy is the presence of PAS-positive, diastase-resistant globules in periportal hepatocytes, adjacent to bands of fibrosis (Figure 1). They appear as magenta-colored inclusions. These globules (which represent aggregated polymers of variant alpha 1-antitrypsin protein) may not be seen during the first 12 weeks of life. In addition, the size of the globules increases with age, but neither the size nor the amount of accumulated polymers correlates with the extent of liver disease. Lymphocytes are found in areas of PAS-positive globules. The process begins with low grade inflammation, starting in the portal tracts. Fibrosis characteristically increases as the disease progresses [6].

5. MANAGEMENT

Management goals for patients with alpha 1-antitrypsin deficiency include:

1. preventing progression of emphysema;
2. preventing liver damage;
3. optimizing the quality and length of affected individuals' lives.

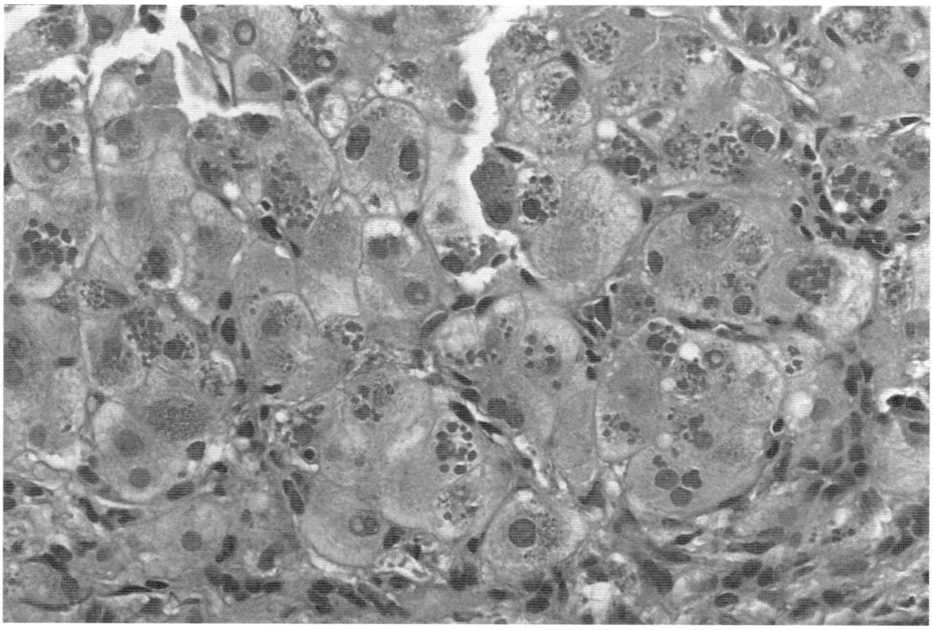

Figure 1. DPAS stain showing PAS-positive, diastase-resistant globules within the cytoplasm of numerous hepatocytes. Mild hepatocyte ballooning and a mild degree of lymphocytic interface hepatitis are also noted. (Photomicrograph courtesy of Terry Gramlich, MD, AmeriPath Inc., Oakwood Village, OH, USA.) (*For colored version, see Plate XX on page 575 at the end of the book.*)

General therapy for emphysema due to alpha 1-antitrypsin deficiency is identical to that for patients with alpha 1-antitrypsin-replete emphysema. Specifically, judicious use of bronchodilators, supplemental oxygen, pulmonary rehabilitation, and preventive strategies, such as influenza and pneumococcal vaccinations, is recommended [21]. Specific therapy for COPD due to alpha 1-antitrypsin deficiency involves the infusion of pooled human plasma alpha 1-antiprotease, the so-called "intravenous augmentation therapy". The goal of intravenous augmentation therapy is to obtain serum levels above the protective threshold of 11 μM/L, so as to interdict progression of emphysema. Available evidence supports the biochemical efficacy of intravenous augmentation therapy, in that serum levels can be brought and maintained above 11 μM/L for almost the entire dosing interval (e.g., once weekly) [22], while the infused serum protein maintains its functional activity, including in the lung. While no definitive randomized controlled trial of augmentation therapy is available [23], observational clinical studies suggest that intravenous augmentation therapy is associated with a slowed rate of decline of lung function in individuals with established emphysema of moderate severity [24–26]. Also, observational studies do suggest a survival advantage among intravenous augmentation therapy recipients [24].

In addition to the three currently available drugs for intravenous augmentation therapy, which is purified AAT from pooled human plasma, other approaches are being actively investigated. Specifically, work is under way to administer augmentation therapy by alternate routes, e.g., by inhalation. Though still under development, the appeal of inhalation augmentation therapy is that a drug can be delivered to the direct site of neutrophil elastase in an efficient and cost-effective manner. Candidate drugs for inhalation augmentation therapy include other pooled human plasma antiprotease preparations as well as recombinant alpha 1-antitrypsin, manufactured both in yeast and in transgenic sheep.

Other promising therapeutic approaches include gene therapy, in which a normal human gene is transfected into a site of AAT manufacture, whether muscle, liver cells, or lung itself. Current approaches use the adeno-associated virus vector.

Current treatment guidelines for AAT deficiency endorse the use of intravenous augmentation therapy in individuals with established emphysema of moderate degree [27,28]. Active smoking is considered a contraindication to intravenous augmentation therapy by some. Certainly, smoking cessation is actively encouraged, as cigarette smoke can inactivate alpha 1-antitrypsin by direct oxidation.

Current estimates suggest that approximately 3000 individuals are receiving regular intravenous augmentation in the United States. Supply limitations exist at times and invite the development of alternative agents and approaches. Other shortcomings of the current approach of intravenous augmentation therapy include a potential risk for transmissible diseases (e.g., prion diseases, etc.), the morbidity of receiving regular intravenous infusions (e.g., weekly or monthly for life), and the considerable expense of intravenous augmentation therapy (approximately \$30,000–\$40,000 of drug expenses per year).

Currently, specific therapy for the liver disease is unavailable, though investigational approaches include the administration of drugs that stabilize the intrahepatocyte variant AAT protein (e.g., 4-phenylbutyric acid) to encourage secretion [29]. Liver transplantation, which has been reserved for individuals with end-stage liver disease, is curative in that transplant recipients have normal type and amounts of circulating AAT.

Optimal management of the patient with AAT deficiency should also involve genetic counseling. The pattern of inheritance is autosomal co-dominant. As an instructive scenario, each child of a marriage of two PI*MZ parents has a 50% chance of inheriting one Z allele. On average, 25% of the offspring of this parentage will be PI*ZZ and PI*MM, with 50% as PI*MZ. As another common scenario, a PI*ZZ parent may wish to assess his/her child's risk for being a homozygote. In the context that genetic discrimination can affect those with established carriage of the Z allele, parents may wish to spare their children from being tested. If the spouse of a PI*ZZ individual is found to be PI*MM, each child of that pair can be predicted to be PI*MZ without their being tested. On the other hand, if the spouse is found to be PI*MZ (as are 3% of Americans), then each child has a 50% chance of being either PI*ZZ or PI*MZ and must be phenotyped to determine disease risk.

6. PROGNOSIS

Patients with severe alpha 1-antitrypsin deficiency typically experience an accelerated yearly decline in their FEV1, reflecting worsening obstructive airway disease. Liver disease can progress in a subset of patients, with cirrhosis ultimately occurring in 11.2% of patients. Without liver transplantation, the prognosis of these patients is poor. In an 11-year follow-up study of PI*ZZ homozygotes, 37% of the individuals died (~3%/year overall), with 59% of the deaths relating to respiratory failure and 13% due to complications of liver disease [3]. Survival to age 60 has been shown to be significantly lower than that for the general US population (16% survival vs. 85% for age-matched controls) [30].

7. CONCLUSIONS

Although much has been learned in recent years about the molecular and genetic basis of alpha 1-antitrypsin deficiency, many questions remain. The reasons for the wide spectrum of clinical severity are not fully understood. It seems that only 10–30% of patients with the PI*ZZ phenotype develop liver disease. Although genetic factors certainly play a role, a number of environmental factors, and possibly some yet to be defined unlinked genetic traits, may affect this rate of progression. Further research into this fascinating class of diseases, known as the "conformational diseases", will hopefully give clinicians and researchers more insight into this complex metabolic process. Clinically, patients should be followed closely and complications of liver and lung disease should be managed appropriately. Currently, patients with liver dysfunction must be followed closely for possible liver transplantation.

REFERENCES

[1] Laurell, C.-B. and Eriksson, A. (1963) The electrophoretic alpha 1-globulin pattern of serum in alpha-1 antitrypsin deficiency. *Scand. J. Clin. Lab. Invest.* **15**, 132.

[2] Potempa, J., Korzus, E. and Travis, J. (1994) The serpin superfamily of proteinase inhibitors: structure, function, and regulation. *J. Biol. Chem.* **269**, 15957–15960.

[3] Stoller, J. (2001) Clinical manifestations and natural history of alpha-1-antitrypsin deficiency. *UpToDate* 12.2.

[4] American Thoracic Society (1989) Guidelines for the approach to the patient with severe hereditary alpha 1-antitrypsin deficiency. *Am. Rev. Respir. Dis.* **140**, 1494–1497.

[5] Carrell, R. and Lomas, D. (2002) Alpha-1 antitrypsin deficiency – a model for conformational diseases. *N. Engl. J. Med.* **346**(1), 45–53.

[6] Sapienza, M.S. and Porayko, M. (2002) Alpha-1 antitrypsin deficiency and liver disease. *Clin. Perspect. Gastroenterol.* **5**, 40–48.

[7] Callea, F., Brisigotti, M., Fabbretti, G., Bonino, F. and Desmet, V.J. (1992) Hepatic endoplasmic reticulum storage diseases. *Liver* **12**, 357–362.

[8] Lomas, D.A., Finch, J.T., Seyama, K., Nukiwa, T. and Carrell, R.W. (1993) Alpha-1-antitrypsin Siiyama. Further evidence for intracellular loop-sheet polymerization. *J. Biol. Chem.* **268**, 15333.

[9] Sveger, T. (1976) Liver disease in alpha-1 antitrypsin deficiency detected by screening of 200,000 infants. *N. Engl. J. Med.* **294**, 1316.

[10] Hussain, M., Mieli-Vergani, G. and Mowat, A.P. (1991) Alpha-1 antitrypsin deficiency and liver disease: clinical presentation, diagnosis and treatment. *J. Inher. Metab. Dis.* **14**, 497.

[11] Stoller, J.K., Smith, P., Yang, P. and Spray, J. (1994) Physical and social impact of alpha 1-antitrypsin deficiency: results of a mail survey of the readership of a national newsletter. *Cleveland Clin. J. Med.* **61**, 461.

[12] Lieberman, J., Winter, B. and Sastre, A. (1986) Alpha 1-antitrypsin PI-types in 965 COPD patients. *Chest* **89**, 370.

[13] Stoller, J.K. (2004) Extrapulmonary manifestations of alpha-1-antitrypsin deficiency. *UpToDate* 12.2.

[14] Eriksson, S. (1964) Pulmonary emphysema and alpha 1-antitrypsin deficiency. *Acta Med. Scand.* **175**, 197.

[15] Wewers, M. (1989) Pathogenesis of emphysema. Assessment of basic science concepts through clinical investigation. *Chest* **95**, 190.

[16] Janoff, A. (1985) Elastases and emphysema. Current assessment of the protease–antiprotease hypothesis. *Am. Rev. Respir. Dis.* **132**, 417.

[17] Silverman, E.K., Pierce, J.A., Province, M.A., Rao, D.C. and Campbell, E.J. (1989) Variability of pulmonary function in alpha-1 antitrypsin deficiency: clinical correlates. *Ann. Intern. Med.* **111** 982.

[18] Larsson, C. (1978) Natural history and life expectancy in severe alpha-1 antitrypsin deficiency, PIZ. *Acta Med. Scand.* **204**, 345.

[19] Turino, G.M., Barker, A.F., Brantly, M.L., Cohen, A.B., Connelly, R.P., Crystal, R.G., Eden, E., Schluchter, M.D. and Stoller, J.K. (1996) Clinical features of individuals with PISZ phenotype of alpha-1 antitrypsin deficiency. *Am. J. Respir. Crit. Care Med.* **154**, 1718.

[20] The Alpha 1-Antitrypsin Deficiency Registry Study Group, Schlucter, M.D., Barker, A.F., Crystal, R.G., Robbins, R.A., Stocks, J.M., Stoller, J.K. and Wu, M.C. (1994) A registry of patients with severe deficiency of alpha-1 antitrypsin: design and methods. *Chest* **106**, 1223.

[21] Pauwels, R.A., Buist, A.S., Calverley, P.M.A., Jenkins, C.R. and Hurd, S.S. (2001) Global strategy for the diagnosis, management, and prevention of chronic obstructive pulmonary disease: NHLBI/WHO global initiative for chronic obstructive lung disease (GOLD) workshop summary. *Am. J. Respir. Crit. Care Med.* **163**, 1256–1276.

[22] Wewers, M.D., Casolaro, M.A., Sellers, S.E., Swayze, S., McPhaul, K.M., Wittes, J.T. and Crystal, R.G. (1987) Replacement therapy for alpha 1-antitrypsin deficiency associated with emphysema. *N. Engl. J. Med.* **316**, 1055–1062.

[23] Dirksen, A., Dijkman, J.H., Madesen, F., Stoel, B., Hutchison, D.C.S., Ulrik, C.S., Skovgaars, L.T., Kok-Jensen, A., Rudolphus, A., Seersholm, N., Vrooman, H.A., Reiber, J.H.C., Hansen, N.C., Hecksher, T., Viskum, K. and Stolk, J. (1999) A randomized clinical trial of alpha 1-antitrypsin augmentation therapy. *Am. J. Respir. Crit. Care Med.* **160**, 1468–1472.

[24] The Alpha 1-Antitrypsin Deficiency Registry Study Group (1998) Survival and FEV1 decline in individuals with severe deficiency of alpha 1-antitrypsin. *Am. J. Respir. Crit. Care Med.* **158**, 49–59.

[25] Seersholm, N., Wencker, M., Banik, N., Viskum, K., Dirksen, A., Kok-Jensen, A. and Konietzko, N. (1997) Does alpha 1-antitrypsin augmentation therapy slow the annual decline in FEV1 in patients with severe hereditary alpha 1-antitrypsin deficiency?. *Eur. Respir. J.* **10** 2260–2263.

[26] Wencker, M., Fuhrmann, B., Banik, N. and Konietzko, N. (2001) Wissenschaftliche Arbeitsgemeinschaft zur Therapie von Lungenerkrankungen. Longitudinal follow-up of patients with alpha (1)-protease inhibitor deficiency before and during therapy with IV alpha(1)-protease inhibitor. *Chest* **119**, 737–744.

[27] American Thoracic Society/European Respiratory Society Statement: Standards for the Diagnosis and Management of Individuals with Alpha-1 Antitrypsin Deficiency. *Am. J. Respir. Crit. Care.* **168**, 818–900.

[28] Abboud, R., Ford, G.T., Chapman, K.R. and Standards Committee of the Canadian Thoracic Society (2001) Alpha 1-antitrypsin deficiency: a position statement of the Canadian Thoracic Society. *Can. Respir. J.* **8**, 81–88.

[29] Burrows, J.A., Willis, L.K. and Perlmutter, D.H. (2000) Chemical chaperones mediate increased secretion of mutant alpha 1-antitrypsin (alpha 1-AT) Z: a potential pharmacological strategy for prevention of liver injury and emphysema in alpha 1-AT deficiency. *Proc. Natl Acad. Sci. USA* **97**, 1796–1801.

[30] Brantly, M.L., Paul, L.D., Miller, B.H., Falk, R.T., Wu, M. and Crystal, R.G. (1988) Clinical features and history of the destructive lung disease associated with alpha-1 antitrypsin deficiency of adults with pulmonary symptoms. *Am. Rev. Respir. Dis.* **138**, 327.

Hepatology: A Practical Approach
B. Al Knawy, M.L. Shiffman, R.H. Wiesner (editors)

Chapter 12

Hereditary Hemochromatosis

Bruce R. Bacon

Saint Louis University School of Medicine, 3635 Vista Avenue at Grand Blvd., St. Louis, MO 63110-0250, USA

1. Introduction 211
2. Classification of Iron Overload Syndromes 211
3. Incidence and Prevalence 212
4. Genetics of Hemochromatosis 212
5. Pathophysiologic Mechanisms 213
6. Clinical Features 213
7. Diagnosis of HH 214
8. Treatment 216
9. Family Screening 218
10. Population Screening For Hemochromatosis 218
11. Hemochromatosis Screening in Patients with Liver Disease 219
12. Summary 220
References 220

1. INTRODUCTION

This chapter will review certain aspects of the diagnosis and management of patients with hereditary hemochromatosis (HH) as well as the role of iron in other liver diseases. With the recent discovery of the hemochromatosis gene, *HFE*, our understanding of the physiology of normal iron uptake by the gastrointestinal tract has been enhanced, and accordingly, our understanding of the pathophysiology of HH has improved considerably.

HH is a common disorder of iron metabolism that is characterized by an increased absorption of iron from the proximal small intestine [1]. Excess absorbed iron is subsequently deposited in the parenchymal cells of the liver, pancreas and other endocrine organs, the heart, joints, and the skin. If undiagnosed and untreated, cirrhosis of the liver and hepatocellular cancer can result. Additionally, diabetes, heart failure, arthropathy, and an increase in skin pigmentation may occur. Definitive proof of the genetic nature of hemochromatosis was demonstrated by Simon and colleagues in the mid-1970s by determining the close linkage of the disease to the short arm of chromosome 6 in the region of HLA A3. In 1996, a group of molecular geneticists used a positional cloning technique to identify the gene responsible for hemochromatosis [2]. This gene was found to be a novel major histocompatibility complex (MHC) class 1-like gene; it was initially named *HLA-H* and was later renamed *HFE*. Several studies from groups of HH patients from around the world showed that about 85–90% of those typical patients had a single missense mutation in *HFE* resulting in the substitution of a tyrosine for a cysteine at amino acid position 282 (C282Y). Since this discovery in 1996, numerous clinical and basic studies have been completed increasing our understanding of this common disorder.

2. CLASSIFICATION OF IRON OVERLOAD SYNDROMES

The term *hemochromatosis* should be reserved for the *HFE*-linked inherited disease that is determined by the inappropriately high absorption of iron by the gastrointestinal mucosa leading to the pathologic deposition of iron in parenchymal cells of the liver, heart, pancreas, and other organs. There are several other distinct clinical syndromes of iron overload that should be differentiated from *HFE*-linked hemochromatosis (Table 1). These include *secondary iron overload* where there is a stimulus to iron absorption by an underlying condition other than that caused by mutant *HFE* and results in parenchymal deposition of excess iron. Examples of such underlying conditions are anemia from ineffective erythropoiesis such as that seen in thalassemia, aplastic anemia, sickle cell anemia, some liver diseases and congenital atransferrinemia. *Parenteral iron overload* is that syndrome which occurs as a result of administration of iron either by packed red blood cells by transfusion or by giving iron dextran by injection. Some patients who have ineffective erythropoiesis with increased iron absorption also receive excessive amounts of iron from blood transfusions; thus, they can become quite heavily iron loaded by both secondary and parenteral iron overload. *Neonatal iron overload* is a rare disorder that has been recognized over the last 20 years. It usually results in liver failure and can be fatal without liver transplantation. *African iron overload* is thought to be caused by a genetic abnormality that is not linked to chromosome 6 that is seen in addition to the well-known dietary factor related to the ingestion of iron-enriched home-brewed beer.

Table 1. Classification of iron overload syndromes.

- Hereditary hemochromatosis
  - *HFE*-linked: C282Y/C282Y, C282Y/H63D, C282Y/S65C
- Secondary iron overload
  - Anemia due to ineffective erythropoiesis
    - Thalassemia
    - Aplastic anemia
    - Sickle cell anemia
  - Liver disease
    - Hepatitis C
    - Alcoholic
    - Nonalcoholic steatohepatitis
    - Porphyria cutanea tarda
  - Increased oral intake of iron
  - Congenital atransferrinemia
- Parenteral iron overload
  - RBC transfusions
  - Iron dextran injections
- Neonatal iron overload
- African iron overload

3. INCIDENCE AND PREVALENCE

Numerous prospective population studies from around the world have shown that homozygosity for the principle mutation in *HFE* (C282Y) is found in about 1 in 250–300 individuals of Northern European descent (Table 2). Identification of asymptomatic probands before they have any significant end organ damage is easily available. Additionally, asymptomatic relatives of probands can be identified by *HFE* mutation analysis. This opportunity has lead to some question amongst experts in the field as to what constitutes a diagnosis of hemochromatosis. For example, if someone is a C282Y homozygote, does that mean that they have hemochromatosis even if they have a normal transferrin saturation and a normal ferritin level? Conversely, should we reserve the term *hemochromatosis* only for those patients who have a significant degree of tissue iron overload with liver damage (i.e., cirrhosis)? Investigators are increasingly using a genetic diagnosis with or without phenotypic expression. It may well be that at some time in the future we will understand why some patients who are C282Y homozygotes show significant phenotypic expression and others do not. Most likely this is on the basis of other genetic factors affecting other proteins of iron uptake.

4. GENETICS OF HEMOCHROMATOSIS

HH is inherited in an autosomal recessive manner. Simple C282Y heterozygotes are not at an increased risk for developing iron overload in the absence of other liver disease (e.g., alcohol, hepatitis C). The hemochromatosis gene, *HFE*, encodes a MHC class 1-like molecule that requires interaction with β2-microglobulin (β2M) for normal presentation to the exterior surface of the cell and for interaction with transferrin receptor (TfR) [3]. The protein has a peptide-binding domain, an immunoglobulin-like domain, a single transmembrane region, and a short cytoplasmic tail. At least three missense mutations have been identified in *HFE*. One results in a substitution of cysteine for tyrosine at amino acid

Table 2. Population studies.

Population sample	Country	*n*	Prevalence of homozygotes	C282Y homozygotes with a normal ferritin (%)
Electoral roll	New Zealand	1064	1 in 213	40
Primary care	USA	1653	1 in 276	50
Epidemiological survey	Australia	3011	1 in 188	25
Blood donors	Canada	4211	1 in 327	81
General public	USA	41,083	1 in 270	33

282 (C282Y), the second results in a change of aspartate for histidine at amino acid 63 (H63D), and the third results in a serine that is replaced by a cysteine at amino acid 65 (S65C). The latter two mutations differ in frequency with H63D being very common and S65C less so. Neither of these mutations results in a significant degree of iron loading, except when they are found in conjunction with C282Y (i.e., compound heterozygote), and in this situation, patients can become iron loaded. C282Y homozygosity is found in the vast majority (85–90%) of patients with typical phenotypic hemochromatosis. However, when population studies are done prospectively, not all C282Y homozygotes have evidence of phenotypic expression (Table 2). Compound heterozygotes (C282Y/H63D, C282Y/S65C) can result in some increase in iron loading but not to the degree seen in C282Y homozygotes.

5. PATHOPHYSIOLOGIC MECHANISMS

Several years ago, when *HFE* was first described, some investigators questioned the role of an MHC class 1-like protein in iron metabolism. Shortly after the initial discovery, it was found that the HFE/β2M complex interacts with TfR and is necessary for transferrin-mediated iron uptake into cells [4]. Further confirmation of the significance of *HFE* mutations leading to iron overload has been provided by the creation of several *HFE* knockout mouse models that have recapitulated the phenotypic expression of the disease [5]. Current hypotheses explaining the mechanism(s) whereby the C282Y mutation in *HFE* results in iron overload are that in crypt enterocytes, the HFE/β2M/TfR complex impairs TfR-mediated iron uptake in the presence of the C282Y mutation in *HFE* resulting in crypt cells becoming "relatively" iron deficient [6]. This in turn leads to an increase in the expression of the divalent metal ion transporter-1 (DMT-1, also called Nramp 2 and DCT-1) which has increased expression in villus cells resulting in increased iron absorption. With increased iron absorption, iron is then bound to apotransferrin in the portal circulation. Excess iron and iron bound to transferrin is quickly taken up by hepatocytes in a periportal distribution. As iron deposition gets to a certain critical concentration, mechanisms for maintaining iron in a nontoxic protein-bound state are exceeded and iron-induced oxidative damage occurs ultimately leading to hepatocellular death with phagocytosis by Kupffer cells. These iron-loaded Kupffer cells produce profibrogenic cytokines which stimulate stellate cells to produce increased amounts of collagen leading to the fibrosis and cirrhosis that can occur in hemochromatosis [7].

6. CLINICAL FEATURES

HH is still frequently undiagnosed and unrecognized because of a lack of awareness of the disease by physicians and patients. Awareness of the disease has improved over recent years with population studies and educational information produced by national organizations. It is rare to see a patient with the classical triad of cirrhosis, diabetes, and bronze pigmentation of the skin, and physicians who are waiting for that presentation will miss the diagnosis in many patients. More commonly, patients are identified by family screening or in the work-up of elevated liver enzymes. Prospective population studies have shown that the homozygote frequency is approximately 1 in 250 in populations of Northern European descent. These studies have been done in Australia, New Zealand, Canada, the United States, and Western Europe (see Table 2). The highest prevalence of C282Y homozygosity is in Ireland where it is approximately 1 in 70.

Currently, many patients present without any symptoms or clinical findings at all, because they are identified by population screening, family studies, or evaluation for nonspecific symptoms. On the other hand, when patients do have symptoms of hemochromatosis, they are often nonspecific and include fatigue, malaise, right upper quadrant abdominal pain, and arthralgias. Common physical findings (when present) include a characteristic arthropathy of the second and third metacarpophalangeal joints, a bronzed/grayish pigmentation of the skin, and hepatomegaly. Common symptoms and physical findings are summarized in Table 3.

Table 3. Symptoms and physical findings in patients with hereditary hemochromatosis.

Symptoms
Asymptomatic
Abnormal serum iron studies on routine screening chemistry panel
Evaluation of abnormal liver tests
Identified by family screening
Identified by population screening
Nonspecific, systemic symptoms
Weakness
Fatigue
Lethargy
Apathy
Weight loss
Specific, organ-related symptoms
Abdominal pain (hepatomegaly)
Arthralgias (arthritis)
Diabetes (pancreas)
Amenorrhea (cirrhosis)
Loss of libido, impotence (pituitary, cirrhosis)
Congestive heart failure (heart)
Arrhythmias (heart)
Physical findings
Asymptomatic
No physical findings
Hepatomegaly
Symptomatic
Liver
Hepatomegaly
Cutaneous stigmata of chronic liver disease
Splenomegaly
Liver failure: ascites, encephalopathy, etc.
Joints
Arthritis
Joint swelling
Heart
Dilated cardiomyopathy
Congestive heart failure
Skin
Increased pigmentation
Endocrine
Testicular atrophy
Hypogonadism
Hypothyroidism

Table 4 summarizes the typical laboratory findings in patients with symptomatic or asymptomatic HH. Recent population studies have found that about half of patients who are C282Y homozygotes have normal ferritin levels and thus do not have evidence of phenotypic expression in terms of increased iron stores (see Table 2). Some of these patients have elevated transferrin saturation levels and as such, have phenotypic evidence of the disease. When the diagnosis of HH is identified by family studies, population screening studies, or by evaluation of routine screening chemistry panels, then most patients (>75%) are without symptoms and have a low frequency (<25%) of cirrhosis, diabetes, or skin pigmentation [8]. Obviously, in the face of abnormal iron studies, a physician should not wait for the typical symptoms and disease manifestations of hemochromatosis to present prior to definitively considering the diagnosis and requesting appropriate studies.

7. DIAGNOSIS OF HH

The diagnosis of HH is relatively straightforward once it is considered. If patients have any of the symptoms or physical findings mentioned in Table 3, or if they are identified as having elevated iron studies on screening chemistry panels, if they are identified by the evaluation of elevated liver enzymes, or as a part of family studies or population surveys, then fasting transferrin saturation and ferritin levels should be obtained. If iron studies are abnormal, then *HFE* mutation analysis should be obtained. An elevated transferrin saturation is usually the earliest phenotypic marker of HH; however, ferritin levels can be elevated in other necroinflammatory disorders or may be normal in young female patients with the disease. Thus, the sensitivity and specificity of these tests become problematic when

Table 4. Laboratory findings in patients with hereditary hemochromatosis.

Measurements	Normal subjects	Patients with hereditary hemochromatosis	
		Asymptomatic	Symptomatic
Blood (fasting)			
Serum iron level (μg/dl)	60–180	150–280	180–300
Serum transferrin level (mg/dl)	220–410	200–280	200–300
Transferrin saturation (%)	20–45	45–100	80–100
Serum ferritin level (ng/ml)			
Men	20–200	150–1000	500–6000
Women	15–150	120–1000	500–6000
Genetic (*HFE* mutation analysis)			
C282Y/C282Y	wt/wt	C282Y/C282Y	C282Y/C282Y
C282Y/H63D[a]	wt/wt	C282Y/H63D	C282Y/H63D
C282Y/S65C[a]	wt/wt	C282Y/S65C	C282Y/S65C
Liver			
Hepatic iron concentration			
μg/g dry weight	300–1500	2000–10,000	8000–30,000
μmol/g dry weight	5–27	36–179	140–550
Hepatic iron index[b]	<1.0	1.0 to >1.9	>1.9
Liver histology			
Perls' Prussian blue stain	0, 1 +	2 + to 4 +	3 +, 4 +

[a]Compound heterozygote.

[b]Hepatic iron index (HII) is calculated by dividing the hepatic iron concentration (in μmol/g dry weight) by the age of the patient (in years). With increased knowledge of genetic testing results in patients with iron overload, the specificity of HII has diminished.

young individuals are being evaluated or when patients have abnormal iron studies which may be due to other diseases. Numerous population surveys from around the world have shown that about 50% of C282Y homozygotes have normal ferritin levels (Table 2). It is unknown whether these individuals will eventually go on to develop increased iron stores. Conversely, it is known that about 50% of patients with chronic hepatitis C, nonalcoholic steatohepatitis (NASH), and alcoholic liver disease will have elevated serum ferritin levels. Other inflammatory disorders (e.g., rheumatoid arthritis), and various neoplastic diseases (e.g., lymphoma) can cause elevated ferritin levels. Thus, there may be many false negative and false positive results of serum iron studies, and in this situation, genetic testing is extremely useful. In these patients with liver disease, presence of C282Y homozygosity or the compound heterozygote genotype (C282Y/H63D) provides definitive evidence that these patients will have at least a component of their iron overload from the genetic disorder.

The role of liver biopsy has become less important in evaluating patients for hemochromatosis since the development of genetic testing. Nonetheless, it is important to know what the liver biopsy changes are in patients with typical HH. The histochemical stain that is used for identifying tissue storage iron is Perls' Prussian blue stain. Also, a portion of liver tissue may be taken for biochemical determination of hepatic iron concentration (HIC) with subsequent calculation of the hepatic iron index (HII). The HII is based on the observation in the mid-1980s that patients with HH had a progressive increase in HIC with increasing age [9]. The HII is calculated by taking the HIC (in μmol/g dry wt) and dividing by the patient's age (in years). In the past, an HII of >1.9 was considered diagnostic of HH. We now know that many patients (perhaps more than 50%) who have HH by genetic testing (C282Y/C282Y) do not have an elevated HII. Accordingly, the HII is very seldom used any more. When liver biopsy is performed, iron deposition is found predominantly in a periportal (acinar zone 1) region of the lobule with a decrease in grading to acinar zones 2 and 3 (pericentral). With significant iron loading, iron may be found in Kupffer cells, in bile duct epithelium, and in fibrous tissue in portal tracts or septa. With very heavy iron overload, the lobular and cellular distribution of iron deposition from HH is sometimes not distinguished from that of other forms of secondary iron overload. However, in the early stages of the disease, the cellular and lobular distribution is quite distinct. Thus, histologic evaluation of iron staining can provide supportive evidence adding to the traditional biochemical tests for iron overload and genetic testing. Our group has shown that a non-HH pattern of iron distribution reliably predicts the absence of homozygosity for C282Y or C282Y/H63D [10]. Conversely, the HH pattern can be seen in other forms of liver disease in the absence of C282Y/C282Y.

Several recent studies have defined the indications for liver biopsy in patients who are being considered for HH. In studies from Brisbane, Rennes, and St. Louis, the parameters of age >40 years, serum ferritin >1000 ng/ml, elevated liver enzymes, or hepatomegaly should lead one to perform a liver biopsy [11]. If a patient had none of these factors, was a C282Y homozygote, and had elevated serum studies indicative of iron overload, then a biopsy was not necessary (Figure 1). Using these guidelines, no patients with a significant amount of fibrosis were missed by not doing a biopsy. Currently, the significance of age <40 years seems less important, and most investigators now only recommend liver biopsy if the ferritin level is >1000 ng/ml or if patients have elevated liver enzymes.

8. TREATMENT

With the advent of genetic screening for hemochromatosis using *HFE* mutation analysis, many patients who are homozygous for the C282Y mutation or who are compound heterozygotes (C282Y/H63D), are identified who have very mild degrees of iron overload. These patients are usually identified by family screening or by population studies and do not present *per se* with disease manifestations of hemochromatosis. The question of whether or not to initiate therapeutic phlebotomy in these patients is often raised. For example, a 25-year-old female who is a C282Y homozygote with a ferritin of 98 ng/ml and a transferrin saturation of 46% does not need to be treated with phlebotomy. The recommendation for such a patient would be to get yearly ferritin and transferrin saturation levels and if the ferritin level goes above the upper limit of normal and/or if the transferrin saturation is increased, phlebotomy can be initiated. In this setting, all that is required is usually the initiation of maintenance phlebotomy rather than a requirement for regular therapeutic phlebotomy. Patients who present with high levels of serum ferritin and/or disease manifestations of hemochromatosis should be committed to a regular therapeutic phlebotomy regimen to deplete excess iron stores.

Treatment of HH is straightforward, simple, inexpensive, and safe. Even though there have been significant advances in the understanding of the pathophysiology of hemochromatosis at a molecular level, these advances have not been translated into new treatments. Patients should be encouraged to have weekly therapeutic phlebotomy of approximately 500 ml of whole blood which is equivalent to 200–250 mg of iron depending on the level of the hemoglobin. Some patients can tolerate two phlebotomies per week and rarely as many as three per week; most patients find weekly phlebotomy tolerable and convenient. The purpose of therapeutic phlebotomy is to deplete excess iron stores, not to create iron deficiency anemia. Therefore, it is not necessary for patients to develop microcytosis or serum levels of iron or ferritin below the low normal range. It is useful to monitor transferrin saturation and ferritin levels every 3 months during a course of therapeutic phlebotomy in order to let patients know how they are doing and to encourage them to continue with their phlebotomy. Therapeutic phlebotomy should be continued until ferritin levels are below 50 ng/ml and transferrin saturation is $<50\%$. This can usually be achieved in most patients but occasionally some patients will have an elevated transferrin saturation in the presence of a ferritin level that is clearly in the iron-deficient range (e.g., <10 ng/ml).

In an otherwise uncomplicated patient, where ferritin levels are not increased for other reasons such as other inflammatory processes, the ferritin level will usually drop by about 30 ng/ml per unit of whole blood removed. This is a convenient way to predict therapeutic phlebotomy requirements.

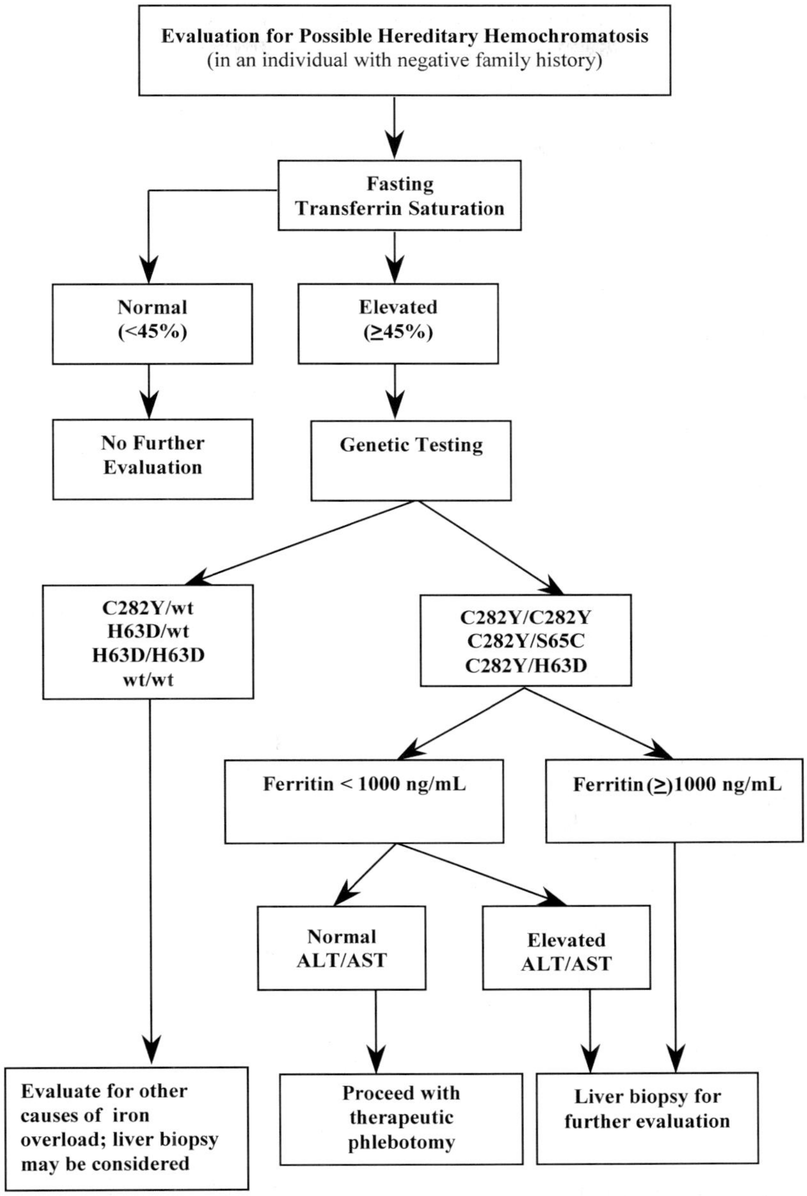

Figure 1. Algorithm for evaluating patients with possible hereditary hemochromatosis being considered for liver biopsy.

Once the initial therapeutic phlebotomy has been completed, it is necessary to switch to maintenance phlebotomy. Most patients require a unit of blood removed every 2–3 months to maintain normal iron status. Since most patients with HH absorb 2–3 mg of iron per day in excess of their metabolic requirements, over a 3-month period of time they will accumulate the amount of iron found in a unit of blood (about 250 mg). Occasionally, following initial therapeutic phlebotomy, some patients do not re-accumulate excess iron stores. These patients do not need maintenance phlebotomy, but should have yearly monitoring of ferritin levels. If the ferritin level shows signs of iron re-accumulation, then maintenance phlebotomy should be instituted.

In addition to depleting excess iron stores, therapeutic phlebotomy generally results in an improved sense of well-being, less fatigue, reduction in right upper quadrant abdominal pain, improved control of diabetes, normalization of abnormal liver enzymes, and if patients are identified prior to the development of cirrhosis, a significant reduction in the risk for the development of hepatocellular cancer. On the other hand, arthralgias and arthropathy as well as testicular atrophy do not improve. Whether or not fibrosis reverses is debated; although, in the absence of fully established cirrhosis it is likely that there is some remodeling with reversal of hepatic fibrosis once phlebotomy has been successful.

There is no reason why the blood from a patient with HH cannot be used for transfusion. However, blood banking societies in the United States have been resistant to this concept, because these patients are achieving a therapeutic gain and thus are not true volunteers. Once testing for blood-borne pathogens has been performed and it is found that the blood is safe, these patients are excellent donors because they come regularly and thus have repeated testing for safety and they have a stimulated bone marrow producing young erythrocytes which should have a longer shelf life. Use of blood for transfusion from hemochromatosis patients has been approved in some countries in Europe and in Canada, and is FDA approved in the United States, although the practice is not widely adopted by the United States blood banking societies. Perhaps this will change over the upcoming years.

9. FAMILY SCREENING

Once a proband has been identified, it is obviously important to realize that this is an inherited disorder and that appropriate family screening should be performed. It is recommended that all first-degree relatives be tested. The availability of genetic testing using *HFE* mutation analysis has greatly improved our ability to do family screening; accordingly, *HLA* typing is no longer done. With *HFE* mutation analysis, both the C282Y and the H63D mutations should be analyzed; the S65C mutation is probably not prevalent enough to warrant routine testing. Occasionally, if there is a patient who is a C282Y heterozygote who has a significant degree of iron loading, it might be reasonable to test for the S65C mutation on the allele not affected by C282Y or H63D [12]. In young probands who have children, it is useful to perform *HFE* mutation analysis on the other parent to assess the likelihood of the child being affected. If the other parent has neither mutation, then the children will be obligate heterozygotes and will not be at increased risk for serious iron overload [13]. Currently, there are questions about whether or not genetic testing should be done in children. The issue of insurance discrimination or job discrimination is real and parents should be appropriately counseled about these concerns prior to performing genetic testing on children [14]. On the other hand, the knowledge gained from genetic testing for HH is so powerful that knowledge of the potential for possible iron storage disease may outweigh the theoretical concern about societal discrimination. These issues must be handled individually. Because C282Y and H63D are such common mutations occurring in approximately one-third of individuals singly or in combination, there is approximately a one in three chance that the child's other parent will have a mutation in *HFE*. If an adult relative is found to be a C282Y homozygote or a compound heterozygote (C282Y/H63D), then iron studies should be performed including a fasting transferrin saturation and ferritin level. If either of these is abnormal, then therapeutic phlebotomy should be proposed to deplete excess iron stores. If liver enzymes are normal and if the ferritin level is < 1000 ng/ml, then liver biopsy is not necessary.

10. POPULATION SCREENING FOR HEMOCHROMATOSIS

Soon after the gene for hemochromatosis was discovered in 1996, it was suggested that this would be an ideal disease for wide scale population screening. This was because the genetic abnormality is common, tests are readily available to determine the presence of a phenotype (transferrin saturation and ferritin), treatment is simple, safe, and effective (phlebotomy), and there is a long latent period before the development of life-threatening complications. However, certain complications in this "straightforward" plan became apparent, as investigators grappled with what exactly constituted phenotypic expression (elevated transferrin saturation or liver disease). Also, some investigators raised the question of genetic discrimination in the form of insurance or job discrimination for individuals who had a genetic diagnosis. Some countries have dealt with this legislatively but that has not yet occurred in the United States. With the recent completion of the human genome project, genetic diagnoses will become increasingly common and it is expected that legislatures will create appropriate laws to prevent this type of genetic discrimination. Another important question relating to population screening is whether all individuals of the population should be studied. It is well known that hemochromatosis is a disorder of Northern European descent with the highest prevalence found in Ireland, the United Kingdom, Germany, Portugal, and France. While there is some genetic admixture in individuals of African or Asian descent, it is rare to find a non-Caucasian patient with the C282Y mutation. Thus, screening programs ideally would be limited to Caucasian populations when looking for the genetic abnormality but it may well be that when screening for iron overload it would be reasonable to screen people of all races. Finally, since phenotypic expression of any kind usually does not occur before adulthood, it would be reasonable to limit population studies to adults. Results of general population screening programs that have been performed are listed in Table 2. The importance of these findings relates to the fact that about 50% of C282Y homozygotes have phenotypic expression with evidence of an increase in iron stores identified as an increased ferritin level. At the present time, arguments for widespread population screening cannot be fully supported.

11. HEMOCHROMATOSIS SCREENING IN PATIENTS WITH LIVER DISEASE

Abnormalities in serum iron studies are commonly identified in patients with a variety of hepatocellular liver diseases. Approximately 50% of patients with alcoholic liver disease, NASH, and chronic viral hepatitis have serum abnormalities of iron metabolism [15–17]. These usually relate to an increase in serum ferritin level but some patients may have an elevated transferrin saturation as well. *HFE* mutation analysis has been performed in groups of patients with alcoholic liver disease, NASH, chronic hepatitis C, and porphyria cutanea tarda (PCT). In patients with alcoholic liver disease, there was no increased prevalence of C282Y heterozygosity in patients who have increased hepatic fibrosis. Similarly, when evaluating patients with alcoholic liver disease who had $>1+$ iron stores, there was no enrichment of C282Y [15]. Accordingly, it has been concluded that most patients with increased iron stores who also have alcoholic liver disease have mild secondary iron overload rather than a component of HH.

In patients with chronic hepatitis C, the relationship between HIC and response to therapy with interferon monotherapy has been well studied [18]. Numerous investigators have shown that patients who failed to respond to interferon monotherapy have a higher HIC than those who do not. This difference is lost when ribavirin is added and the resultant overall response to antiviral therapy improved. Therapeutic phlebotomy has been used to deplete excess iron stores in patients with chronic hepatitis C and that was shown to improve liver enzyme values and in some studies there was some improvement in histology. More recent studies in which *HFE* mutation analysis has been performed in patients with chronic hepatitis C have generally shown no difference in the prevalence of C282Y or H63D mutations in patients with chronic hepatitis C when compared to control populations. Some studies have shown an increase in fibrosis when C282Y was present but other studies have not confirmed this association [19,20]. It is not clear whether long-term chronic phlebotomy therapy might be beneficial to patients with chronic hepatitis C.

In patients with NASH, there are studies that show an increased prevalence of C282Y in NASH patients and other studies that do not support this association. Some patients with NASH have elevated iron studies in the absence of the C282Y mutation. The role of phlebotomy in NASH has been considered and may be of some benefit because of a role of iron in the regulation of insulin resistance [21]. More studies on the interactions of iron in NASH should be performed.

Finally, in PCT, it has been well established for many years that there is a role of increased iron in the presentation of this disease [22]. Studies from both

Europe and the United States have shown that about 40% of patients who have PCT are C282Y heterozygotes or homozygotes. Accordingly, it is recommended that all patients who present with PCT have *HFE* mutation analysis performed. Skin lesions of PCT respond to phlebotomy and removal of other inciting factors such as certain medications and alcohol use. Also, there is a strong association between PCT and the presence of hepatitis C. Treatment of PCT includes phlebotomy to deplete excess iron stores and is usually successful.

12. SUMMARY

It is important to distinguish HH from other syndromes of iron overload and to realize that not all patients with HH have a genetic mutation found in *HFE*. Now that genetic testing is readily available, it is clear that the vast majority of patients with hemochromatosis do not develop endstage manifestations and can be identified and treated prior to the development of any complications. The role of liver biopsy is less important in making the diagnosis and abnormalities in iron metabolism associated with *HFE* mutations clearly play an important role in PCT but may also be important in NASH and in hepatitis C, although the evidence supporting this is diminishing. Generalized population screening may not be appropriate given the realities of phenotypic expression in those patients with either the C282Y/C282Y or the C282Y/H63D genotype. Finally, the unraveling of the mechanisms of iron uptake in the small intestine that are altered in HH has become much better understood since the discovery of *HFE*. All of this important information has become apparent over the last 5–6 years since the discovery of *HFE*.

REFERENCES

[1] Bacon, B.R. and Britton, R.S. (2002) Hereditary hemochromatosis, in *Sleisenger and Fordtran's Gastrointestinal and Liver Disease*, vol. 2, eds. Feldman, M., Friedman, L. and Sleisenger, M., 7th edition (Harcourt Health Sciences, Philadelphia, PA) pp. 1261–1268.

[2] Feder, J.N., Gnirke, A., Thomas, W., Tsuchihashi, Z., Ruddy, D.A., Basava, A., Dormishian, F., Domingo, Jr., R., Ellis, M.C., Fullan, A., Hinton, L.M., Jones, N.L., Kimmel, B.E., Kronmal, G.S., Lauer, P., Lee, V.K., Loeb, D.B., Mapa, F.A., McClelland, E., Meyer, M.C., Mintier, G.A., Moeller, N., Moore, T., Morikang, E., Prass, C.E., Quintana, L., Starnes, S.M., Schatzman, R.C., Brunke, K.J., Drayna, D.T., Risch, N.J., Bacon, B.R. and Wolff, R.K. (1996) A novel MHC class I-like gene is mutated in patients with hereditary haemochromatosis. *Nat. Genet.* **13**, 399–408.

[3] Waheed, A., Parkkila, S., Zhou, X.Y., Tomatsu, S., Tsuchihashi, Z., Feder, J.N., Schatzman, R.C., Britton, R.S., Bacon, B.R. and Sly, W.S. (1997) Hereditary hemochromatosis: effects of C282Y and H63D mutations on association with beta$_2$-microglobulin, intracellular processing, and cell surface expression of the HFE protein in COS-7 cells. *Proc. Natl Acad. Sci. USA* **94**, 12384–12389.

[4] Parkkila, S., Waheed, A., Britton, R.S., Bacon, B.R., Zhou, X.Y., Tomatsu, S., Fleming, R.E. and Sly, W.S. (1997) Association of the transferrin receptor in human placenta with HFE, the protein defective in hereditary hemochromatosis. *Proc. Natl Acad. Sci. USA* **94**, 13198–13202.

[5] Zhou, X.Y., Tomatsu, S., Fleming, R.E., Parkkila, S., Waheed, A., Jiang, J., Fei, Y., Brunt, E.M., Ruddy, D.A., Prass, C.E., Schatzman, R.C., O'Neill, R., Britton, R.S., Bacon, B.R. and Sly, W.S. (1998) *HFE* gene knockout produces mouse model of hereditary hemochromatosis. *Proc. Natl Acad. Sci. USA* **95**, 2492–2497.

[6] Fleming, R.E., Britton, R.S., Waheed, A., Sly, W.S. and Bacon, B.R. (2002) Molecular and cellular iron transport, vol. 8, ed. Templeton, D.M. (Marcel Dekker, Inc., New York, Basel) pp. 189–205.

[7] Britton, R.S., Leicester, K.L. and Bacon, B.R. (2002) Iron toxicity and chelation therapy. *Int. J. Hematol.* **76**, 219–228.

[8] Bacon, B.R. and Sadiq, S.A. (1997) Hereditary hemochromatosis: presentation and diagnosis in the 1990s. *Am. J. Gastroenterol.* **92**, 784–789.

[9] Bassett, M.L., Halliday, J.W. and Powell, L.W. (1986) Value of hepatic iron measurements in early hemochromatosis and determination of the critical iron level associated with fibrosis. *Hepatology* **6**, 24–29.

[10] Brunt, E.M., Olynyk, J.K., Britton, R.S., Janney, C.G., Di Bisceglie, A.M. and Bacon, B.R. (2000) Histological evaluation of iron in liver biopsies: relationship to *HFE* mutations. *Am. J. Gastroenterol.* **95**, 1788–1793.

[11] Bacon, B.R., Olynyk, J.K., Brunt, E.M., Britton, R.S. and Wolff, R.K. (1999) *HFE* genotype in patients with

hemochromatosis and other liver diseases. *Ann. Intern. Med.* **130**, 953–962.

[12] Wallace, D.F., Walker, A.P., Pietrangelo, A., Clare, M., Bomford, A.B., Dixon, J.L., Powell, L.W., Subramaniam, N. and Dooley, J.S. (2002) Frequency of the S65C mutation of *HFE* and iron overload in 309 subjects heterozygous for C822Y. *J. Hepatol.* **36**, 474–479.

[13] Adams, P.C. (1998) Implications of genotyping of spouses to limit investigation of children in genetic hemochromatosis. *Clin. Genet.* **53**, 176–178.

[14] Shaheen, N.J., Lawrence, L.B., Bacon, B.R., Barton, J.C., Barton, N.H., Galanko, J., Martin, C.F., Burnett,, C.K. and Sandler, R.S. (2003) Insurance, employment, and psychosocial consequences of a diagnosis of hereditary hemochromatosis in subjects without end organ damage. *Am. J. Gastroenterol.* **98**, 1175–1180.

[15] Grove, J., Daly, A.K., Burt, A.D., Guzail, M., James, O.F., Bassendine, M.F. and Day, C.P. (1998) Heterozygotes for HFE mutations have no increased risk of advanced alcoholic liver disease. *Gut* **43**, 262–266.

[16] Bacon, B.R., Farahvash, M.J., Janney, C.G. and Neuschwander-Tetri, B.A. (1994) Nonalcoholic steatohepatitis: an expanded clinical entity. *Gastroenterology* **107**, 1103–1109.

[17] Smith, B.C., Grove, J., Guzail, M.A., Day, C.P., Daly, A.K., Burt, A.D. and Bassendine, M.F. (1998) Heterozygosity for hereditary hemochromatosis is associated with more fibrosis in chronic hepatitis C. *Hepatology* **27**, 1695–1699.

[18] Di Bisceglie, A.M., Bonkovsky, H.L., Chopra, S., Flamm, S., Reddy, R.K., Grace, N., Killenberg, P., Hunt, C., Tamburro, C., Tavill, A.S., Ferguson, R., Krawitt, E., Banner, B. and Bacon, B.R. (2000) Iron reduction as an adjuvant to interferon therapy in patients with chronic hepatitis C who have previously not responded to interferon: a multi-center; prospective, randomized, controlled trial. *Hepatology* **32**, 135–138.

[19] George, D.K., Goldwurm, S., MacDonald, G.A., Cowley, L.L., Walker, N.I., Ward, P.J., Jazwinska, E.C. and Powell, L.W. (1998) Increased hepatic iron concentration in nonalcoholic steatohepatitis is associated with increased fibrosis. *Gastroenterology* **114**, 311–318.

[20] Younossi, Z.M., Gramlich, T., Bacon, B.R., Matteoni, C.A., Boparai, N., O'Neill, R. and McCullough, A.J. (1999) Hepatic iron and nonalcoholic fatty liver disease. *Hepatology* **30**, 847–850.

[21] Facchini, F.S., Hua, N.W. and Stoohs, R.A. (2002) Effect of iron depletion in carbohydrate-intolerant patients with clinical evidence of nonalcoholic fatty liver disease. *Gastroenterology* **122**, 931–939.

[22] Bonkovsky, H.L., Poh-Fitzpatrick, M., Pimstone, N., Obando, J., Di Bisceglie, A., Tattrie, C., Tortorelli, K., LeClair, P., Mercurio, M.G. and Lambrecht, R.W. (1998) Porphyria cutanea tarda, hepatitis C, and HFE gene mutations in North America. *Hepatology* **27**, 1661–1669.

Hepatology: A Practical Approach
B. Al Knawy, M.L. Shiffman, R.H. Wiesner (editors)

Chapter 13

Wilson's Disease

Hisham O. Akbar

King Abdulaziz University Hospital, P.O. Box 80215, Jeddah 21589, Saudi Arabia

1. Introduction 223
   1.1 Definition 223
   1.2 Prevalence 223
2. Pathophysiology 223
3. Clinical Features 224
   3.1 Hepatic form 224
   3.2 Neuropsychiatric form 225
   3.3 Mixed form 225
4. Diagnosis 226
5. Management 228
6. Prognosis 230
References 230

1. INTRODUCTION

In 1912 Kinnear Wilson reported the syndrome of familial progressive hepatolenticular degeneration with neurological and hepatic manifestation; corneal involvement and impaired copper metabolism were not included.

1.1 Definition

Wilson's disease is an autosomal recessive metabolic disorder characterized by progressive accumulation of copper in the liver, brain, cornea, erythrocytes, kidneys and joints as a result of defective cellular copper transport and impaired biliary copper excretion [1].

1.2 Prevalence

Wilson's disease is rare, although occurring throughout the world in all races and nationalities, affecting one case in 30,000–100,000 live births with gene frequency of 1:200–1:400 [2]. Consanguinity and interfamilial marriages, which are common in certain communities and countries, are associated with higher incidence particularly in Jews of eastern European origin, Arabs, Indians and Chinese. It typically presents during childhood and the teenage period (5–20 years); however, late presentation at the age of 50 years has been reported. Twenty-five percent of siblings are usually detected in presymptomatic stage during the recommended screening procedure. Relatives are at increased risk as compared to the general population.

2. PATHOPHYSIOLOGY

Copper is a component of many enzymes and plasma proteins such as ceruloplasmin, dopa hydroxylase, superoxide dismutase, tyrosinase, and lysine oxidase and is required in trace amounts for oxidative metabolism, free radical detoxification and neurotransmitter synthesis.

Total body copper is approximately 50–150 mg. Daily copper requirement for adults is 2–3 mg and is commonly available in shellfish, liver, chocolate, nuts, mushrooms and legumes.

40–60% of copper is absorbed in the proximal small intestine, transported bound to albumin and cleared by the liver. In the enterocytes copper is bound to metallothionein and exported to the portal circulation by the Menke's protein. Absorption is reduced by zinc and ascorbate. In the hepatocytic cytosol, copper binds to glutathione and metallothione in which constitutes 80% of hepatic copper. Copper is then incorporated by the liver into copper-containing enzymes, ceruloplasmin (blue copper) and secreted into plasma, or excreted in bile [3]. This is controlled by Wilson's disease protein predominantly present in trans-Golgi vesicles [4]. The bulk of ingested copper is excreted in normal individuals by the liver in bile and subsequently in stool, which in turn is responsible for copper balance. Intestinal reabsorption of biliary copper is negligible. Urinary copper excretion is minimal and accounts for only 10% of daily excretion (<30 mcg/day).

Biliary excretion of copper as well as ceruloplasmin synthesis is impaired in Wilson's disease leading to the accumulation of copper in the liver and other organs. As a result of the above, patients with Wilson's disease characteristically have a decrease in plasma ceruloplasmin levels and increase in hepatic copper concentration [5]. This finding is similar to that in normal fetus and neonates which reverts to normal adult levels during the first 2 years of life probably through stimulation of a controller gene after birth.

In 1985 the abnormal gene in Wilson's disease was assigned to the long arm of chromosome 13 and subsequently in 1993 it was identified, cloned and designated ATP7B [6,7]. This is a copper transporting P type ATPase responsible for copper transport across the cell membrane by removing copper from cytosol ligands, delivering copper to apoceruloplasmin and biliary excretion. ATP7B is expressed mainly in the liver and a few other tissues including the kidney, brain, heart, lung, placenta, pancreas and muscles. Currently more than 100 different disease-specific gene mutations have been reported. Frequency of gene mutation differs among different countries; His1069Gln was reported in 60–70% of Polish and Austrian patients and rarely among Indian and Asian patients with Wilson's disease [8,9]. His1069Gln results from substitution of histidine at amino acid position 1069 to glutamine. Homozygote individuals may carry two different mutations.

Impaired biliary excretion and decrease in ceruloplasmin synthesis result in positive copper balance with progressive accumulation of copper in the hepatic cytoplasm bound to metallothionein. As copper accumulation progresses, metallothionein saturation is exceeded, intracellular redistribution of copper occurs with deposition in the mitochondria and lysozymes. Excessive copper deposition acting as pro-oxidant will lead to the production of hydroxyl free radicals, depletion of glutathione stores, decrease in mitochondrial enzymes, accumulation of lipid peroxides and triglycerides in the hepatocytes and hepatic dysfunction. Excessive copper leaks from necrotic hepatocytes into the circulation result in increase of free serum copper concentration and subsequently increased copper deposition in other tissues (brain, cornea, kidneys, etc.) [2,3,10].

3. CLINICAL FEATURES

Clinical presentation tends to be variable depending on the age of presentation, degree and extent of copper deposition. No definite association was found between the mode of presentation or subsequent clinical course and gene mutation type [11]. In general, the commonest modes of presentation are [2,12,13] (Figure 1):

(1) *Subclinical*: detected during investigation of increased liver enzymes in a young individual or during screening of siblings.
(2) *Clinical*:
  (a) hepatic form,
  (b) neuropsychiatric form,
  (c) mixed form.

3.1 Hepatic form

The hepatic form usually occurs at an earlier age during childhood or adolescence as compared to the neuropsychiatric form. 40–50% of patients with

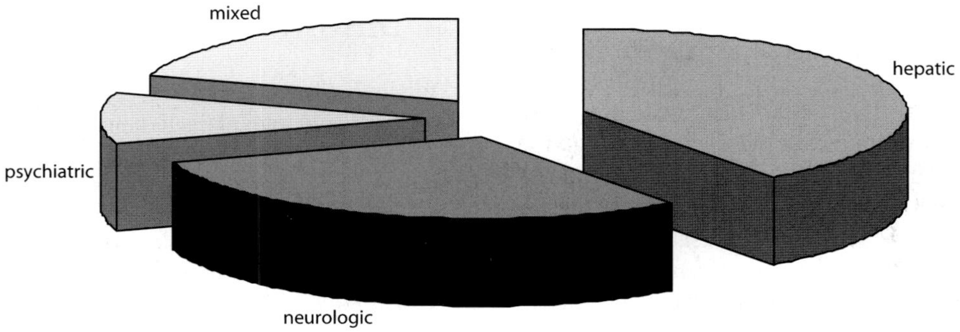

Figure 1. Wilson's disease clinical presentation. (*For colored version, see Plate XXI on page 575 at the end of the book.*)

Wilson's disease present with hepatic manifestation either as:

(a) *Acute fulminant hepatitis*: characterized by rapidly progressive deterioration of liver function as a result of massive hepatic necrosis with progressive jaundice, ascites, hepatic encephalopathy, renal impairment and acute intravascular hemolysis secondarily to sudden release of copper from damaged hepatocytes. It also may complicate noncompliance in previously controlled patients.

(b) *Chronic hepatitis*: this is usually the typical hepatic presentation, which is nonspecific and mimics manifestations of chronic liver disease due to other causes. Patients complain of fatigue, lassitude, anorexia and myalgia. As the disease progress features of portal hypertension, hypersplenism and liver failure may develop.

3.2 Neuropsychiatric form

Patients usually present at a later age after puberty (>20 years) where liver disease is passed unnoticed during early life. Neurological and psychiatric presentations occur in 30 and 10%, respectively. Features include:

(1) *Neurological*:
  (a) deterioration of school performance
  (b) dysarthia, hoarseness, slurred speech, drooling and dysphagia
  (c) hypokinesia, tremors and rigidity (Parkinsonian)
  (d) incoordination, dysdiadokinesia and ataxic gait
  (e) dystonia and mask face
  (f) risus sardonicus and seizures

(2) *Psychiatric*:
  (a) behavioral changes (irritability, emotional lability)
  (b) psychosis (mania, depression, schizophrenia)
  (c) dementia
  (d) delusions and suicidal attempts.

3.3 Mixed form

20–25% of patients with Wilson's disease may present with features related to hepatic and neuropsychiatric evolvement.

Other manifestations may develop during clinical course include (Table 1):

Table 1. Clinical manifestation of Wilson's disease.

Hepatic	Acute fulminant hepatitis, steatosis, chronic hepatitis, liver failure
Neurological	Extrapyramidal, cerebellar manifestation
Psychiatric	Depression, mania, delusions
Ocular	Kayser–Fleischer ring, sunflower cataract
Hematological	Hemolysis, thrombocytopenia, leucopenia
Musculoskeletal	Osteoporosis, rickets, chondrocalcinosis
Renal	Renal tubular acidosis, nephrolithiasis
Cardiac	Arrhythmias, cardiomyopathy
Endocrine	Hypoparathyroidism, delayed puberty
Miscellaneous	Cholilithiasis, drug reactions

(1) *Ophthalmic*:
   (a) *Kayser–Fleischer ring*: is greenish yellow coloration of the limbus of the cornea. It is best identified using slit lamp examination. The ring that starts at the superior pole is due to deposition of sulfur rich copper granules in the Descemet's membrane. It is usually associated with neurological manifestation and may be absent in acute fulminant hepatitis or early hepatic disease.
   (b) *Sunflower cataract*: is greyish brown coloration in the anterior lense capsule that does not interfere with vision and best examined using slit lamp.
(2) *Hematological*:
   (a) *Acute hemolysis* (*Coomb's negative*): this could be isolated transient presentation or associated with acute fulminant hepatitis.
   (b) *Hypersplenism*: usually complicating liver cirrhosis with portal hypertension and characterized by thrombocytopenia and leucopenia.
   (c) *Bleeding tendency*: either due to thrombocytopenia or to impaired coagulation factors synthesis in advanced liver disease leading to increase in prothrombin and partial thromboplastin time.
(3) *Musculoskeletal*:
   (a) osteoporosis
   (b) rickets or osteomalacia
   (c) osteoarthritis
   (d) chondrocalcinosis
   (e) azure or blue lunulae of the finger nails
(4) *Renal*:
   (a) *Fanconi syndrome*: characterized by glycosuria, aminoaciduria, uricosuria, hypouricemia, hypercalciuria and phosphaturia
   (b) Distal renal tubular acidosis
   (c) nephrolithiasis
   (d) nephrotic syndrome and Goodpasture-like syndrome secondary to treatment with penicillamine
(5) *Cardiac*: arrhythmias, cardiomyopathy and autonomic dysfunction.
(6) *Miscellaneous*: cholilithiasis, hypoparathyroidism and delayed puberty.

4. DIAGNOSIS

Wilson's disease should be considered in any young patient with unexplained hepatic, neuropsychiatric disease or hemolysis, so that lifelong treatment is initiated to prevent complications [3] (Figure 2). Diagnosis requires a high index of suspicion and is divided into the following [12,14]:

1. *Clinical evaluation*:

(a) signs and symptoms of liver disease
(b) cerebellar or extrapyramidal manifestation
(c) psychiatric disturbances
(d) *Kayser–Fleischer ring*: present in 55% of patients with Wilson's disease and in 91% with neurological presentation. It has also been reported in patients with chronic cholestatic disease.

2. *Biochemical tests*: no single biochemical abnormality is completely reliable to make a diagnosis (Table 2).

(a) *Increased liver enzymes*: mild-to-moderate increase in serum aminotransferases including patients with acute fulminant hepatitis (<500 IU/ml).
(b) *Serum ceruloplasmin level*: serum level (20–40 mg/dl) is reduced in more than 80% of patients with Wilson's disease to less than 20 mg/dl. False normal ceruloplasmin levels can occur with acute inflammation including acute fulminant hepatitis (acute phase protein), pregnancy, estrogen administration and measurements using immunoprecipitation method rather than oxidative method which measures both blue copper containing ceruloplasmin and colorless apoceruloplasmin. 10–20% of heterozygote have low serum ceruloplasmin. Low levels of ceruloplasmin could also be found in patients with severe malnutrition, nephrotic syndrome, protein loosing enteropathy, aceruloplasminaemia and other chronic liver disease with low protein.
(c) *Free serum copper level*: ceruloplasmin accounts for more than 90% of serum copper and the rest is free or bound to albumin (nonceruloplasmin bound-NCB copper). Total serum copper in Wilson's disease is reduced (<700 mcg/l); however, measured free serum

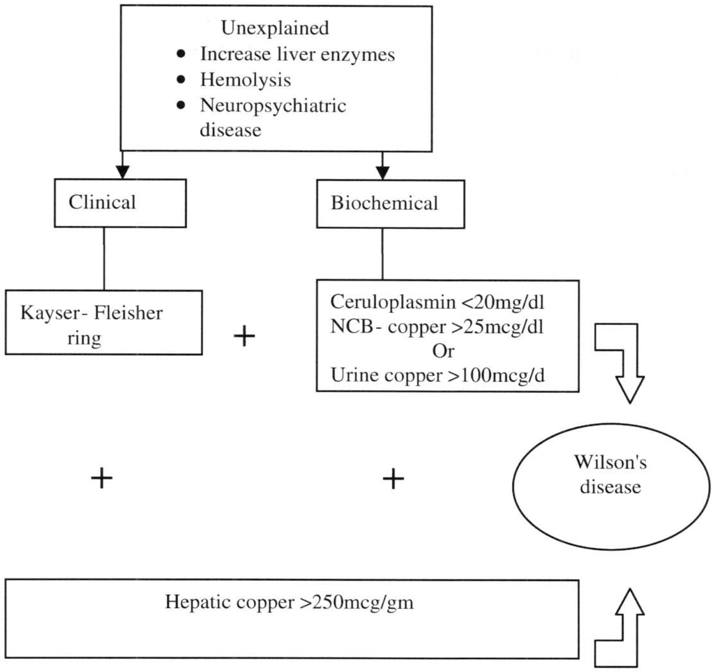

Figure 2. Diagnosis of Wilson's disease.

copper concentration (50–100 mcg/l) or calculated (total serum copper − 3.15 × serum ceruloplasmin (mg/l)) is more than 250 mcg/l (25 mcg/dl).

(d) *24 h urine collection for copper*: urinary copper excretion in normal individuals is less than 30 mcg/day. In Wilson's disease with impaired copper biliary excretion, urinary copper excretion increases to more than 100 mcg/day as a reflection of increase in body copper load. Other causes of chronic liver diseases could be associated with increase in copper excretion. Specificity of urine collection could be improved using a single dose (500 mg) of penicillamine which increases excretion in Wilson's disease to more than 1200 mcg/day as compared to less than 500 mcg/day in a normal person. However, overlap in urinary copper excretion between Wilson's disease and other chronic liver disease may still exist.

3. *Pathological studies*:

(a) *Liver histology*: is nonspecific where histological findings could be shared by other causes of chronic liver disease. In general, liver biopsy may show moderate fatty infiltration, glycogen vacuolation of the nuclei in periportal hepatocytes, Mallory's hyaline bodies and

Table 2. Copper levels in Wilson's disease compared to normal.

Copper level	Normal	Wilson's disease
Ceruloplasmin	20–40 mg/dl	<20 mg/dl
Nonceruloplasmin copper (NCB-copper)	50–100 mcg/l	>250 mcg/l
24 h urine collection	30–70 mcg/day	>100 mcg/day
Post-penicillamine urinary copper	<500 mcg/day	>1200 mcg/day
Hepatic copper	<50 mcg/g	>250 mcg/g

features of chronic active hepatitis or macronodular cirrhosis. Copper staining using rubeanic acid or rhodamine is usually unreliable for diagnosis since copper tends to be periportal with patchy distribution, may be absent from regenerating nodules and may be seen in cholestatic liver disease.

(b) *Hepatic copper concentration*: to avoid false increase in copper level in the liver biopsy, the liver biopsy needle should be washed with EDTA and rinsed with 5% dextrose. Liver specimen should be placed in a copper-free dry container and dried before copper analysis. Normally copper concentration is 20–50 mcg/g and above 250 mcg/g in patients with Wilson's disease. Heterozygote tends to have a high copper concentration but less than that of homozygote.

4. *Imaging studies*:

(a) *Abdominal imaging*: may show features of cirrhotic liver, gallstones, renal stones, splenomegaly or ascites.
(b) *Bone X-ray and bone densitometry*: changes suggestive of osteoporosis and occasionally subarticular cysts.
(c) *Brain MRI*: this is more sensitive than computed tomography of the brain. Though nonspecific it may show changes before development of neurological manifestations, which include brain atrophy, ventricular enlargement and high T2 signal in the basal ganglion.

5. *Others*:

(a) *Genetic testing*: using haplotype analysis is not common except for research purposes due to extensive mutation of ATP7B gene.
(b) *Radio labeled copper plasma clearance*: may be used in difficult cases where a 24/4 h activity ratio of more than 1 makes diagnosis of Wilson's disease unlikely.
(c) *Reitan trial test*: for assessment of cognitive function.

5. MANAGEMENT

The aim of therapy in patients with Wilson's disease is to remove already accumulated copper in the tissues and subsequent maintenance of negative copper balance to reverse clinicopathological manifestation and prevent development of complications (Figure 3). Historically intramuscular BAL injection was the first drug used for treatment of Wilson's disease.

(a) *Medical therapeutics*: This includes a low copper diet and drugs that act as chelating agents or to maintain negative copper balance (Table 3) [3,15,16]:

(1) *Penicillamine* (*Cuprimine*): First used for treatment of Wilson's disease in 1956, it is the most commonly used drug. It acts by reductive chelation and enhances copper urinary excretion with further decrease in serum ceruloplasmin and reversal of most of the signs and symptoms of Wilson's disease. Deterioration of neurological symptoms can occur after 2–6 weeks as a result of increase in brain copper or shift in intraneuronal copper. Initial daily dose is 1–2 g in divided doses on an empty stomach. Treatment should be continued until the patient's clinical status and laboratory tests normalize and stabilize monitored by decrease in urinary copper excretions (50–70 mcg/day) indicating adequate de-coppering state, which may take several years. This also could be accessed by decrease in necro-inflammatory changes and hepatic copper concentration. Dose can be decreased (1 g/day) to maintain negative copper balance and continued indefinitely. Penicillamine usually is well tolerated but several side effects may occur including bone marrow suppression, pyridoxine deficiency, nephrotic syndrome, drug-induced lupus and Good–Pasteur like syndrome. Hypersensitivity reaction occurring with the initiation of treatment (20%) can be treated by reintroduction of the drug with a smaller dose and gradual dose increase to achieve therapeutic effect or concomitant use of corticosteroids. It is reported to be unsafe during pregnancy; however, after weighing pros and cons of treatment, it should be continued during pregnancy and is unlikely to produce teratogenic effect [17].
(2) *Trientine* (*Syprine*): effect is similar to penicillamine and is used sometimes in patients who could not tolerate penicillamine. It is more expensive and can also initially worsen

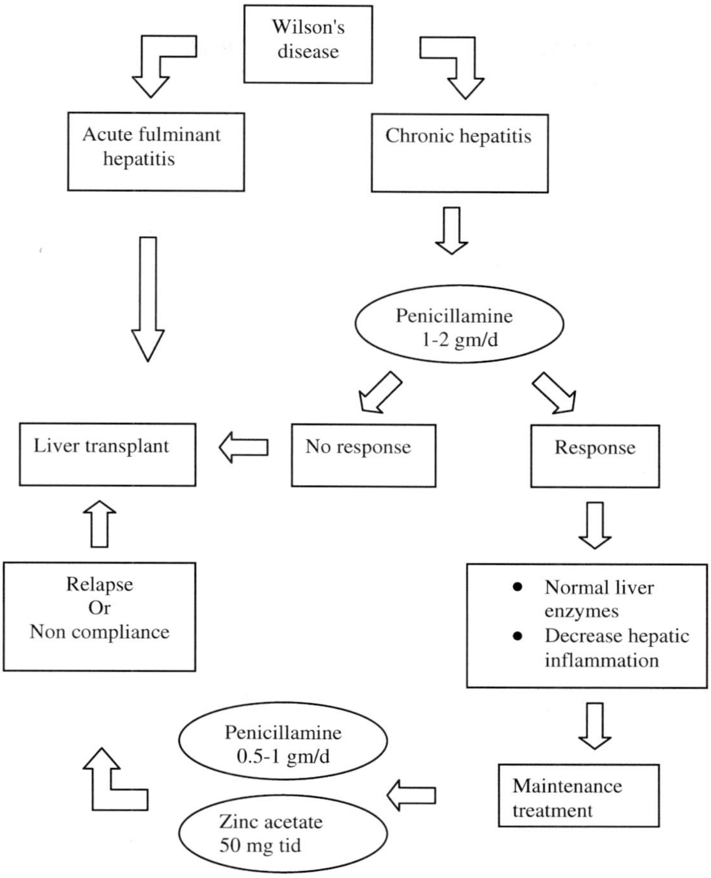

Figure 3. Treatment of Wilson's disease.

neurological manifestation. Sideroplastic anemia, colitis and drug-induced lupus are possible complications.

(3) *Tetrathiomolybdate* (*TM*): inhibits copper absorption and binds tissue copper to form an inert complex. Adequate response is achieved when equilibrium occurs between molybdenum level and nonceruloplasmin copper. It may be helpful in patients with neurological manifestation. Its clinical use is limited by its toxicity.

(4) *Zinc acetate* (*Galzin*): approved for maintenance treatment of Wilson's disease in 1997 and was also found to be effective as an initial treatment. It decreases copper intestinal absorption through

Table 3. Drugs used for treatment of Wilson's disease.

Drug	Dose	Side effect
Penicillamine	1–2 g/day	Hypersensitivity reaction, bone marrow suppression, SLE, nephrotic syndrome
Trientine	1–2 g/day	Sideroblastic anemia, worsening neurological manifestation, teratogenic
Tetrathiomolybdate	60–120 mg/day	Bone marrow suppression
Zinc acetate	150–300 mg/day	Dyspepsia

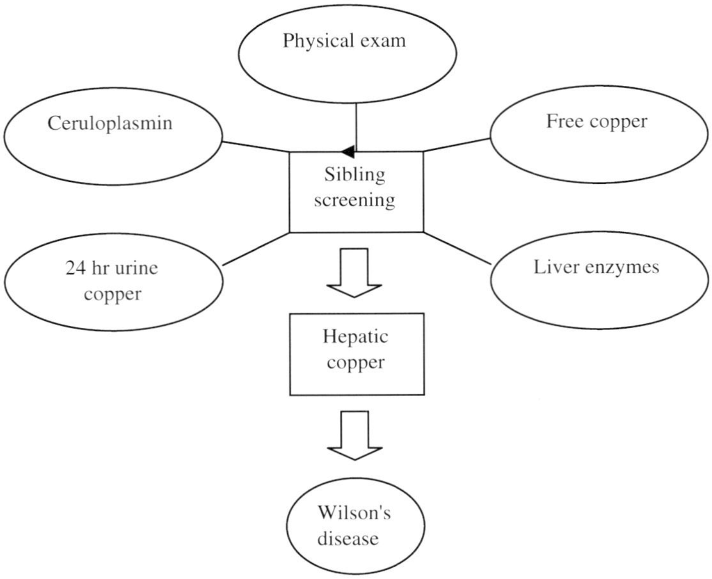

Figure 4. Screening of siblings of patients with Wilson's disease.

induction of enterocytes metallothionein which binds to copper and is excreted in stool with cellular desquamation. Daily 150 mg in divided doses in between meals is recommended to decrease urinary copper to <100 mcg/day and decrease nonceruloplasmin bound copper to <200 mcg/l. Hepatic copper concentration after several years of therapy is variable and cannot be used for therapy response. Compliance can be accessed by zinc urinary excretion of more than 2 mg/day. It is safe during pregnancy and well tolerated except for mild gastrointestinal disturbances. Acute hepatitis has been reported after starting zinc through competitive binding with metallothionein and copper displacement in the hepatocytes.

(b) *Surgical procedures*: liver transplantation is indicated in patients with Wilson's disease who fail medical therapy or with advanced liver failure [18]. It is the only effective treatment for acute fulminant hepatitis. Neuropsychiatric manifestations have been reported to improve in a few patients post-liver transplant; however, its indication with exclusive neurological involvement is controversial [19].

(c) *Prevention*: Siblings should be screened using clinical and laboratory assessments to detect homozygote in the presymptomatic stage and treated using penicillamine or zinc (Figure 4).

6. PROGNOSIS

Wilson's disease is fatal if left untreated. Treated patients who are compliant and respond to treatment have a good prognosis. Response to medical treatment may be delayed for several months (4–12 months). Resolving of neurological manifestation may be delayed for 2 years provided there is no irreversible damage. Patients presenting with acute fulminant hepatitis have a poor prognosis with a high mortality rate (>80%). Development of hepatocellular carcinoma is uncommon probably due to the copper protective effect. A high index of suspicion aided by laboratory assessment will result in early diagnosis, prompt treatment and better prognosis.

REFERENCES

[1] Brewer, G.J. and Yuzbasiyan-Gurkan, V. (1992) Wilson disease. *Medicine (Baltimore)* **71**, 139–164.

[2] Sheinberg, J.H. and Sternlieb, I. (1996) Wilson disease and idiopathic copper toxicosis. *Am. J. Clin. Nutr.* **63**, 842S–845S.

[3] Gollan, J.L. and Gollan, T.J. (1998) Wilson disease in 1998: genetic, diagnostic, and therapeutic aspects. *J. Hepatol.* **28**(Suppl. 1), 28–36.

[4] Schaefer, M., Roelofsen, H., Wolters, H., Hofmann, W.J., Muller, M., Kuipers, F., Stremmel, W. and Vonk, R.J. (1999) Localization of the Wilson's disease protein in human live. *Gastroenterology* **117**, 1380–1385.

[5] Ferenci, P., Gilliam, T.C., Gitlin, J.D., Packman, S., Schilsky, M.L., Sokol, R.J. and Sternleib, I. (1996) An international symposium on Wilson's and Menkes' diseases. *Hepatology* **24**(4), 952–958.

[6] Bull, P.C., Thomas, G.R., Rommers, J.M., Fobres, J.R. and Cox, D.W. (1993) The Wilson disease gene is a putative copper transporting P-type ATPase similar to the Menkes gene. *Nat. Genet.* **5**, 327–337.

[7] Tanzi, R.E., Petrukhin, K., Chernov, I., Pellequer, J.L., Wasco, W., Ross, B., Romano, D.M., Parano, E., Pavone, L. and Brzustowicz, L.M. (1993) The Wilson disease gene is a copper transporting ATPase with homology to the Menkes disease gene. *Nat. Genet.* **5**, 344–350.

[8] Maier-Dobersberger, T., Fenenci, P., Polli, C., Balac, P., Dienes, H.P., Kaserer, K., Datz, C., Vogel, W. and Gangl, A. (1997) Detection of the His1069Gln mutation in Wilson disease by rapid polymerase chain reaction. *Ann. Intern. Med.* **127**, 21–26.

[9] Czlonkowska, A., Rodo, M., Gajda, J., Ploos van Amstel, H.K., Juyn, J. and Houwen, R.H. (1997) Very high frequency of the His1069Gln mutation in Polish Wilson disease patients. *J. Neurol.* **244**, 591–599.

[10] Riordan, S.M. and Williams, R. (2001) The Wilson's disease gene and phenotypic diversity. *J. Hepatol.* **34**, 165–171.

[11] Gow, P.J., Smallwood, R.A., Angus, P.W., Smith, A.L., Wall, A.J. and Sewell, R.B. (2000) Diagnosis of Wilson's disease: an experience over three decades. *Gut* **46**, 415–419.

[12] Steindl, P., Ferenci, P., Dienes, H.P., Grimm, G., Pabinger, I., Madl, C., Maier-Dobersberger, T., Herneth, A., Dragosics, B., Meryn, S., Knoflach, P., Granditsch, G. and Gangl, A. (1997) Wilson's disease in patients presenting with liver disease a diagnostic challenge. *Gastroenterology* **113**(1), 212–218.

[13] Jackson, G.H., Meyer, A. and Lipmann, S. (1994) Wilson's disease. Psychiatric manifestations may be the clinical presentation. *Postgrad. Med.* **95**(8), 135–138.

[14] Sanchez-Albisua, I., Garde, T., Hierro, L., Camarena, C., Frauca, E., de la Vega, A., Diaz, M.C., Larrauri, J. and Jara, P. (1999) A high index of suspicion: the key to an early diagnosis of Wilson's disease in childhood. *J. Paediatr. Gastroenterol. Nutr.* **28**, 186–190.

[15] Walshe, J.M. (1999) Penicillamine: the treatment of first choice for patients with Wilson's disease. *Mov. Disord.* **14**, 545–550.

[16] Brewer, G.J., Dick, R.D., Johnson, V.D., Brunberg, J.A., Kluin, J. and Fink, J. (1998) Treatment of Wilson's disease with zinc: XV long-term follow-up studies. *J. Lab. Clin. Med.* **132**(4), 264–277.

[17] Sternlieb, I. (2000) Wilson's disease and pregnancy. *Hepatology* **31**(2), 531–532.

[18] Brewer, G.J. and Askari, F. (2000) Transplant livers in Wilson's disease for hepatic, not neurologic, indications. *Liver Transpl.* **6**(5), 662–664.

[19] Guarino, M., Stracciari, A., D'Alessandro, R. and Pazzaglia, P. (1995) No neurological improvement after liver transplantation for Wilson's disease. *Acta Neurol. Scand.* **92**, 405–408.

Hepatology: A Practical Approach
B. Al Knawy, M.L. Shiffman, R.H. Wiesner (editors)

Chapter 14
Autoimmune Hepatitis and Overlap Syndromes

Albert J. Czaja

Division of Gastroenterology and Hepatology, Mayo Clinic, 200 First Street SW, Rochester, MN 55905, USA

1. Introduction 233
   1.1 Disease definition 233
   1.2 Disease prevalence and incidence 236
   1.3 General demographics 236
2. Pathophysiology 236
   2.1 Cell-mediated cytotoxicity 236
   2.2 Antibody-dependent cell-mediated cytotoxicity 237
   2.3 Autoantigens 238
   2.4 Genetic factors 238
   2.5 Overlap syndromes 238
3. Clinical Features 239
   3.1 Serologic distinctions in AIH 239
   3.2 Symptoms of AIH 240
   3.3 Physical findings of AIH 240
   3.4 Laboratory features of AIH 240
   3.5 Histological findings in AIH 240
   3.6 Features of an overlap syndrome 240
4. Diagnosis 241
   4.1 Blood tests 241
   4.2 Imaging studies 241
   4.3 Pathological studies 242
   4.4 Promising new autoantibodies 243
5. Management 244
   5.1 Medical therapeutics of AIH 244
   5.2 Medical therapeutics of the overlap syndromes 245
   5.3 Prevention and screening 245
   5.4 Emerging therapies 246
6. Prognosis 246
References 246

1. INTRODUCTION

1.1 Disease definition

Autoimmune hepatitis (AIH) is an unresolving inflammation of the liver of unknown cause that is characterized by interface hepatitis on histological examination, hypergammaglobulinemia, and autoantibodies [1]. Criteria for the definite and probable diagnoses have been codified by an international panel, and these criteria define the disease (Table 1) [2]. Diseases that resemble AIH must be excluded, and cholestatic features preclude the diagnosis. Interface hepatitis (Figure 1) is the histological hallmark of AIH, and portal plasma cell infiltration

Table 1. International diagnostic criteria for autoimmune hepatitis.

Definite autoimmune hepatitis	Probable autoimmune hepatitis
Abnormally increased serum aminotransferase level	Abnormally increased serum aminotransferase level
Serum globulin, γ-globulin, or immunoglobulin G level >1.5 × UNL	Serum globulin, γ-globulin, or immunoglobulin G level >1.0 × UNL
ANA, SMA, or anti-LKM1 >1:80	ANA, SMA, or anti-LKM1 >1:40 or presence of any AIH-related autoantibody
AMA negative	AMA negative
Negative HBsAg, anti-HCV, and IgM anti-HAV	Negative HBsAg, anti-HCV, and IgM anti-HAV
Interface hepatitis (moderate-severe), possibly in association with acinar hepatitis or bridging necrosis	Interface hepatitis (moderate–severe), possibly in association with acinar hepatitis or bridging necrosis
No biliary lesions, granulomas, or other prominent changes suggestive of another disease	No biliary lesions, granulomas, or other prominent changes suggestive of another disease
Normal serum α_1-anti-trypsin and ceruloplasmin levels	Abnormal ceruloplasmin level unassociated with Wilson disease
No recent hepatotoxic drugs and average alcohol consumption <25 g/d	No recent hepatotoxic drugs and average alcohol consumption <50 g/d or persistent AIH despite discontinuation of drug and/or abstinence from alcohol

UNL, upper normal limit; ANA, antinuclear antibodies; SMA, smooth muscle antibodies; anti-LKM1, antibodies to liver/kidney microsome type 1; AIH, autoimmune hepatitis; AMA, antimitochondrial antibodies; HBsAg, hepatitis B surface antigen; anti-HCV, antibodies to hepatitis C virus; and IgM anti-HAV, immunoglobulin M antibodies to hepatitis A virus.

(Figure 2) is a characteristic but not a requisite feature. Neither histological finding is specific for AIH, and the diagnosis is based on a constellation of findings.

Syndromes with mixed features that resemble AIH and other classical conditions constitute the *overlap syndromes* (Table 2) [2]. These syndromes refer to any condition in which the clinical features suggest a mixture of diseases. Typically, they include patients with AIH and cholestatic clinical, laboratory, and/or histological features. Disorders with intermingled manifestations of AIH and primary biliary cirrhosis (PBC) [4], AIH and primary sclerosing cholangitis

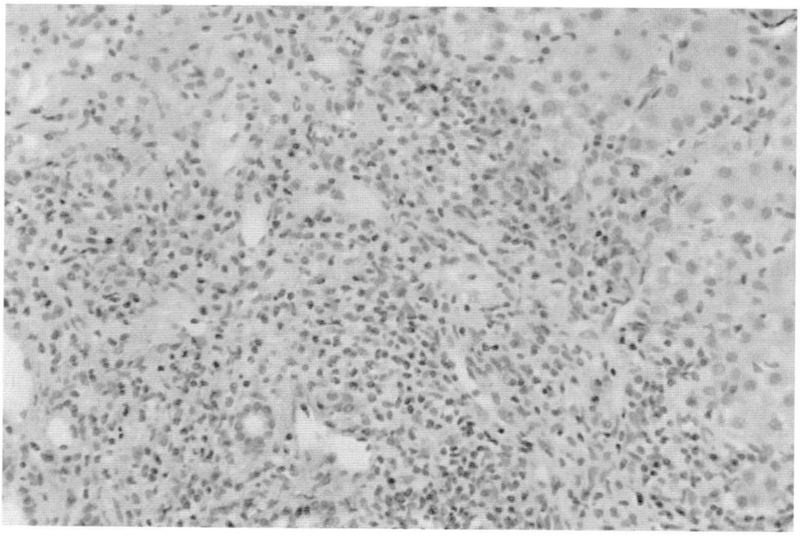

Figure 1. *Interface hepatitis.* The limiting plate of the portal tract is disrupted by an inflammatory infiltrate in association with hepatocyte damage. Hematoxylin and eosin; original magnification, ×200. (*For colored version, see Plate XXII on page 576 at the end of the book.*)

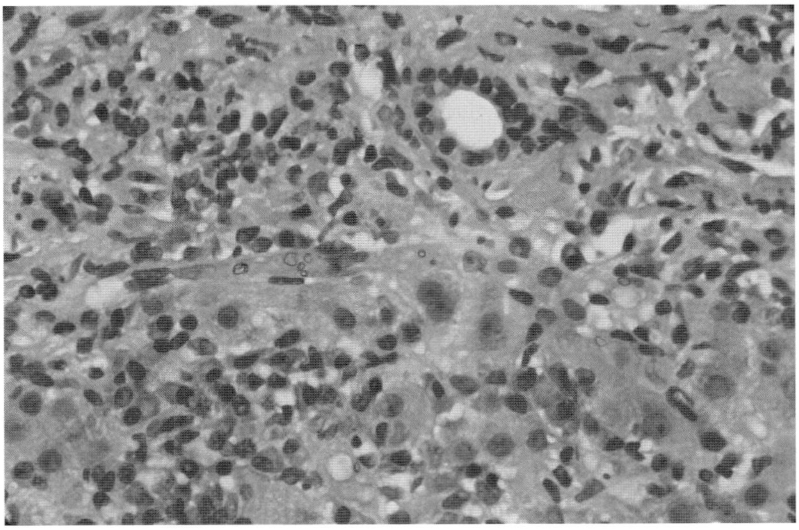

Figure 2. *Plasma cell infiltration.* Plasma cells, which are characterized by a perinuclear cytoplasmic halo, are present within the inflammatory infiltrate of the portal tract. Hematoxylin and eosin; original magnification, ×400. (*For colored version, see Plate XXIII on page 576 at the end of the book.*)

(PSC) [5], and cholestatic hepatitis in the absence of PBC and PSC (autoimmune cholangitis) are the principal overlap forms [6]. Rarely, patients with AIH may have a co-infection with hepatitis C virus (HCV), and the two concurrent disorders suggest a hybrid syndrome [7].

The diagnostic criteria of the overlap syndromes have not been standardized nor do these variant forms have confident treatment strategies [8]. The validity of the overlap syndromes requires a clear definition of the boundaries of presentation for classical disease. Overlap syndromes of AIH should be

Table 2. Distinctive features and treatment options for overlap syndromes.

Distinctive aspects	AIH + PBC	AIH + PSC	AIC	AIH + HCV
Clinical findings	Pruritus pigmentation	Pruritus CUC	Pruritus no CUC	None
Laboratory findings	AMA positive, AP > 3 × UNL, abnormal IgM	AMA negative, no HLA DR4, AP > 3 × UNL	AMA negative, ANA positive, AP > 3 × UNL	HCV RNA in blood, SMA or ANA ≥ 1:320
Imaging studies	None	Abnormal cholangiogram	Normal cholangiogram	None
Histological findings	Cholestasis, bile duct injury, florid duct lesion, copper deposition	Ductopenia, portal edema, portal fibrosis, fibrous obliterative cholangitis	Ductopenia, portal edema, bile duct injury, florid duct lesion	Interface hepatitis with or without plasma cells, no steatosis or lymphoid aggregates
Treatment options	Prednisone alone or with azathioprine, UDA and prednisone	Prednisone and UDA	Prednisone, prednisone and azathioprine, prednisone and UDA	Prednisone alone or with azathioprine

AIH, autoimmune hepatitis; PBC, primary biliary cirrhosis; PSC, primary sclerosing cholangitis; AIC, autoimmune cholangitis; HCV, hepatitis C virus; CUC, chronic ulcerative colitis; AMA, antimitochondrial antibodies; AP, serum alkaline phosphatase level; UNL, upper normal limit; HLA, human leukocyte antigen; ANA, antinuclear antibodies; SMA, smooth muscle antibodies; UDA, ursodeoxycholic acid.

restricted to disorders that have mixed clinical expressions rather than isolated atypical findings. Patients with isolated atypical findings (antimitochondrial antibodies (AMA) or sporadic bile duct injury on histological examination) may have subclinical overlap syndromes, but the background findings are insufficient to compel an alternative diagnosis or treatment schedule [9].

A scoring system developed by the International AIH Group has been refined to exclude viral and cholestatic syndromes with high specificity, and it can assess the strength of the diagnosis of AIH and the degree of resemblance of an overlap syndrome to the classical disease (Table 3) [2].

1.2 Disease prevalence and incidence

The mean annual incidence of AIH among Caucasoid North Americans and Northern Europeans is 1.9 per 100,000, and its point prevalence is 16.9 per 100,000 [10]. AIH affects 100,000–200,000 individuals in the US, and it accounts for 2.6% of the liver transplants in the European Liver Transplant Registry and 5.9% of the liver transplants in the US [1].

The frequency of the overlap syndromes has been estimated by retrospective analyses based on the presence of cholestatic features or atypical findings in patients with classical AIH [11]. Under these circumstances, 5% of patients with AIH can be reclassified as having AIH and PBC, and 7% can be re-designated as having autoimmune cholangitis ("AMA-negative PBC"). Inflammatory bowel disease occurs in 16% of patients with classical AIH, and 44% of these individuals have cholangiographic changes of PSC. These findings suggest that 7% of patients with AIH may have concurrent PSC. The overall frequency that cholestatic syndromes overlap with AIH is 12%. Eleven percent of patients with classical AIH may be co-infected with HCV.

1.3 General demographics

Seventy percent of patients with AIH are female, and 50% are less than 40 years [1,3]. The onset of illness is usually between the third and fifth decade, but patients may range in age from 9 months to 77 years. Forty percent have an abrupt, rarely fulminant, presentation, and the disease may resemble an acute viral or toxic hepatitis. Thirty-eight percent have concurrent immune diseases, especially autoimmune thyroiditis, Graves' disease, synovitis, or ulcerative colitis. Diverse ethnic groups are susceptible to AIH, and it has been reported in Australia, Japan, Mexico, Kuwait, the Indian subcontinent, Europe, South America, and the US. African Americans may have an especially aggressive form of the disease. Familial occurrences are rare, but the disease has been reported in siblings, parents, and grandparents of afflicted individuals.

The overlap syndromes of AIH typically occur in adulthood, and the clinical demographics are usually those of AIH [3,6,8,11]. An exception to this adult predilection is the occurrence of "autoimmune sclerosing cholangitis" in the AIH of childhood [12].

2. PATHOPHYSIOLOGY

2.1 Cell-mediated cytotoxicity

The pathogenesis of AIH and the overlap syndromes is unknown. The most popular hypothesis is that viruses, drugs, or environmental factors trigger a cell-mediated form of cytotoxicity in a genetically susceptible host [13]. This hypothesis predicts that self-antigens or foreign antigens, which resemble self-antigens are expressed by class II molecules of the major histocompatibility complex (MHC). CD4 T helper cells are activated, and these cells are the principal effectors of the disease. Cytokines characteristic of a type 1 cytokine response orchestrate the differentiation of the CD4 T helper cells into cytotoxic T cells that accomplish liver cell destruction through the release of lymphokines. Disease non-specific autoimmune promoter genes facilitate the clonal expansion of the cytotoxic T cells through synergisms with the principal susceptibility alleles. This hypothesis has been supported by the demonstration of antigen-sensitized, disease-specific, cytotoxic T cells within the liver of patients with AIH. Furthermore, polymorphisms of the tumor

Table 3. International scoring system for diagnosis of autoimmune hepatitis.

Category	Factor	Score	Category	Factor	Score
Gender	Female	+2	Immune disease	Thyroiditis, colitis, synovitis, others	+2
AP:AST (or ALT) ratio	<1.5	+2	Other liver-defined autoantibody	Anti-SLA/LP, anti-actin, anti-LC1, pANCA	+2
	1.5–3.0	0			
	>3.0	−2			
γ-globulin or IgG levels × UNL	>2.0	+3	Histological features	Interface hepatitis	+3
	1.5–2.0	+2		Plasma cells	+1
	1.0–1.5	+1		Rosettes	+1
	<1.0	0		None of above	−5
				Biliary changes	−3
				Other features	−3
ANA, SMA, or anti-LKM1 titers	>1:80	+3	Treatment response	Complete	+2
	1:80	+2		Relapse	+3
	1:40	+1			
	<1:40	0			
AMA	Positive	−4			
HBsAg, anti-HCV, IgM anti-HAV	Positive	−3			
	Negative	+3			
Hepatotoxic drug exposure	Yes	−4	*Pretreatment score*		
	No	+1	Definite diagnosis		>15
			Probable diagnosis		10–15
Alcohol	<25 g/day	+2	*Posttreatment score*		
	>60 g/day	−2	Definite diagnosis		>17
			Probable diagnosis		12–17
HLA	DR3 or DR4	+1			

AP, serum alkaline phosphatase level; AST, serum aspartate aminotransferase level; ALT, serum alanine aminotransferase level; ANA, antinuclear antibodies; SMA, smooth muscle antibodies; anti-LKM1, antibodies to liver kidney/microsome type 1; AMA, antimitochondrial antibodies; anti-SLA/LP, antibodies to soluble liver antigen/liver pancreas; anti-LC1, antibodies to liver cytosol type 1; pANCA, perinuclear anti-neutrophil cytoplasmic antibodies; IgG, immunoglobulin G; UNL, upper normal limit; HBsAg, hepatitis B surface antigen; anti-HCV, antibodies to hepatitis C virus; and IgM anti-HAV, immunoglobulin M antibodies to hepatitis A virus.

necrosis factor-α gene (*TNF-A*) [14] and the cytotoxic T lymphocyte antigen-4 gene (*CTLA*-4) [15] have been described in Caucasoid North American and Northern European patients that can promote a type 1 cytokine response and favor immunocyte activation.

2.2 Antibody-dependent cell-mediated cytotoxicity

An antibody-dependent, cell-mediated form of cytotoxicity has also been proposed [13]. According to this hypothesis, the activated CD4 T helper cells result in unmodulated production of immunoglobulin G by plasma cells through a defect in suppressor function. The excess immunoglobulin G binds with normal constituents of the hepatocyte membrane, and natural killer cells with Fc receptors target the antigen–antibody complex on the membrane surface. Liver cell injury ensues as a result of cytolysis. The antibody-dependent, cell-mediated mechanism of AIH has been supported by the demonstration of antigen–antibody complexes on the surface of hepatocytes and by the over-expression of interleukin 10 in some patients. Excess interleukin 10 favors a type 2 cytokine response that promotes the antibody-dependent pathogenic pathway. Both mechanisms of liver cell injury may be important at different stages of the disease and depend on the prevailing cytokine milieu.

2.3 Autoantigens

The cytochrome mono-oxygenase, P450 2D6 (CYP2D6), has been proposed as the target autoantigen of AIH associated with antibodies to liver/kidney microsome type 1 (anti-LKM1) [1,3,16]. This antigen has been sequenced, cloned and mapped for epitopes, and anti-LKM1 react to four antigenic sites located between peptides 257–269, 321–351, 373–389, and 410–429. The main antigenic site is the peptide sequence, 257–269, which is highly specific for AIH, and the second most recognized sequence is 321–351. P450 2D6 (CYP2D6) shares homologies with the genomes of HCV and herpes simplex type 1, and this molecular mimicry may result in cross-reacting antibodies in rare instances. AIH has also been described in 15% of patients with autoimmune polyendocrinopathy-candidiasis-ectodermal dystrophy, and P450 (CYP) 1A2 and P450 (CYP) 2A6 have been implicated as the target autoantigens [1,3]. The asialoglycoprotein receptor on the hepatocyte membrane is a promising candidate autoantigen for other forms of AIH.

2.4 Genetic factors

AIH has a strong genetic basis, which contributes to susceptibility, clinical expression, and treatment outcome [17]. The human leukocyte antigen (HLA) DR3 is the principal susceptibility factor in Caucasoid North American and Northern European populations, and HLA DR4 is a secondary but independent risk factor. Eighty-five percent of white patients with AIH in the US have HLA DR3, DR4, or DR3 and DR4. High-resolution DNA-based techniques have indicated that susceptibility in this population resides on the *DRB1* gene and that the susceptibility alleles are *DRB1*0301* and *DRB1*0401* [17].

*DRB1*0301* and *DRB1*0401* each encode an identical six amino acid sequence between positions 67 and 72 on the DRβ polypeptide chain ("shared motif hypothesis") [17]. This amino acid sequence is represented by the amino acid code, LLEQKR, in which lysine (K) is at position DRβ71. Lysine is at a critical contact point of the antigen binding groove of the class II MHC molecule, and its physical and electrostatic properties can affect antigen presentation and immunocyte recognition. *DRB1*0404* and *DRB1*0405* are the susceptibility alleles for AIH in Mexico (Mestizos), Japan, and South America (adult patients), and they each encode a similar core motif at positions DRβ67–72 (LLEQRR). These alleles encode an arginine (R) for a lysine (K) at DRβ71, and arginine is a positively charged, polar amino acid that is structurally similar to lysine. In contrast, *DRB1*1501* protects against AIH in Caucasoid patients, and this allele encodes the sequence, ILEQAR, between DRβ67–72. The substitution of isoleucine (I) for leucine (L) at position DRβ67 is a neutral substitution and would not affect antigen presentation. The substitution of a negatively charged alanine (A) for lysine (K) at DRβ71, however, would greatly alter the antigen binding properties of the DR molecule. In this fashion, the substitution of a single amino acid in a critical location could protect against the disease [17].

Recent studies from Brazil and Argentina have indicated that AIH, especially in children, is associated with *DRB1*1301* [18]. This allele encodes ILEDER as the critical motif in the class II MHC molecule, and the substitution of the negatively charged glutamic acid (E) for lysine (K) at DRβ71 defeats the shared motif hypothesis of pathogenesis. *DRB1*1301* has been associated with protracted infection with the hepatitis A virus (HAV), and HAV has been implicated as a trigger for AIH. South American children with *DRB1*1301*, therefore, may be naturally selected by protracted HAV infection to develop AIH. Genetic susceptibility to region-specific etiologic agents is another explanation for AIH in ethnically and genetically diverse populations ("molecular foot print hypothesis") [18].

2.5 Overlap syndromes

The bases for the concurrence of features typical of different diseases in the same patient are unknown [3–8]. The overlap syndromes may reflect coincidental disorders ("serendipitous mishap") or the extreme end of the normal spectrum of a single disease ("hepatitic PBC" versus "cholestatic AIH"). They may represent transitional states as one disease emerges from another, or they may reflect a promiscuous, poorly modulated immune response to homologous self and foreign antigens (molecular mimicry). AIH and PSC share HLA similarities in that both disorders are associated with HLA DR3. *DRB3*0101* is the principal susceptibility allele of PSC, and it encodes for HLA DR52. HLA DR52 and the A1-B8-DR3-DR52 phenotype occur as frequently in AIH as PSC, and this similarity suggests that a shared genetic predisposition between the diseases may favor their coexistence [17].

3. CLINICAL FEATURES

3.1 Serologic distinctions in AIH

Three types of AIH have been proposed based on distinctive autoantibodies (Table 4) [16]. None of these types has been established as a valid clinical entity, but each designation has entered the clinical jargon as a descriptive term. *Type 1 AIH* is the most common form of the disease worldwide, and it is associated with antinuclear antibodies (ANA) and/or smooth muscle antibodies (SMA) [16]. Type 1 AIH affects all ages, ethnic groups, and genders, and it frequently has an acute presentation. *DRB1*0301* and *DRB1*0401* are the principal susceptibility alleles for type 1 AIH. Patients with *DRB1*0301* have a younger age of disease onset than patients with other alleles, and they have a higher frequency of treatment failure, relapse after drug withdrawal, and requirement for liver transplantation. Patients with *DRB1*0401* are typically older, more commonly female, frequently afflicted with other concurrent autoimmune diseases, and more often responsive to corticosteroid therapy than patients with *DRB1*0301* [16].

Type 2 AIH affects mainly children, and it is characterized by anti-LKM1 (Table 4) [16]. Twenty percent of adults with type 2 AIH in Europe are adults, whereas only 4% of Caucasoid adults with AIH in the US have anti-LKM1. The target autoantigen of type 2 AIH is the cytochrome monooxygenase, P450 IID6 (CYP2D6) [16], and *DRB1*0701*, HLA B14, HLA DR3 and *C4A-QO* have been implicated as susceptibility factors [1,16,17]. Immune diseases (especially vitiligo, autoimmune thyroiditis, and insulin-dependent diabetes mellitus) and organ-specific autoantibodies (antibodies to thyroid, parietal cell, and/or islets of Langerhans) occur commonly. Like type 1 AIH, type 2 disease can have an acute, even fulminant, presentation.

Type 3 AIH is the least established form, and it is associated with antibodies to soluble liver antigen/liver pancreas (anti-SLA/LP) (Table 4) [1,16]. The target autoantigen is a 50 kDa liver cytosolic protein that is likely to be a transfer ribonucleoprotein complex (tRNP$^{(Ser)Sec}$ complex)

Table 4. Types of autoimmune hepatitis based on serological findings.

Type 1 AIH	Type 2 AIH	Type 3 AIH
Children and adults	Mainly children	Children and adults
Female predominance	Female predominance	Female predominance
Most common form	Rare in the US	Present in 16% of AIH
Acute, rarely fulminant, onset possible	Acute, rarely fulminant, onset possible	Acute, rarely fulminant, onset possible
ANA and/or SMA positive	Anti-LKM1 positive	Anti-SLA/LP positive
Autoimmune thyroiditis, synovitis, ulcerative colitis common	Insulin-dependent diabetes, vitiligo, autoimmune thyroiditis common	Autoimmune thyroiditis common
Associated with *DRB1*0301* and **0401*	Associated with *DRB1*0701*, HLA B14, HLA DR3, and *C4A-QO*	Associated with *DRB1*0301*
Unknown target autoantigen	P450 2D6 (CYP2D6) is target antigen	Unknown target autoantigen
pANCA common	May be associated with APECED	Indistinct from type 1 AIH
Responds to corticosteroids	Responds to corticosteroids	Responds to corticosteroids

AIH, autoimmune hepatitis; ANA, antinuclear antibodies; SMA, smooth muscle antibodies; anti-LKM1, antibodies to liver/kidney microsome type 1; anti-SLA/LP, antibodies to soluble liver antigen/liver pancreas; HLA, human leukocyte antigen; and APECED, autoimmune polyendocrinopathy candidiasis ectodermal dystrophy.

or a serine hydroxymethyltransferase involved in the selenocysteine metabolic pathway [19]. Patients typically lack anti-LKM1, but they commonly have other autoantibodies, including SMA, ANA, and AMA. Indeed, only 26% of patients with type 3 AIH have anti-SLA/LP as their sole serological markers. Patients with anti-SLA/LP have clinical and laboratory features that are indistinguishable from patients with type 1 AIH, and they respond well to corticosteroids. The frequency of type 3 AIH among Caucasoid adult patients with chronic hepatitis of unknown cause is 3% [1].

3.2 Symptoms of AIH

Fatigue is the most common symptom of AIH, and it occurs in 85% of patients. Right upper quadrant discomfort is experienced by 48%, and jaundice is recognized in 46%. Polymyalgias [30%], diminished appetite (30%), bowel disturbance (28%), cushingoid features (19%), delayed menarche or amenorrhea, and obscure fever (to as high as 40°C) are also possible. Intense pruritus and weight loss are atypical manifestations, and they suggest an alternative diagnosis or an overlap syndrome. Patients with severe inflammatory activity, especially children, can be asymptomatic.

3.3 Physical findings of AIH

Hepatomegaly is the most common physical finding at presentation (≤78%), and mild hepatic punch tenderness is also common. Splenomegaly is detected in 36%, even in the absence of histological cirrhosis, and spider nevi can be found in 58%. Ascites and hepatic encephalopathy are rare manifestations at presentation, and hyperpigmentation and xanthelasmas are incompatible with the diagnosis. Patients with AIH rarely have the stereotypic findings of facial rounding, hirsutism, and acne described in the original descriptions of "lupoid hepatitis," and 26% have normal physical examinations.

3.4 Laboratory features of AIH

Predominant abnormalities in the serum aminotransferase and γ-globulin levels characterize AIH, and the diagnosis is suspect without these findings (Table 1). Typically, the serum aspartate aminotransferase (AST) level ranges from 200 to 500 U/l at accession, and hypergammaglobulinemia is present in over 80%. Immunoglobulin levels are usually increased in a polyclonal fashion, and a predominant increase in the immunoglobulin G component is characteristic. Eighty-three percent of patients have hyperbilirubinemia, but only 46% have serum bilirubin levels that exceed 3 mg/dl. Serum alkaline phosphatase concentrations are abnormal in 81%, but only 33% have levels more than 2-fold the upper limit of normal and only 10% have values more than fourfold normal. The magnitude of the serum alkaline phosphatase elevation at presentation is commonly the most important finding that suggests the existence of an overlap syndrome, and serum levels above 3-fold normal justify serious efforts to exclude this possibility [11].

3.5 Histological findings in AIH

Interface hepatitis is the *sine qua non* of AIH (Figure 1), but it does not differentiate the disease from viral-related or drug-induced conditions [1]. Plasma cells can be seen at the interface and in the acinus in 66% of patients (Figure 2). Panacinar (lobular) hepatitis is usually seen in acute onset disease or relapse after treatment withdrawal, and panacinar hepatitis with bridging necrosis or multiacinar collapse is indicative of severe disease with a high frequency of progression to cirrhosis. Other histological findings that have been described in AIH include acinar zone 3 perivenular (centrilobular) necrosis with and without sparing of the portal tracts and giant syncytial multinucleated hepatocytes. Granulomas, copper deposits, siderosis, and steatosis are incompatible with the diagnosis, and ductopenia and/or destructive cholangitis indicate a cholestatic syndrome rather than AIH. Bile duct changes that coexist with the characteristic features of AIH connote an overlap syndrome.

3.6 Features of an overlap syndrome

The features of an overlap syndrome are those of AIH and another, usually cholestatic, disorder (Table 2) [3,8]. Symptoms of pruritus, physical findings of hyperpigmentation or xanthelasma, abnormal elevation of the serum alkaline phosphatase level to more than 3-fold the upper limit of normal, and histological changes of ductopenia and/or destructive cholangitis are features that suggest these syndromes. The presence of inflammatory bowel disease in a patient with AIH justifies cholangiography to exclude PSC, and recalcitrance to corticosteroid therapy warrants reassessment to exclude an active viral infection or subclinical cholestatic disorder.

Patients with AIH and PBC typically have lower serum levels of immunoglobulin G and higher serum concentrations of immunoglobulin M than patients with classical AIH (Table 2) [11]. SMA are present less commonly, and seropositivity for AMA is required for the diagnosis. Serum AST and alkaline phosphatase levels are comparable to those of AIH, but histological features of bile duct injury are present in conjunction with findings of interface hepatitis. The biliary changes may include a florid duct lesion [4].

Patients with AIH and PSC have lower serum AST and γ-globulin levels than patients with AIH, lower frequencies of SMA seropositivity and HLA DR4, and higher serum concentrations of alkaline phosphatase (Table 2) [11]. They typically have inflammatory bowel disease, and cholangiography discloses changes of PSC. Histological findings include ductopenia, portal tract edema and fibrosis, cholangiolar proliferation, and rarely, fibrous obliterative cholangitis, in association with interface hepatitis.

Patients with autoimmune cholangitis lack AMA, have lower serum levels of AST, γ-globulin and immunoglobulin G, lower frequencies of SMA seropositivity, and higher serum concentrations of alkaline phosphatase than patients with AIH (Table 2) [6,11]. Inflammatory bowel disease is absent, and cholangiography is normal. The histological changes of AIH are accompanied by features of PBC (florid duct lesion) or PSC (ductopenia, portal tract edema, and/or cholangiolar proliferation) [6].

Patients with AIH and HCV have high serum titers [≥1:320] of SMA and/or ANA, hypergammaglobulinemia, and abnormally increased serum concentrations of immunoglobulin G. HCV RNA is detectable in serum, and histological examination discloses features of interface hepatitis with or without plasma cell infiltration and minimal or no steatosis or portal lymphoid aggregation (Table 2) [3]. Syndromes in which the viral manifestations of the disease predominate have chronic hepatitis C with autoimmune features. These latter patients typically have low serum titers (≤1:160) of SMA or ANA (not both), and histological findings of steatosis and portal lymphoid aggregation without plasma cell infiltration [3].

4. DIAGNOSIS

4.1 Blood tests

The essential laboratory tests to evaluate AIH and its overlap syndromes are the serum AST, total bilirubin, alkaline phosphatase, γ-globulin, immunoglobulin, and albumin levels (Figures 3 and 4). The core battery of serologic tests includes assays for ANA, SMA, anti-LKM1, AMA, and antibodies to HCV. Antibodies to SLA/LP are not generally available.

4.2 Imaging studies

Hepatic ultrasonography is useful to evaluate features of cirrhosis and portal hypertension and to exclude biliary obstruction and hepatic mass. It may also indicate biliary obstruction or thickening of the extrahepatic bile ducts and in this fashion, suggest the possibility of concurrent PSC. Its non-interventional nature and easy availability justify its use in all patients with AIH at presentation.

Endoscopic retrograde cholangiography is warranted in all patients with AIH and inflammatory bowel disease and in those individuals with unexplained cholestatic features. Magnetic resonance cholangiography is associated with fewer complications than cholangiography, but its preference over the endoscopic procedure must be based on each institution's experience.

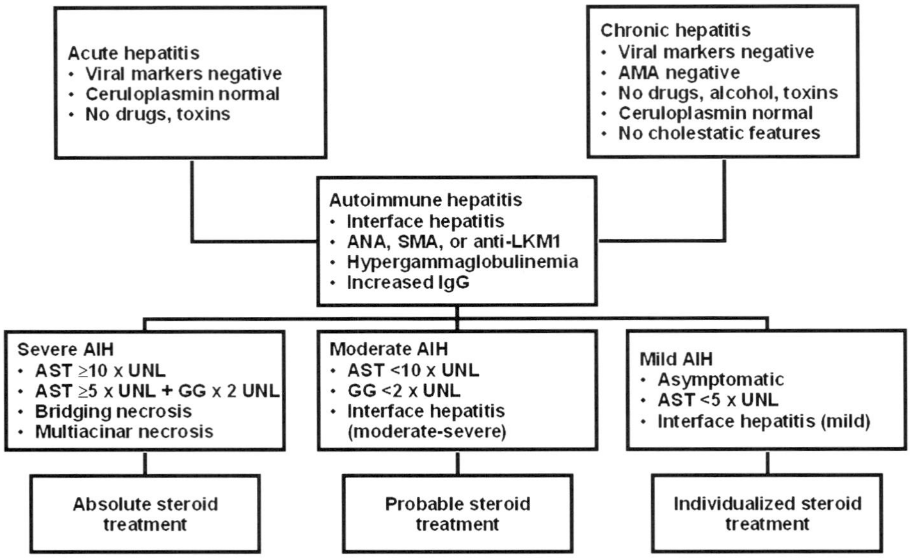

Figure 3. Diagnostic and treatment algorithms for autoimmune hepatitis. Presentations can be acute (rarely fulminant) or chronic (indolent). Viral infections, drug toxicities, toxic and alcohol exposures, and cholestatic syndromes must be excluded. Antimitochondrial antibodies (AMA) must be absent for a definite diagnosis, and autoantibodies such as antinuclear antibodies (ANA), smooth muscle antibodies (SMA), or antibodies to liver/kidney microsome type 1 (anti-LKM1) must be present. An abnormally increased serum level of immunoglobulin G (IgG) is characteristic of the disease. Treatment decisions are based on the severity of symptoms and inflammatory activity as assessed by laboratory tests and liver tissue examination. The degree of elevation of the serum aspartate aminotransferase (AST) or γ-globulin (GG) levels above the upper normal limit (UNL) and the severity of liver tissue injury judged by liver biopsy evaluation are key determinants of the treatment decision. Therapy must be individualized in patients who do not have severe disease.

Ulcerative colitis occurs in 16% of patients with AIH, and 44% of these individuals have cholangiographic changes of PSC. The clinical and prognostic value of discovering asymptomatic or clinically mild inflammatory bowel disease in adult patients with AIH justify at least flexible sigmoidoscopy and mucosal biopsies in all patients at presentation. Colonoscopy with mucosal biopsies is the preferred method to exclude inflammatory bowel disease in individuals with cholestatic features.

Upper tract endoscopy or contrast studies of the esophagus and stomach are appropriate at presentation to evaluate the presence of portal hypertension and cirrhosis. Sampling variation may limit the accuracy of liver biopsy examination in detecting cirrhosis, and the demonstration of varices at presentation can be useful to stage the disease and determine the need for prophylactic β-blockade. Esophageal varices occur in 15% of patients with AIH.

4.3 Pathological studies

Liver tissue examination is a requisite for the diagnosis of AIH and the overlap syndromes (Figures 3 and 4). Histological findings of ductopenia and/or destructive cholangitis in conjunction with features of interface hepatitis and plasma cell infiltration are indicative of a mixed hepatitic and cholestatic disorder that could represent autoimmune cholangitis or the overlap syndromes of AIH and PBC or AIH and PSC [6,8]. Histological changes of steatosis and portal lymphoid aggregates in a patient with features of AIH and active HCV infection indicate a viral-predominant disorder that should be managed with anti-viral agents. Histological changes of interface hepatitis and plasma cell infiltration in the absence of steatosis in a patient with features of AIH and active HCV infection indicate an autoimmune-predominant disorder that should be managed with immunosuppressive drugs [3].

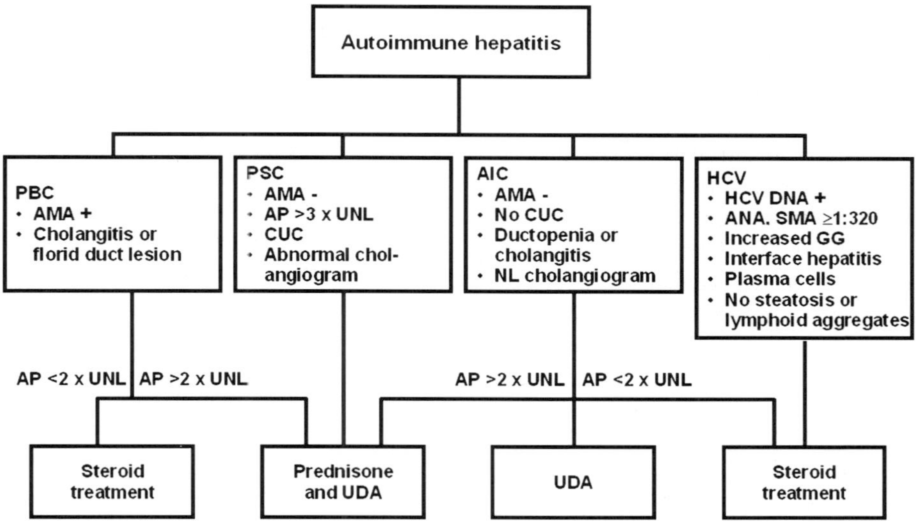

Figure 4. Diagnostic and treatment algorithms for overlap syndromes. The overlap syndromes of autoimmune hepatitis have predominant features of autoimmune hepatitis intermixed with features of primary biliary cirrhosis (PBC), primary sclerosing cholangitis (PSC), autoimmune cholangitis (AIC), and true hepatitis C virus (HCV) infection. Treatment is based on the predominant manifestations of the disease as reflected in the degree of elevation of the serum alkaline phosphatase (AP) level above the upper normal limit (UNL) for the cholestatic syndromes and the resemblance of the overlapping HCV syndrome to classical autoimmune hepatitis. The presence or absence of antimitochondrial antibodies (AMA) and chronic ulcerative colitis (CUC) is important in distinguishing the cholestatic disorders. Cholangiography is essential to diagnose the PSC variant, and a normal (NL) cholangiogram is useful in securing the diagnosis of AIC. The overlap syndrome with HCV should be indistinguishable from classical autoimmune hepatitis and characterized by high titers of antinuclear antibodies (ANA) and/or smooth muscle antibodies (SMA) and abnormally increased serum γ-globulin (GG) levels. Therapy consists of corticosteroid regimens standard for autoimmune hepatitis (steroid treatment), prednisone in combination with ursodeoxycholic acid (UDA), or ursodeoxychlic acid alone for predominant cholestatic features.

Variations in tissue sampling and interpretation affect the consistency and significance of the histological findings. Cirrhosis is the most difficult diagnosis to establish by needle biopsy. Multiple biopsy specimens from the same liver at the same time show cirrhosis in only 33% of samples, and the reproducibility of an interpretation of cirrhosis by the same observer is 78%. Inconsistencies in tissue sampling and interpretation are less pronounced in assessing inflammatory changes, and the reproducibility of these interpretations is 90%. The composite histological findings of interface hepatitis and plasma cell infiltration in the absence of steatosis, portal lymphoid aggregates, and bile duct injury have a specificity of 81% and predictability of 62% for AIH. The histological findings, however, have a low sensitivity for the disease, and the characteristic features of interface hepatitis and plasma cell infiltration in the absence of other confounding features occur in only 40% of patients with AIH.

4.4 Promising new autoantibodies

Autoantibodies continue to be characterized in the hope of improving their diagnostic specificity and prognostic value [19]. None of the pathologic autoantibodies in AIH is pathogenic, but each may be an imprint of an important pathogenic mechanism and clue to a target autoantigen. Antibodies to actin (anti-actin) are associated with early age onset of disease and higher frequencies of treatment failure, death from liver failure, and requirement for liver transplantation than patients without anti-actin. Antibodies to asialoglycoprotein receptor (anti-ASGPR) are associated with histological activity and a propensity to relapse after drug withdrawal. Antibodies to SLA/LP are highly specific for AIH and associated with relapse after drug withdrawal and *DRB1*0301*. Their sensitivity for AIH is only 16%, but they may be surrogate markers of a genetic propensity to relapse.

Antibodies to liver cytosol type 1 (anti-LC1) are commonly associated with anti-LKM1, and they occur mainly in young patients (≤20 years). They have been associated with severe inflammatory activity and progression to cirrhosis. Antibodies to LC1 fluctuate with disease activity and reduce in titer or disappear during corticosteroid therapy. As such, they are barometers of the disease and possibly involved in the pathogenic mechanisms of liver cell injury. None of these promising new autoantibodies is currently available in the clinical arena, but each has a commercial assay in development. Detection of these autoantibodies in otherwise seronegative patients indicates probable AIH if other features support that diagnosis. Their role in the delineation of overlap syndromes is to support the presence of AIH in the hybrid form.

5. MANAGEMENT

5.1 Medical therapeutics of AIH

Prednisone alone or a lower dose of prednisone in combination with azathioprine is effective in treating AIH (Table 5) [1]. The presence of severe symptoms, serum AST elevations above 10-fold normal, serum AST elevations above 5-fold normal in conjunction with serum γ-globulin levels above twice normal, and the presence of bridging necrosis or multiacinar necrosis on liver biopsy assessment are absolute indications for treatment (Figure 3). Patients with less severe abnormalities do not have an established benefit–risk ratio that favors therapy, and treatment must be individualized. In these patients with mild–moderate disease, the treatment decision is typically driven by the severity of associated symptoms.

The combination regimen of prednisone and azathioprine is preferred because of the corticosteroid-sparing effects of azathioprine (Table 5) [1]. Contraindications to its use are severe cytopenia, homozygous deficiency of thiopurine methyltransferase, and active malignancy. Azathioprine has been used successfully during pregnancy, but its theoretical teratogenic effects and the availability of an alternative treatment regimen of comparable efficacy (prednisone alone at higher dose) justify its discontinuation during this period. Determination of

Table 5. Standard Treatment Regimens for Autoimmune Hepatitis.

Clinical setting	Treatment regimens		
	Prednisone schedule	Combination schedule	
	Prednisone	Prednisone	Azathioprine
Initial treatment			
Week 1	60 mg daily	30 mg daily	50 mg daily
Week 2	40 mg daily	20 mg daily	50 mg daily
Week 3	30 mg daily	15 mg daily	50 mg daily
Week 4	30 mg daily	15 mg daily	50 mg daily
Until end point	20 mg daily	10 mg daily	50 mg daily
Treatment failure	60 mg daily × 1 mo 10 mg/mo reduction until 20 mg daily	30 mg daily × 1 mo 10 mg/mo reduction until 10 mg daily	150 mg daily 50 mg/mo reduction until 50 mg daily
Relapse	Same as initial treatment	Same as initial treatment	Same as initial treatment
Multiple relapses	2.5 mg reduction/mo until lowest level to control AST < 5 × UNL	Tapered discontinuation over 6 weeks	Sole drug at 2 mg/kg daily
Incomplete response	Same as for multiple relapses	Same as for multiple relapses	Same as for multiple relapses
Drug toxicity	Dose reduction or withdrawal Azathioprine only in titrated dose	Dose reduction or withdrawal Azathioprine only in titrated dose	Dose reduction or withdrawal Prednisone only in titrated dose

AST, serum aspartate aminotransferase level; UNL, upper normal limit; mo, month.

thiopurine methyltransferase activity prior to the institution of azathioprine therapy is a sensible precaution in all patients.

Initial therapy is finite and not intended to be administered forever [1]. The medications are given in a fixed daily dose until disappearance of symptoms, resolution of laboratory abnormalities, and improvement of the liver tissue to normal, portal hepatitis, or inactive cirrhosis. Improvement of the serum AST level to less than 2-fold normal is an acceptable biochemical end point if other criteria for remission are satisfied. Alternate day therapies and variable doses of medication adjusted according to biochemical indices do not induce histological remission and should be avoided in adults during the first course of treatment.

Histological improvement lags behind clinical and laboratory improvement by 3–8 months, and treatment should be continued for at least this period [1]. The average duration of treatment until remission in patients with severe disease is 22 months. Liver biopsy evaluation prior to drug withdrawal is the only mechanism to ensure remission of the disease and avoid an exacerbation due to premature withdrawal of the medication. Treatment is withdrawn in a gradual fashion over a 6 week period, and serum AST and γ-globulin levels are monitored for relapse at 3 week intervals for at least 3 months (Table 5). Follow-up studies at 3–6 month intervals are then appropriate.

Adjunctive therapies are based on perceptions of the risk that prednisone will exacerbate diabetes, hypertension, and osteopenia. Postmenopausal women should be considered for supplemental therapies that include vitamin D (400 units daily), calcium (1–1.5 g daily), and bisphosphonates (alendronate, 70 mg each week). Bone mineral density assessments should be performed each year of therapy in these individuals.

5.2 Medical therapeutics of the overlap syndromes

Treatment of the overlap syndromes is empiric and based on the predominant manifestations of the disease (Table 2) [3]. Only patients with the overlap syndrome of AIH and PBC respond as well to corticosteroid therapy as patients with classical AIH [11]. These patients commonly have serum AST and alkaline phosphatase levels that are similar to patients with AIH, and this resemblance may explain the similarities of their treatment response. Patients with AIH and PBC who have serum alkaline phosphatase levels more than twofold normal, serum γ-glutamyl transpeptidase levels more than fivefold normal, and/or florid duct lesions on histological examination frequently respond to a combination of prednisone and ursodeoxycholic acid [4] (Figure 4).

Patients with autoimmune cholangitis or the overlap syndrome of AIH and PSC respond poorly to corticosteroid therapy, and they are typically treated with a combination regimen of prednisone (20 mg daily) and ursodeoxycholic acid (13–15 mg per kg daily) (Table 2) [3,11]. This regimen has not been shown to consistently improve histological features or prognosis, and the success of treatment in these patients is measured by improvements in symptoms and laboratory indices. The major predictor of response to corticosteroid treatment for the cholestatic variant forms of AIH is the degree of serum alkaline phosphatase elevation at presentation. Patients with serum alkaline phosphatase levels above twofold the upper limit of normal do not respond to this treatment [11] (Figure 4).

Patients with the definite diagnosis of AIH who have concurrent HCV viremia respond to conventional corticosteroid regimens as commonly as uninfected counterparts (Table 2 and Figure 4) [3,7]. Relapse is common after corticosteroid therapy, and these patients may require long-term indefinite treatment. The HCV burden increases with immunosuppressive therapy, but the viral disease typically lacks significant clinical expression. The emergence of a viral-predominant disorder during corticosteroid treatment warrants discontinuation of the medication and institution of anti-viral agents [7]. Patients with chronic hepatitis C with autoimmune features have viral-predominant disease, and they should be treated with conventional anti-viral regimens.

5.3 Prevention and screening

AIH is probably triggered by a variety of viruses, medications, and environmental factors that have antigenic homologies, and susceptibility does have a genetic basis. Preventive measures, however, have not been established nor has the familial occurrence been sufficiently strong or detailed to warrant family screening. The triggering antigenic epitope is probably a common, short amino acid motif, but it remains undefined. Furthermore, the genetic risk factors are common in the general population. HLA DR3 occurs in 19% of healthy Caucasoid individuals in the US, and HLA DR4 is present in 35%.

5.4 Emerging therapies

New drugs are emerging from the transplantation arena that promise to provide greater blanket immunosuppression than prednisone and azathioprine [20]. Budesonide, cyclosporine, tacrolimus, rapamycin, and mycophenolate mofetil await controlled clinical trials that can rigorously evaluate their theoretical advantages and corroborate their anecdotal successes. Cyclosporine (5–6 mg/kg daily) and mycophenolate (1 g twice daily) have shown the most promise in limited clinical studies as first-line and salvage therapies.

6. PROGNOSIS

Sixty-five percent of patients with AIH enter remission within 18 months of therapy [1,20]. Ten- and 20-year life expectancies of treated patients exceed 80%, and their survival is similar to that of age- and sex-matched normal individuals from the same geographical region. Treatment-related complications result in premature discontinuation of the drugs in 13%; deterioration despite compliance with therapy (treatment failure) occurs in 9%; and 13% improve but not to a degree to satisfy remission criteria after 3 years (incomplete response). The most common management problem after treatment is relapse after drug withdrawal, and this outcome occurs in 50–86% of patients.

Treatment failure is managed by high dose prednisone alone (60 mg daily) or prednisone (30 mg daily) in combination with azathioprine (150 mg daily) [1,20]. These regimens improve the clinical manifestations, but histological resolution is achieved in only 20%. Patients who have failed conventional treatment must be assessed for variant syndromes or alternative diagnoses, and they may become candidates for liver transplantation. Other empiric drug therapies for treatment failure include 6-mercaptopurine (1.5 mg per kg daily), cyclosporine (5–6 mg/kg daily), and mycophenolate mofetil (2 g daily) [20].

Liver transplantation is effective in the treatment of decompensated patients with AIH [20]. There are no features at presentation that predict prognosis after therapy, and all patients with severe AIH should be treated, if possible, with corticosteroids before making the transplantation decision. Five-year survival of patient and graft after transplantation is 83–92%, and the actuarial 10-year survival is 75%.

AIH recurs in at least 17% of patients after transplantation [20]. Usually it develops in individuals who have been inadequately immunosuppressed, and the recurrence is easily managed by adjustments in the immunosuppressive regimen. In rare instances, progression to cirrhosis and graft failure can occur. Acute and chronic rejection may occur more commonly in patients transplanted for AIH than in other recipients, and they may be more difficult to remove from corticosteroids.

Relapse after corticosteroid withdrawal is defined mainly by an increase in serum AST level to more than threefold normal [1,20]. Relapse requires reinstitution of the original treatment regimen and maintenance of fixed dose therapy until clinical and laboratory resolution. Treatment can then be adjusted to reduce medication to the lowest level possible to control manifestations and maintain serum AST levels below fivefold normal (low dose prednisone regimen). Alternatively, azathioprine (2 mg per kg daily) can be used to replace prednisone, and the azathioprine only regimen continued indefinitely.

The frequencies of death from liver failure or requirement for liver transplantation are similar between re-treatment schedules based on conventional dose regimens and maintenance dose schedules. The major basis for a re-treatment preference is patient tolerance. The low dose prednisone and the azathioprine only schedules are superior to the original, full-dose treatment schedules in their prevention of side effects. No treatments after relapse should be continued without an intention of subsequent drug withdrawal.

An effort to reduce the dose or discontinue the therapy should be made each year of stable, inactive disease regardless of the regimen. Twenty-eight percent of patients who have relapsed and been re-treated can be ultimately withdrawn from their medication.

The outcomes of patients with overlap syndromes are uncertain and depend on their responses to empiric treatments with prednisone alone, prednisone and azathioprine, or combinations of these regimens with ursodeoxycholic acid. The responses of these syndromes to drugs such as cyclosporine and mycophenolate mofetil are unknown.

REFERENCES

[1] Czaja, A.J. and Freese, D.K. (2002) Diagnosis and treatment of autoimmune hepatitis. *Hepatology* **36**, 479–497.

[2] Alvarez, F., Berg, P.A., Bianchi, F.B., Bianchi, L., Burroughs, A.K., Cancado, E.L., Chapman, R.W., Cooksley, W.G.E., Czaja, A.J., Desmet, V.J., Donaldson, P.T., Eddleston, A.L.W.F., Fainboim, L., Heathcote, J., Homberg, J.-C., Hoofnagle, J.H., Kakumu, S., Krawitt, E.L., Mackay, I.R., MacSween, R.N.M., Maddrey, W.C., Manns, M.P., McFarlane, I.G., Meyer zum Buschenfelde, K.-H., Mieli-Vergani, G., Nakanuma, Y., Nishioka, M., Penner, E., Porta, G., Portmann, B.C., Reed, W.D., Rodes, J., Schalm, S.W., Scheuer, P.J., Schrumpf, E., Seki, T., Toda, G., Tsuji, T., Tygstrup, N., Vergani, D. and Zeniya, M. (1999) International Autoimmune Hepatitis Group report: review of criteria for diagnosis of autoimmune hepatitis. *J. Hepatol.* **31** 929–938.

[3] Ben-Ari, Z. and Czaja, A.J. (2001) Autoimmune hepatitis and its variant syndromes. *Gut* **49**, 589–594.

[4] Chazouilleres, O., Wendum, D., Serfaty, L., Montebault, S., Rosmorduc, O. and Poupon, R. (1998) Primary biliary cirrhosis-autoimmune hepatitis overlap syndrome: clinical features and response to therapy. *Hepatology* **28**, 296–301.

[5] McNair, A.N., Moloney, M., Portmann, B.C., Williams, R. and McFarlane, I.G. (1998) Autoimmune hepatitis overlapping primary sclerosing cholangitis in five cases. *Am. J. Gastroenterol.* **93**, 777–784.

[6] Czaja, A.J., Carpenter, H.A., Santrach, P.J. and Moore, S.B. (2000) Autoimmune cholangitis within the spectrum of autoimmune liver disease. *Hepatology* **31**, 1231–1238.

[7] Bellary, S., Schiano, T., Hartman, G. and Black, M. (1995) Chronic hepatitis with combined features of autoimmune chronic hepatitis and chronic hepatitis C: favorable response to prednisone and azathioprine. *Ann. Intern. Med.* **123**, 32–34.

[8] Czaja, A.J. (1996) The variant forms of autoimmune hepatitis. *Ann. Intern. Med.* **125**, 588–598.

[9] Czaja, A.J. and Carpenter, H.A. (2001) Autoimmune hepatitis with incidental histological features of bile duct injury. *Hepatology* **34**, 659–665.

[10] Boberg, K.M., Aadland, E., Jahnsen, J., Raknerud, N., Stiris, M. and Bell, H. (1998) Incidence and prevalence of primary biliary cirrhosis, primary sclerosing cholangitis, and autoimmune hepatitis in a Norwegian population. *Scand. J. Gastroenterol.* **33**, 99–103.

[11] Czaja, A.J. (1998) Frequency and nature of the variant syndromes of autoimmune liver disease. *Hepatology* **28**, 360–365.

[12] Gregorio, G.V., Portmann, B., Karani, J., Harrison, P., Donaldson, P.T., Vergani, D. and Mieli-Vergani, G. (2001) Autoimmune hepatitis/sclerosing cholangitis overlap syndrome in childhood: a 16-year prospective study. *Hepatology* **33**, 544–553.

[13] Czaja, A.J. (2001) Understanding the pathogenesis of autoimmune hepatitis. *Am. J. Gastroenterol.* **96**, 1224–1231.

[14] Czaja, A.J., Cookson, S., Constantini, P.K., Clare, M., Underhill, J.A. and Donaldson, P.T. (1999) Cytokine polymorphisms associated with clinical features and treatment outcome in type 1 autoimmune hepatitis. *Gastroenterology* **117**, 645–652.

[15] Agarwal, K., Czaja, A.J., Jones, D.E.J. and Donaldson, P.T. (2000) CTLA-4 gene polymorphism and susceptibility to type 1 autoimmune hepatitis. *Hepatology* **31**, 49–53.

[16] Czaja, A.J. and Manns, M.P. (1995) The validity and importance of subtypes in autoimmune hepatitis – a point of view. *Am. J. Gastroenterol.* **90**, 1206–1211.

[17] Czaja, A.J., Doherty, D.G. and Donaldson, P.T. (2002) Genetic bases of autoimmune hepatitis. *Dig. Dis. Sci.* **47**, 2139–2150.

[18] Czaja, A.J., Souto, E.O., Bittencourt, P.L., Cancado, E.L.R., Porto, G., Goldberg, A.C. and Donaldson, P.T. (2002) Clinical distinctions and pathogenic implications of type 1 autoimmune hepatitis in Brazil and the United States. *J. Hepatol.* **37**, 302–308.

[19] Czaja, A.J. and Homburger, H.A. (2001) Autoantibodies in liver disease. *Gastroenterology* **120**, 239–249.

[20] Czaja, A.J. (2002) Treatment of autoimmune hepatitis. *Semin. Liver Dis.* **22**, 365–377.

Hepatology: A Practical Approach
B. Al Knawy, M.L. Shiffman, R.H. Wiesner (editors)

Chapter 15
Primary Biliary Cirrhosis

Jenny Heathcote

Toronto Western Hospital, University of Toronto, 399 Bathurst St., Toronto, Ont., Canada M5T 2S8

1. Introduction 249
2. Demography 250
3. Pathophysiology 250
4. Pathogenesis 251
5. Clinical Features 251
   5.1 Asymptomatic PBC 251
   5.2 Symptomatic PBC 251
6. Natural History 252
7. Diagnostic Workup 252
8. Variant Forms of PBC 254
   8.1 AMA negative PBC 254
   8.2 PBC/AIH overlap syndromes 254
9. Management 254
   9.1 Symptomatic treatment 254
   9.2 Preventative therapy 255
   9.3 Specific therapy 256
References 257

1. INTRODUCTION

The term primary biliary cirrhosis (PBC) is often a misnomer, as many patients do not have cirrhosis, at least not at the time of initial presentation. This disease is a chronic cholestatic disease of the liver which predominantly affects adult women. It is characterized by gradual destruction of the interlobular bile ducts which leads to the retention of bile within hepatocytes. The impaired flow of bile (cholestasis) is associated with pruritus and promotes the development of fibrosis, which progresses over time to cirrhosis and terminally results in liver failure. The rate of disease progression varies considerably between affected individuals.

The hallmark for PBC is the serum antimitochondrial antibody (AMA) [1]. This antibody, easily detected using immunofluorescence techniques, is found in nearly all individuals with PBC. Studies indicate that AMA may be present in serum many years before any changes in liver biochemical tests. Biochemical abnormalities when present are characterized by an elevation (2- to 10-fold) in the serum alkaline phosphatase (ALP). Elevations in the gamma-glutamyl transpeptidase (GGT) and 5′ nucleotidase (5′NT) are generally also present. Less often, the serum aminotransferase levels are elevated, rarely more than 2- or 3-fold. Conjugated hyperbilirubinemia is typical of end stage disease but the majority of affected individuals are anicteric at diagnosis and asymptomatic.

The differential diagnosis, once the elevation in ALP has been established to be hepatic in origin includes PBC as well as other chronic cholestatic conditions, e.g., primary sclerosing cholangitis (PSC), as well as infiltrative conditions, e.g., lymphoma. However, serum AMA is absent in all these conditions. This autoantibody is very specific for PBC, only rarely being detected in individuals with chronic granulomatous infections such as tuberculosis and syphilis.

2. DEMOGRAPHY

PBC has been best described in populations from Northern Europe, Japan, North America and Australia, i.e., from temperate climates. But there are case reports from warmer places, e.g., India. The disease affects all racial groups amongst persons living and diagnosed in the Northern Hemisphere [2]. It is possible that the rate of PBC increases with emigration from warm to cooler climates.

The reported incidence of PBC varies. This is in part due to different case retrieval methods employed. In Northern England it has been estimated that the incidence of PBC is 14–32 cases/million/year and in the United States perhaps more [3,4]. If one examines only the female population over 40, then the annual incidence is considerably higher (91–110 per million) [3]. Whereas the incidence of this disease appears to be relatively stable [4], its prevalence is increasing. The likely explanation is that the disease is now being diagnosed at an earlier stage; however, it is also possible that affected individuals are living longer.

Although most individuals are between 35 and 65 years old when diagnosed, the youngest cases described have been teenagers, and this disease may also occur *de novo* in the 8th or 9th decade! Affected individuals may have other diseases considered autoimmune in nature and there is frequently a family history of autoimmune disease. The female predominance (F:M 9–14:1) supports the concept of PBC having an autoimmune basis. The risk of other family members having PBC is greatest in the daughters of affected women but the risk is low, 2.3% [5].

3. PATHOPHYSIOLOGY

The *bile duct damage* in PBC is caused by the invasion of the portal tracts and the bile ducts therein by chronic inflammatory cells. This inflammation may be granulomatous in nature and eosinophils may also be observed (Figure 1).

The consequent ductopenia causes *progressive cholestasis* and *liver fibrosis*. Portal hypertension

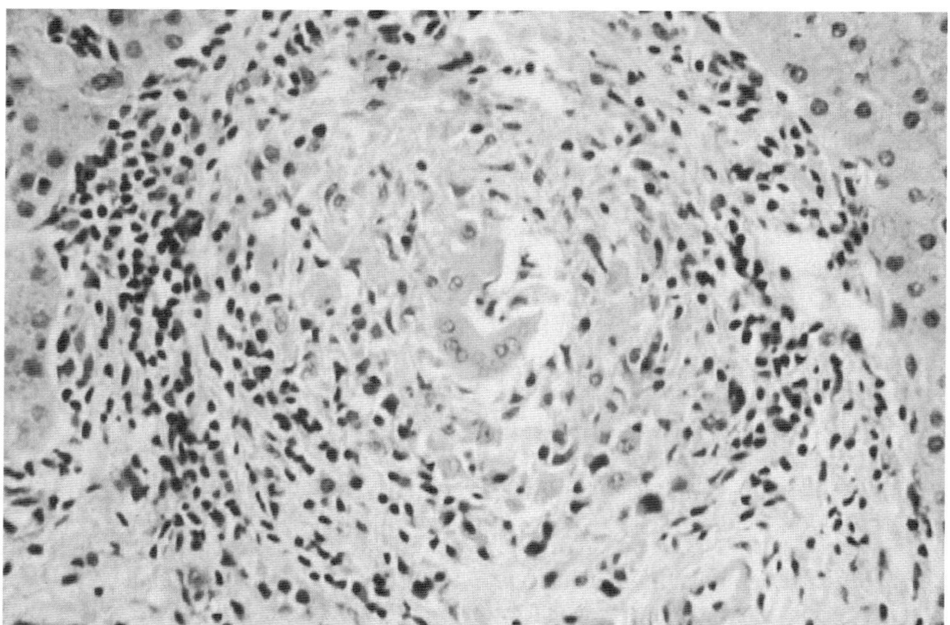

Figure 1. Typical bile duct lesion in PBC. (*For colored version, see Plate XXIV on page 577 at the end of the book.*)

occasionally occurs early in the course of PBC secondary to the destruction of the small portal venous radicals within the inflamed portal tracts (nodular regenerative hyperplasia causing pre-sinusoidal portal hypertension), but most often portal hypertension is secondary to full blown cirrhosis. As with all individuals who have cirrhosis, primary hepatocellular carcinoma may complicate the disease.

4. PATHOGENESIS

Even in individuals who have normal biochemical tests, but who test positive for AMA, some interlobular bile duct destruction can be found on liver biopsy. This bile duct destruction is likely an autoimmune-mediated process. The initiating factor remains a mystery, but recent evidence suggests that infection and/or xenobiotic induced damage to host proteins may initiate what becomes a self-perpetuating process, confined to interlobular and septal ducts. Serum AMA reacts not only with enzymes located on the inner membrane of mitochondria but also with antigens expressed in the cytoplasm and on the apical membrane of biliary epithelial cells (BEC) of individuals with PBC (not seen in healthy or liver disease controls, e.g., PSC). This may be an example of "molecular mimicry" by bacterial antigens with nucleotide sequences similar to mitochondrial enzymes. For the expression of these molecular mimics to be part of the pathogenesis of PBC it presupposes that BEC can become antigen-presenting cells. In fact aberrant expression of HLA can be seen on BEC in PBC. Lymphocytes found in the liver of patients with PBC are sensitized to these antigens and are probably responsible for bile duct necrosis. In addition, apoptosis of BEC can be observed if special techniques are employed so likely death of BEC occurs by both these immune-mediated mechanisms. Thus, PBC is likely due to an immune response to altered host or foreign proteins, altered by some infectious and/or toxic injury [6].

5. CLINICAL FEATURES

5.1 Asymptomatic PBC

As many as 60% of individuals with PBC have no symptoms attributable to liver disease at the time of presentation (Table 1). Quite often abnormal liver biochemistry is found at the time of workup for another condition, e.g., osteoporosis. Persons may be diagnosed following the detection of an elevated serum cholesterol at the time of a general checkup. PBC may remain asymptomatic for many years, and a few affected individuals may never develop symptoms. No factors predictive for the development of symptomatic disease have been identified [7].

Table 1. PBC: clinical manifestations.

Complications	Associated diseases
Fatigue	Hashimotos thyroiditis
Pruritus	Secondary Sjorgens's (sicca, CREST)
Xanthelasma	Rheumatoid arthritis
Osteoporosis	Pulmonary fibrosis
Jaundice	Celiac disease
Pigmented skin	Sarcoidosis
Variceal hemorrhage	Hypertrophic pulmonary osteoarthropathy
Ascites	Glomerulonephritis
Hepatic encephalopathy	Myesthenia gravis polymyositis

5.2 Symptomatic PBC

The most common symptom reported by persons with PBC is *fatigue*. This is not present in all, and the severity of fatigue does not correlate with the severity of underlying liver disease or with the age of the individual. Some patients are so fatigued that their quality of life is significantly impaired. The cause is unknown. *Pruritus* is the next most common symptom. It is usually generalized and most noticeable at night. Again, this symptom can vary in severity; from mild to so severe it can make the person almost suicidal. It is worsened by pregnancy and sometimes by use of the oral contraceptive pill. *Xanthelasma* around the eyes and occasionally xanthomatous deposits on the palms of the hands and on tendons are seen, predominantly in those with early disease. Both xanthelasma and pruritus tend to lessen with progression of disease. Jaundice is a late manifestation of PBC and is usually present when signs of hepatic decompensation are noted, e.g., ascites. Prolonged cholestasis leads to increasing pigmentation of the skin, suntans no longer fade in the winter. *Osteoporosis* is common particularly with late stage liver disease, other risk factors may be present, e.g., post-menopausal status [8].

There are many non-hepatic diseases which may be seen in association with PBC and individuals may present with symptoms secondary to these diseases even prior to the onset of overt liver disease [9]. The most common associations are with Hashimoto's thyroiditis and with various manifestations of secondary Sjorgren's syndrome. These may be limited to sicca syndrome involving the eyes, mouth and/or vagina, Raynauds disease or include the complete CREST (Calcinosis, Raynauds, Esophageal dysmotility, Sclerodactyly and Telangiectasia) syndrome. Many patients test positive for rheumatoid factor and some may suffer rheumatoid arthritis. Other conditions which are less often seen in patients with PBC include pulmonary fibrosis, sarcoidosis, hypertrophic pulmonary osteoarthropathy, glomerulonephritis, myesthenia gravis and polymyositis. Some would argue that celiac disease and ulcerative colitis may also be associated with PBC – the coexistence of one or other may further promote any osteoporosis.

6. NATURAL HISTORY

The course of PBC is not the same in all individuals. As mentioned previously, some may never progress from an asymptomatic state, although most do become symptomatic with time [7]. Fortunately, only a few may develop rapidly progressive bile duct loss progressing to liver failure even before they have developed cirrhosis. The median survival for untreated asymptomatic disease is 16 years and for symptomatic disease 7.5 years (Figure 2) [10]. The cause of death if due to liver disease is most commonly due to liver failure, less often due to liver cancer. Not unexpectedly death in asymptomatic individuals is due to non-hepatic causes. Despite hyperlipidemia being common in PBC, there appears to be no increased risk of death from coronary artery disease, or from any other cancer aside from hepatocellular carcinoma.

7. DIAGNOSTIC WORKUP

As already mentioned, the hallmark for this disease is the AMA (Figure 3). At least one-third of patients will also test positive for antinuclear antibody and some even test positive for smooth muscle antibody. The *biochemical abnormalities* observed in PBC include elevation (often marked) in ALP, GGT and 5′NT, either with or without an elevation in total cholesterol and/or bilirubin. In the early stages of this disease, the lipid pattern is predominantly an elevation in HDL, but as the liver disease progresses

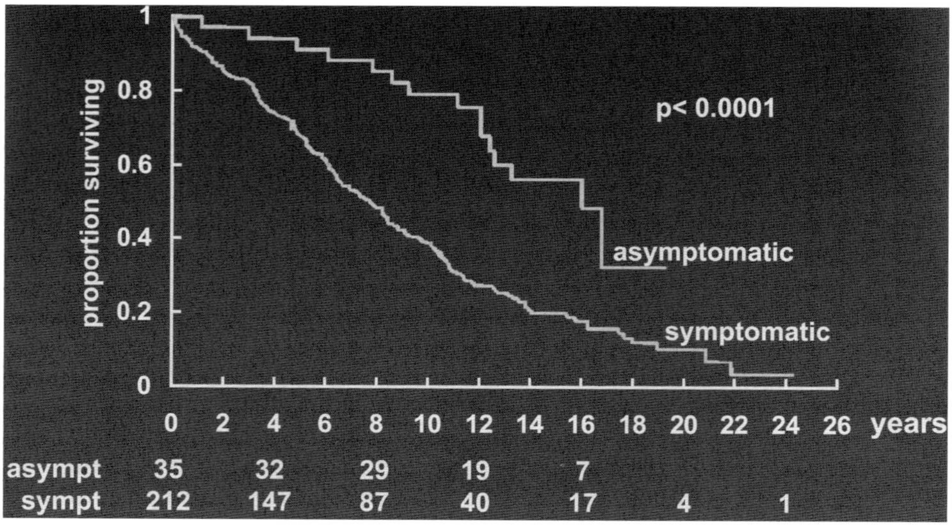

Figure 2. PBC: long-term survival. (*For colored version, see Plate XXV on page 577 at the end of the book.*)

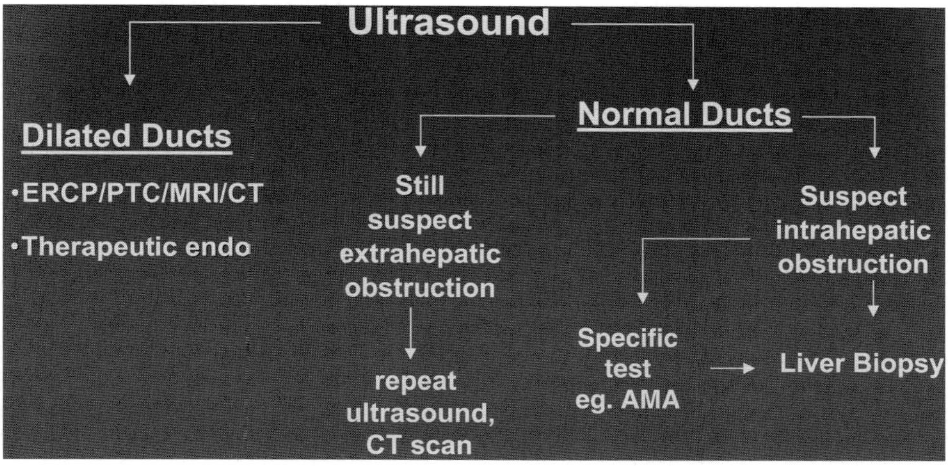

Figure 3. Diagnostic workup of the cholestatic patient. *(For colored version, see Plate XXVI on page 578 at the end of the book.)*

an elevation in LDL becomes predominant. *Hyperbilirubinemia* when present should be mostly in the conjugated fraction if jaundice is due to cholestasis. It is important in those with a persistently mildly elevated bilirubin to check the conjugation status of the bilirubin as some patients may have Gilbert's syndrome (quite innocuous) in which case the bilirubin levels tend to fluctuate and do not reflect progressive liver disease. In Gilbert's, the elevation in bilirubin is in the unconjugated fraction. In PBC, a typical pattern of *immunoglobulins* is seen, predominantly the IgM is elevated although the IgG is often elevated as well – rarely IgA deficiency is described.

The *hematological picture* in individuals with PBC is generally normal unless there is concomitant celiac disease when anemia both from iron and/or folate deficiency may be present. As portal hypertension progresses, hypersplenism develops causing mainly thrombocytopenia. Rarely an autoimmune thrombocytopenia, or an autoimmune hemolytic anemia is reported in individuals with PBC. *Renal function* is generally normal, and although renal tubular acidosis may be detected in almost half of patients with PBC, most are asymptomatic. It is not unusual for patients with PBC to have asymptomatic urinary tract infections. *Thyroid function* should be checked regularly as thyroid antibodies are common (>40%). Thyroid disease may affect 25% and if untreated, may be a cause for fatigue. It is important, at least at the time of diagnosis to conduct an *ultrasound examination of the liver and biliary system* in order to rule out biliary obstruction. Marked intra-abdominal lymphadenopathy is common in PBC – the nodes when examined are full of granulomas.

The AMA test is so specific one could argue against the need for performing a *liver biopsy* to confirm the diagnosis. Certainly in the elderly, liver biopsy is probably unnecessary but in those under 65 a liver biopsy may be helpful for prognostic purposes. If cirrhosis or marked fibrosis is present, one can be confident that even (as is often the case) there are no symptoms at the time of biopsy, that individual will progress more rapidly than if no cirrhosis were present.

Careful examination of liver histology is required paying particular attention to all of the usual portal tract contents – particularly the bile ducts and venous radicals. Chronic inflammatory cells are seen surrounding and invading the bile ducts (Figure 1). Sometimes granulomas are seen in the portal tracts often surrounding a damaged bile duct. Eosinophils are common in PBC. An interface hepatitis, lymphoplasmacytic in nature is quite common but a pan lobular inflammatory component is rare. Biopsies are generally described as showing stage 1, 2, 3, or 4, stage 1 being bile duct destruction, stage 2 bile duct proliferation, stage 3 septal fibrosis and stage 4 cirrhosis [11]. It is usual, however, for more than one stage to be present in a single liver biopsy specimen and final staging is based on the most advanced lesion seen in the biopsy.

8. VARIANT FORMS OF PBC

8.1 AMA negative PBC

The antigenic targets for AMA have now been identified as members of the 2-oxo acid dehydrogenase complex of enzymes located on the inner membrane of mitochondria. Although immunofluorescence techniques remain reliable and sensitive for the detection of AMA, highly specific and sensitive ELISA and immunoblotting tests have been developed now that the target antigens have been identified. However, even when using these very specific tests, there are some individuals who have all the features of PBC but who test consistently negative for AMA even when these highly specific tests are employed. Such cases have been referred to by some as autoimmune cholangitis [12]. Most likely they have the same disease as AMA positive PBC patients, as their natural history is no different.

8.2 PBC/AIH overlap syndromes

Approximately 10% of patients who have all the features of PBC have additional features of autoimmune hepatitis. These features include other autoantibodies such as smooth muscle antibody, hypergammaglobulinemia predominantly in the IgG fraction and a 5-fold elevation or more in serum aminotransferase values. On liver biopsy, in addition to the classical bile duct lesions of PBC there may be noted some features more typical of autoimmune hepatitis, namely a lymphoplasmacytic interface hepatitis [13]. Recent observations suggest that progression to cirrhosis is faster when the latter is present, however, the overall survival of those with PBC/AIH overlap syndromes seems to be no different from PBC uncomplicated by features of AIH [14].

9. MANAGEMENT

The management of individuals given a diagnosis of PBC must include symptomatic relief, preventative measures, as well as specific therapies.

9.1 Symptomatic treatment

(a) The *fatigue* associated with PBC is not restored by a good night's sleep. It is not related to physical activity, and it does not correlate with the severity of the liver disease (Table 2). This symptom is extremely frustrating for the patient, their families, friends and employers. Hence, counseling is required so as household members understand that the affected individual is not malingering! It is essential to ensure that there are no other possible precipitating factors for their fatigue, e.g., hypothyroidism, medications (antihistamines), obesity, lack of exercise or poor sleep hygiene. Fatigue may be associated with symptoms of depression [15], and if the depression warrants treatment, treatment should be given but this rarely alters the severity of the fatigue.

(b) *Pruritus* – The patient is the one who decides how inconvenient the pruritus has become but the physician must listen and react appropriately – too often this complaint is ignored by doctors! Sometimes itching can be tolerated without the addition of medical therapy. However, it is important not to neglect or underestimate this symptom, which may cause marked sleep disturbance, social embarrassment and when extremely severe, suicidal ideation. The first line of treatment is the anion exchange resin, cholestyramine. This rather unpleasant tasting powder binds bile intraluminally. There is some agent in bile which acts as a pruritogen. When the gallbladder is intact, cholestyramine is most effective when given before and after breakfast (4 g each time). As it binds other agents, e.g., thyroxin, digoxin, oral

Table 2. PBC: symptomatic therapy.

Fatigue	Good sleep hygiene ± antidepressants
Pruritus	Cholestyramine 4–12 g/d
	Rifampicin 150 mg bid
	Naltrexone 10–50 mg/d
Xanthoma	Leave alone except for palmar

contraceptive pill, it is important that no medications be taken at least 2 h, and preferably 4 h after taking this powder. This agent is very effective in controlling pruritus in about 80% of patients, but its use is associated with unpleasant side effects, mostly abdominal bloating and constipation. In a patient with steatorrhoea secondary to marked jaundice in end stage PBC, cholestyramine will worsen this condition. The second line of therapy is the antibiotic rifampin [16]. The mechanism whereby this affects its anti-pruritic activity is unclear. Crossover trials have indicated that it dramatically improves the pruritus associated with cholestasis in half of those treated, when the drug is prescribed in a dose of 150 mg BID. Rifampin is an enzyme inducer, and therefore needs to be used with caution with other drugs. Patients should be warned that it stains the urine dark brown/orange. Rifampin can cause hepatitis (although this is most often seen when given together with INH), renal impairment and hemolysis. So patients should be monitored closely when taking this drug. If neither of these agents is effective, exposure to ultraviolet light without sun block (under the direction of a dermatologist) may bring relief. The mechanism whereby this works is unclear. Several studies indicate that administration of opioid antagonists effects a dramatic relief from pruritus secondary to cholestasis. Experiments have shown that serum from pruritic patients with PBC when injected into the ventricles of animals induces intense itching. Thus, it would appear that the pruritus of PBC is of central origin and possibly related to elevated levels of endogenous opioids. Introduction of opioid antagonists causes immediate cessation of pruritus, but is accompanied by symptoms of opioid "withdrawal", which may be very profound [17]. Hence, opioid antagonist treatment needs to be started in very small doses, generally given initially intravenously as naloxone and gradually switched to small oral doses of naltrexone. Tolerance may develop. If it is impossible to control pruritus by any of these measures, then plasmaphoresis can bring about short-term symptom relief, but the patient should be considered for liver transplantation. If a patient with PBC becomes pregnant it is likely that pruritus will either develop or worsen during the second trimester. If cholestyramine is used, particular care to avoid vitamin K depletion is required to avoid an *antepartum* hemorrhage.

(c) *Xanthelasma* – When present generally occur in individuals with early PBC, and their presence is not always associated with hypercholesterolemia. Surgical removal may be followed by rapid recurrence and thus is not advised.

9.2 Preventative therapy

(a) There is some controversy as to whether or not osteoporosis is associated with PBC. The controversy is likely because osteoporosis is most common in individuals with late stage PBC who are often post-menopausal women (thus already at risk for osteoporosis) (Table 3). It is less often found in pre-menopausal women with early disease. Vitamin D and calcium metabolism are normal in PBC unless jaundice is present. Nevertheless, it is wise to verify that adequate calcium (1500 mg daily) and vitamin D (1000 U/d) are taken by all individuals with PBC. Bone mineral density should be checked at baseline, and at two yearly intervals thereafter unless osteoporosis is present in which case more frequent monitoring to follow the effects of therapy is advised. The usual therapeutic measures taken for osteoporosis may be tried, i.e., hormone replacement therapy (HRT) for post-menopausal women ± a bisphosphonate. There are no data to suggest that HRT causes any worsening of cholestasis in women with PBC, but it is probably safer to give it transdermally. Patients should be encouraged to exercise and abstain from smoking and imbibing excess alcohol.

(b) *Portal hypertension* – Portal hypertension may develop early in this disease and therefore waiting to perform screening endoscopy for esophageal varices until there is clear-cut evidence of hypersplenism, e.g., platelet count less than

Table 3. Preventative therapy: PBC.

Osteoporosis	Avoid risk factors Ca 1500 mg, vitamin D 1000 IU/d HRT when appropriate (transdermal) Bisphosphonates
Portal hypertension	Non-selective β blockers
Hypothyroidism	Thyroid replacement
Malabsorption	Fat soluble vitamins
Sicca syndrome	Regular dentist, false tears, careful pill swallowing, lubricating jelly for vagina

100 × 10^6 may be inadvisable. Certainly all patients known to have cirrhosis need to have screening endoscopy and if varices grade 2 or greater are found, prophylactic treatment with non-selective beta blocker therapy is required. To date, there is no evidence to suggest that prophylactic banding of varices is any better than medical therapy for the prevention of variceal hemorrhage.

(c) *Thyroid disease* – Regular checks of thyroid function should be conducted particularly if patients complain of excessive of fatigue.

(d) *Fat soluble vitamin administration* – It is only required once patients become icteric.

(e) *Sicca syndrome* – Patients should be advised to have regular dental checkups, swallow all medications standing with plenty of water, place false tears in their eyes regularly and use a lubricating jelly prior to sexual intercourse. Zylogen spray may be used to facilitate speech in those with marked xerostomia.

9.3 Specific therapy

(a) *Ursodeoxycholic acid* (UDCA) is the current standard of care for PBC. Randomized, controlled trials have shown that treatment with this dihydroxy, hydrophilic bile acid leads to a marked improvement in all the biochemical (including serum cholesterol) and serological markers of cholestasis, a delay in the development of fibrosis [18] and in the complications of liver disease, e.g., ascites, development of varices and hepatic encephalopathy. An analysis of more than 500 patients treated for up to 4 years initially with either UDCA (13–15 mg/kg/d) or placebo, with most placebo patients rolling over to UDCA after 2 years of therapy indicates that this treatment was associated with a delay in the need for transplantation or of death, using an intent to treat analysis [19] (Figure 4). If the patients who were initially randomized to placebo had been maintained on placebo the full 4 years, an even greater effect of UDCA would likely have been observed. In a meta-analysis which included all studies employing UDCA regardless of dose, no survival advantage was observed but this was assessed after only 2 years of follow-up [20]. In general, PBC is a slowly progressive disease and thus to assess any therapeutic benefit it is necessary to study many patients for a long time. UDCA has few side effects. Patients may notice a slight increase in weight after the introduction of treatment and some complain of thinning hair, though baldness has never been described. Occasionally the introduction of therapy with UDCA may be associated with frequent bowel movements. If this occurs the dose should be reduced and then slowly increased over weeks to months so as to finally arrive at a dose of 13–15 mg/kg/d. In a few patients UDCA seems to worsen pruritus – in others this symptom diminishes with UDCA therapy!

(b) *Immunosuppressive therapy* – Even though it is thought that PBC is an autoimmune disease the results of treatment with immunosuppressive therapy have been disappointing. Large studies of azathioprine and cyclosporine have shown no benefit. Smaller studies

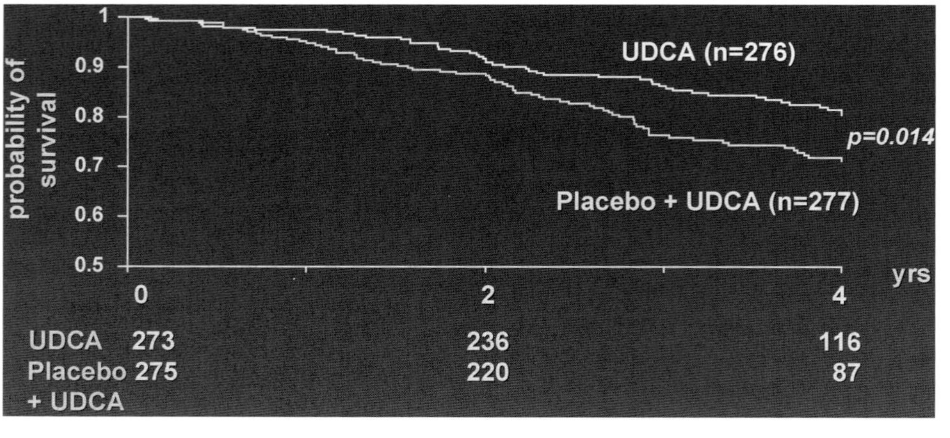

Figure 4. Combined analysis of RCT of UDCA in PBC. Probability of survival free of transplantation. (*For colored version, see Plate XXVII on page 578 at the end of the book.*)

employing prednisone or budesonide suggest this treatment improves liver biochemistry, but there are no long-term data and the studies were too small to indicate whether it has an effect on survival. One randomized controlled trial of methotrexate which involved 60 patients suggested no survival benefit at 6 years using this drug as monotherapy [21]. A large trial of its combination with UDCA in the USA has not shown any benefit of MTX either.

(c) *Other therapies* – A number of other agents have been tried, many in combination with UDCA but all studies have been too small and of too short a duration to reliably assess efficacy. Other agents that have been evaluated include cholesterol lowering drugs, e.g., bezafibrate which seems to be associated with an improvement in liver biochemistry as well as in cholesterol.

At the present time, the mainstay of therapy remains UDCA, but this does not prevent terminal disease, and liver transplantation may still be required for decompensated liver disease.

(d) *Liver transplantation* remains the ultimate treatment, although recurrence of PBC in the transplanted liver occurs in some. But this recurrent disease is rarely symptomatic, and has not been shown to progress to end stage liver disease requiring a second transplant. Patients with cholestatic liver disease have the highest survival rate following liver transplantation maintained at greater than 70% at 5 years and thus this procedure offers a definite benefit to individuals with end stage PBC [22].

A better understanding of the pathogenesis of this disease will allow for specific therapeutic targets to be developed. In order for any treatment to have its greatest effects, it needs to be initiated at the start of the disease, however, in PBC this is when most patients have no symptoms and may have no markers of disease aside from a positive AMA. This poses a dilemma as very early PBC is only slowly progressive and thus survival cannot be used as a measure of outcome. Better surrogate markers for disease progression need to be developed to monitor treatment effects. The markers currently used, namely the height of the serum bilirubin and the Mayo Score [23] (Table 4) are of value only once an individual has symptomatic, progressive disease. However, the current therapy, namely, UDCA is already making a mark – as considerably fewer cases of PBC have been referred for liver transplantation since the mid-1990s [24].

Table 4. Mayo Risk Score calculation.

Components of Mayo Risk Score
- Age (years)
- Serum bilirubin (mg/dl)
- Serum albumin (g/dl)
- Prothrombin time (PT) (s)
- Edema score (see below)

Edema and diuretic status	Edema score
No edema and no diuretic therapy	0
Edema present for which no diuretic therapy given	0.5
Edema resolved with diuretic therapy	0.5
Edema present despite diuretic therapy	1

Mayo risk score = (0.871 × (ln(bilirubin in mg/dl))) − (2.53 × (ln(albumin in g/dl))) + (0.039 × (age in years)) + (2.38 × (ln(PT time in seconds))) + (0.859 × (edema score)).

REFERENCES

[1] Walker, J.G., Doniach, D., Roitt, I.M. and Sherlock, S. (1965) Serological tests in diagnosis of primary biliary cirrhosis. *Lancet* **39**, 827–31.

[2] Witt-Sullivan, H., Heathcote, J., Cauch, K., Blendis, L., Ghent, C., Katz, A., Milner, R., Pappas, S.C., Rankin, J. and Wanless, I.R. (1990) The demography of primary biliary cirrhosis in Ontario, Canada. *Hepatology* **12**, 98–105.

[3] James, O.F., Bhopal, R., Howel, D., Gray, J., Burt, A.D. and Metcalf, J.V. (1999) Primary biliary cirrhosis once rare, now common in the United Kingdom? *Hepatology* **30**(2), 390–4.

[4] Kim, W.R., Lindor, K.D., Locke, III, G.R., Therneau, T.M., Homburger, H.A., Batts, K.P., Yawn, B.P., Petz, J.L., Melton, III, L.J. and Dickson, E.R. (2000) Epidemiology and natural history of primary biliary cirrhosis in a US community. *Gastroenterology* **119**(6), 1631–6.

[5] Jones, D.E.J., Watt, F.E., Metcalf, J.V. *et al.* (1999) Familial primary biliary cirrhosis reassessed: a

geographically based population study. *J. Hepatol.* **30**, 402.

[6] Gershwin, M.E. (2001) The natural history of primary biliary cirrhosis: of genes and cooperation. *J. Hepatol.* **35**, 412–415.

[7] Springer, J., Cauch-Dudek, K., O'Rourke, K., Wanless, I.R. and Heathcote, E.J. (1999) Asymptomatic primary biliary cirrhosis: a study of its natural history and prognosis. *Am. J. Gastroenterol.* **94**(1), 47–53.

[8] Menon, K.V.N., Angulo, P., Weston, S., Dickson, E.R. and Lindor, K.D. (2001) Bone disease in primary biliary cirrhosis: independent indicators and rate of progression. *J. Hepatol.* **35**, 316–323.

[9] Culp, K.S., Fleming, C.R., Duffy, J., Baldus, W.P. and Dickson, E.R. (1982) Autoimmune associations in primary biliary cirrhosis. *Mayo Clin. Proc.* **57**(6), 365–70.

[10] Mahl, T., Shockcor, W. and Boyer, J.L. (1994) Primary biliary cirrhosis: survival of a large cohort of symptomatic and asymptomatic patients followed for 24 years. *J. Hepatol.* **20**, 707.

[11] Scheuer, P.J. (1967) Primary biliary cirrhosis. *Proc. R. Soc. Med.* **60**, 1257.

[12] Michieletti, P., Wanless, I.R., Katz, A., Scheuer, P.J., Yeaman, S.J., Bassendine, M.F., Palmer, J.M. and Heathcote, E.J. (1994) Antimitochondrial antibody negative primary biliary cirrhosis: a distinct syndrome of autoimmune cholangitis. *Gut* **35**, 260–265.

[13] Corpechot, C., Carrat, F., Poupon, R. and Poupon, R.E. (2002) Primary biliary cirrhosis: incidence and predictive factors of cirrhosis development in ursodiol-treated patients. *Gastroenterology* **122**, 652–658.

[14] Joshi, S., Cauch-Dudek, K., Wanless, I.R., Lindor, K.D., Jorgensen, R., Batts, K. and Heathcote, E.J. (2002) Primary biliary cirrhosis with additional features of autoimmune hepatitis: response to therapy with ursodeoxycholic acid. *Hepatology* **35**, 409–413.

[15] Cauch-Dudek, K., Abbey, S., Stewart, D.E. and Heathcote, E.J. (1998) Fatigue in primary biliary cirrhosis. *Gut* **43**, 705–710.

[16] Ghent, C.N. and Carruthers, S.G. (1988) Treatment of pruritus in primary biliary cirrhosis with rifampin. Results of a double-blind, crossover, randomized trial. *Gastroenterology* **94**, 488–493.

[17] Wolfhagen, F.H.J., Sternieri, E., Hop, W.C.J., Vitale, G., Bertolotti, M. and Van Buuren, H.R. (1997) Oral naltrexone treatment for cholestatic pruritus: a double-blind, placebo-controlled study. *Gastroenterology* **113**, 1264–1269.

[18] Parés, A., Caballería, L., Rodés, J., Bruguera, M., Rodrigo, L., García-Plaza, A., Berenguer, J., Rodríguez-Martínez, D., Mercader, J., Velicia, R. and UDCA-Cooperative Group from the Spanish Association for the Study of the Liver. (2000) Long-term effects of ursodeoxycholic acid in primary biliary cirrhosis: results of a double-blind controlled multicentric trial. *J. Hepatol.* **32**, 561–566.

[19] Poupon, R.E., Lindor, K.D., Cauch-Dudek, K., Dickson, E.R., Poupon, R. and Heathcote, E.J. (1997) Combined analysis of randomized controlled trials of ursodeoxycholic acid in primary biliary cirrhosis. *Gastroenterology* **113**, 884–890.

[20] Goulis, J., Leandro, G. and Burroughs, A.K. (1999) Randomised controlled trials of ursodeoxycholic-acid therapy for primary biliary cirrhosis: a meta-analysis. *Lancet* **354**, 1053–1060.

[21] Hendrickse, M., Rigney, E., Giaffer, M.H., Soomro, I., Triger, D.R., Underwood, J.C. and Gleeson, D. (1999) Low-dose methotrexate is ineffective in primary biliary cirrhosis: long-term results of a placebo-controlled trial. *Gastroenterology* **117**, 400–407.

[22] Markus, B.H., Dickson, E., Grambsch, P., Fleming, T.R., Mazzaferro, V., Klintmalm, G.B.G., Wiesner, R.H., Van Thiel, D.H. and Starzl, T.E. (1989) Efficacy of liver transplantation in patients with primary biliary cirrhosis. *N. Engl. J. Med.* **320**, 1709–1713.

[23] Dickson, E., Grambsch, P.M., Fleming, T.R., Fisher, L.O. and Langworthy, A. (1989) Prognosis in primary biliary cirrhosis: model for decision making. *Hepatology* **10**, 1–7.

[24] Liermann Garcia, R.F., Evangelista Garcia, C., McMaster, P. and Neuberger, J. (2001) Transplantation for primary biliary cirrhosis: retrospective analysis of 400 patients in a single center. *Hepatology* **33**, 22–27.

Hepatology: A Practical Approach
B. Al Knawy, M.L. Shiffman, R.H. Wiesner (editors)

Chapter 16
Primary Sclerosing Cholangitis

Annika Bergquist and Ulrika Broomé

Department of Gastroenterology and Hepatology, Huddinge University Hospital, Karolinska Institute, Huddinge, Sweden

1. Introduction	259
2. Definition of Disease	259
3. Prevalence	260
4. General Demographics	260
5. Pathophysiology	260
6. Clinical Features	261
7. Complications in PSC	262
8. Cholangiocarcinoma	262
9. Associated Diseases	263
10. Diagnosis – Blood Tests	264
11. Diagnosis – Imaging	265
12. Diagnosis – Histology	265
13. Management	265
13.1 Medical therapeutics	265
13.2 Endoscopic and surgical treatment	267
13.3 Orthotopic liver transplantation	267
14. Prognosis – Natural History of PSC	269
References	270

1. INTRODUCTION

Primary sclerosing cholangitis (PSC) is a chronic, progressive, destructive biliary disease of unknown aetiology, characterized by multiple fibrosing inflammatory strictures of the extra- and intrahepatic bile ducts. The disease often progresses to cirrhosis and leads to premature death due to liver failure or cholangiocarcinoma. PSC has become a major indication for liver transplantation. PSC is closely associated with inflammatory bowel disease (IBD), above all ulcerative colitis (UC).

2. DEFINITION OF DISEASE

The diagnosis of PSC is based on characteristic clinical, biochemical, histological and, most important, radiological features, with irregularity and beading of the intra- and/or extrahepatic bile ducts (Figure 1). Secondary causes of sclerosing cholangitis, such as previous biliary surgery, biliary stone disease, ischemic bile-duct damage due to treatment with floxuridine, congenital biliary-tree abnormalities, cholangiopathy associated with acquired immunodeficiency syndrome or bile duct neoplasms must be excluded. Cholangiographic features simulating intrahepatic PSC can also be seen in patients with cirrhosis, hepatocellular carcinoma, polycystic liver disease, submassive hepatic necrosis, amyloidosis, intrahepatic portal thrombosis, liver metastases, leukaemia and lymphoma, pointing to the importance of combining clinical, histological and cholangiographic features when diagnosing PSC. Some patients with IBD have cholestatic biochemical abnormalities and liver histology consistent with PSC but a normal cholangiogram. These patients are considered to have small bile duct sclerosing

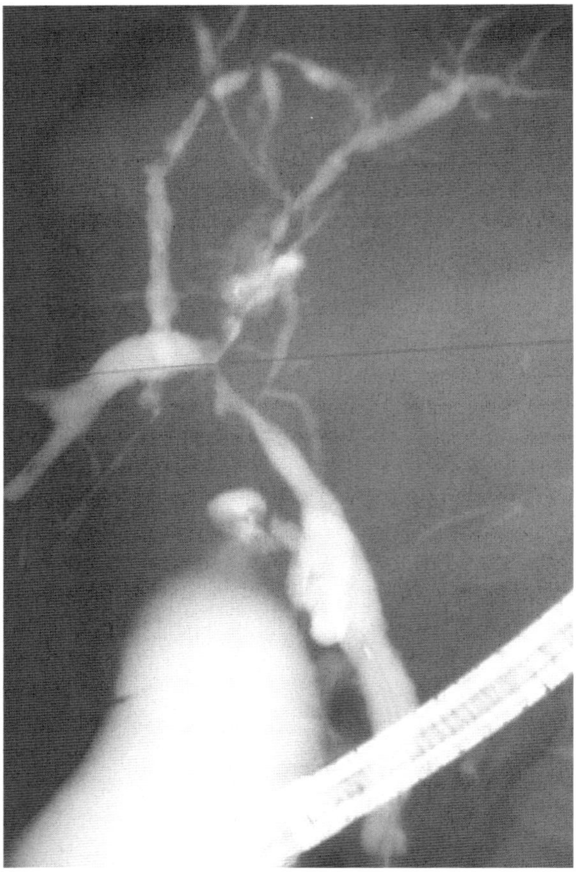

Figure 1. Characteristic intra- and extrahepatic changes in a cholangiogram with multiple strictures and dilatations of the biliary tree from a patient with primary sclerosing cholangitis. It is impossible to rule out or prove the presence of a cholangiocarcinoma.

cholangitis which may be part of the spectrum of PSC. In a recent study including 32 Swedish patients with small bile duct PSC, it was shown that the majority of patients with small bile duct PSC do not progress to large bile duct PSC [1]. Moreover, the prognosis seems better for these patients compared to those having large duct PSC. Similar results have also been presented from Oxford and the Mayo Clinic.

3. PREVALENCE

The first case of PSC was presented in the English literature in 1927. Over the next 50 years, the disease remained a medical rarity. With the increased use of endoscopic retrograde cholangiography (ERCP) more cases are identified, especially among IBD patients, suggesting that PSC is more common than was previously believed. The true prevalence of PSC is not known. A real population based study has only been reported from Norway, where the prevalence was 8.5 per 100,000 inhabitants. This is higher than figures reported from other countries. In a Spanish study, the point prevalence in 1988 was found to be 2.24 cases per million, indicating that the prevalence of PSC may be lower in the southern part of Europe. The frequency of PSC in patients with UC may be underestimated since some patients with PSC may not undergo cholangiography for reasons of only minimal rises in liver function tests and lack of symptoms.

4. GENERAL DEMOGRAPHICS

PSC has been reported in all races and may affect any age group but is predominantly seen in young and middle-aged men. The mean age at diagnosis is 32–42 years and about two-thirds of the patients are men. There are global differences in presentation of the disease, but age, gender and a strong association to IBD seem to be consistent around the world. Family occurrence of PSC is reported but is probably rare. Two recent studies have shown that a large number of PSC patients are non-smokers and it seems that smoking in UC patients is associated with a decreased risk of acquiring PSC. PSC is also seen in children but less frequent than in adults. Sclerosing cholangitis in childhood is a heterogeneous condition, which has different aetiologies and may be inherited and diagnosed in the neonatal period or present later with features of autoimmunity. The term autoimmune sclerosing cholangitis has been suggested for this group.

5. PATHOPHYSIOLOGY

The aetiology and pathogenesis of PSC has not yet been clearly established. There is strong evidence to suggest that immune mechanisms play an essential role in the pathogenesis of this disease. This is supported by associations with certain HLA haplotypes, the presence of autoantibodies, lymphocytes in the portal tracts, increased levels of total serum immunoglobulins and the association with other autoimmune diseases. Controversies exist whether the HLA association has any prognostic importance. The strong HLA associations particularly with HLA1-B8-DR3 have been well replicated and this allele is in turn associated with other autoimmune diseases. The majority of patients have serum-autoantibodies mostly ANCAs, but there is no current evidence that they act as a driving force in the pathogenic process. We have recently shown that the majority of PSC patients have antibodies directed against the biliary epithelium. Whether the immune reactions seen in PSC are the cause or consequence of the tissue destruction is still not known. PSC patients lack some of the classical characteristics of autoimmunity, such as the usual female preponderance of the disease and lack of a good response to immunosuppression. Non-immune mechanisms such as bacterial infection, ischaemia and toxicity have been suggested to play an important role in the development of the disease and these factors may trigger peribiliary inflammation and cytokine-induced hepatic fibrosis. PSC may be triggered in genetically susceptible individuals by toxic or infectious agents that reach the liver via colon because of increased colonic permeability due to colitis.

6. CLINICAL FEATURES

The clinical presentation of PSC can vary greatly, and the patients may be either asymptomatic or symptomatic. The presentation of symptoms and signs has changed during the last 10–20 years. PSC was commonly seen as a symptomatic disease in the early 1980s, with jaundice, pruritus and abdominal pain present in about two-thirds of all patients at the time of diagnosis; asymptomatic patients were rare (7–10%). As ERCP has come into frequent use and the knowledge of PSC has increased, the number of patients with asymptomatic disease at diagnosis has risen. Today, 15–45% of all PSC patients are asymptomatic at the time of diagnosis. Many asymptomatic patients remain completely well despite progression of cholangiographic and histology changes. As much as 17% of the asymptomatic patients and 50% of the symptomatic ones are reported as having cirrhosis at the time of diagnosis. In the symptomatic group, the disease is characterized by periodic remissions and exacerbations. The most common symptoms in patients with PSC are fatigue, jaundice, pruritus and abdominal pain, whereas ascites, bleeding from oesophageal varices and acute cholangitis are much less frequent (Table 1). Fatigue is a common complaint in patients with PSC. The cause of fatigue in cholestatic liver disease is unknown although it was recently suggested that altered serotoninergic transmission in the brain could account for this symptom. Pruritus is present in approximately 30% of the PSC patients. The severity of pruritus is not closely linked to the severity of the underlying liver disease. Evidence has emerged to support the role of central nervous system in the pathogenesis of cholestatic pruritus. Osteopenia due to osteoporosis is a common complication of cholestatic liver disease. Angulo *et al.* studied 81 PSC patients with bone mineral density of the lumbar spine and found significantly less values than expected when compared with normal individuals. Moreover, seven patients (8.6%) had a bone mineral density below the fracture threshold. These patients were older, had a longer duration of IBD and a more advanced PSC. Pathologic fractures after liver transplantation occur in one-third of patients with PSC and almost exclusively in those patients who already had osteopenia at the time of liver transplantation. The cause of osteoporosis in PSC is multifactorial and pathophysiological mechanisms specifically related to cholestatic disease have not been identified. Fat-soluble vitamin deficiency is a common feature in PSC patients with advanced disease. The patient's fat-soluble vitamin level should therefore be monitored and those found to have decreased levels are recommended replacement therapy. In patients having malabsorption it is of

Table 1. Symptoms in patients with primary sclerosing cholangitis.

Symptoms	Frequency (%)
Asymptomatic disease	15–44
Pruritus	25–59
Jaundice	30–69
Abdominal pain	16–37
Hepatomegaly	34–62
Weight loss	10–34
Acute cholangitis	5–28
Ascites	2–10
Variceal bleeding	2–14

importance to exclude chronic pancreatitis as well as Celiac disease since both are found to be over-represented in PSC. Hyperpigmentation, xanthomas and xantelasma do occur, but are rare and are found less frequently than in primary biliary cirrhosis. Signs of portal hypertension and cirrhosis in PSC – such as oesophageal varices, ascites and encephalopathy – do not differ from other liver disorders. However, a special complication of portal hypertension in PSC patients with a history of colectomy with an ileal stoma is the development of peristomal varices. The majority of the patients developing peristomal varices also suffer from oesophageal varices.

7. COMPLICATIONS IN PSC

Complications specific for PSC include fever, bacterial cholangitis, gallbladder and biliary stones, dominant biliary tract strictures and cholangiocarcinoma. Episodes of fever may occur without an association to bacterial cholangitis and disappear spontaneously without antibiotic treatment. Ascending cholangitis, secondary to bacterial infections of the biliary system, is uncommon unless the biliary tree has been surgically manipulated. There are obvious problems when trying to distinguish between episodes of idiopathic fever and chills, and those produced by acute bacterial cholangitis. The actual benefit from prophylactic antibiotic therapy to prevent recurrent bouts of cholangitis noticed in these patients has not been properly documented. If acute cholangitis does occur in patients who have not been operated upon, presence of cholelithiasis, a dominant stricture or a bile duct cancer should be considered.

Chronic cholelithiasis is associated with the development of cholesterol gallstones, and recurrent cholangitis may lead to the development of pigment gallstones. Most stones in PSC patients are confined to the gall bladder, and are reported in up to one-third of the patients with PSC. In patients with known PSC presenting with symptoms, especially cholangitis, it is important to search for stones. Patients with PSC and biliary tract calculi have more symptoms, especially ascending cholangitis, than those without. Dominant strictures affect 15–20% of all PSC patients at some time during the course of the disease. The strictures are located in the common bile duct or common hepatic duct in the liver hilum. The patient often presents with an acute onset of jaundice, pruritus and fever; in these cases, a cholangiogram should be made. It is usually difficult to differentiate between a dominant benign stricture and a stenosis due to cholangiocarcinoma. Whenever a dominant stricture occurs, brush cytology and/or fine needle biopsy should be performed in order to exclude a malignant change in the biliary tree. Although the sensitivity of brushings may be low, the specificity is usually high [2].

8. CHOLANGIOCARCINOMA

The increased risk for cholangiocarcinoma in PSC is well established, but the factors responsible for the malignant development in the bile ducts are unknown. The differences in reported risk are probably related to the length of follow-up, stage of disease and under-recognition in studies with low autopsy rate. The largest study that has evaluated the risk of CC in PSC includes 604 Swedish PSC patients [3]. The prevalence of CC in this study was 13%. Thirty-seven per cent of the patients with CC developed the tumour within 1 year after PSC diagnosis. The incidence rate of CC was 1.5% per year in PSC patients with a duration of PSC more than 1 year. It is very difficult to diagnose cholangiocarcinoma in patients with PSC and also patients without cirrhosis may develop CC. The unsuspected finding of cholangiocarcinoma in the liver explant following liver transplantation has been observed in 8–18% despite a careful pre-transplant investigation. Once the cholangiocarcinoma has developed, the prognosis is poor with a median time of survival of less than 6 months. Several diagnostic tools have been evaluated in order to diagnose CC in patients with PSC (Table 2). It has been suggested that PSC patients with a concomitant cholangiocarcinoma present with more rapid clinical and biochemical deterioration than patients without CC. However, this has not been confirmed in a recent case-control study including PSC patients with and without cholangiocarcinoma. It is difficult to demonstrate or rule out the presence of a cholangiocarcinoma in PSC on a cholangiogram (Figure 1). Comparisons with previous imaging are essential to signal fast progression of disease or development of malignancy. In a case–control study cholangiography and computer tomography (CT) were

Table 2. Diagnostic tools for detecting cholangiocarcinoma in PSC.

Method	Sensitivity	Specificity
Mayo model risk score	Moderate	Moderate
Ultrasound/computer tomography/ERCP	Poor	Poor
Tumour markers (CA19-9, CEA)	Moderate	Moderate
PET	Excellent (?)[a]	Excellent (?)[a]
Brush cytology	Poor	Excellent

[a]Needs to be confirmed.

evaluated as diagnostic tool for detecting CC in PSC showing a sensitivity and specificity of around 50 and 80%, respectively [4]. New techniques such as positron emission tomography (PET) may become useful in the diagnosis of cholangiocarcinoma in patients with PSC. Even if this interesting finding will be confirmed in new studies PET is expensive and not widely available.

Several tumour markers such as CA19-9, CEA, CA50, CA125 and CA242 have been evaluated in the diagnostic evaluation of suspected cholangiocarcinoma in patients with PSC. The most studied are CA19-9 and with an index using the formula CA19-9 + (CEA × 40) > 400 U an accuracy of 86% was obtained [5]. However, the sensitivity was much lower for detecting CC and incidental cholangiocarcinomas were even more difficult to diagnose. Moreover, CA19-9 may also rise due to episodes of cholangitis. In a recent prospective study evaluating tumour markers taken repeatedly every 6 months the markers failed to identify all patients developing cholangiocarcinoma. In some patients without malignancy a rise in tumour markers was also seen without signs of bacterial cholangitis. Thus, the use of tumour markers in patients with PSC has several limitations. In summary, serum levels of CA19-9 can be of some value in suspecting cholangiocarcinoma, although it has failed as a screening measure to detect early neoplastic changes.

Due to the high rate of cholangiocarcinoma in PSC patients and the poor prognosis after tumour development, it is of importance to identify which patients are at high risk for CC development so these patients could undergo liver transplantation at an early stage. Biliary dysplasia as an early stage of CC is controversial. In a recent study the concept of biliary dysplasia was defined and evaluated. The presence of biliary dysplasia in liver biopsies from patients with PSC seems to increase the possibility that CC is present in another part of the liver [6]. Therefore, if biliary dysplasia is found much effort should be made to diagnose or rule out CC. In single studies it has been suggested that risk factors for CC development in PSC are smoking, alcohol consumption, history of colorectal dysplasia/cancer, biliary dysplasia or presence of K-ras mutations in the bile. These findings need, however, to be verified.

In addition, PSC patients with cirrhosis are also at risk for developing hepatocellular carcinoma and should be included in surveillance programs.

9. ASSOCIATED DISEASES

PSC is associated with a number of diseases, the most important being IBD. The majority of patients with PSC who have an associated IBD suffer from UC. Although an association with Crohn's disease was suggested by Atkinson and Caroll already in 1964, this association has been less well recognized. In recent studies, 1.3–13% of patients with Crohn's disease also have PSC. It was suggested in a study from Norway that PSC may be seen as commonly in colonic Crohn's disease as in UC. IBD can be diagnosed at any time during the course of PSC, and PSC can occur at any time during the course of IBD. PSC may also develop after proctocolectomy in colitis. Proctocolectomy for UC appears to have little or no effect on the progression of PSC and there seems to be no correlation between the severity of UC and that of PSC. There is a wide global range in the prevalence of UC in patients with PSC, varying from 23% (reported from Japan) to as much as 100% (in Norway). The prevalence of PSC in patients with IBD can vary between 2.4 and 7.5%. The reason for the variation in PSC prevalence can possibly be explained by the fact that PSC can be asymptomatic with only a mild elevation of liver function tests, and that these abnormalities may fluctuate, so that episodes of normal liver function may occur. Therefore, the prevalence of PSC in patients with

IBD will depend on the number of patients being screened with liver function tests, and how frequently these tests are made. Other causes to elevation of liver function tests besides PSC, such as autoimmune hepatitis and fatty change, may be present in IBD patients. Furthermore, elevated liver enzymes may be seen during colonic disease activity, treatment with steroids and total parenteral nutrition. Most UC patients having PSC suffer from substantial colitis. The prevalence of PSC is 5.5% in patients with substantial and 0.5% in patients with distal colitis. The colitis in PSC generally runs a quiescent course compared to that in UC patients without PSC. Furthermore, the subclinical time span of IBD in PSC patients may be as long as 7 years before onset of clinical symptoms. Thus, the quiescent course of the colitis in PSC may lead to an underestimation of the colitis in PSC unless all patients undergo colonoscopic investigation with multiple biopsies. Furthermore, proctosigmoidoscopy as the sole means of investigation is insufficient in diagnosing UC in patients with PSC, since one study has shown that in 23% of the PSC and UC patients the rectum was spared. In PSC patients with UC requiring a proctocolectomy, an ileal pouch-anal anastomosis has proven to be the most appropriate definite operation for the majority of these patients. Non-specific inflammation of the pouch (pouchitis) is the most frequent long-term complication in UC patients operated on with an ileal pouch-anal anastomosis. Patients with PSC are more likely to have chronic pouchitis (60%) than UC patients without PSC (15%). The risk of pouchitis is not related to the severity of the liver disease. In PSC patients having pouchitis before liver transplantation, most continue to have pouchitis after transplantation in spite of triple immunosuppression treatment, suggesting that antibiotic, rather than immune modifying therapy, is the treatment of choice for pouchitis.

It is well known that patients with UC have an increased risk of developing colorectal carcinoma. The two major risk factors for this complication are long duration of disease and extensive colitis. The cause of neoplastic change in UC remains unexplained. Lately, the presence of PSC has been shown to increase the risk of colorectal cancer/dysplasia in patients with UC [7]. PSC patients with UC remain at an increased risk of developing colon cancer/dysplasia even after they have undergone liver transplantation. It is therefore of importance to emphasize the necessity that all patients with PSC and UC should be included into colonoscopic surveillance programs, probably at an earlier time than UC patients without PSC. Also after transplantation, an annual colonoscopy of these patients is suggested. It has been speculated that secondary bile acids play a role as carcinogenic agents in the colorectal mucosa. This theory is supported by the observation that right-sided colorectal cancer seems to be more common in patients with PSC than in patients with UC alone. This is also suggested by a recent report showing that treatment with ursodeoxycholic acid (UDCA) decreased the risk for developing colorectal dysplasia in patients with PSC and UC [8].

A number of other diseases besides UC are associated with PSC. Whether there are true associations to PSC itself or just parallel phenomena are not clear. Pancreatitis, appears to be the second most common disorder associated with PSC affecting 15–50% of all patients with PSC. Asymptomatic pancreatitic changes are often seen on ERCP although clinically important, pancreatic exocrine failure is rare. The diagnosis of chronic pancreatitis should be considered in patients with inappropriate steatorrhea or loss of weight, especially in PSC patients who are not jaundiced and who have an early stage of the disease. The diagnosis is of importance since pancreatic enzyme supplements may be of benefit. In addition, it has recently been suggested that PSC patients have an increased risk of developing pancreatic cancer [3]. The relationship between Celiac disease and PSC remains unknown, although an immunological connection is suspected. The clinical awareness of possible coexistence is important, and if patients with PSC present with severe steatorrhea and weight loss, Celiac disease must be considered. Other PSC associated autoimmune disorders are among others, insulin dependent diabetes, autoimmune hemolytic anaemia, Sjögren's syndrome, thyreoditis, systemic sclerosis, SLE, alopecia and polymyositis.

10. DIAGNOSIS – BLOOD TESTS

The classic laboratory finding in patients with PSC is an increased ALP level. Most patients also have raised aminotransaminase (AST/ALT) levels. In many studies, a two-fold increase of the ALP level is used as one of the diagnostic criteria for PSC. The range of the increase is – for practical clinical use – not of much help, as also a normal ALP level has been reported in approximately 10% of all PSC patients. The liver enzymes often run a fluctuating course. It is therefore important to follow patients with UC with repeated measurements of liver function tests to make sure that they do not suffer from PSC. Accordingly, it is advisable not only to take liver function tests in UC patients regularly, but also to do magnetic resonance cholangiographies (MRCP) on wide indications whenever symptoms or signs indicate liver disease in these patients. The level of serum albumin and prothrombin time are normal in early PSC. In patients suffering from both PSC and UC, a decrease in albumin may be related to an active IBD. Serum bilirubin levels are usually normal in the early stages of PSC, but gradually increasing as the disease progresses. Striking fluctuations in bilirubin levels may occur, even in the early stages of the disease when significant extrahepatic biliary strictures, stones, sludge formation or infections occur. Positive titres of antinuclear antibodies (ANA) or smooth muscle antibodies have been detected in 22% of PSC patients. The anti-neutrophil antibody (ANCA) is raised in around 80% of the PSC patients and may have a fluctuating course.

11. DIAGNOSIS – IMAGING

The "gold standard" for the diagnosis of PSC is ERCP showing localized or multifocal strictures and intervening segments of normal or diverticulum-like outpouchings or ectatic ducts (Figure 1). However, MRCP has been progressively tested in patients with PSC and can usually equal ERCP [9]. With further improvements MRCP will replace ERCP to diagnose PSC and be used to select patients for endoscopic interventions. CT and ultrasound is of no or little value to diagnose PSC but have a role to identify complications of the disease such as biliary stones and cholangiocarcinoma.

12. DIAGNOSIS – HISTOLOGY

The liver histology in PSC is variable and often unspecific, and is diagnostic in less than half of all cases. Characteristic features in liver biopsies from patients with PSC are: bile duct proliferation, periportal inflammation and fibrosis, and obliteration and finally loss of bile ducts. The extent of fibrosis is often scored into four stages, where stage IV represents cirrhosis. Sampling variability do occur and among 56 PSC patients undergoing two liver biopsies at the same occasion 11% differed by more than one stage and cirrhosis was missed in 37%. Overlapping features of autoimmune hepatitis are frequently seen in patients with PSC. However, with the revised scoring system for autoimmune hepatitis recently published the possibility of excluding autoimmune hepatitis in patients with PSC has improved considerably. Nevertheless, approximately 10% of all PSC patients will fulfil the criteria for definite or probable autoimmune hepatitis.

13. MANAGEMENT

The treatment of PSC has been limited by the lack of knowledge about the pathogenic process. There are several options for treatment namely, medical, endoscopic and surgical therapy including liver transplantation. A summary of management of patients with PSC is given in Figure 2.

13.1 Medical therapeutics

There are few prospective randomized controlled treatment studies in PSC. In many studies patients with advanced disease are included. Since the major target in PSC are the bile ducts and they lack the capacity to regenerate, the disease process will lead to the development of ductopenia and a progressive irreversible failure of hepatic biliary excretion. Therefore, specific treatment would likely be more effective in the early disease course. Several medical treatments with different mechanisms of action including immunosuppressants, anti-inflammatory, anti-fibrotic as well as bile acids have been evaluated in PSC. None of them have shown a convincing evidence of benefit and to date an effective medical treatment for PSC is lacking. UDCA at a dose of 10–15 mg/kg is the most tested drug and has been evaluated in several studies. The studies have shown an improvement in biochemical tests, but no effect on progression of disease or survival has been documented. The largest study including 105 patients did

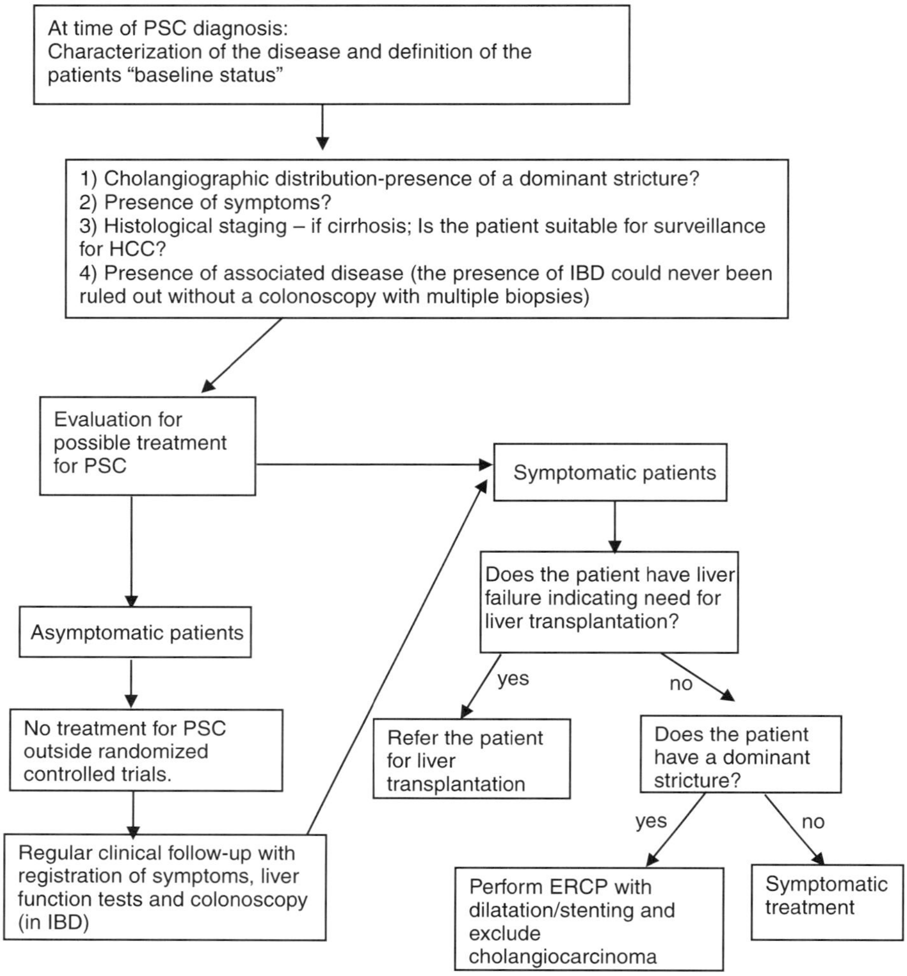

Figure 2. The management of patients with primary sclerosing cholangitis.

not demonstrate any clinical benefit and did not alter disease progression or time to transplantation [10]. In a recent small randomized study it was shown that high dose UDCA (20 mg/kg) given for 2 years significantly improved both histology and cholangiographic features [11]. Controlled studies with methotrexate, colchicine, penicillamine and cyclosporin have not demonstrated any favourable effects. Tacrolimus (FK506), corticosteroids, budesonide, nicotine patches and pentoxifyllin have all been studied in small often uncontrolled trials without convincing effects. However, all these studies are hampered by few patients included and short follow-up. UDCA have also been tested in combination with other drugs such as prednisolone, azathioprine and methotrexate. In one study evaluating combination treatment with UDCA, prednisolone and azathioprine in 6 out of 10 patients, who had follow-up liver biopsies showed histological improvement. However, changes in liver histology in such a small group of patients should be interpreted cautiously. The value of combining UDCA treatment with bile duct strictures dilation was evaluated in a non-randomized study indicating that the combination was more effective than the predicted survival calculated from their baseline status [12]. Maybe, the most effective future therapy in PSC will be to combine different treatment modalities. However, future studies will have to assess not only the efficacy of the treatments but since all therapies most likely will be given for many years an acceptable benefit–risk ratio has to be proven.

Since no effective treatment is available to stop disease progression in PSC, therapy has to focus on treating complications and symptoms of PSC. The treatment of pruritus in PSC is the same as for other cholestatic patients. The general principles for handling osteoporosis in PSC are similar to those followed for post-menopausal osteoporosis. In all patients optimal conditions for preventing bone loss should be established. Attention should focus on adequate calcium and vitamin D intake and physical exercise. It has been suggested that PSC patients should receive prophylactic therapy with calcium and vitamin D in an oral dose daily of 800 μg vitamin D and 1 g of calcium. Antiresorptive agents such as biphosphonates appear to be the most rational choice if a PSC patient needs treatment for osteoporosis. Treatment of end stage disease and portal hypertension – such as oesophageal varices, ascites and encephalopathy – do not differ from other liver disorders. However, patients that have developed peristomal varices often present with recurrent hemorrhagic episodes. Local treatments to control bleeding are usually unsuccessful. In the long run liver transplantation should be considered in these cases. It has been suggested that ileostomy should be avoided in PSC patients requiring proctocolectomy and that ileoanal, ileorectal or ileal pouch-anal anastomosis, which are less susceptible to variceal formation and bleeding are to be preferred in these patients.

13.2 Endoscopic and surgical treatment

Dominant bile duct strictures may cause rapid and clinical deterioration in some patients with PSC and can be treated endoscopically or surgically. Endoscopic treatment involves balloon dilatation of the strictures and/or placement of a biliary stent. In some centres also nasobiliary drainage with or without lavage is used. Many of these reports also include sphincterotomy to facilitate further interventions. If mainly intrahepatic changes are present treatment is less effective. Patients that most likely will benefit from endoscopic therapy are those with progressive rise of liver enzymes, jaundice or cholangitis and dominant strictures should only be treated endoscopically in symptomatic patients. Indeed, findings in several uncontrolled studies suggest that the symptomatic patients may have prolonged biochemical and clinical response for several years after endoscopic therapy. However, end stage patients in need of a liver transplant should preferably not undergo endoscopic therapy since deterioration of the liver function has been described after ERCP. Placement of a stent is associated with recurrent occlusion and bacterial cholangitis and therefore the stents have to be changed regularly. Cholangitis can be a serious complication in PSC because of the presence of poorly drained ducts. If bacterial cholangitis occurs, it is best treated with broad-spectrum antibiotics. Giving antibiotic before endoscopic interventions can reduce the risk of cholangitis. Due to the risk of cholangitis, Johnson *et al.* suggest that stents should be avoided in PSC and only balloon dilations should be undertaken. However, Ponsioen *et al.* treated 32 patients with short-term stenting (mean 11 days). In 83% of the patients cholestatic complaints improved and during follow-up only 20% needed new interventions during the first year [13]. It is of importance to point out that only skilled endoscopists should perform endoscopic therapy in patients with PSC. Several cases of bile duct perforation during ERCP have been described in these patients, which may be due to a weakened bile duct wall or due to technical reasons. Small biliary stones and pigment debris can also effectively be treated endoscopically. Although it seems as if endoscopic therapy in selected PSC patients is of clinical importance optimal regimes have not been defined and it has not been proved to have any significant effect on survival. It must be emphasized that endoscopic interventions should never delay referral for liver transplantation. Biliary tract reconstructive procedures have been used to bypass dominant strictures not amenable to endoscopic or percutaneous drainage. Non-randomized studies suggest that bilioenteric bypass may reduce symptoms in non-cirrhotic PSC patients and prolong survival. However, previous abdominal operations may also have a negative influence on the outcome after liver transplantation.

13.3 Orthotopic liver transplantation

Since, there is no current treatment, which effectively halts the progression of PSC, liver transplantation remains the only option for patients who progress to end stage disease. In Scandinavia, PSC is the most common indication for liver transplantation and in the North America PSC the fourth most common indication accounting for approximately 10% of liver transplants. If the patient does not have cholangiocarcinoma the results of liver transplantation in PSC are excellent and several recent studies have reported 1-year survival of 90–97% and 5-year survival rates of 80–85% [14]. To assess optimal timing of liver transplantation, several natural history risk scores have been developed and utilized. These risk scores are developed using sophisticated statistical approaches, mostly Cox multivariate regression tests. Survival can be predicted based on independent clinical, biochemical and histological features (Table 3). Probably the most widely used prognostic model is the Mayo Model Risk Score which recently has been presented in a revised version [15]. This model includes age, AST, albumin, bilirubin and history of variceal bleeding. One advantage of this model is the absence of liver histology and no invasive investigation is needed. It has also been shown to be superior to the Child classification. However, the timing of liver transplantation in PSC is difficult and none of these prognostic models are able to predict the appearance of cholangiocarcinoma. In a recent study including 118 patients different pre-transplant variables associated with survival after liver transplantation were investigated [16]. It was shown that the presence of IBD, previous upper abdominal surgery, ascites, increased creatinine and presence of malignancy all had a negative impact on survival after liver transplantation. Data from the Mayo Clinic have demonstrated that the post-transplant survival rate is clearly related to the pre-transplant Child–Pugh stage. The 1-year survival rate in Child–Pugh A was 98.1%, Child–Pugh B; 89% and in Child–Pugh C; 73%, respectively. It seems therefore advisable not to wait too long to refer PSC patients for evaluation for liver transplantation.

10–20% of all PSC patients develop cholangiocarcinoma and liver transplantation is not an effective treatment because of the high probability of tumour recurrence. Therefore, cholangiocarcinoma is usually a contraindication for liver transplantation. However, incidentally diagnosed cholangiocarcinoma in the explanted liver less than 1 cm may not have any impact on outcome after transplantation [17]. In a study from the Mayo Clinic it was demonstrated that a small subgroup of patients with cholangiocarcinoma, meeting strict selection criteria, who undergo radiation and chemotherapy prior to liver transplantation, appear to have acceptable long-term liver transplant results.

There is accumulating evidence that PSC recurs after liver transplantation. However, the diagnosis of post-transplant PSC has not been widely accepted largely due to problems with non-anastomotic biliary strictures that also occur after liver transplantation in several other conditions. Therefore, other causes to biliary strictures after liver transplantation have to be excluded, such as hepatic artery thrombosis, established ductopenic disease, anastomotic strictures alone, non-anastomotic strictures before post-transplant day 90 and ABO incompatibility between donor and recipient. With the use of strict criteria Graziadei reported that 24 of 120 PSC patients (20%) had recurrent PSC after liver transplantation [18]. The median time for the development of non-anastomotic biliary strictures was 360 days. The survival was, however, not different in the group with recurrent disease compared to those without.

Besides problems with recurrence of PSC it seems as if PSC patients have an increased incidence of both acute and chronic rejection and hepatic artery thrombosis.

Table 3. Factors found to be of prognostic importance in primary sclerosing cholangitis.

Dickson *et al.* [20] ($n = 426$)	Kim *et al.* [15] ($n = 405$)	Broomé *et al.* [19] ($n = 305$)	Shetty *et al.* [21] ($n = 208$)
Age Bilirubin Histological stage Splenomegaly	Age Bilirubin Albumin AST history of variceal bleeding	Age Bilirubin Histological stage	Age Child–Turcotte–Pugh Score

14. PROGNOSIS – NATURAL HISTORY OF PSC

As described previously, the clinical course of patients with PSC is variable, and PSC is frequently a progressive disease leading to complications due to chronic cholestasis, cirrhosis, hepatic failure, portal hypertension or cholangiocarcinoma. Some patients have a long standing silent disease without progression lasting for decades while others have a rapid progression of symptoms and signs ending with manifest liver failure and a need for liver transplantation within a few years. Moreover, many patients have exacerbations and remissions. Both histological and cholangiographic progression of the hepatic changes may occur without the development of new symptoms or signs. Therefore, the natural history has been difficult to describe, with conflicting reports of the prognosis appearing in the literature. The natural history of PSC is described in a number of studies; the median survival time from diagnosis to death or transplantation is reported to be around 12 years, but may be as high as 21 years. Differences in survival time between the various studies may have many reasons, one being the variation in definition of the onset of the disease. It is difficult to accurately determine the onset of PSC because the disease usually begins insidiously. Early detection of PSC can only be made with prospective regular follow-ups of liver function tests in patients with IBD. Whether the onset of the disease is defined as the time of the first symptom consistent with PSC, the time of the first abnormal liver function test, the time for cholangiography or the time for referral to a tertial centre, the definition will lead to differences in the overall survival time. Furthermore, if termination of the disease is defined as the time of death or time for liver transplantation will also influence survival time. One of the largest studies, including 305 PSC patients, showed that 44% of the patients were asymptomatic at diagnosis; 22% of the asymptomatic patients developed symptoms during a median of 5 years follow-up [19]. The study also shows that patients with an asymptomatic PSC disease at diagnosis have a more favourable prognosis than patients with symptoms as confirmed by others. Comparison of survival in symptomatic and asymptomatic patients is shown in Figure 3. As discussed before, asymptomatic patients with PSC are diagnosed with increasing frequency. Forty-five asymptomatic PSC patients were analysed by Porayko *et al.* for evaluation of progression and natural history of asymptomatic PSC disease. The majority of these

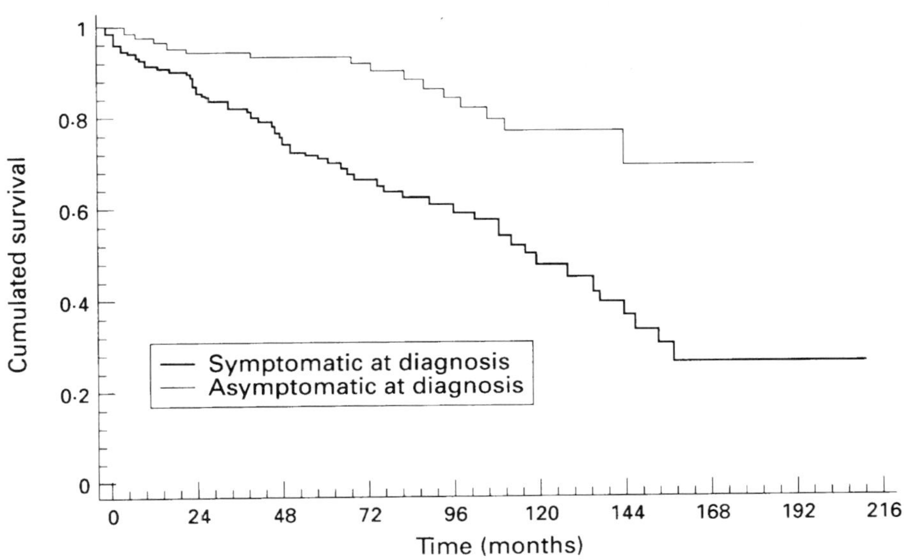

Figure 3. Comparison of survival in 305 symptomatic and asymptomatic Swedish PSC patients. Patients with symptomatic disease have a significantly decreased survival compared to asymptomatic patients ($p < 0.001$) [19].

patients had minimal histological changes (stage I–II) at liver biopsy, none with cirrhosis. During a mean follow-up of 6 years, 76% showed progression of the liver disease, i.e., development of signs or symptoms, and 31% of the asymptomatic patients died or were transplanted because of liver failure. Even though asymptomatic patients seem to have a more favourable prognosis, and there are reports of patients with long-term survival, PSC must be regarded as a progressive disease frequently leading to complications of cholestasis, cirrhosis, liver failure and cholangiocarcinoma. Factors found to be of prognostic importance in PSC are presented in Table 3. Today, the chances of predicting cholangiocarcinoma in the setting of PSC are very small and it is important to stress that so far no factor has been singled out to identify patients who will later develop cholangiocarcinoma. Once the cholangiocarcinoma has developed, the prognosis is poor, currently curative treatment is not available. The prognostic value of cholangiography has also been investigated by Olsson *et al.* High-grade intrahepatic strictures on the first diagnostic cholangiogram indicate early jaundice, while short and high-grade extrahepatic strictures indicate early pruritus, abdominal pain and fever. Since PSC is a disease of young people the question sometimes rises concerning the risk for progression secondary to pregnancy. This matter is addressed in only one study of 13 pregnancies in 10 patients with PSC. The pregnancy did not seem to have a negative effect on the progression of the PSC disease and the outcome for both babies and mothers was favourable. However, in two pregnant patients, the pruritus was so intense as to bring on premature delivery.

In conclusion, although PSC is a rare disease with limited possibilities to halt the progression of the disease, it is important to identify these patients. They benefit from active treatment of symptoms, complications and should be continuously evaluated for optimal timing for liver transplantation.

REFERENCES

[1] Broomé, U., Glaumann, H., Lindström, E., Lööf, L., Almer, S., Prytz, H., Sandberg-Gertzén, H., Lindgren, S., Fork, T., Järnerot, G., Olsson, R. and Lindberg, G. (2002) Natural history and outcome in 32 Swedish patients with small duct primary sclerosing cholangitis (PSC). *J. Hepatol.* **36**, 586–589.

[2] Ponsioen, C.Y., Vrouenraets, S.M., Van Milligen de Wit, A.W., Sturm, P., Tascilar, M., Offerhaus, G.J., Prins, M., Huibregtse, K. and Tytgat, G.N. (1999) Value of brush cytology for dominant strictures in primary sclerosing cholangitis. *Endoscopy* **31**, 305–309.

[3] Bergquist, A., Ekbom, A., Olsson, R., Kornfelt, D., Lööf, L., Danilesson, Å., Hultcrantz, R., Lindgren, S., Prytz, H., Sandberg-Gertzén, H., Almer, S., Granath, F. and Broomé, U. (2002) Hepatic and extrahepatic malignancies in primary sclerosing cholangitis. *J. Hepatol.* **36**, 321–327.

[4] Campbell, W.L., Peterson, M.S., Federle, M.P., Siqueira, E.S., Slivka, A., Grazioli, L., Ichikawa, T., Oliver, J.H., Kim, T. and Li, W. (2001) Using CT and cholangiography to diagnose biliary tract carcinoma complicating primary sclerosing cholangitis. *Am. J. Gastroenterol.* **177**, 1095–1100.

[5] Ramage, J., Donaghy, A., Farrant, J., Iorns, R. and Williams, R. (1995) Serum tumor markers for the diagnosis of cholangiocarcinoma in primary sclerosing cholangitis. *Gastroenterology* **108**, 865–869.

[6] Fleming, K., Boberg, K., Glaumann, H., Bergquist, A., Smith, D. and Clausen, O. (2001) Biliary dysplasia as a marker of cholangiocarcinoma in primary sclerosing cholangitis. *J. Hepatol.* **34**, 360–365.

[7] Broomé, U., Löfberg, R., Veress, B. and Eriksson, S. (1995) Primary sclerosing cholangitis and ulcerative colitis: evidence for increased neoplastic potential. *Hepatology* **22**, 1404–1408.

[8] Tung, B.Y., Emond, M.J., Haggitt, R.C., Bronner, M.P., Kimmey, M.B., Kowdley, K.V. and Brentnall, T.A. (2001) Ursodiol use is associated with lower prevalence of colonic neoplasia in patients with ulcerative colitis and primary sclerosing cholangitis. *Ann. Int. Med.* **134**, 89–95.

[9] Angulo, P., Pearce, D.H., Johnson, C.D., Henry, J.J., LaRusso, N.F., Petersen, B.T. and Lindor, K.D. (2000) Magnetic resonance cholangiography in patients with biliary disease: its role in primary sclerosing cholangitis. *J. Hepatol.* **33**, 520–527.

[10] Harnois, D., Angulo, P., Jorgensen, R., LaRusso, N. and Lindor, K. (2001) High-dose ursodeoxycholic acid as a therapy for patients with primary sclerosing cholangitis. *Am. J. Gastroenterol.* **96**, 1558–1562.

[11] Mitchell, M., Bansi, D., Hunt, N., Von Bergmann, K., Fleming, K. and Chapman, R. (2001) A preliminary trial of high-dose ursodeoxycholic acid in primary

sclerosing cholangitis. *Gastroenterology* **121**, 900–907.

[12] Stiehl, A., Rudolph, G., Koters-Plachky, P., Sauer, P. and Walker, S. (2002) Development of bile duct stenosis in patients with primary sclerosing cholangitis treated with ursodeoxycholic acid: outcome after endoscopic treatment. *J. Hepatol.* **36**, 151–156.

[13] Ponsioen, C., Lam, K., van de Milligan de Wit, W., Huigbregtse, K. and Tytgat, G. (1999) Four year experience with short term stenting in primary sclerosing cholangitis. *Am. J. Gastroenterol.* **94**, 2403–2407.

[14] Seaberg, E.C., Belle, S.H., Beringer, K.C., Schivins, J.L. and Detre, K.M. (1998) Liver transplantation in the United States from 1987–1998: updated results from the Pitt-UNOS Liver Transplant Registry. *Clin. Transpl.* **12**, 17–37.

[15] Kim, W.R., Therneau, T.M., Wiesner, R.H., Poterucha, J.J., Benson, J.T., Malinchoc, M., LaRusso, N.F., Lindor, K.D. and Dickson, E.R. (2000) A revised natural history model for primary sclerosing cholangitis. *Mayo Clin. Proc.* **75**, 688–694.

[16] Neuberger, J., Gunson, B., Komolmit, P., Davies, M. and Christensen, E. (1999) Pretransplant prediction of prognosis after liver transplantation in primary sclerosing cholangitis using a Cox regression model. *Hepatology* **29**, 1375–1379.

[17] Goss, J.A., Shackleton, C.R., Farmer, D.G., Arnaout, W.S., Seu, P., Markowitz, J.S., Martin, P., Stribling, R.J., Goldstein, L.I. and Busuttil, R.W. (1997) Orthotopic liver transplantation for primary sclerosing cholangitis. *Ann. Surg.* **225**, 472–483.

[18] Graziadei, I.W., Wiesner, R.H., Batts, K.P., Marotta, P.J., LaRusso, N.F., Porayko, M.K., Hay, J.E., Gores, G.J., Charlton, M.R., Ludwig, J., Poterucha, J.J., Steers, J.L. and Krom, R.A. (1999) Recurrence or primary sclerosing cholangitis following liver transplantation. *Hepatology* **29**, 1050–1056.

[19] Broomé, U., Glaumann, H., Lindström, E., Lööf, L., Almer, S., Prytz, H., Sandberg-Gertzén, H., Lindgren, S., Fork, T., Järnerot, G., Olsson, R. and Lindberg, G. (1996) Natural history and prognostic factors in 305 Swedish patients with primary sclerosing cholangitis. *Gut* **38**, 610–615.

[20] Dickson, E.R., Murtaugh, P.A., Wiesner, R.H., Grambsch, P.M., Fleming, T.R., Ludwig, J., LaRusso, N.F., Malinchoc, M., Chapman, R.W., Kaplan, M.M. (1992) Primary sclerosing cholangitis: refinement and validation of survival models. *Gastroenterology* **102**, 1893–1901.

[21] Shetty, K., Rybicki, L. and Carey, W. (1997) The Child–Pugh classification as a prognostic indicator for survival in primary sclerosing cholangitis. *Hepatology* **25**, 1049–1053.

Hepatology: A Practical Approach
B. Al Knawy, M.L. Shiffman, R.H. Wiesner (editors)

Chapter 17

Hepatic Vascular Disorders

Michael P. Curry and Sanjiv Chopra

Harvard Medical School, Boston, MA, USA

1. Introduction 273
2. The Hepatic Arterial Circulation 274
   2.1 Ischemic hepatitis 274
   2.2 Hepatic artery occlusion 275
   2.3 Hepatic artery aneurysms 276
3. The Hepatic Venous Circulation 276
   3.1 Congestive hepatopathy 276
   3.2 Hepatic vein thrombosis 278
   3.3 Membranous obstruction of the vena cava 282
   3.4 Veno-occlusive disease 283
   3.5 Peliosis hepatis 284
4. The Portal Venous Circulation 285
   4.1 Portal vein thrombosis 285
References 287

1. INTRODUCTION

The liver comprises one-fiftieth of the total adult body weight and has three vascular systems – the hepatic artery (HA), portal vein (PV) and hepatic vein (HV). Although it makes up only 2% of the total adult body weight, it receives 25% of the cardiac output. The PV carries two-thirds of the blood flow to the liver. This blood is rich in nutrients absorbed from the intestinal tract but is relatively lacking in oxygen. In contrast, the HA supplies the remaining one-third of the total hepatic blood supply and carries 50% of the liver's oxygen supply. The HA and PV carry the inflow of both arterial blood from the aorta and venous blood from the intestines and spleen to the liver. These vessels enter the liver through a fissure at the *porta hepatis* and both vessels divide into branches that supply the right and left lobes of the liver. The venous drainage of the liver is comprised of the right, middle and left HVs which enter the inferior vena cava (IVC) from the back of the liver near its point of entry into the right atrium. The functional unit of the liver is the hepatic acinus, which consists of a cluster of liver cells grouped around terminal branches of the hepatic arteriole and portal venule. The hepatic sinusoids lack basement membrane and contain fenestrae, which allow close contact and free flow of blood with the hepatic parenchyma. Blood entering through the HA and PV track to these vessels and flows through the hepatic sinusoid, eventually draining into the hepatic venule. Rappaport's classification divides the hepatic acinus into a zonal distribution each centered on a portal triad and its surrounding cells: zone 1 occupies the periportal area and so receives blood with high levels of oxygen and nutrients, whereas zone 3 occupies the peripheral area around the HV and receives relatively hypoxic blood. Zone 2 is interposed between zone 1 and 3 (Figure 1). This unique blood supply and the high level of metabolic activity of the liver make it vulnerable to a broad spectrum of circulatory disturbances. The resultant hepatic injury is dependent on the particular blood vessel involved.

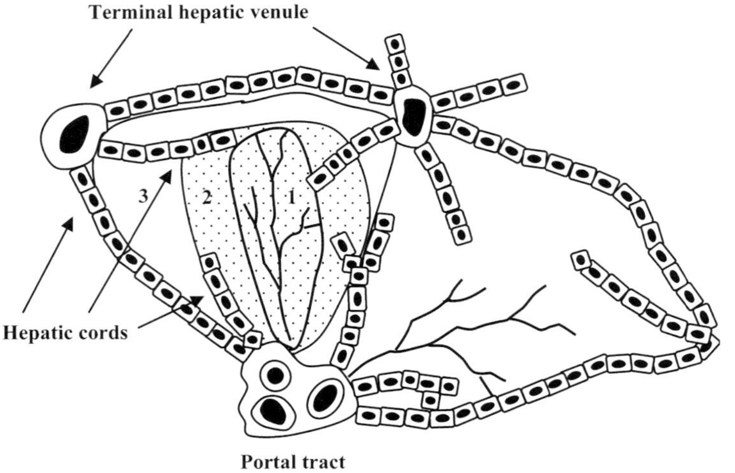

Figure 1. Blood supply of the simple hepatic acinus and the zonal arrangement of cells. The hepatic acinus occupies the adjacent of neighboring hexagonal fields. Zone 1 is supplied by the most oxygenated blood while zone 3 being furthest from the hepatic artery and portal vein receives blood with the lowest oxygen tension and so is subject to damage by low perfusion and congestion states.

In addition, cirrhosis often results in significant portal hypertension and the development of a remarkable collateral circulation designed to carry portal blood into the systemic veins. In this chapter we address the consequences of pathologic alterations in the vascular supply to the liver.

2. THE HEPATIC ARTERIAL CIRCULATION

The HA arises from the celiac axis to form the gastroduodenal artery and the HA proper, which enters the liver at the *porta hepatis* and divides into the right and left branches. Hepatic ischemia results from an imbalance between oxygen supply and consumption. Hepatic arterial flow is quite constant and is regulated by the smooth muscle cells of the hepatic arterioles. When portal venous flow decreases such as in cirrhosis, the hepatic arterioles relax resulting in increased hepatic arterial flow. Because the metabolic activity of the liver is relatively constant, oxygen supply and not demand is the critical determinant of hepatic ischemia. Neither systemic hypoxia nor anemia is sufficient to cause hepatic injury in the absence of compromised blood supply. Reduction in blood supply is compensated by an increase in the extraction of oxygen by the liver parenchyma thereby maintaining tissue oxygenation. While this is sufficient for zone 1 and 2, the low oxygen tension in zone 3 can result in liver damage.

2.1 Ischemic hepatitis

Ischemic hepatitis refers to diffuse injury resulting from acute hypoperfusion such as is seen in acute heart failure or shock due to trauma, burns, hemorrhage, sepsis, and following arterial interruption during transplantation. Common synonyms include *shock liver*, *hypoxic hepatitis* and *hepatic infarction*. A decrease in blood pressure leads to a reduction in liver blood flow, hepatic arterial vasoconstriction and reduced oxygen tension in zone 3 resulting in anoxia, and necrosis of hepatocytes. Ischemic hepatitis is particularly frequent in patients in coronary care units where it affects about 20% of patients with a low cardiac output resulting in both decreased hepatic arterial flow (ischemic hepatitis) and passive venous congestion (congestive hepatopathy).

Clinical features: Virtually any systemic cause of shock can result in ischemic hepatitis and in general the hemodynamic insult is clinically apparent. Other causes, which may be less apparent, include transient circulatory disturbances, sickle cell crisis and hepatic arterial occlusion after liver transplantation. Most cases are recognized as an asymptomatic and dramatic rise in serum aminotransaminases after a hypotensive episode. Rarely, patients present with nausea, right upper quadrant pain, jaundice and encephalopathy. Prolongation of the prothrombin time beyond 3 seconds is rare and mental status changes are usually due to cerebral anoxia rather than hepatic encephalopathy. Fulminant hepatic failure is rare in patients without pre-existing liver disease. In patients with cirrhosis complicated by ischemic hepatitis the mortality rates range from 60 to 100%.

Diagnosis: The widespread use of liver function testing is probably responsible for the recent increase in recognition of ischemic hepatitis. The typical laboratory pattern noted is a striking rise in serum aminotransaminases (25–250 times the upper limit of normal (ULN)) and lactate dehydrogenase (LDH) within 3 days of the hemodynamic insult. Serum bilirubin and alkaline phosphatase values increase slightly. With restoration of blood pressure, serum aminotransaminases rapidly return to baseline values within 7 days. The rapid rise and fall of aminotransaminases, the associated early elevation of LDH and other consequences of the hemodynamic insult such as acute tubular necrosis are helpful clinical indicators in making the diagnosis of ischemic hepatitis.

The hallmark pathological finding is that of zone 3 necrosis, which may extend into the midzone if ischemia is severe or prolonged. In the event of concomitant passive congestion caused by right heart failure, there may be sinusoidal congestion, hemorrhagic necrosis of zone 3 and variable degrees of cholestasis. However, a liver biopsy is usually not necessary to confirm the diagnosis. Additionally, in the appropriate clinical setting, serological tests for viral and autoimmune hepatitis or metabolic liver disease are rarely necessary in the diagnostic work-up.

Management: Treatment is aimed at restoring blood pressure, treating the underlying disease and monitoring and treating other organ systems at risk of end-organ damage. Administration of pressor agents to support blood pressure should be guided by the overall hemodynamic situation. The use of therapies to deplete reactive oxygen radicals has not been studied.

2.2 Hepatic artery occlusion

HA occlusion is a relatively uncommon occurrence. It can give rise to a variety of clinical sequelae, ranging from an asymptomatic condition to hepatic infarction and death. This variability depends on the site of occlusion, speed of occlusion and the presence or absence of an adequate collateral circulation.

Etiology: It is most commonly seen after liver transplantation and is usually related to an anomalous donor HA. Other etiologies include therapeutic intervention for treatment of focal neoplasms such as embolization/chemoembolization, unintended ligation at surgery (laparoscopic cholecystectomy), atheromatous disease, giant cell arteritis, polyarteritis nodosa or embolism in patients with bacterial endocarditis (see Table 1). Hepatic infarction differs from hepatic ischemia in that it is usually a focal lesion that is well demarcated. Additionally, the involvement of all three zones by coagulative necrosis of the hepatic acinus is distinct from the zone 3 necrosis characteristic of ischemic hepatitis.

Clinical features: The classical features of hepatic arterial occlusion and resultant infarction include severe epigastric or right upper quadrant pain, back or shoulder tip pain, fever, nausea, vomiting,

Table 1. Causes of hepatic infarction.

Hepatic artery thrombosis
Following liver transplantation
Hypercoagulable disease
Severe atherosclerosis
Hepatic artery ligation at surgery
Hepatic artery embolism
Bacterial endocarditis
Therapeutic embolization/chemoembolization
Tumor emboli
Polyarteritis nodosa
Aortic dissection
Eclampsia
Cocaine intoxication
Sickle cell crisis

jaundice, tachycardia and hypotension. If liver damage is severe, fulminant hepatic failure may ensue. In the post-transplant setting, acute HA occlusion usually results in a rapid deterioration in the patient's condition with the development of acute liver failure and the need for re-transplantation. In patients with a gradual occlusion, a collateral circulation develops and biliary strictures secondary to ischemia ensue.

Diagnosis: The diagnosis of HA occlusion can be suggested by Doppler ultrasonography and confirmed by hepatic arteriography. Computed tomography (CT) scans are important in evaluating the extent and following the progress of infarction and these lesions are best evaluated after administration of intravenous contrast. In cases of HA occlusion due to embolic disease, infarcts may also be seen in the spleen and kidneys. Additionally the CT scan is useful in ascertaining the development of abscess formation. While the presence of gas in the lesion is suggestive, its absence does not reliably exclude abscess formation and needle aspiration may be necessary to arrive at the correct diagnosis. The gold standard for HAT is an HA angiogram. In addition to being diagnostic, thrombolytic agents can be administered locally by placement of a catheter in the HA and angioplasty can be performed.

Management: The management of HA occlusion is dependent on the clinical situation. In patients with an asymptomatic presentation, a work-up for an underlying illness or hypercoagulable condition is necessary. In cases that complicate liver transplantation, urgent re-transplantation may be necessary. There are a few case reports of the use of thrombolytic agents with or without angioplasty and stent placement.

2.3 Hepatic artery aneurysms

The authors of a recent review of splanchnic aneurysms suggest that the rise in the incidence of HA aneurysms is related to the increase in percutaneous procedures and also the increased use of CT imaging in the evaluation of blunt hepatic trauma [1].

Etiology: Aneurysms of the HA are rare lesions that constitute 20% of all splanchnic artery aneurysms. They occur in the setting of atheromatous disease, polyarteritis nodosa, and abdominal or systemic sepsis. Pseudoaneurysms can occur after liver injury including liver biopsy. The aneurysms can be both intra- and extra-hepatic and show considerable variation in size.

Clinical features: They are commonest in middle-aged males and are often asymptomatic for long periods. Unlike splenic artery aneurysms, there does not appear to be a strong association with rupture and pregnancy with only one case report of HA aneurysm rupture during pregnancy reported in the literature. Complications include dissection and rupture. Fistulization into an intra-hepatic bile duct can result in pain, jaundice and gastrointestinal (GI) bleeding (hematobilia).

Management: A high level of suspicion is required in patients with unexplained GI bleeding and a history of recent hepatic trauma or needle biopsy. Surgical intervention is generally required for extra-hepatic aneurysms. The mortality is high if emergency surgery is required for rupture and intra-abdominal bleeding (80%). Rupture into a bile duct can be treated with arteriography and embolization. If unsuccessful, a hepatic resection may be necessary.

3. THE HEPATIC VENOUS CIRCULATION

The hepatic venous circulation begins in zone 3 of the hepatic acinus. These vessels join the sublobular veins and drain into larger HVs, which enter the IVC (Figure 2).

3.1 Congestive hepatopathy

Passive congestion of the liver results because of right heart failure. It is sometimes associated with ischemic hepatitis as a consequence of reduced cardiac output (Figure 3).

Clinical features: Liver dysfunction arising in the setting of congestion is usually mild and is most commonly diagnosed by detecting abnormalities of liver function on routine testing. Patients are

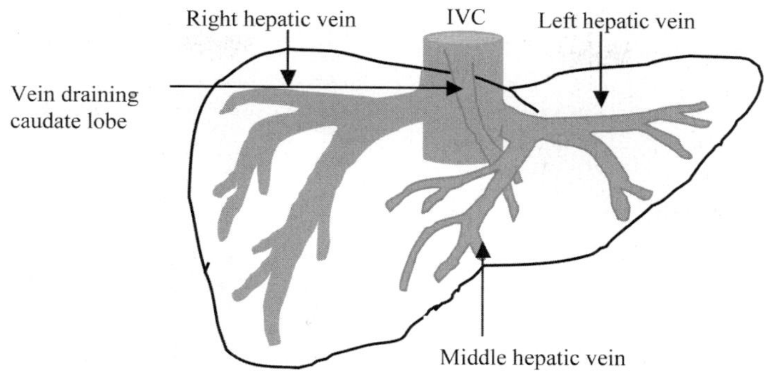

Figure 2. Anatomy of the venous drainage of the liver. Note the separate cephalad insertion of the vein draining the caudate lobe.

usually asymptomatic but a minority may present with right upper quadrant discomfort that can be severe enough to mimic acute cholecystitis. The liver is often enlarged, firm and smooth and may reach the umbilicus. The liver may be pulsatile in patients with significant tricuspid regurgitation and the presence of hepatojugular reflux is useful to confirm patency of the HVs. Splenomegaly is frequent and high protein ascites may be present as a manifestation of right heart failure rather than liver dysfunction. Jaundice is frequent (70%).

Diagnosis: Diagnosis is suspected on the basis of the clinical findings. The serum bilirubin level corresponds to the degree of right heart failure, is predominantly unconjugated and rarely exceeds 4 mg/dl. Minor elevations of alkaline phosphatase are seen. Serum aminotransaminases are usually 2–3 times the ULN in chronic heart failure; however, in acute heart failure with zone 3 necrosis, they may be high enough to simulate acute viral hepatitis. Serum albumin is decreased in up to 50% of patients with chronic heart failure. Doppler ultrasound examination will confirm patency of the HVs and the IVC. In addition, the HVs may appear distended on ultrasound. HV distension occurs because the elevated right atrial pressure is readily transmitted to the HVs. CT scan of liver may give an appearance of "nutmeg liver" due to hepatic congestion (Figure 4). Echocardiography can confirm the presence of right heart dysfunction.

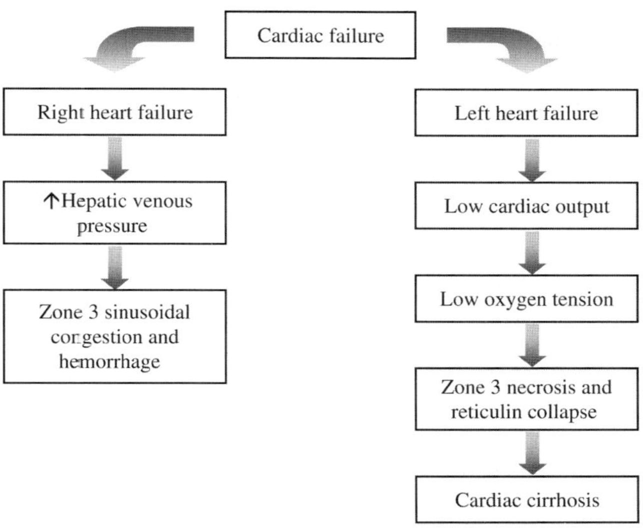

Figure 3. A schema to show the consequences of right, left and congestive cardiac failure.

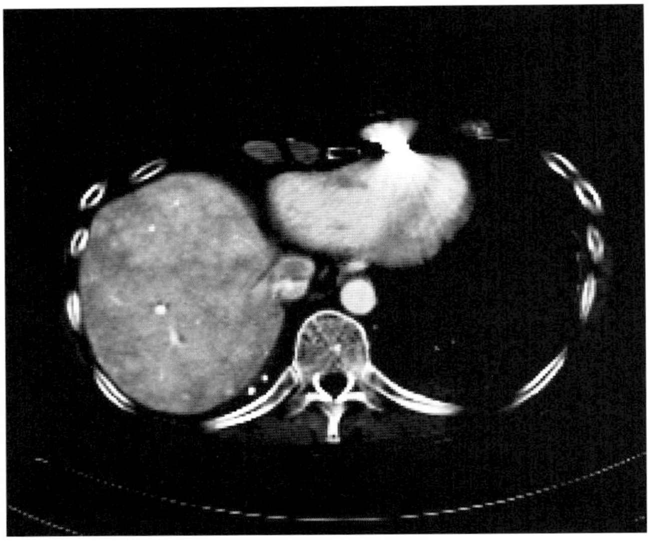

Figure 4. The characteristic "nutmeg" appearance of the liver in congestive hepatopathy on a contrast enhanced CT scan.

The classical pathological features usually reveal an enlarged liver with prominent HVs. Microscopically, the hepatic venule is dilated and there is sinusoidal congestion with frank hemorrhage and necrosis in severe cases in zone 3. Bile pigment is often noted in jaundiced patients. Collagen deposition can be seen around the central veins. The prognosis is that of the underlying heart disease. The presence of longstanding hyperbilirubinemia is a poor prognostic sign.

Diuretic therapy is the mainstay of treatment, however, care must be taken to avoid over vigorous diuresis, which may result in decreased cardiac output and further accentuate zone 3 ischemia.

3.2 Hepatic vein thrombosis

Budd–Chiari syndrome is the generic term for hepatic venous outflow obstruction, which results in a clinical spectrum of abdominal pain, ascites and hepatomegaly [2]. In 1845, Budd described three cases of HV thrombosis related to abscess-induced phlebitis. This was followed by Chiari's descriptions of both HV thrombosis and IVC thrombosis. In 1911, Pleasant reviewed 296 cases in the literature of both HV thromboses and IVC thromboses and the term Budd–Chiari syndrome became synonymous with both types of thrombosis. Obstruction of the IVC at its hepatic portion results in a similar presentation but is classified as a separate entity from Budd–Chiari syndrome and is known as membranous obstruction of the vena cava (MOVC) [2,3]. Primary obstruction of the hepatic venules by a non-thrombotic fibrous obliteration, the so-called veno-occlusive disease (VOD), differs from Budd–Chiari syndrome in etiology and is discussed separately [3].

The obstruction of a single HV is usually clinically silent. However, obstruction of two or three main HV results in significant hemodynamic changes including an increase in sinusoidal pressure resulting in pain and hepatomegaly. The increased sinusoidal pressure causes sinusoidal dilatation and central congestion. The filtration of interstitial fluid increases, which leads to passage of fluid through the surface of the liver, and results in the formation of high protein ascites. Reduction of flow through the hepatic sinusoids causes hepatocellular ischemia and necrosis and when thrombosis occurs rapidly, acute liver failure may ensue. When occlusion is more gradual, collateral vessels form and centrilobular fibrosis develops leading to cirrhosis. The caudate lobe is drained independently by a venous system that drains directly into the vena cava and is often spared in the thrombotic process (Figure 3). In these cases

Table 2a. Major causes of Budd–Chiari syndrome.

Myeloproliferative disease
Hepatic neoplasms
Hepatic infection
Pregnancy
Oral contraceptives
Hypercoagulable states
Behcet's disease
Membranous webs of the IVC
Idiopathic

the caudate lobe undergoes compensatory hypertrophy.

Etiology: An underlying disorder can be identified in over 80% of patients presenting with Budd–Chiari syndrome (Tables 2a and 2b). In Western countries, the vast majority of cases are associated with hypercoagulable conditions. Therefore, a systematic search for thrombogenic conditions is recommended (Table 2b). An estimated 1% of patient with myeloproliferative disorders present with a symptomatic HV thrombosis and 6% are found to have thrombosis of large HVs at autopsy. As many as 50% of the patients presenting with Budd–Chiari syndrome have an underlying myeloproliferative disorder, which can be recognized by traditional hematological investigations. In some cases the myeloproliferative disorders may be occult because the increase in red cell volume normally seen in polycythemia rubra vera may be masked by a parallel increase in plasma volume or by red cell destruction as a consequence of hypersplenism. In these cases, the presence of spontaneous erythroid colony formation, increased megakaryocyte colony growth and clonal karyotypic abnormalities are strongly suggestive of the presence of occult myeloproliferative disease. In addition, the combination of a myeloproliferative disorder and a hypercoagulable states has been described.

Another important predisposing risk is the use of the oral contraceptive pill. There is an estimated twofold increased risk of HV thrombosis in an individual taking oral contraceptive, which is similar to the risk of other thrombotic events.

Table 2b. Prevalence of the hypercoagulable causes of hepatic vein thrombosis presenting to a single hospital in Belgium.

Thrombogenic disorder	% of all patients
Primary myeloproliferative disorder (all)	50
Polycythemia rubra vera	
Chronic myelogenous leukemia	
Essential thrombocythemia	
Agnogenic myeloid metaplasia	
Primary myeloproliferative disorder (overt from)	25
Primary myeloproliferative disorder (occult from)	25
Primary myeloproliferative disorder plus another thrombogenic disorder	25
Antiphospholipid syndrome	15
Paroxysmal nocturnal hemoglobinuria	5
Antithrombin III deficiency	<1
Protein S deficiency	5
Protein C deficiency	20
Factor V Leiden mutation	30
Factor V Leiden mutation plus another thrombogenic disorder	20
Prothrombin gene mutations	5
Current oral contraceptive use/pregnancy	55
Combination of thrombogenic disorders	25

Adapted from Deltenre *et al.* (2001) *Gut* **48**, 264–268.

Recently, factor V Leiden gene mutation, which induces a state of protein C resistance, has been shown to account for 20–30% of cases of HV or IVC thrombosis. This mutation is present in the majority of patient with pregnancy or oral contraceptive associated HV thrombosis.

HV thrombosis occurs in approximately 12% of patients with paroxysmal nocturnal hemoglobinuria and is the leading cause of death in patients with this disorder.

Neoplasms associated with the development of HV thrombosis include hepatocellular, renal cell, adrenal, pancreatic, pulmonary carcinomas and right atrial myxomas.

Clinical features: The clinical presentation of patients with Budd–Chiari is variable ranging from an asymptomatic state to fulminant hepatic failure depending on the rate and extent of venous obstruction. Approximately 20% of patients present with fulminant liver failure, 40% with subacute presentation with symptoms for less than 6 months and 40% present with symptoms for longer than 6 months and features of cirrhosis and portal hypertension. Some asymptomatic patients are found to have HV thrombosis or routine scanning or after evaluation for asymptomatic elevations of abnormal liver function test. The finding of collateral blood flow or flow within one or more of the HV probably explains the absence of symptoms. The classical triad of abdominal pain, ascites and hepatomegaly occurs in patients with the fulminant or acute presentation, which usually occurs with rapid and complete occlusions of all HVs. The natural history is one of rapid deterioration, progressive encephalopathy and death within 8 weeks if not treated. These presentations are fortunately rare. Transaminases are characteristically very high, the liver is enlarged and tender and ascites and renal dysfunction are common. The subacute presentation is more commonly seen and patients present with a vague right upper quadrant discomfort, mild to moderate ascites, which is usually resistant to medical therapy, hepatosplenomegaly and mild jaundice. The chronic form is characterized by progressive fatigue, abdominal distension, and mild elevations of liver function, coagulopathy, encephalopathy and possible variceal bleeding.

Diagnosis: Standard laboratory tests are rarely helpful in the diagnosis of Budd–Chiari syndrome. However, routine hematologic studies may point to an underlying diagnosis of a myeloproliferative or procoagulant disorder. Doppler ultrasonography can confirm the diagnosis of HV thrombosis in 75% of cases. It is the best screening test for evaluating the HVs with results comparable to selective venography. Echogenic material can be seen in the lumen of the enlarged HVs devoid of a flow signal. In addition, the following findings may be seen: turbulent or reversed flow; subcapsular collateral vessels connecting HVs or diaphragmatic veins are seen in 80% of cases; and a spider web appearance of veins usually located at the HV ostia. CT findings include non-visualization of veins following contrast administration, the presence of HV thrombus and compression of the IVC by an enlarged caudate lobe. Magnetic resonance imaging (MRI) with gadolinium enhancement allows visualization of the obstructed HV but also shows the large intra-hepatic "comma-shaped" collaterals. Angiography remains the "gold standard" for the diagnosis of Budd–Chiari syndrome. Inferior venacavography must be accompanied by retrograde HV cannulation to determine the location and cause of obstruction (Table 3). In addition, pressure measurements taken at the time of venography will provide important information when planning for surgical decompression.

Table 3. The "C's" of Budd–Chiari syndrome.

Causes
Clotting disorder
Cancer
Conception
Contraception
Congenital web
Cryptogenic
Imaging
Compensatory hypertrophy of the Caudate lobe
Clot on Cavogram
Comma-shaped Collaterals
Pathology
Candy cane appearance of the liver biopsy (macroscopic)
Centrilobular Congestion (microscopic)

Liver biopsy is an important test in the assessment of patients with Budd–Chiari. Indirect evidence showing centrilobular congestion, cell loss and fibrosis can be obtained to support the diagnosis. Additionally, therapeutic decisions can be altered depending on the histological severity. It must be remembered that some cases may not involve all HVs equally and therefore some authors advocate for biopsies of the right and left lobes because of an uneven distribution of hepatic lesions.

Prognosis: The natural history of Budd–Chiari syndrome is variable and depends on the initial presentation. Patients presenting with the acute form will rapidly deteriorate and die within a few days if not transplanted. In patients with a chronic presentation the overall 3-year survival rate is 50%. Patients with incomplete venous occlusion can exhibit a good prognosis. A recently published multivariate analysis revealed that young age, low Child–Pugh's score, diuretic sensitive ascites and a normal creatinine were good prognostic signs. The presence of PVT is associated with a poor prognosis.

Management: The aim of treatment is to alleviate venous congestion and preserve hepatic function and to address the underlying hypercoagulable state. A combination of medical, radiological and/or surgical interventions is often required for a favorable outcome. Therapy depends on the severity of the underlying hepatocellular dysfunction. In patients presenting with fulminant liver failure, urgent liver transplantation may be required. Three- and 10-year survival rates of 88 and 69% have been reported in two separate studies.

Diuretic therapy, dietary sodium restrictions and paracentesis may be required for management of ascites. In approximately 30% of patients, ascites is diuretic resistant from the outset and these patients may benefit from a portosystemic shunt. Thrombolytic therapy has been used effectively in a small number of cases and when combined with angioplasty may be more effective than when used alone. Angioplasty and placement of vascular stents are more commonly used in cases of IVC thrombosis secondary to IVC webs and membranes (Figure 5). There are no large controlled studies that have evaluated the efficacy of thrombolytic agents and therefore it should only be used in selected circumstances. Thrombolytic therapy should be reserved for patients in whom there is a venogram documented recent localized thrombosis and where there is no evidence of portal hypertension.

Transjugular intra-hepatic portosystemic shunts (TIPSS) placement provides another alternative treatment for patients with Budd–Chiari syndrome and serves to decompress the venous circulation by providing an alternative venous outflow tract. Unfortunately, the number of patients undergoing TIPSS treatment is small and there is limited follow-up available to evaluate long-term liver function and survival.

Surgical therapies include thrombectomy and dorsocranial liver resection, portosystemic shunts, and liver transplantation. Thrombectomy and liver resection have largely been abandoned since the advent of percutaneous angioplasty except for patients with a thrombosed portal and mesenteric system. In these patients, dorsocranial liver resection, thrombectomy and anastomosis of the veins to the right atrium is the only option if medical therapy has failed. A variety of surgical shunts are available and they serve to decompress the centrilobular congestion and relieve

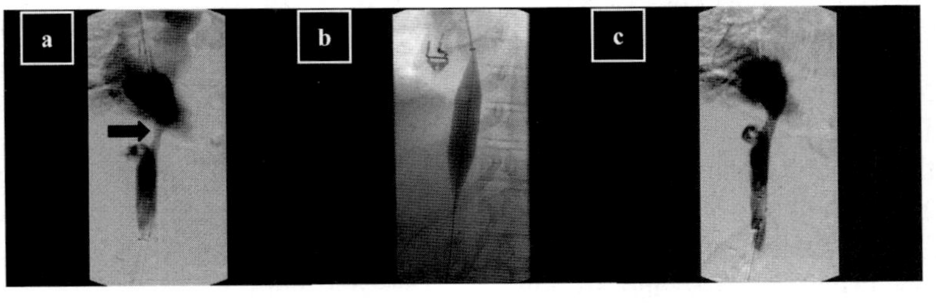

Figure 5. Cavograms demonstrate an IVC stenosis that resulted in hepatic congestion and zone 3 necrosis (black arrow) (a). The patient underwent successful transvenous angioplasty, which resulted in dilatation of the stenosis (b,c).

hepatocellular necrosis. These should be considered in patients with acute or subacute presentations with resultant preservation of hepatic synthetic function. Post-operative anticoagulation is necessary as the shunt thrombosis rate is as high as 25%. Side-to-side portocaval shunts convert the PV into the outflow tract and are the procedure of choice. However, the presence of caval thrombosis or compression from an enlarged caudate lobe prohibits adequate flow and predisposes to thrombosis. While the level of pressure in the IVC has not been shown to be of much value in predicting surgical outcome, it is generally accepted that a pressure greater than 20 mm Hg would preclude a portocaval or mesocaval shunt unless the IVC is stented or a cavo-atrial shunt is placed. Recently, a multivariate analyses adjusting for confounding factors have shown no significant survival advantage of surgical shunt over medical management. In contrast, the largest experience from a single center reports 85% long-term survival of all patients undergoing portosystemic shunt with significant improvement in hepatic function, hepatic histology and ascites. This group has also reported that deterioration in liver function is observed in patients with marginal liver function after shunt surgery.

Behcet's disease, a systemic vasculitis, is frequently complicated by HV thrombosis. In most cases there is associated thrombosis or either the IVC or the PV. Involvement of the IVC appears to be more common in patients with Behcet's disease than in those without. The clinical course of HV thrombosis associated with Behcet's disease is poor, but is probably related to the involvement of additional vessels [4].

3.3 Membranous obstruction of the vena cava

Thrombosis of the IVC occurs in association with various systemic and local conditions, as discussed above, but idiopathic thrombosis at the hepatic portions of the IVC is the most common. MOVC was first described by Osler in 1879 and is now thought to be a distinct disorder from HV thrombosis [5].

Etiology: Until recently, the membranous obstruction was thought to be congenital abnormality, but it is now widely regarded to be acquired and may occur as a consequence of the thrombosis itself. For this reason it may be more appropriately termed *obliterative hepatocavopathy* [3,5]. These membranous webs occur just cephalad to the entrance of the right HV into the IVC.

For reasons that are unknown, Budd–Chiari syndrome (HV thrombosis) is more common in Western countries whereas IVC thrombosis is more common in the East and Indian sub-continent.

In contrast to classical Budd–Chiari syndrome, hypercoagulable disorders are generally uncommon in obliterative hepatocavopathy. Thrombosis of the hepatic portion of the IVC slowly organizes into fibrotic tissue and produces a variety of stenotic an occluding lesions, which may consist of a membrane with a central hole, a thin membrane, a thick membrane or an occlusion affecting a long stretch of IVC (Figure 5).

Because IVC thrombosis is more common in developing countries than in the West, infection has been considered to be a major etiological factor. In reports form Nepal, inferior cavography has been associated with the development of fever suggesting a possible phlebothrombosis. In India, pericaval filariasis is considered to be an important etiological factor.

Clinical features: HV and IVC occlusion can occur at any age; however, adults are much more frequently affected by IVC thrombosis. Another difference between HV thrombosis and obliterative hepatocavopathy is that clinical manifestations develop more slowly with the latter. This may be related to the sequential thrombosis that causes HV ostia occlusion. Occlusion of the IVC results in a rise in sinusoidal pressure similar to classical Budd–Chiari syndrome with centrilobular congestion, sinusoidal dilatation resulting in hepatomegaly, right upper quadrant pain. Ascites is seen less commonly than with HV thrombosis. Some patients present with associated intermittent or prolonged fever. The severity of disease depends on the extent of occlusion of the HV orifices with less severe symptoms in those with incomplete obstruction. Complete obstruction of the IVC will result in the development of lower limb edema and marked venous dilatation over the trunk. The caudally located inferior HV that drains the caudate lobe often remains patent and results in caudate lobe enlargement. The development of chronic occlusion results in cirrhosis and portal hypertension. The clinical course of IVC thrombosis is variable and dependent on the extent of thrombosis and whether the HV is involved or not. The short-term prognosis is good. However, there are little data available regarding the long-term outcome of patients with obliterative hepatocavopathy.

The incidence of hepatocellular carcinoma (HCC) as a complication of obliterative hepatocavopathy is increased over the general public. This appears to be distinctly related to the obstruction and not a feature of viral infection. The highest incidence is reported in South Africa (45–50%). In contrast HCC is not a complication of HV thrombosis.

Diagnosis and pathology: The diagnostic algorithm for obliterative hepatocavopathy is similar to that outlined for Budd–Chiari syndrome. Venography is important in determining the location and extent of the obstruction and the pressure gradient across the web [3,6].

Management: Transvenous and transhepatic angioplasty have been used to dilate venous webs that have resulted in occlusion (Figure 5). Metal wall stents have been placed in cases of stenosis after angioplasty with good results. Thrombolytic therapy has not been well studied in IVC thrombosis. Occlusion of the main HVs may require portoatrial or mesoatrial shunts with prosthetic graft to reduce portal pressure. However, there is a high incidence of graft thrombosis.

3.4 Veno-occlusive disease

The term veno-occlusive disease refers to a form of non-thrombotic, obliterative phlebitis of the small intra-HVs characterized clinically by the development of hepatomegaly, right upper quadrant pain, ascites and jaundice.

Etiology: Initial reports of VOD were related to the ingestion of pyrrolizidine alkaloids in the form of herbal tea in Jamaica. The introduction of chemotherapy agents in the 1950s was associated with a number of associated cases of VOD. The use of azathioprine as an immunosuppressive agent in renal transplantation is also associated with a VOD, but there has often been co-existent peliosis hepatis or nodular regenerative hyperplasia. The commonest cause of VOD is the use of combinations of chemotherapeutic drugs or chemotherapeutic drugs and irradiation therapy. Chemotherapeutic drugs associated with VOD at conventional doses include actinomycin D, dacarbazine, cytosine arabinoside, mithramycin, 6-thioguanine, urethane and indicine N-oxide. VOD develops in 5–60% of patients during the first 3 weeks after bone marrow transplantation and varies in severity from mild reversible disease to severe disease associated with multi-organ failure (Table 4).

Clinical features: The clinical features resemble those of Budd–Chiari syndrome and obliterative hepatocavopathy; however, the hepatic venous

Table 4. Etiology of veno-occlusive disease.

- Poisoning with pyrrolizidine alkaloids
- Hepatic irradiation
- Medications and toxins
  - Alcohol
  - Arsenic poisoning
  - Azathioprine
  - Cytoreductive therapy
    - Cyclophosphamide
    - Cytosine arabinoside
    - Dacarbazine
    - Dimethylbusulfan
    - Floxuridine
    - Urethane
  - Oral contraceptive medication
  - Vitamin A
  - Thorotrast
  - Insecticides
- Cirrhosis
  - Alcohol
  - Hepatitis B
- Alcoholic hepatitis
- Liver transplantation
- HIV infection
- Systemic lupus erythematosis

outflow obstruction is due to occlusion of the hepatic sinusoids and terminal hepatic venules rather than the HVs and IVC. The clinical syndrome of tender hepatomegaly, fluid retention and weight gain, and elevation of the serum bilirubin define VOD associated with cytoreductive therapy in the absence of other possible causes. It usually occurs within 30 days of transplant and is classified as mild (VOD that resolves without need for treatment), moderate (symptomatic VOD requiring diuretic or pain medications) or severe (VOD requiring treatment that does not resolve before death or within 100 days of transplant).

Elevation in serum bilirubin is a feature of VOD and usually occurs within 20 days. Elevation in bilirubin to level of 12–18 mg/dl tends to occur after the weight gain and hepatomegaly. Elevation of serum aminotransaminases occurs early and probably reflects zone 3-hepatocyte necrosis. A serum AST level greater than 750 IU/l is associated with a poor prognosis. Early elevation in bilirubin is more commonly seen in patients with a poor outcome as is the presence of ascites and edema.

Diagnosis: Doppler ultrasonography is useful in confirming the patency of IVC and HVs. In addition, it can confirm the presence of hepatomegaly and ascites and rule out extra-hepatic biliary obstruction as a cause of jaundice. Doppler studies may show reversal of portal venous flow in advanced VOD; however, this is not a sensitive marker for early disease. Enhanced CT studies should be avoided if possible because of the possibility of precipitating renal failure following contrast administration.

Liver biopsy is useful in cases where the diagnosis is unclear. Transvenous biopsies may be performed in patients with thrombocytopenia following myeloablative therapy. Measurement of hepatic venous pressure gradients can also be performed at the time of the biopsy. A hepatic venous pressure gradient greater than 10 mm Hg is highly specific for VOD. Early pathological changes include the deposition of fibrinogen and factor VIII within the sinusoids and venular walls. Hepatic sinusoids are dilated and congested with erythrocytes. Progressive venular occlusion results in hemorrhagic necrosis of the centrilobular region. Later changes include venular sclerosis, fibrosis of venular lumens and occlusion of the terminal hepatic venules.

Management: Management of VOD requires identification and discontinuation of the underlying cause. Supportive care is the mainstay of therapy. Renal and pulmonary failures in patients with severe VOD are appropriately managed with hemodialysis and mechanical ventilation. Published case mortality rates for VOD complicating hematopoietic stem cell transplantation vary from 0 to 67%. Patients succumb to renal and cardiopulmonary disease. Avoidance of hepatotoxic regimens should be employed in those patients with known risks for VOD which include a previous non-fatal episode of VOD, second transplant with myeloablative therapy, hepatic inflammation as evidenced by elevated ALT, AST or hepatic fibrosis/cirrhosis on liver biopsy. In addition, the administration of ursodeoxycholic acid has been shown to reduce the risk of post-transplant VOD. No significant beneficial effects have been attributed to pentoxifylline. Tissue plasminogen activator has been evaluated in numerous studies but is not beneficial in patients with renal or pulmonary failure. Defibrotide, a polydeoxyribonucleotide derived from animal tissue, has shown promise in uncontrolled trials of patient with moderate VOD with complete resolution in 35–55% of patients. In patients who present with acute liver failure, liver transplantation may be required. Guidelines for liver transplantation exist for patients with severe VOD and liver failure complicating hematopoietic stem cell transplantation [7].

3.5 Peliosis hepatis

Peliosis hepatis is an uncommon condition characterized by large blood filled cavities not lined by sinusoidal cells. It usually presents in adults and is associated with anabolic steroid use for chronic wasting conditions. It has become increasingly recognized recently, particularly in immunocompromised individuals.

Etiology: Peliosis hepatis has been attributed to steroid therapy, immunosuppressive therapy such as azathioprine and in patients with chronic infections. In patients with acquired immunodeficiency syndrome (AIDS), infection with *Bartonella quintana* and *Bartonella henselae* has been associated with peliosis hepatis.

Clinical features: Patients may be asymptomatic or present with hepatomegaly, fever, portal hypertension, and ascites or liver failure. Rupture of the vascular lesion may result in intra-hepatic or intraperitoneal hemorrhage.

Diagnosis: Ultrasonography shows multiple hypoechoic areas of different sizes. Enhanced CT scanning will reveal multiple low-density regions with foci of spontaneous high density suggesting the presence of blood within the lesions. On MRI, the multiple lesions are hypointense on T1-weighted and hyperdense on T2-weighted images, with bright foci on all sequences suggesting blood-filled cavities. Laparoscopy shows multiple dark blebs on the surface of the liver.

Management: Where possible, the cause should be identified and treated appropriately. Suspected medication should be withdrawn. In immunosuppressed individuals, the bacillary form should be treated with erythromycin.

4. THE PORTAL VENOUS CIRCULATION

The portal system includes all the veins that carry blood from the alimentary tract, the spleen, pancreas and gall bladder to the liver. The PV proper is formed by the union of the superior mesenteric (SMV) and splenic veins (SV) posterior to the head of the pancreas. It enters the liver at the porta hepatis and has a segmental intra-hepatic distribution, which accompanies the HA. The portal venous system develops at 5–10 weeks of embryonic life from paired vitelline and umbilical veins, which drain the yolk sac and placenta, respectively. These veins intercommunicate around the embryonic duodenum and supply the developing hepatic sinusoids. The ductus venosus is a remnant of the communication between the portal and HVs and empties directly into the right heart. Development of these structures results in a single postduodenal PV. The umbilical vein atrophies to become the ligamentum teres, which maintains its connection at the left PV. When the portal circulation is obstructed, a collateral circulation is formed to carry blood into the systemic circulation. These collateral blood vessels form varices along the GI tract, at the falciform ligament, in the retroperitoneum and with the left renal vein.

4.1 Portal vein thrombosis

Etiology: Portal vein thrombosis (PVT) occurs in a number of settings with the etiology varying with the patient's age. It is more commonly seen in children and among this group, the commonest cause for PVT is thrombophlebitis of the PV. A predisposing illness can be documented in 40% of cases. In adults approximately 25% have associated cirrhosis. The etiology for cirrhosis-induced PVT may relate to the development of retrograde flow in the PV. In addition, the presence of HCC may result in PVT either due to a hypercoagulable cause or due to direct invasion of the PV by tumor thrombus (Figure 6). Other causes of PVT in non-cirrhotic patients include abdominal surgery, pancreatobiliary disease, intra-abdominal sepsis (diverticulitis or appendicitis), and single or concurrent hypercoagulable disorders [8,9]. Acute PVT is often a clinically silent disease and is usually diagnosed on radiological imaging performed for other reasons such as acute pancreatitis. Thrombi usually resolve within days to weeks. Chronic PVT develops in patients in whom the acute thrombosis does not resolve. This may result in a non-cavernous thrombosis or a cavernous transformation (Figure 7) (collateral circulation carrying blood toward the liver).

Clinical features: The clinical features and consequences of portal hypertension are outlined elsewhere in the text and will not be discussed in great detail.

The most common clinical manifestation of PVT is the development of varices (90%) and variceal hemorrhage, which occurs in up to 70% of individuals. However, in contrast to portal hypertension related to cirrhosis, the risk of death and liver failure is significantly less because of preserved hepatic synthetic function.

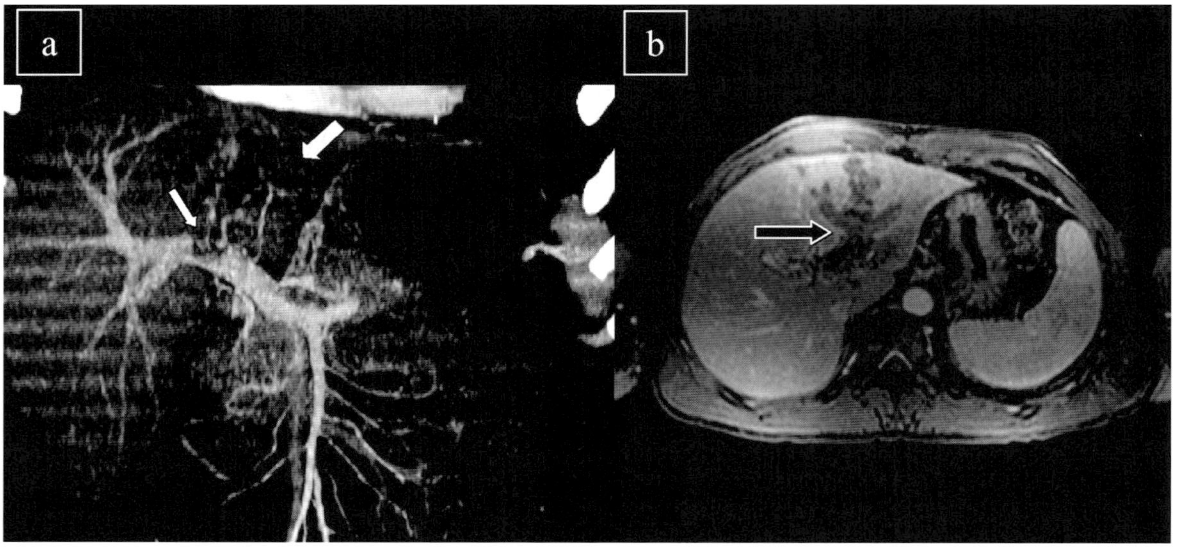

Figure 6. (a) CT reconstruction demonstrating a tumor thrombus at the confluence of the left and right portal vein (small arrow). The tumor is located in the left lob of the liver by the large arrow. (b) MRI demonstrating lack of visualization of the portal vein because it contains tumor thrombus (black arrow).

Similarly jaundice is rare in patients with extra-hepatic PVT and when present is usually due to the consequences of the concomitant hepatobiliary disease. The presence of fever should alert one to the possibility of portal pyemia especially in patients with intra-abdominal sepsis. Serum aminotransaminases are usually normal or mildly elevated and liver failure should not be present unless there is underlying cirrhosis.

In addition to the features of portal hypertension as outlined above, children that suffer from extra-hepatic PVT are at risk of significant growth retardation. In a prospective study of children with PVT, short stature and a reduction in growth velocity were observed in 50% of children when compared with normal controls. Possible explanations for this include decreased hepatotrophic growth hormones as a consequence of the decreased portal blood flow.

The outcome of extra-hepatic PVT is generally very good. A recent series from the Netherlands of 172 patients showed an overall 1-, 5- and 10-year survival of 70, 61 and 54%, respectively. In the absence of cirrhosis and mesenteric vein thrombosis, survival was better at 95, 89 and 81%, respectively. Variables at diagnosis that were noted to be associated with reduced survival included advanced age, malignancy, cirrhosis, mesenteric vein thrombosis, absence of abdominal inflammation, and serum levels of amino-transaminase and albumin. Interestingly, the presence of variceal hemorrhage did not adversely affect overall outcome [8].

Management: The diagnosis should be confirmed by appropriate imaging. Doppler ultrasound and multi-phase contrast enhanced CT or MRI have now replaced venous phase angiography in detailing the vascular anatomy of the liver. All patients should undergo endoscopy to evaluate for the presence of esophageal and gastric varices. If esophageal varices are present, eradication with band ligation is appropriate prior to commencing anticoagulation. During the eradication program, a hematologist should evaluate the patient for the possibility of an underlying hypercoagulable condition. Chronic anticoagulation has been evaluated in a retrospective study and appears to be an effective and safe option for patients with acute PVT as diagnosed by recent abdominal pain and absence of clinical or radiological evidence of chronic portal hypertension. While this retrospective data should be interpreted with caution, it seems prudent to anticoagulate

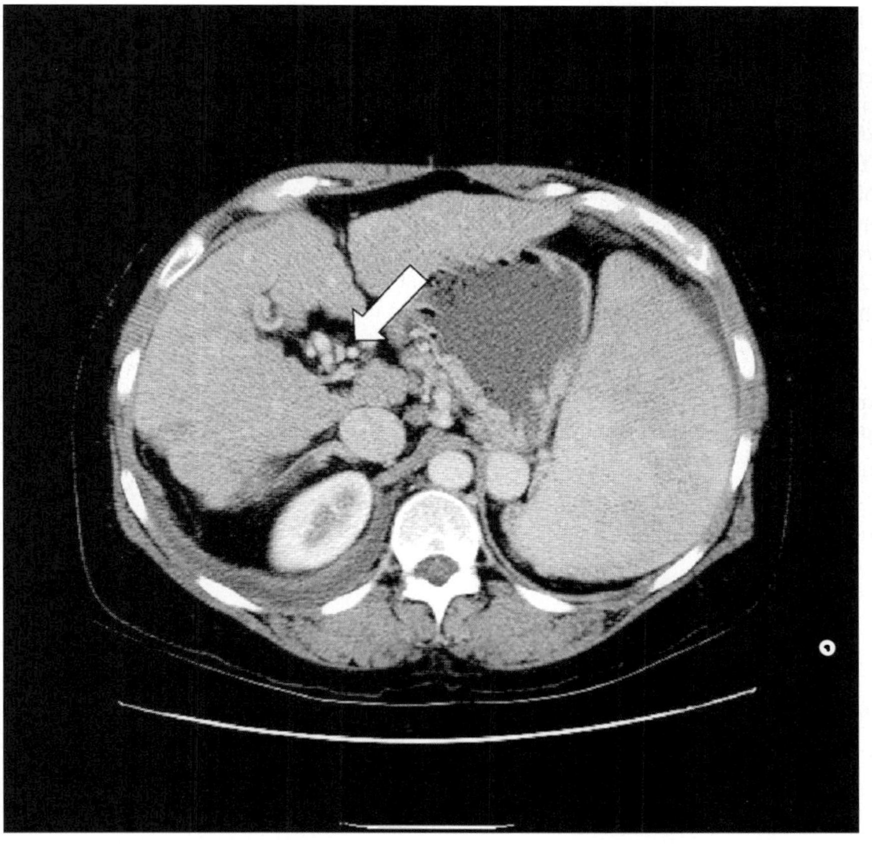

Figure 7. Portal venous phase of a contrast enhanced CT scan demonstrating cavernous transformation of the portal vein. A number of tubular structures can be seen in the expected region of the portal vein.

patients with hypercoagulable disease to prevent further thrombosis. Thrombolytic agents have been used to treat patients with acute PVT; however, it is not known whether this is an effective practice as the natural history of these thromboses is not known. For patients who develop chronic PVT, there is very little to offer. The use of non-selective β-blocker therapy to reduce the risk of variceal bleeding, which is well studied in cirrhosis, has not been studied in extra-hepatic PVT. Anticoagulation of patient with chronic PVT carries the risk of increase in bleeding from gastrointestinal varices. A recent retrospective review of anticoagulation of non-cirrhotic PVT patients demonstrated no significant increase in the number of bleeding episodes or difference in blood loss in patients receiving anticoagulation versus those who did not. However, caution must be used when interpreting this retrospective data and further prospective trials are necessary to address this question. Acute hemorrhage from varices should be managed with variceal sclerotherapy or ligation. Repeated bleeding should be treated with a definitive surgical procedure depending on the available options. If the mesenteric vein is patent, a mesocaval shunt should be placed. If bleeding is from gastric varices, a splenectomy and devascularization procedure is curative.

REFERENCES

[1] Roh, L.S. and LeSher, A. (1989) Dissecting aneurysm of the hepatic artery. *Am. J. Forensic Med. Pathol.* **10**(1), 67–70.

[2] Valla, D.C. (2002) Hepatic vein thrombosis (Budd–Chiari syndrome). *Semin. Liver Dis. Vasc. Coagul. Disord. Liver* **22**, 5–14.

[3] Okuda, K., Kage, M. and Shrestha, S.M. (1998) Proposal of a new nomenclature for Budd–Chiari syndrome: hepatic vein thrombosis versus thrombosis of the inferior vena cava at its hepatic portion. *Hepatology* **28**, 1191–1198.

[4] Bayraktar, Y., Balkanci, F., Bayraktar, M. and Calguneri, M. (1997) Budd–Chiari syndrome: a common complication of Behcet's disease. *Am. J. Gastroenterol.* **92**(5), 858–862.

[5] Okuda, K. (2002) Inferior vena cava thrombosis at its hepatic portion (obliterative hepatocavopathy). *Semin. Liver Dis. Vasc. Coagul. Disord. Liver* **22**, 15–26.

[6] Kage, M., Arakawa, M., Kojiro, M. and Okuda, K. (1992) Histopathology of membranous obstruction of the inferior vena cava in the Budd–Chiari syndrome. *Gastroenterology* **102**, 2081–2090.

[7] Richardson, P. and Bearman, S.I. (1998) Prevention and treatment of hepatic veno-occlusive disease after high dose cytoreductive therapy. *Leuk. Lymphoma* **31**, 266–277.

[8] Janssen, H.L., Wijnhoud, A., Haagsma, E.B., van Uum, S.H., van Nieuwkerk, C.M., Adang, R.P., Chamuleau, R.A., van Hattum, J., Vleggaar, F.P., Hansen, B.E., Rosendaal, F.R. and van Hoek, B. (2001) Extrahepatic portal vein thrombosis: aetiology and determinants of survival. *Gut* **49**, 720–724.

[9] Cohen, J., Edelman, R.R. and Chopra, S. (1992) Portal vein thrombosis: a review. *Am. J. Med.* **92**(2), 173–182.

Hepatology: A Practical Approach
B. Al Knawy, M.L. Shiffman, R.H. Wiesner (editors)

Chapter 18
Liver Disorders of Pregnancy

Qurrat-Ul-Ain Nawab and Caroline A. Riely

Gastroenterology Division, University of Tennessee, Memphis, 951 Court Ave., Room 555 D, Memphis, TN 38163, USA

1. Normal Physiologic Variations in Pregnancy 289
 1.1 Physical examination 290
2. Liver Diseases Unique to Pregnancy 291
 2.1 Hyperemesis gravidarum 291
 2.2 Cholestasis of pregnancy 291
 2.3 Acute fatty liver of pregnancy 292
 2.4 Pre-eclamptic liver disease 293
3. Pregnancy and Chronic Liver Disease 295
 3.1 Portal hypertension 295
 3.2 Autoimmune hepatitis 296
 3.3 Primary biliary cirrhosis 296
 3.4 Wilson's disease 296
 3.5 Hepatic masses 296
4. Liver Diseases Exacerbated by Pregnancy 296
 4.1 Hepatitis E 296
 4.2 Herpes simplex hepatitis 296
 4.3 Budd–Chiari syndrome 297
 4.4 Malignancy 297
References 297

Many internal medicine practitioners poorly understand liver disease in pregnancy. Most of the conditions are of unknown pathogenesis, and have little if any similarity to liver diseases in non-pregnant patients. Liver disease can have an ominous prognosis for both the mother and her unborn child. Early recognition and understanding of these diseases are vital, as potentially two lives can be saved. The differential diagnosis of these conditions is aided by knowledge of their characteristic time of onset in the progress of gestation (Table 1).

1. NORMAL PHYSIOLOGIC VARIATIONS IN PREGNANCY

Normal pregnancy is associated with various physiologic changes. It is very important to keep these changes in mind when we deal with pregnant mothers in order to recognize a normal variant state from abnormal. These changes are outlined in Table 2. Most women experience an increase in appetite beginning early in first trimester and persisting throughout pregnancy. There is usually an overall decrease in tone and motility of gastrointestinal tract thought to be secondary to the effect of progesterone and, as a result, there is an increase in transit time. There is a decrease in lower esophageal sphincter tone, which may be the cause of the heartburn frequently seen in pregnant women. The function of the gall bladder is markedly altered. There is an increase in fasting and residual gall bladder volumes. In the second and third trimesters, these volumes are twice as great as in non-pregnant controls. Biliary cholesterol saturation is increased and the proportion of

Table 1. Liver diseases unique to pregnancy.

First trimester
Hyperemesis gravidarum
Second or third trimester
Cholestasis of pregnancy
Third trimester
HELLP syndrome
Acute fatty liver of pregnancy

chenodeoxycholic acid is decreased, resulting in a predisposition to gallstone formation. The gall bladder in pregnancy still contracts appropriately, emptying 40% of its contents, as it does in the non-pregnant state. Hepatic blood flow does not change compared with pre-pregnancy levels, but fractional blood flow to the liver drops from 35% in non-pregnant state to 29% during pregnancy [1]. The blood volume increases on an average by 48%. Plasma volume increases by 1500 ml^{-1}. There is an increase in cardiac output by 35% and decrease in peripheral resistance by 50%. Red blood cell volume, total iron-binding capacity, and iron absorption increase. Other systems also undergo variation and there is an increase in total minute ventilation and an increase in oxygen consumption. Total cholesterol is increased in pregnant state, as is the thyroid binding globulin. Pregnant women are at higher risk for thromboembolic events. Most of these alterations revert to normal after delivery.

1.1 Physical examination

There are also some physical exam changes noted in pregnant women. The presence of palmar erythema and spider angiomas may mimic chronic liver disease. Pulse rate usually increases. On the other hand, there is usually a drop in blood pressure, more pronounced in second trimester, which returns to normal by term. The presence of an enlarged uterus makes it difficult to palpate the liver.

Table 2. Normal physiologic variations in pregnancy.

GI tract	Renal	CVS	Hematology	Endocrinology	Pulmonary
↓ Muscle tone	↓ Serum creatinine	↑ Stroke volume	↑↑ Plasma volume	↑ Total cholesterol	↑ Minute ventilation by 0–50%
↓ Motility	↓ Serum uric acid	↑ Heart rate by 15–20 min^{-1}	↑ RBC mass	↑ Total T3	↑ Oxygen consumption by 20%
↓ Lower esophageal sphincter tone	↓ BUN	↑ CO by 35%	↑ ESR	↑ Total T4	↑ Tidal volume by 40%
↓ Cheno/cholate synthesis	↑ Creatinine clearance	↓ BP, returns to normal at term	↑ Fe absorption	↑ Thyroid binding globulin	↑ Functional residual volume
↓ Rate of enterohepatic circulation	↑ GFR	↓ Peripheral vascular resistance by 50%	↑ TIBC		■ Forced vital capacity
↑ Cholesterol secretion in bile	↑ Kidney size		↑ WBC and polymorphs		■ Respiratory rate
↑ Lithogenicity of bile	↑ Renal plasma flow		↑ Thromboembolic risk		■ Peak expiratory flow rate
↑ Gall bladder volume	Glycosuria Aminoaciduria		↑ Fibrinogen ↓ Hg and HCT		

↑, increase; ↓, decrease; ■, unchanged.

2. LIVER DISEASES UNIQUE TO PREGNANCY

Liver diseases that occur only in pregnancy are unique. It is vital to understand these diseases, as most of them are reversible if promptly recognized.

2.1 Hyperemesis gravidarum

Hyperemesis gravidarum can be defined as intractable nausea and vomiting during pregnancy, necessitating hospitalization. It begins in the first trimester. Only the rare case persists into the second half of gestation. It can lead to severe dehydration and ketosis. It can complicate 1.0–1.5% of pregnancies. This is a clinical diagnosis that rests on the typical presentation and the absence of other diseases [2]. A number of risk factors are associated with hyperemesis gravidarum. These include increased body weight, twin pregnancy, and nulliparity. Advanced maternal age and cigarette smoking are associated with decreased risk for this condition.

Pathophysiology: The pathogenesis of this disorder is unclear. It has been attributed to the increase in gestational hormones which normally peak in early gestation. Other postulates include the presence of *Helicobacter pylori* infection or of a female fetus [3]. Occurrence of hyperthyroidism and liver dysfunction has been well documented, presumably due to an effect of increased gestational hormones. Liver biopsy, which is not generally necessary, shows modest changes in zone 3, vacuolization, necrosis, and cholestasis without inflammation [4].

Clinical features: This condition usually begins in the first trimester, with onset between the 4th and 10th week of gestation. Affected patients are present with severe nausea and vomiting. They can have signs of volume depletion. Many patients report weight loss. Ptyalism (excessive salivation) occurs frequently. Laboratory findings include increased hematocrit and urea nitrogen indicating volume contraction. There are increased ketones and specific gravity of the urine. Electrolyte abnormalities include a decrease in serum sodium, potassium and chloride. In about two out of three affected patients, elevated aminotransferases are associated with this disorder. Hyperbilirubinemia is less common.

Differential diagnosis: The differential diagnosis of intractable vomiting in early gestation can be difficult. Infections like hepatitis and gastritis must be ruled out. A past medical history of gastroparesis in diabetics, renal failure, or hyperparathyroidism may help to narrow the differential. Severe abdominal pain is not a typical feature of this disorder, and if present may require prompt upper endoscopy to rule out peptic ulcer. Drug-induced hepatitis must be included in the differential diagnosis if hyperemesis gravidarum is associated with elevated liver enzymes.

Management: These patients require volume replacement. Fluids can be given to an outpatient. If symptoms get worse then they may need hospitalization. In rare cases, enteral or parenteral hyperalimentation may be necessary to maintain proper nutrition for mother and fetus [5].

Maternal and fetal outcome: There are no known or suspected hepatic sequelae of hyperemesis gravidarum, and, as is the case with other liver diseases unique to pregnancy, complete recovery is anticipated. Usually fetal outcome is favorable. When severe this condition has significant consequences. Women who are unable to maintain their weight are at increased risk for intrauterine fetal growth retardation, still births, and fetal anomalies.

2.2 Cholestasis of pregnancy

Cholestasis of pregnancy usually begins late in the second trimester or in the third trimester. This condition was previously known as pruritus gravidarum, intrahepatic jaundice of pregnancy or obstetric hepatosis. Epidemiologic studies have shown that this syndrome is most common in certain ethnic groups, including Scandinavians and the Araucanian Indians of Chile, who have a prevalence of 27% for this syndrome [6].

Pathophysiology: The pathogenic mechanisms underlying cholestasis of pregnancy are not fully understood. Studies have suggested that this inherited disorder is an autosomal dominant trait that may be transmitted by phenotypically normal men.

Clinical features: The most common symptom is pruritus of palms and soles, which in a few cases may progress to intolerable degree. It is usually worse at nighttime. In severe cases there is progression to frank jaundice. The serum alkaline phosphatase is usually high, which can be a normal occurrence in pregnancy secondary to placental alkaline phosphatase. Serum GGT level is normal or near normal. In severe cases bilirubin levels are elevated. In the absence of jaundice, bilirubin can be found in urine and blood. Other important laboratory values include elevated aminotransferases levels, which can occasionally rise up to 600–1000 IU. Steatorrhea occurs, but the prothrombin time is usually normal. Liver biopsy is rarely indicated, but when performed, it shows bland cholestasis without inflammation.

Differential diagnosis: Cholestatic diseases like primary biliary cirrhosis can be exacerbated by pregnancy, so past medical history can help to rule out other cholestatic diseases. The differential diagnosis can also include viral- and drug-induced hepatitis.

Management: The clinical course is progressive. Alleviating pruritus before delivery is not easy. Antipruritic agents like hydroxyzine may provide some relief. The bile acid-binding resin cholestyramine has been used, but it can aggravate fat malabsorption. If steatorrhea is present, the patient should receive parenteral vitamin K supplementation [7].

Maternal and fetal outcome: These pregnancies are high risk and require careful monitoring of mother and fetus. Pruritus and elevated liver function tests remit to normal shortly after delivery. Studies show small but significant increases in rates of stillbirth and prematurity.

2.3 Acute fatty liver of pregnancy

Acute fatty liver of pregnancy (AFLP) is a rare disorder. Patients usually present in the third trimester. Sheehan first described this disease in 1940. In 1956, the term AFLP was proposed by Moore and has been universally used. The incidence of AFLP is not clearly established but was estimated to be one case per 13,328 deliveries at the Los Angeles County-University of Southern California Medical Center [8]. Multiple gestational pregnancies are associated with an increased risk of AFLP. AFLP can present in the postpartum period.

Pathophysiology: The pathogenesis of AFLP has been an enigma. Recent reports show that at least some women with AFLP are heterozygous carriers for a defect in long-chain 3-hydroxyl-acyl CoA dehydrogenase (LCHAD), an enzyme involved in beta oxidation of fatty acids. It is amitochondrial enzyme. The gene defects that result in LCHAD deficiency are known, and DNA testing for them is available [9]. Such women are asymptomatic except when they are pregnant with an affected infant who may be well but may cause AFLP during gestation. It is important to test the infant of any affected pregnancy as they later may develop Reye-like syndrome, which can result in non-ketotic hypoglycemia and may lead to death. Liver biopsy shows microvesicular fatty infiltration that is most prominent in the central region. These changes are similar to those seen in cases of Reye syndrome, or Jamaican vomiting sickness, disorders known to result from poisoning of mitochondrial function.

Clinical presentation: Affected patients present at any time from the 28th to the 40th week of pregnancy, with mean gestation close to the term (36 weeks) (see Table 3). Presenting symptoms of AFLP are very varied, ranging from none to typical acute hepatic failure. The most common complaints include nausea, vomiting and abdominal pain. Jaundice may be the presenting complaint. Few patients may present with symptoms of hepatic failure such as somnolence or bleeding. Many patients with AFLP also have pre-eclampsia but AFLP can be differentiated from HELLP. Physical examination is usually not very helpful. Patients with AFLP often manifest the physical signs of pre-eclampsia, including hypertension, edema, agitation and hyperreflexia. A clinical hallmark is coagulopathy with low fibrinogen level, which is striking because fibrinogen levels are usually high during pregnancy. Aminotransferase levels are elevated but are usually less than 1000 U.

Table 3. Acute fatty liver of pregnancy.

Most common symptoms	
Nausea or vomiting	76%
Epigastric pain	43%
Anorexia	21%
Jaundice	16%
Polyuria and polydipsia	<5%
Most common signs	
High blood pressure (>140/90)	50%
Proteinuria	66%
Peripheral edema	56%
Fever	40%
Hepatic encephalopathy	~5%
Abnormal lab values	
Hyperbilirubinemia	
Hyponatremia	
Hyperuricemia	
Hypoglycemia	
Increased transaminase levels (ALT, AST)	
Increased prothrombin time	
Increased serum creatinine	
Thrombocytopenia	
Differential diagnosis	
Pre-eclampsia	
Intrahepatic cholestasis of pregnancy	
Viral hepatitis	
Drug-induced hepatitis	

Differential diagnosis: The clinical picture can be similar to HELLP syndrome, eclampsia or disseminated intravascular coagulation (Algorithm 1). Other causes of acute hepatic failure like drugs or viral hepatitis should be ruled out. History and laboratory work-up help to exclude these causes.

Management: Prompt recognition of AFLP is vital in order to save the mother and her fetus. Care includes prompt delivery and maximum supportive care. This usually requires intensive care unit admission. Improvement begins with delivery and is reflected by improvement in the coagulation profile. In severe cases, there may be a variety of complications such as acute respiratory failure, acute pancreatitis, renal failure, gastrointestinal hemorrhage or diabetes insipidus.

Maternal and fetal outcome: Women improve after prompt delivery. Surviving mothers return to full health with no hepatic sequelae. Liver transplantation has been done for affected patients, but prompt recognition of AFLP should make transplantation unnecessary. Fetal demise occurs. Prompt intervention may save the fetus. AFLP may reoccur in subsequent pregnancies [10].

2.4 Pre-eclamptic liver disease

Pre-eclampsia is a multi-system disorder affecting from 3 to 10% of pregnancies. It complicates 30% of multiple gestational pregnancies [11]. Patients usually present in their third trimester. Hepatic involvement in pre-eclampsia spreads over a wide spectrum, ranging from fibrinogen deposits seen in patients with no symptoms of liver disease through the life-threatening complications of hepatic rupture or infarct in pre-eclampsia. Risk factors include nulliparity, maternal age greater than 40 years, family history of pregnancy-induced hypertension, chronic hypertension, chronic renal failure, diabetes and multiple gestation.

Clinical presentation: Patients may present with a clinical spectrum (see Algorithm 2). They can present with abdominal pain, nausea and vomiting, blurry vision, sudden increase in body weight or more complicated picture such as shock, seizures, or renal failure. Hallmarks of this disease include hypertension with pressures of 140/90 or greater, or an increase in systolic blood pressure of with 30 mm Hg or increase in diastolic blood pressure of 15 mm Hg over mid-trimester levels, with proteinuria and edema. Complications of severe pre-eclampsia are eclampsia, HELLP, hepatic rupture and hepatic infarction.

Eclampsia: It is pre-eclampsia with seizures. Twenty-five percent of seizures can occur before labor, 50% during labor and 25% occur in first 72 h *postpartum*.

HELLP: Patients with pre-eclampsia or eclampsia who have *hemolysis*, presence of schistocytes and burr cells on peripheral smear, *elevated liver enzymes*, primarily aminotransferase levels, and low platelet counts (<100,000 cm^{-1}) are defined as having HELLP syndrome. Liver biopsy in affected patients often demonstrates the periportal hemorrhage and fibrin deposition that classically have been associated with severe pre-eclampsia and are unique to it. The differential diagnosis in this setting is difficult.

Assess severity of disease

Markedly elevated liver enzymes
Hypoglycemia
Prolonged protime
Shock
Signs of fetal distress

Absent

Observe
Prepare mom for delivery
Continous fetal monitoring

Present

Transfer to ICU
Supportive care
Early delivery

Algorithm 1. Acute fatty liver of pregnancy.

Causes of severe abdominal pain should be ruled out. Other diagnoses in the differential include thrombotic thrombocytopenia and other causes of thrombocytopenia.

Hepatic infarction: Affected patients have pre-eclampsia and present, often after delivery, with abdominal pain, prolonged spiking fevers suggestive of abscess, anemia due to blood loss into the substance of the liver, and strikingly elevated aminotransferase levels (3000–6000 IU). Transient hepatic failure with prolongation of the prothrombin time and disseminated intravascular coagulation may occur. The best imaging techniques for detection of these infarcts are computed tomographic (CT) scan or magnetic resonance imaging (MRI). They appear as well demarcated, geographic infarcts of liver, most prominent in the left lobe of the liver. Liver biopsy is not indicated, but when it is done, it shows hemorrhagic necrosis with an infiltrate of polymorphonuclear cells in the adjacent viable liver. A similar CT scan appearance has been reported in association with the presence of a lupus anti-coagulant, anticardiolipin, during gestation. Presumed small arteriole thrombosis with resulting localized infarction also has been reported in pregnancy in women with ulcerative colitis. The clinical history help clinicians rule out these diseases.

Hepatic hematoma and spontaneous rupture of the liver: This condition is more common in older women who are multiparous but also occurs in primigravidas. Patients usually present with severe abdominal pain and have pre-eclampsia. CT scan is very helpful. If it shows a distended but intact liver capsule then the patient can be observed in the intensive care unit and does not require any surgical intervention. The patient with hepatic rupture presents in severe shock. The diagnosis can be confirmed be angiography [12].

Management: Once the diagnosis of pre-eclampsia is confirmed, it is very important to rule out all the possibly fatal complications (see Algorithm 2). The mainstay of treatment is supportive care in the intensive care unit and prompt delivery. Steroids have been useful to tide over patients with HELLP who are too early in gestation to deliver. Plasmapheresis has been advocated in HELLP syndrome but has not been shown to be effective. Hepatic infarction patients require supportive care. Spontaneous rupture requires prompt surgical intervention, with packing with gel foam or with an omental pedicle, hepatic artery ligation, or lobectomy [13].

Material and fetal outcome: Early recognition is vital to save fetal and maternal life. In mild cases of pre-eclampsia, mothers can be stabilized and delivery can be postponed till fetal maturity. But in patients with severe complications, prompt delivery as the only way to save the mother's life. In hepatic rupture and severe cases of HELLP, fetal demise may occur.

Fetuses are at higher risk for prematurity. Patients who survive the initial episode of hepatic infarction go on to complete resolution, often after several weeks of fever.

3. PREGNANCY AND CHRONIC LIVER DISEASE

Most women with chronic liver disease are infertile because of the associated anovulatory state. Pregnancy can occur in women with portal hypertension without cirrhosis or in women with some successfully treated chronic liver diseases. Such pregnancies present special problems for both patient and clinician. Women with liver disease do not have an increased risk for bearing children with congenital anomalies. On the other hand, they do have more maternal problems with pregnancy, and a greater risk for prematurity or stillbirth.

3.1 Portal hypertension

Portal hypertension can occur in the absence of chronic liver diseases as in portal vein thrombosis, hepatoportal sclerosis or congenital hepatic fibrosis. These patients do not have diminished fertility. Worsening of pre-existing portal hypertension might be anticipated in the setting of the marked increase in blood volume and in azygous flow seen in pregnancy. Such patients are at risk of variceal hemorrhage or ascites formation, or splenic artery aneurysm rupture [14].

Management: In the above clinical settings, shunt surgery and sclerotherapy have been successful.

Maternal and fetal outcome: Women with portal hypertension should be advised early about the increased risk of variceal bleeding, and worsening ascites. Upper endoscopy may be advisable to determine whether varices are present or not.

Third trimester
Hypertension
Proteinuria
Nulliparous
Multiple gestation

↓

Assess for complications

↓

Hemolytic anemia Elevated liver enzymes Thrombocytopenia	Abdominal pain CT-scan-distended liver capsule	Abdominal pain Signs of shock CT-scan-hemopertonium	Markedly elevated LFT's Fever CT-scan-infarction
↓	↓	↓	↓
HELLP	Hepatic hematoma	Hepatic rupture	Hepatic infarction
↓	↓	↓	↓
Admit to ICU Supportive care Prepare for early delivery	Admit to ICU Supportive care Observe Prepare for early delivery	Maintain airway supprt volume Prepare for surgery	Aggressive fluids Early delivery observe

Algorithm 2. Preeclampsia–eclampsia.

Women may benefit from beta blockers. These mothers are at higher risk of giving birth to premature babies, or stillbirth. An expert in maternal–fetal medicine should monitor these women during pregnancy.

3.2 Autoimmune hepatitis

Autoimmune hepatitis improves dramatically with immunosuppression. Affected women when treated appropriately with azathioprine and prednisone regain fertility.

Management: Immunosuppression should be continued because relapse is associated with progression of the liver disease. Low doses of azathioprine used are not known to be teratogenic [15].

Maternal and fetal outcome: Like any other liver disease in pregnancy, obstetric complications include prematurity. The disease may flare in the postnatal period. These patients should be followed with care for the first 4–6 months after delivery.

3.3 Primary biliary cirrhosis

Pregnancy in women affected with this disease may not have any complications except for increased cholestasis. Ursodeoxycholic acid has been successfully used to treat this cholestatic condition.

3.4 Wilson's disease

Women successfully treated for Wilson's disease can regain fertility. Chelation should be continued through out the pregnancy because discontinuation can lead to a sudden increase in copper levels, fulminant hepatic failure and death.

3.5 Hepatic masses

Hepatic masses are usually benign neoplasms, which may be discovered during pregnancy. These may include adenomas, focal nodular hyperplasia and hemangiomas. These neoplasms may bleed into the abdomen and may cause complications. Serial ultrasounds are advised to watch their size cautiously. If these tumors are discovered before pregnancy then should be removed if they are of significant size.

4. LIVER DISEASES EXACERBATED BY PREGNANCY

Some diseases are worse when they occur during pregnancy, as normal physiologic changes in pregnant women make them more susceptible to complicated clinical course.

4.1 Hepatitis E

Hepatitis E is a single-stranded RNA virus of the Calciviridae family. It is usually transmitted by fecal–oral route. This usually occurs in epidemics associated with contaminated water supplies. It is very common in densely populated parts of the developing world, such as Africa, India, Pakistan and Mexico [16]. Hepatitis E is usually mild except in pregnant women in their third trimester.

Clinical presentation: Patients are usually in their third trimester. They can present with nausea and vomiting or in fulminant hepatic failure. Transaminases are generally very high and the prothrombin time is usually elevated. This virus has been isolated from the stool of infected people and it has been cloned. Serologic testing will be available soon.

Management: Like patients with any other type of hepatitis, affected patients require supportive care. If they are not in fulminant hepatic failure, then the baby can be delivered when mature.

Maternal and fetal outcome: Up to 20% of women with hepatitis E in the third trimester die secondary to fulminant hepatic failure [17]. Hepatitis can spread to the fetus *in utero*, resulting in symptomatic hepatitis [18].

4.2 Herpes simplex hepatitis

When it occurs in third trimester of pregnancy, hepatitis due to systemic infection with herpes simplex virus is likely to be severe, and in half of the cases hepatic failure due to herpes simplex has occurred in pregnant women.

Clinical presentation: Affected patients generally have a viral prodrome, including fever and upper respiratory tract symptoms. A vesicular rash is diagnostically helpful but may not present visibly. Encephalopathy may develop as a result of hepatitis or encephalitis. Patients generally have elevated transaminases, and prolonged prothrombin time. They usually have anicteric hepatitis, and have a bilirubin level of 3 mg/dl or less. Positive serologies are diagnostic but on an emergent basis they may not be available. Liver biopsy, which is generally not indicated, shows punched-out areas with typical inclusion bodies [19].

Management: Once again management includes supportive care and acyclovir. Patients respond promptly to acyclovir. Prompt delivery is not necessary.

Maternal and fetal outcome: If diagnosed promptly, women do well with appropriate therapy. Herpes can be transmitted vertically to the fetus, but acyclovir that treats mother serves to treat the baby.

4.3 Budd–Chiari syndrome

Pregnancy represents a hypercoagulable state and may be associated with the acute onset of Budd–Chiari syndrome. Most affected patients have another underlying hypercoagulable state, such as deficiency of protein C or S or the presence of an anticardiolipin antibody or some myeloproliferative disorder [20]. This presents more frequently in late pregnancy or in the immediate *postpartum* period. The prognosis is usually ominous when it occurs in the setting of pregnancy. Treatment includes anticoagulation and delivery and rarely liver transplantation.

4.4 Malignancy

The modest immunosuppression of pregnancy may promote tumor growth. Although rare, metastases to the liver may be present in pregnancy. Possible primary sites include the colon, pancreas, and breast [21].

REFERENCES

[1] Schrier, R.W. (1990) Body fluid volume regulation in health and disease: a unifying hypothesis. *Ann. Intern. Med.* **113**, 155.

[2] Abell, T.L. and Riely, C.A. (1992) Hyperemesis gravidarum. *Gastroenterol. Clin. N. Am.* **21**, 835–849.

[3] Jacoby, E. and Porter, K. (1999) *Helicobacter pylori* infection and persistent hyperemesis gravidarum. *Am. J. Perinatol.* **16**, 85–88.

[4] Abell, T. (1992) Nausea and vomiting of pregnancy and the electrogastrogram: old disease, new technology. *Am. J. Gastroenterol.* **87**, 689–691.

[5] Hsu, J., Clark-Glena, R., Nelson, D. and Kim, C.H. (1996) Nasogastric enteral feeding in the management of hyperemesis gravidarum. *Obstet. Gynecol.* **88**, 343–346.

[6] Reyes, H., Gonzalez, M., Ribalta, J., Aburto, H., Matus, C., Schramm, G., Katz, R. and Medina, E. (1978) Prevalence of intrahepatic cholestasis of pregnancy in Chile. *Ann. Intern. Med.* **88**, 487–493.

[7] Rioseco, A., Ivankovic, M., Manzur, A., Hamed, F., Kato, S.R., Parer, J.T. and Germain, A.M. (1994) Intrahepatic cholestasis of pregnancy: a retrospective case control of perinatal outcome. *Am. J. Obstet. Gynecol.* **170**, 890–895.

[8] Pockros, P.J., Peters, R.L. and Reynolds, T.B. (1984) Idiopathic fatty liver of pregnancy: findings in ten cases. *Medicine* **68**, 1–11.

[9] Sims, H., Brackett, J., Powell, C., Treem, W.R., Hale, D.E., Bennett, M.J., Gibson, B., Shapiro, S. and Strauss, A.W. (1995) The molecular basis of pediatric long chain 3-hydroxyacyl-CoA dehydrogenase deficiency associated with maternal acute fatty liver of pregnancy. *Proc. Natl Acad. Sci. USA* **92**, 841–845.

[10] Reyes, H., Sandoval, L., Wainstein, A., Ribalta, J., Donoso, S., Smok, G., Rosenberg, H. and Meneses, M. (1994) Acute fatty liver of pregnancy: a clinical study of 12 episodes in 11 patients. *Gut* **35**, 101–106.

[11] Saftlas, A.F., Olson, D.R., Franks, A.L. Atrash, H.K. and Pokras, R. (1990) Epidemiology of preeclampsia and eclampsia in United States, 1979–1986. *Am. J. Obstet. Gynecol.* **162**, 460–465.

[12] Sommer, D.G., Greenway, G.D., Bookstein, J.J. and Orloff, M.J. (1979) Hepatic rupture with toxemia of pregnancy: angiographic diagnosis. *Am. J. Roentgenol.* **132**, 455–456.

[13] Henny, C.P., Lim, A.E., Brummelkamp, W.H., Buller, H.R. and Ten Cate, J.W. (1983) Review of the importance of acute multidisciplinary treatment following spontaneous rupture of the liver capsule during pregnancy. *Surg. Gynecol. Obstet.* **156**, 593–598.

[14] Hillemanns, P., Knitza, R. and Muller-Hocker, J. (1996) Rupture of splenic artery aneurysm in a pregnant patient with portal hypertension. *Am. J. Obstet. Gynecol.* **174**, 1665–1666.

[15] Steven, M.M., Buckley, J. and Mackay, I. (1979) Pregnancy in chronic active hepatitis. *Q. J. Med.* **48**, 519–531.

[16] Hamid, S., Jafri, S., Khan, H., Shah, H., Abbas, Z. and Fields, H. (1996) Fulminant hepatic failure in pregnant women: acute fatty liver or acute viral hepatitis. *J. Hepatol.* **25**, 20–27.

[17] Rab, M., Bile, M., Mubarik, M., Asghar, H., Sami, Z., Siddiqi, S., Dil, A.S., Barzgar, M.A., Chaudhry, M.A. and Burney, M.I. (1997) Water borne hepatitis E virus epidemic in Islamabad, Pakistan: a common source outbreak traced to the malfunction of a modern water treatment plant. *Am. J. Trop. Med.* **57**, 151–157.

[18] Khuroo, M., Kamili, S. and Jameel, S. (1995) Vertical transmission of hepatitis E virus. *Lancet* **345**, 1025–1026.

[19] Klein, N., Mabie, W., Shaver, D.C., Latham, P.S., Adamec, T.S., Pinstein, M.L. and Riely, C.A. (1991) Herpes simplex virus hepatitis in pregnancy. Two patients sucessfully treated with acyclovir. *Gastroenterology* **100**, 239–244.

[20] Ouwendijk, R., Koster, J., Wilson, J., Stibbe, J., Lameris, J.S., Visser, W. and Benhamou, J.P. (1994) Budd–Chiari syndrome in a young patient with anticardiolipin antibodies: need for prolonged anticoagulant treatment. *Gut* **35**, 1004–1006.

[21] Maeta, M., Yamashiro, H., Oka, A., Tsujitani, S., Ikeguchi, M. and Kaibara, N. (1995) Gastric cancer in the young, with special reference to 14 pregnancy-associated cases: analysis based on 2,325 consecutive cases of gastric cancer. *J. Surg. Oncol.* **58**, 191–195.

Hepatology: A Practical Approach
B. Al Knawy, M.L. Shiffman, R.H. Wiesner (editors)

Chapter 19
Drug-Induced Liver Disease

Mitchell L. Shiffman

Hepatology Section, Liver Transplant Program, Virginia Commonwealth University Health System, Richmond, VA, USA

1. Introduction 299
2. Epidemiology 300
   2.1 Risk factors associated with drug-induced liver injury 300
3. Clinical Presentation 301
   3.1 Cholestasis 301
   3.2 Hepatitis 303
   3.3 Granulomas 303
   3.4 Steatosis 303
   3.5 Fibrosis 304
   3.6 Vascular lesions 304
   3.7 Tumors 304
4. Pathophysiology 304
   4.1 Mechanisms of drug-induced liver injury 305
      4.1.1 The cytochrome system 305
      4.1.2 Intrinsic toxicity of hepatic metabolites 305
      4.1.3 Idiosyncratic toxicity of hepatic metabolites 306
      4.1.4 Toxicity secondary to drug interactions 307
   4.2 Hepatotoxicity secondary to selected common medications 308
      4.2.1 Acetaminophen and ethanol 308
      4.2.2 Isoniazid 309
      4.2.3 Anti-seizure medications 309
      4.2.4 Lipid lowering drugs 309
      4.2.5 Oral diabetic agents 310
      4.2.6 Non-steroidal anti-inflammatory drugs 310
      4.2.7 Herbs and health food supplements 310
   4.3 Subclinical hepatotoxicity 311
5. Management and Treatment 311
   5.1 Treatment of acetaminophen toxicity 312
References 313

1. INTRODUCTION

Pharmaceuticals and environmental or occupational toxins are one of the most common causes of liver test abnormalities. These agents are the etiology for jaundice in 2–5% of hospitalized patients, and are found to be causative in 10% of patients with elevated liver chemistries and 25–33% of patients with fulminant hepatic liver failure. In addition to acute liver failure, some medications and chemicals are known to cause progressive liver fibrosis and cirrhosis with prolonged use over many years, induce fatty liver disease, lead to thrombosis of the hepatic vasculature and induce both benign and/or malignant tumors within the liver. In contrast, medications may also cause stable asymptomatic elevations in liver transaminases or alkaline phosphatase (ALP), which are of no long-term clinical significance. It is important to recognize that nearly every prescription medication and many natural health food supplements are capable of causing liver injury. Genetic differences in the way medications and toxins are metabolized are responsible for the various patterns and severity of liver injury which can be induced by the same agent in various persons.

Drug-induced liver injury has increased in frequency over the past decade [1]. This is both secondary to the increased development of new medications by the pharmaceutical industry and the increased use of nutritional and health food supplements. It is important to keep in mind that clinical trials of potentially new medications are performed in only a few hundred to a few thousand patients prior to their approval by the United States Food and Drug Administration and the health regulatory bodies of other countries. Assuming the incidence of hepatotoxicity is less than 1%; less than 1–5 patients would develop liver chemistry abnormalities when a potential new medication is developed through various phases of testing. As a result, the hepatotoxic potential of most drugs is only realized after they are approved for general use and utilized in large numbers of patients worldwide. It is therefore important for physicians to both recognize and understand the inherent risks of the medications they prescribe and other non-prescription medicinal agents that patients may consume. This chapter will review the various mechanisms by which chemicals cause liver injury and provide an algorithm for physicians to evaluate patients suspected of drug-induced liver disease.

2. EPIDEMIOLOGY

Abnormalities in liver chemistries are the single most common toxicity associated with the use of prescription medications and nutritional health food supplements [1]. However, the risk of developing hepatotoxicity varies significantly with various medications from a high of 5–20/1000 persons exposed for INH to a low of 1–10/1,000,000 exposed for minocycline. As will be discussed below, most drug-induced hepatotoxicity is idiosyncratic and cannot be predicted [2,3]. However, many patient characteristics increase the risk of developing drug-induced hepatotoxicity.

2.1 Risk factors associated with drug-induced liver injury

Specific groups of persons are at increased risk for the development of liver toxicity following exposure to various pharmaceuticals, health food supplements or environmental chemicals. The most important of these risk factors are summarized in Table 1. Drug-induced liver injury is nearly three times as common in persons over the age of 50 years compared to younger persons. Persons who are either obese or malnourished and women are at increased risk to develop drug-induced liver injury. Nearly 60% of all reported cases of drug-induced hepatotoxicity occur in women. Patients with a previous history of hepatotoxicity are also at increased risk to develop hepatotoxicity from other medications. Finally, the more medications a patient is taking the more likely they will develop abnormalities in serum liver chemistries.

Regular alcohol consumption also increases the risk of liver injury from pharmaceuticals and environmental toxins. Alcohol contributes to drug-induced liver injury by enhancing the metabolism of chemicals by the liver; and this leads to the more rapid production of toxic intermediary metabolites. The increased risk of hepatotoxicity resolves when persons become abstinent from alcohol, even if the patient has developed alcohol-induced cirrhosis. The most important clinical interaction between any single medication and alcohol occurs with acetaminophen. Regular alcohol use significantly increases

Table 1. Factors which increase the risk of drug-induced liver disease.

Age: more common and severe in persons >50 years
Gender: women > men
Obesity
Chronic alcohol use
Malnutrition
Patients with previous hepatotoxicity
Use of multiple drugs

the risk of acetaminophen toxicity and may lead to acute liver failure even at recommended dosages. It is therefore important that persons who consume alcohol on a regular basis avoid acetaminophen.

It is important to recognize that simply having chronic liver disease does not increase the risk of developing drug-induced liver injury except in rare circumstances and with specific drugs. The same holds true for patients with cirrhosis. In fact, since most drug-induced liver injury is caused by hepatic metabolism of a drug or chemical to a toxic intermediate and patients with cirrhosis have reduced metabolism; having cirrhosis theoretically reduces the risk for developing drug-induced liver disease. The presence of chronic liver disease, including cirrhosis, is therefore not a contraindication to the use of most medications when clinically indicated. This is addressed in more detail in Chapter 20, Section II. Exceptions to this (where chronic liver disease does appear to increase the risk of hepatotoxicity) include methotrexate in patients with fatty liver disease or cirrhosis and the use of chemotherapeutic agents in patients with cirrhosis. However, when a patient with chronic liver disease, especially with cirrhosis, develops drug-induced liver injury this is typically more severe and is associated with a significantly increased risk for developing liver failure.

3. CLINICAL PRESENTATION

Medications and environmental pathogens may cause a wide variety of histopathologic changes to the liver. Histologic examination of the liver is therefore very useful in the evaluation of patients with suspected drug-induced liver disease. In many cases a liver biopsy may confirm that a suspected medication was the cause of the liver injury. Table 2 contains a list of the most common types of drug-induced pathologic changes caused by medications and chemicals. This list is not complete and is provided to demonstrate the vast array of histopathologic lesions caused by various drugs and chemical agents. Several of the most commonly encountered patterns of drug-induced liver injury are discussed in more detail below.

3.1 Cholestasis

The most common manifestation of drug-induced liver disease is cholestasis. Biochemically, this is characterized by an elevation in serum ALP. Other causes for cholestasis are discussed in Chapter 20, Section II. In most cases of drug-induced cholestasis the serum bilirubin is normal; although this may be elevated in severe cases. Patients who develop jaundice are at increased risk to progress to fulminant hepatic failure and need to be monitored closely even after the inciting medication has been discontinued.

Cholestasis may be caused by many commonly utilized over-the-counter and prescription medications including non-steroidal anti-inflammatory drugs (NSAIDs) and H_2 blockers as well as by proton pump inhibitors, anti-hypertensives, antibiotics (particularly erythromycin and related agents), oral anti-fungal agents, oral diabetic agents, anti-seizure medications, contraceptive and other sex steroids and many other classes of pharmaceuticals. Cholestasis is secondary to the production of an intermediate metabolite that is toxic to one or more enzymes located within the canalicular membrane of the hepatocyte. This is typically the result of an idiosyncratic reaction. Thus, other medications within the same category may not necessarily cause hepatotoxicity in this manner or at all.

The rise in serum ALP in patients with drug-induced cholestasis generally occurs 2–8 weeks following exposure. It is generally mild, less than 3-fold above the upper limits of normal and remains relatively stable for prolonged periods of time. In most cases, ALP returns to normal promptly following discontinuation of the offending agent. Occasionally, cholestasis may not resolve and becomes a chronic process. In some cases cholestasis is part of a systemic hypersensitivity reaction induced by a toxic metabolite and is associated with fever, eosinophilia and dermatitis.

Performing a liver biopsy and examining liver histology is frequently helpful in patients with drug-induced cholestasis. The biopsy typically demonstrates bilirubin deposits within canaliculi and is devoid of inflammation except in those cases

Table 2. Histologic changes and common drugs associated with hepatotoxicity.

Type of injury	Medications
Hepatitis	Isoniazid
	Nitrofurantoin
	Methyldopa
	Phenytoin
	Sulfonamides
	Dapsone
	Protease inhibitors
	Cholesterol lowering drugs
	Cocaine
	Ethambutol
	Phosphorous or iron poisoning
	Anesthetic agents
Cholestasis	NSAIDs
	H_2 blockers
	Proton pump inhibitors
	Phenytoin and other anti-seizure medications
	Oral hypoglycemic agents
	Lipid lowering drugs
	Anti-fungal agents
	Sulfonamides
	Erythromycin
	Anti-depressants
	Haldol, thorazine and other anti-psychotic agents
Granulomas	Quinidine
	Hydralazine
	Allopurinol
	Phenytoin
Fibrosis	Ethanol
	Methotrexate
	Vinyl chloride
	Organic solvents
Phospholipidosis	Amiodarone
	Chloroquine
	Parenteral nutrition
	Trimethoprim-sulfamethoxazole
Steatosis	Ethanol
	Tetracycline
	Amiodarone
	Methotrexate
	Valproic acid
	Nifedipine
	Glucocorticoids
Hepatic or venous thrombosis	Estrogens
	Contraceptive steroids
Veno-occlusive disease	Chemotherapeutic agents
	Azathioprine
	Pyrrolizidine alkaloids
	Urethane
	Radiation therapy
Hepatic adenomas	Estrogens
	Contraceptive steroids

where there is an accompanying immunologic reaction. Bile duct injury may be present, particularly when cholestasis has been chronic.

3.2 Hepatitis

Hepatitis is a common manifestation of drug-induced hepatotoxicity and may take on several forms. One form results from an immunologic reaction stimulated by an intermediate metabolite; is associated with serologic markers of autoimmunity including anti-nuclear, anti-smooth muscle and/or microsomal antibodies and histologic features characteristic of autoimmune hepatitis (see Chapter 20, Section II). Pharmaceuticals most commonly implicated in this process include nitrofurantoin, methyldopa, diclofenac, propylthiouracil and halothane. Other drugs can cause hepatitis both biochemically and histologically but rarely induce the formation of autoantibodies. Agents in this category include many of the sulfonamides and trazadone.

In most cases of drug-induced hepatitis the rise in serum liver transaminases is modest, less than 10 times the upper limit of normal and this is not associated with a rise in serum bilirubin. Liver transaminases typically decline and return to normal following discontinuation of the inciting agent. In those patients with autoantibodies or histologic evidence of autoimmune hepatitis in the absence of autoantibodies, treatment with steroids is frequently required before the liver transaminases normalize. Jaundice is a serious consequence of drug-induced hepatitis and significantly increases the risk that the patient will progress and develop acute liver failure, even if the drug is discontinued and steroids are utilized.

3.3 Granulomas

Non-caseating granulomatous reactions may be caused by numerous medications. In some cases granulomas may develop in extrahepatic sites as well. Granulomatous changes within the liver present biochemically as cholestasis; and only rarely cause necrosis, fibrosis or long-term sequella.

3.4 Steatosis

Many medications cause fatty acids to accumulate within the liver. This is secondary to an intermediate metabolite of the inciting drug interfering with mitochondrial lipid metabolism. Two patterns of steatosis have been recognized. Microvesicular steatosis occurs when small fat droplets accumulate uniformly within the hepatocyte. The nucleus therefore remains central. Drugs which have been associated with microvesicular steatosis include tetracycline, amiodarone, cocaine, various NSAIDs and valproic acid. In macrovesicular steatosis a single large fat droplet pushes the nucleus to the periphery of the hepatocyte. The most common drugs or medications associated with macrovesicular steatosis include ethanol, halothane, various chemotherapeutic agents, warfarin, parenteral nutrition and methotrexate.

Drug-induced steatosis is typically recognized when the patient develops elevated serum liver transaminases, ALP or a mixed pattern in which both types of liver chemistries are elevated. These elevations are typically mild, less than 3 times above the upper limit of normal and remain relatively constant. Jaundice develops only rarely; and is typically confined to that small subset of patients with microvesicular steatosis who develop acute liver failure. Liver chemistries may return to normal following discontinuation of the agent although steatosis may remain present for quite some time. Patients with steatosis may also develop hepatomegally or can are recognized by having a fatty liver on various imaging studies (see Chapter 20, Section II).

Most patients with drug-induced fatty liver remain asymptomatic despite having mild elevations in serum liver chemistries. However, microvesicular steatosis, especially when caused by valproic acid, may progress to acute liver failure. Histologically, this is identical to the lesion present in patients with acute fatty liver of pregnancy and Reyes syndrome.

A variant of steatosis is associated with phospholipid rather than fatty acid accumulation within hepatocytes. This syndrome has been associated with use of amiodarone, nifedipine, griseofulvin and tamoxifen; typically causes chronic changes to the hepatocytes and is associated with systemic manifestations of the phospholipidosis syndrome.

3.5 Fibrosis

Some medications and toxins cause progressive hepatic fibrosis and lead to cirrhosis in the absence of liver test abnormalities. The most common drug associated with this pattern of liver injury is alcohol. Fibrosis progression has also been reported with prolonged use of methotrexate, amiodarone, chlorpromazine, vitamin A and exposure to vinyl chloride and various organic solvents.

3.6 Vascular lesions

The hepatic vasculature may be damaged by certain pharmaceuticals, over-the-counter vitamins and herbal supplements; particularly when utilized in large doses over a prolonged period of time. The most common vascular lesion found within the liver is thrombosis of the large hepatic veins also referred to as the Budd–Chiari syndrome. This is associated with the use of oral contraceptive steroid hormones. Veno-occlusive disease is a disorder in which the small hepatic veins become sclerotic and gradually obliterate the lumen. This disorder has developed following treatment with various types of chemotherapeutic agents and from prolonged exposure to azathioprine, arsenic and pyrrolizidine alkaloids. The later is found in leaves utilized to make tea and other beverages in China, the Caribbean islands and other tropical locations. A third type of vascular insult to the liver is peliosis which is characterized by massive dilatation of hepatic sinusoids. This lesion can be caused by prolonged use of high dose vitamin A, contraceptive steroids, anabolic steroid supplements and the anti-estrogen tamoxifen. The clinical presentation, significance and treatment of these three hepatic vascular lesions are discussed in Chapter 20, Section II.

3.7 Tumors

Both benign and malignant liver tumors of the liver have been associated with exposure to various drugs and chemicals. One of the most common tumors of the liver is the benign hepatic adenoma; which both develop and grow under the influence of oral contraceptive steroids. When small (less than 2–4 cm in diameter), these tumors may totally regress following discontinuation of steroid hormones. Large adenomas have a risk of degenerating into a hepatocellular carcinoma, particularly when steroid hormone use continues. Estrogen use also appears to enhance the growth of focal nodular hyperplasia. The use of radiologic studies to characterize such lesions is summarized in Chapter 20, Section II. The evaluation and treatment of hepatic masses is summarized in Chapter 20, Section II. Angiosarcoma developing within the liver has been reported in persons following exposure to various herbicides, arsenic and vinyl chloride.

4. PATHOPHYSIOLOGY

The liver is the most susceptible organ in the body to the toxic effects of medications, xenobiotics and ingested toxins. Once in the circulation these agents are extracted from the circulation via non-selective organ anion transport mechanisms located on the basolateral service of hepatocytes. Within liver cells these agents are metabolized via a series of enzymatic reactions into non-toxic products. These products are then secreted into the circulation or bile and subsequently excreted from the body in breath, urine or stool.

Hepatotoxicity may occur in one of two ways. The parent chemical may be directly hepatotoxic. Although some organic solvents and other chemicals may act in this manner pharmaceuticals are not directly hepatotoxic. The toxicity of potentially new medications is identified shortly after these compounds are developed and tested in animals and/or utilized in clinical trials. The recognition of such toxicity precludes further development and approval of the medication. In contrast, most medications and environmental agents exhibit hepatotoxicity via intermediates which are produced when the parent drug is metabolized by the liver. The development of toxic intermediates is for the most part via an idiosyncratic process which may vary greatly between patients [4–7].

4.1 Mechanisms of drug-induced liver injury

In general, pharmaceuticals, chemicals, xenobiotics and organic herbs are not directly toxic to the liver. One of the few examples of a chemical which causes direct hepatotoxicity is a toxin found in *Amanita phalloides*, a mushroom which grows wild in many countries throughout the word. Exposure to even small amounts of this toxin causes severe necrosis of liver cells and in many cases leads to fulminant liver failure (see Chapter 20, Section II). In contrast, pharmaceuticals and many environmental agents are not directly cytotoxic. Rather, these agents elicit hepatotoxicity via the production of toxic intermediates which are created by hepatic metabolism of the parent drug or chemical.

Drugs and environmental toxins are metabolized by the liver via a two step process. The first step involves the production of an active metabolite. In almost all cases this step occurs in the hepatic cytochromes located on the smooth endoplasmic reticulum. The intermediary compound produced may either be non-toxic, cytotoxic or act as an allergen and stimulate an immune response against the hepatocyte. The second step detoxifies this potentially toxic intermediate to a non-toxic water-soluble product (Figure 1). This step is performed either by hepatic cytochromes or takes place in the cytoplasm by enzymes which covalently link glucuronate, sulfate, glycine, a methyl group or water to the active intermediate.

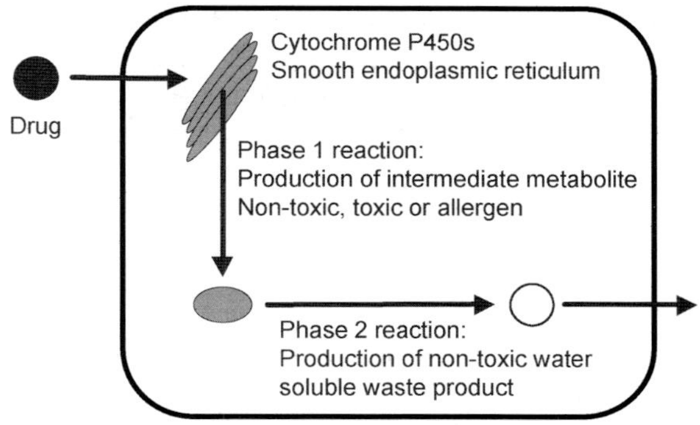

Figure 1. The two step mechanism by which drugs and other compounds are metabolized by the liver. The native compound is first broken down by a cytochrome P450 enzyme located on the smooth endoplasmic reticulum. This intermediate metabolite can be non-toxic, toxic or act as an allergen and precipitate an immunologic reaction. The second step is the detoxification of this intermediate to a water-soluble non-toxic waste product. This is typically accomplished in the cytoplasm by conjugation with glucuronate, sulfate, glycine, a methyl group or water. (*For colored version, see Plate XXVIII on page 579 at the end of the book.*)

4.1.1. The cytochrome system

The cytochrome system is a family of enzymes located on the cytoplasmic side of the smooth endoplasmic reticulum. Also referred to as P450 enzymes, this system evolved with the development of complex multiorgan species and has been relatively conserved over billions of years. The primary function of the cytochrome system is to detoxify chemicals and thereby protect the organism from environmental toxins. Three unique P450 enzyme families designated CYP1, CYP2 and CYP3 have been identified to date. Within each of these CYP families exists a series of enzyme subtypes. Each enzyme subtype is responsible for metabolizing several medications and/or chemicals. A list of some P450 enzyme subtypes and examples of the pharmaceuticals they metabolize is provided in Table 3. Over half of all prescription medications appear to be metabolized by CYP3A4.

Over time, marked genetic heterogeneity has developed within the P450 enzyme family. This has created CYP subtypes which may be subtly different between persons. As a result, the same CYP enzyme in different persons may metabolize the same medication in a slightly different way; and this may produce an intermediary metabolite with slightly different characteristics and potential toxicities. As a result, a toxic metabolite may be produced when a drug is metabolized by one person but not another. This principle explains why toxicity following exposure to any one specific medication or chemical cannot be predicted in any given patient; yet this same toxic reaction may occur within members of the same family.

4.1.2. Intrinsic toxicity of hepatic metabolites

Intrinsic hepatotoxicity results when the metabolite of a pharmaceutical, xenobiotic, natural herb or an

Table 3. Interactions between chemicals, medications and selected cytochrome P450s.

P450 type	Drugs metabolized	Inhibitors	Inducers
CYP1A2	Caffeine Theophylline	Cimetidine Ciprofloxacin	Charcoal-broiled foods Omeprazole
CYP2C8	Rosiglitazone	?	Rifampin Phenytoin
CYP2C9	NSAIDs Phenytoin	Fluvoxamine	Rifampin Phenytoin Phenobarbital
CYP2E1	Acetaminophen Ethanol	Ethanol Disulfiram	Ethanol Isoniazid
CYP3A4	Erythromycin Cyclosporine Corticosteroids Diltiazem Lidocaine Simvastatin	Ethanol Ketoconazole Erythromycin Rotinavir Grapefruit juice	Ethanol Isoniazid Rifampin Phenytoin Phenobarbital Carbamazepine

industrial organ solvent is toxic. In general, it is uncommon for the metabolites of pharmaceuticals to possess intrinsic hepatotoxicity. One such pharmaceutical which does possess intrinsic toxicity is acetaminophen. Within the hepatocyte acetaminophen is metabolized to *N*-acetyl-*p*-benzoquinoneimine (NAPQI) a highly hepatotoxic agent. Fortunately, when acetaminophen is consumed at normal recommended doses only minute amounts of NAPQI are produced and this is rapidly conjugated with glutathione to a non-toxic product. However, when acetaminophen is taken in overdose, NAPQI is produced in excess, the available glutathione necessary to metabolize this toxic intermediate may become depleted, NAPQI accumulates within liver cells and this leads to variable degrees of hepatocyte necrosis. In severe cases of overdose or in the setting of chronic alcohol use, which accelerates the production of NAPQI, acute liver failure may result.

Another common drug in which the primary metabolite possesses intrinsic toxicity is ethanol; which is metabolized to the intermediate product acetaldehyde. Acetaldehyde in turn is rapidly metabolized to CO_2 and H_2O. In most persons, who consume moderate amounts of alcohol or less, there is little to no accumulation of acetaldehyde. In contrast, acetaldehyde may accumulate in some persons who consume alcohol in excess over prolonged periods of time and this may lead to many of the manifestations of alcohol-induced liver injury including, steatosis and fibrosis. Metabolites of INH and carbon tetrachloride also cause intrinsic cytotoxicity. Intrinsic toxicity is predictable, dose dependent and occurs in all patients exposed to sufficient amounts of the toxic agent (Table 4). Biochemically, this form of toxicity presents as a hepatitis with or without jaundice depending upon the severity of the injury. Histologically, variable degrees of necrosis are present depending upon the severity of the insult.

4.1.3. Idiosyncratic toxicity of hepatic metabolites

Most intermediate metabolites are not toxic except in an occasional, rare, individual. In such persons the production of the intermediate metabolite is either toxic via the production of an aberrant toxic metabolite or elicits an immunologic reaction unique to that individual. Idiosyncratic toxicity is responsible for the great majority of liver injury produced by pharmaceuticals and environmental agents. This form of hepatotoxicity is neither predictable nor dose dependent. The toxic metabolite is produced when the parent compound is metabolized by a P450 enzyme that is genetically unique to the individual experiencing the toxic reaction. As a result, idiosyncratic reactions to the same agent may cluster within families. Biochemically there is either

Table 4. Mechanisms of drug-induced liver injury.

	Intrinsic	Idiosyncratic	
		Aberrant metabolite	Hypersensitivity
Dose dependent	Yes	No	No
Predictable	Yes	No	No
Genetic basis	No	Yes	Yes
Enzyme pattern	H	C, H or mixed	C, H or mixed
Cause	Toxic metabolite	Toxic metabolite	Hypersensitivity reaction
Time from rechallenge to toxicity	Similar as primary event 1–2 days	Similar as primary event 1–12 weeks	Immediate 1–2 doses
Examples	Ethanol Acetaminophen Poison mushrooms Carbon tetrachloride	Many drugs	Many drugs

cholestasis, hepatitis or a mixed biochemical pattern. Histologically a wide variety of lesions may be identified depending upon the particular toxic reaction.

Idiosyncratic reactions secondary to the production of aberrant metabolites may require significant time for the toxic metabolite to accumulate and elicit liver injury; in some individuals this may take up to 12 weeks. Toxicity is elicited upon rechallenge, but again this requires weeks to months for the aberrant toxic metabolite to accumulate and cause hepatotoxicity once again. In contrast, some idiosyncratic reactions result from the production of a metabolite that acts as an allergen and stimulates an immunologic response against the hepatocyte. Hypersensitivity idiosyncratic toxicity typically occurs 2–8 weeks following exposure to the pharmaceutical or inciting agent and recurs almost immediately upon rechallenge. In some cases hypersensitivity idiosyncratic hepatotoxicity is associated with a generalized systemic reaction which includes arthralgias, myalgias and/or dermatitis. The various features of intrinsic and idiosyncratic drug hepatotoxicity are contrasted in Table 4.

4.1.4. Toxicity secondary to drug interactions

Since many pharmaceuticals and environmental toxins are metabolized by the same CYP subenzyme, exposure to several drugs at the same time may lead to interactions which could either increase or decrease the metabolism of each drug and thereby alter the potential for hepatotoxicity from each. In addition, some drugs directly inhibit a particular CYP while others enhance the metabolic capacity of the cytochrome. The various ways in which drugs may interact with P450 and the effect this has on hepatotoxicity is illustrated in Figure 2. Knowledge of such interactions is therefore critical when prescribing pharmaceuticals which require their blood level to be maintained within a narrow therapeutic window such as theophylline, cyclosporine and phenytoin.

Some drugs or compounds directly inhibit specific P450 enzymes. On the one hand, this reduces the rate at which toxic metabolite is formed and thereby reduces the potential for drug hepatotoxicity. On the other hand, inhibition of the CYP will delay the clearance of certain drugs from the circulation that are metabolized by that particular cytochrome. This may lead to an increase in the serum level of a pharmaceutical and systemic toxicity. Examples of drugs which inhibit various P450 enzymes include cimetidine, sulfinpyrazone, ciprofloxacin, erythromycin, ketoconazole and an undefined substance in grapefruit juice (Table 3).

In addition to inhibiting a P450 subenzyme, competition may occur between drugs or other compounds which are metabolized by the same CYP. For example, if a patient with a stable blood level of theophylline suddenly starts to consume increased amounts of caffeine, competition for metabolism of these two drugs will lead to reduced metabolism

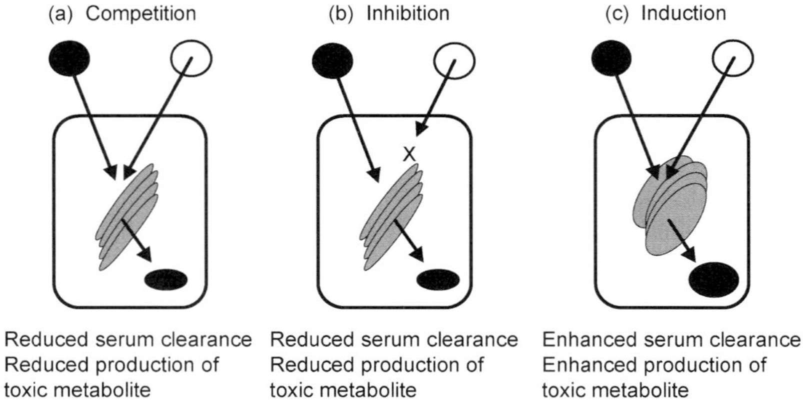

Figure 2. Mechanisms by which the metabolism of a drug is altered by other compounds which interact with cytochrome P450. (a) Competition for the CYP enzyme reduces the metabolism of each drug, (b) inhibition of the CYP slows the metabolism of drugs metabolized by this particular CYP enzyme and (c) induction of the CYP enhances the metabolism of the drug and leads to more rapid production of toxic metabolite. *(For colored version, see Plate XXIX on page 579 at the end of the book.)*

and an increase in the blood level of theophylline. This higher blood level of theophylline may then cause extrahepatic toxicity and its dose must be adjusted downward. It is therefore important to monitor the intake of drugs and environmental chemicals which both compete for and inhibit P450 metabolism.

Chronic exposure to some pharmaceuticals or chemicals may induce P450 enzymes. This increases the mass of the CYP, increases the metabolism of various drugs and leads to a more rapid decline in the serum level of many drugs. Examples of compounds which cause proliferation of P450 enzymes include alcohol, rifampin, phenytoin, phenobarbital omeprazole, smoking and charcoal broiled meats. Thus, if a patient with a stable blood level of cyclosporine is treated with phenytoin, proliferation of the P450 will enhance metabolism and reduce the blood level of cyclosporine below its therapeutic threshold. The dose of cyclosporine must therefore be adjusted upward.

Proliferation of P450 enzymes also enhance the rate at which potentially toxic intermediates are produced. This mechanism significantly increases the risk of hepatotoxicity for many pharmaceuticals with otherwise low hepatotoxic potential. One of the most common and important causes of hepatotoxicity which result from such interactions occurs between alcohol and acetaminophen.

4.2 Hepatotoxicity secondary to selected common medications

Any medication has the potential to elicit hepatotoxicity. Some of the most common medications utilized and the mechanism by which these medications cause hepatotoxicity are discussed below.

4.2.1. Acetaminophen and ethanol

One of the most common and potentially the most serious of all drug–drug interactions occurs between acetaminophen and those agents which induce CYP3A4 [9,10]. These agents include alcohol, phenobarbital, rifampin and phenytoin. Regular alcohol consumption or regular use of these other medications which cause induction of this CYP leads to an increase in the mass of this enzyme. This significantly enhances the rate at which acetaminophen is metabolized to NAPQI. The rapid production of this toxic metabolite rapidly depletes intracellular glutathione stores, the substrate necessary to detoxify NAPQI. This increases the intracellular concentration of NAPQI and leads to cellular necrosis. Given the very rapid rate at which acetaminophen is metabolized to NAPQI in the face of P450 induction; the risk of hepatotoxicity is increased considerably even when only therapeutic amounts of acetaminophen are consumed. As a result, patients who consume alcohol on a regular basis or take medications which are known to cause the proliferation of the P450 cytochromes should avoid acetaminophen.

4.2.2. Isoniazid

Following acetaminophen, isoniazid (INH) is probably the most widely utilized medication with significant potential for hepatotoxicity. Minor elevations in serum liver transaminases (<3-fold the upper limit of normal) occur in 10–20% of persons within the first 3 months of taking INH. However, it is uncommon for these liver test abnormalities to progressively worsen; in most cases the changes actually improve with ongoing treatment. Progressive liver injury and jaundice develops in about 1% of persons taking INH; this doubles in persons over the age of 50 years. The risk of toxicity is also increased in patients taking rifampin, a potent inducer of many P450 subenzymes.

INH is in part metabolized via acetylation; and marked genetic variation in this enzyme has been demonstrated as well. Patients may be either slow or fast acetylators of INH metabolites; and some studies have suggested that slow acetylators are at increased risk for hepatotoxicity secondary to the accumulation of INH metabolites.

4.2.3. Anti-seizure medications

Many anti-seizure medications have a potential to cause hepatotoxicity. The mechanism by which this occurs varies widely. Phenytoin causes hepatotoxicity via an idiosyncratic process and the production of a toxic aberrant metabolite. Such patients typically develop marked elevations in serum liver transaminases which occur 4–6 weeks after the start of this medication. In some patients phenytoin toxicity may cause idiosyncratic immunologic toxicity associated with a cholestatic hepatitis, fever, dermatitis and a Stephens–Johnson reaction.

Valproic acid causes hepatotoxicity in a completely different manner. This agent has been associated with the development of severe microvesicular steatosis which in some cases can progress to acute liver failure. The development of microvesicular steatosis secondary to valproic acid is believed to be secondary to the production of a metabolite which interferes with mitochondrial fatty acid metabolism. As in most other cases of drug-induced hepatotoxicity, serum liver transaminases begin to rise about 4–12 weeks after the start of this medication.

Finally, it is important to keep in mind that many anti-seizure medications are potent inducers of many different CYP enzymes. This may alter the metabolism and increase the potential toxicity of many other medications.

4.2.4. Lipid lowering drugs

As a class of drugs, the statins have proven to have a very low incidence of overt hepatotoxicity [11]. Approximately 3% of patients who were treated with statins during clinical trial were noted to develop mild abnormalities in serum liver transaminases, ALP or a cholestatic hepatitis. However, these values either stabilized, often returned to normal despite continued treatment or normalized soon after the medication was discontinued. In retrospect, the great majority of patients who are noted to have mild elevations in liver chemistries while taking statins probably have underlying non-alcoholic fatty liver disease and these abnormalities are not medication related. Although still recommended by regulatory agencies, monitoring serum liver chemistries in patients who are started on statin therapy for treatment of elevated serum cholesterol is unlikely to either detect drug-induced hepatotoxicity or be cost effective.

In contrast to the statins, dose dependent hepatotoxicity is well documented to occur during treatment with nicotinic acid. Both immediate and sustained release preparations have been associated with cholestasis or a cholestatic hepatitis. Significant elevations in liver chemistries are associated with fatigue, malaise and jaundice which in some cases has progressed to acute liver failure. It is important to keep in mind that hepatotoxicity from niacin can occur anytime, from as little as just a few weeks to as long as years.

4.2.5. Oral diabetic agents

Cholestasis, cholestatic hepatitis and both systemic and dermatologic hypersensitivity reactions have been observed when sulfonylureas are utilized for treatment of type II diabetes mellitus. Most cases resolve promptly following medication withdrawal. The most recent oral hypoglycemic agents are the glitazones. The first such drug in this class, troglitazone, was associated with hepatotoxicity and several cases of acute liver failure. This appears to be the result of an idiosyncratic reaction and the formation of a toxic metabolite which accumulates over time. Although most patients developed severe hepatotoxicity within 4–8 weeks after they started taking this medication, toxicity developing after being on this medication for several months has also been reported. Troglitazone was withdrawn from use by its manufacturer in 1999. Rosiglitazone and pioglitazone appear to be much safer compounds and elicit hepatotoxicity only rarely. Mild elevations in serum liver transaminases and in some cases ALP have been reported, but acute liver failure has not been observed to date. Despite this, drug regulatory bodies have recommended that serum liver chemistries be monitored in all patients treated with glitazones both at baseline and at 2-month intervals during the first year of treatment. As noted above for the statins, the routine monitoring of serum liver chemistries has not been shown to reduce the incidence of severe hepatotoxicity or overt acute liver failure and is unlikely to be a cost-effective approach to this problem.

4.2.6. Non-steroidal anti-inflammatory drugs

Non-steroidal anti-inflammatory agents as a class, are some of the most widely utilized of all prescription and non-prescription medications. Overall, the incidence of hepatotoxicity secondary to these drugs is uncommon. However, given that these compounds are utilized in up to 15% of the general population on a yearly basis; NSAIDs as a group are responsible for 5–10% of all cases of hepatotoxicity. NSAID-induced toxicity is the result of an idiosyncratic reaction caused by the production of a metabolite which is either toxic or which stimulates an immunologic response. Hepatotoxicity may occur during treatment with any of more than 20 different NSAID compounds including aspirin. However, the frequency at which the various NSAID preparations cause hepatotoxicity vary greatly (Table 5). The highest incidence of toxicity is observed with diclofenac, sulindac and phenylbutazone. The lowest incidence appears to be with diflunisal, ketorolac and tolmentin. Hepatotoxicity secondary to NSAIDs is manifested by either an elevation in serum liver transaminases, cholestasis or a mixed cholestatic hepatitis.

Table 5. Relative risk of NSAIDs for hepatotoxicity.

	Relative toxicity
Diclofenac, sulindac or phenylbutazone	100
Naproxen	10
Ibuprofen, indomethacin	5
Diflunisal, ketorolac, tolmentin	1

4.2.7. Herbs and health food supplements

The use of herbs and health food supplements has increased significantly in many developed countries throughout the world. Many of these compounds have been utilized for centuries by certain cultures; they appear to be safe and in some cases they appear to be effective. However, herbal preparations can also cause hepatotoxicity via the same mechanisms as occurs with conventional medications; the production of toxic intermediate metabolites. The lack of regulation and oversight to ensure that

Table 6. Examples of common herbs, health food supplements and vitamins which can be associated with hepatotoxicity.

	Type of toxicity
Chaparell	Hepatitis and necrosis
Chinese or Jamaican tea containing pyrrolizidine compounds	Veno-occlusive disease
Cascara sagrada	Hepatitis
Germander	Hepatitis, necrosis
Jin Bu Huan	Hepatitis and steatosis
Kava	Dose-dependent necrosis
Vitamin A	Dose-dependent hepatitis
Zulu remedy	Dose-dependent necrosis

these compounds are both pure and packaged in appropriate dosages may also increase the hepatotoxic potential for some of these compounds.

Those herbs and food supplements associated with the highest risk for hepatotoxicity are listed in Table 6 [13,14]. Kava has been reported to cause an autoimmune hepatitis-like reaction, but only when taken in high dosages. Other herbal products associated with autoimmune hepatitis-like reactions include Jin Bu Huan, Ma-huang and Dai-saiko-to. Hepatic necrosis has been reported in some persons following the use of Chaparral leaf, Germander and Zulu. Cholestasis has been linked to the use of Cascara sagrada; and veno-occlusive disease following the consumption of large quantities of some Chinese herbal tea which contains pyrrolizidine alkaloids.

Even natural occurring and synthetic vitamins may also cause hepatotoxicity when utilized in excess. This is particularly true of vitamin A, which is well known to be a dose-dependent hepatotoxin [12]. Toxicity may occur after a single large overdose or with prolonged exposure to high doses of this fat-soluble vitamin. The acute injury is characterized by elevations in serum liver transaminases. However, prolonged use of vitamin A may lead to cirrhosis without any abnormalities in liver chemistries.

4.3 Subclinical hepatotoxicity

Many medications cause mild elevations in serum liver chemistries which remain stable for prolonged periods of time. The elevation in serum liver transaminases or ALP in such patients is usually less than three times the upper limit of normal and no systemic symptoms or signs of toxicity are present. Over time these elevations in liver chemistries may resolve. Such medications can usually be continued without risk, especially if the medication is required for treatment of an ongoing medical condition. However, monitoring serum liver chemistries at periodic intervals as long as these tests remain elevated seems prudent. Another approach to these patients is to perform a liver biopsy and evaluate for histologic signs of liver injury. In subacute hepatotoxicity, liver histology is typically either normal or near normal.

5. MANAGEMENT AND TREATMENT

The approach to patients suspected of having drug-induced hepatotoxicity is outlined in Figure 3. Whenever any new medication is started patients should be made aware of the small but real potential that a hepatotoxic reaction may develop.

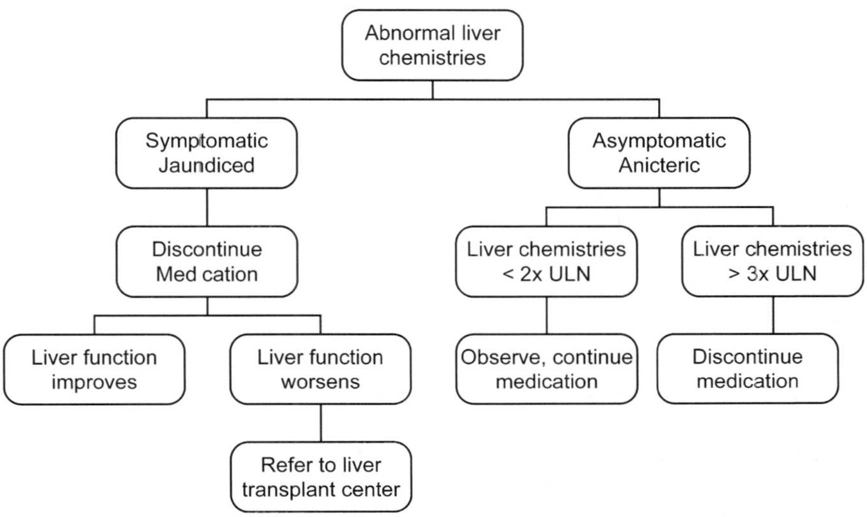

Figure 3. Flow chart for evaluation of a patient with suspected drug-induced elevations in serum liver chemistries.

Such reactions are typically associated with nausea, anorexia, myalgias and arthralgias. Some patients also develop fever and jaundice. Whenever these symptoms develop 4–12 weeks after the start of a new medication drug-induced hepatotoxicity should be suspected; the patient should be evaluated and liver chemistries should be monitored. An elevation in serum liver transaminases, ALP and/or bilirubin should lead to an immediate discontinuation to the medication. In the great majority of cases, the prompt recognition of drug-induced hepatotoxicity and the discontinuation of the inciting agent will lead to complete resolution of the insult and liver chemistries will return to the limits of normal. Unfortunately, these abnormalities in serum liver chemistries may persist or worsen in some patients despite the discontinuation of the inciting medication. Such patients are at high risk for progression to liver failure and should be referred to a center where liver transplantation is available, particularly if jaundice is present or signs of acute liver failure have developed (see Chapter 20, Section II).

One approach to avoid hepatotoxicity is to monitor serum liver chemistries at periodic intervals following the start of a medication. Indeed, the monitoring of serum liver chemistries is recommended for many medications with known hepatotoxic potential. This includes INH, many lipid lowering medications, anti-seizure medications, protease inhibitors and certain oral hypoglycemic agents. However, other studies have demonstrated that simply monitoring patients for symptoms of hepatotoxicity may be a more sensitive way of identifying patients with drug-induced hepatotoxicity sooner than by measuring serum liver chemistries.

One of the limitations in monitoring liver chemistries in patients started on medications is that baseline values, prior to the start of the medication, are frequently not obtained. Thus, when a mild elevation in serum liver transaminases or ALP is identified 1–2 months after starting a new medication it is unknown if this elevation was preexisting and due to some form of underlying liver disorder or secondary to subclinical hepatotoxicity. As long as the abnormality is mild (less than 3 times the upper limit of normal), the patient has no symptoms associated with hepatotoxicity, is not jaundiced and can be monitored; the medication may be continued. If the mild elevation in serum liver chemistries does not worsen the medication may be continued but a complete evaluation for the etiology of the liver chemistry abnormalities should be undertaken (Chapter 20, Section II).

5.1 Treatment of acetaminophen toxicity

Acetaminophen is the most common cause of drug-induced hepatotoxicity in the United States, United Kingdom, Australia and many other countries. In many of these countries acetaminophen is one of the most common causes of acute liver failure and this frequently results from deliberate overdose during a suicide attempt or gesture. However, nearly one-third of all cases of severe acetaminophen hepatotoxicity results when therapeutic amounts of acetaminophen are consumed by susceptible patients. Factors which increase the risk of acetaminophen hepatotoxicity include regular alcohol consumption, use of medications known to induce certain cytochromes (Table 3) and malnutrition.

The management of acetaminophen hepatotoxicity varies with the time of presentation following ingestion and whether liver failure has already developed or not. When patients present within 4 h of ingestion gastric lavage to remove any undigested pill fragments should be performed. Use of activated charcoal has not shown to be effective. The serum acetaminophen level should be determined and the risk for toxicity assessed according to a standardized nomogram at presentation and again 4–6 h later. The principal treatment or antidote for acetaminophen overdose is *N*-acetylcysteine (NAC) [8]. This agent replenishes glutathione which is necessary to metabolize the toxic intermediate of acetaminophen, NAPQI, to a non-toxic product. When the administration of NAC is started within 16 h of ingesting acetaminophen the severity of the hepatotoxicity is limited and this typically resolves within several days. In many countries NAC is administered intravenously; in the United States only an oral formulation is available. Patients with serum levels of acetaminophen which fall within the toxic range according to the nomogram are at increased risk to develop acute liver failure. It is important to keep in mind that liver failure progresses rapidly when it is due to acetaminophen. As a result, transfer of patients to a center where emergent liver transplantation could be performed if necessary should be strongly considered; especially if there is evidence of coagulopathy or mild hepatic encephalopathy.

REFERENCES

[1] Farrell, G.C. and Liddle, C. (2002) Hepatotoxicity in the twenty-first century. *Semin. Liver Dis.* **22**, 109–210.

[2] Bissell, D.M., Gores, G.J., Laskin, D.L. and Hoofnagle, J.H. (2001) Drug-induced liver injury: mechanisms and test systems. *Hepatology* **33** 1009–1013.

[3] Larrey, D. and Pageau, G.P. (1997) Genetic predisposition to drug-induced hepatotoxicity. *J. Hepatol.* **26**(Suppl. 2), 12–21.

[4] Gennis, M.A., Vemuri, R., Burns, E.A., Hill, J.V., Miller, M.A. and Spielberg, S.P. (1991) Familial occurrence of hypersensitivity to phenytoin. *Am. J. Med.* **91** 631–634.

[5] Lee, W.M. (1995) Drug-induced hepatotoxicity. *N. Engl. J. Med.* **333**, 1118–1127.

[6] Lewis, J.H. (2000) Drug-induced liver disease. *Med. Clin. N. Am.* **84**, 1275–1311.

[7] Knowles, S.R., Uetrecht, J. and Shear, N.H. (2000) Idiosyncratic drug reactions: the reactive metabolite syndrome. *Lancet* **356**, 1587–1591.

[8] Keays, R., Harrison, P.M., Wendon, J.A., Forbes, A., Gove, C., Alexander, G.J. and Williams, R. (1991) Intravenous acetylcysteine in paracetamol-induced fulminant liver failure: a prospective controlled trial. *BMJ* **303** 1026–1029.

[9] Zimmerman, H.J. and Maddrey, W.C. (1995) Acetaminophen hepatotoxicity with regular intake of alcohol: analysis of instance of therapeutic misadventure. *Hepatology* **22**, 767–773.

[10] Whitcomb, D.C. and Block, G.D. (1994) Association of acetaminophen hepatotoxicity with fasting and ethanol use. *JAMA* **272**, 1845–1850.

[11] Downs, J.R., Clearfield, M., Tyroler, H.A., Whitney, E.J., Kruyer, W., Langendorfer, A., Zagrebelsky, V., Weis, S., Shapiro, D.R., Beere, P.A. and Gotto, A.M. (2001) Air Force/Texas Coronary Atherosclerosis Prevention Study: additional perspectives on tolerability of long term treatment with lovastatin. *Am. J. Cardiol.* **87** 1074–1079.

[12] Geubel, A.P., De Galocsy, C., Alves, N., Rahier, J. and Dive, C. (1991) Liver damage caused by therapeutic vitamin A administration: estimation of dose related toxicity in 41 cases. *Gastroenterology* **100** 1701–1709.

[13] Larrey, D. and Pageaux, G.P. (1995) Hepatolotoxicity of herbal remedies and mushrooms. *Semin. Liver Dis.* **15**, 183–188.

[14] Seeff, L.B., Lindsay, K.L., Bacon, B.R., Kresina, T.F. and Hoofnagle, J.H. (2001) Complementary and alternative medicine in chronic liver disease. *Hepatology* **34** 595–603.

Hepatology: A Practical Approach
B. Al Knawy, M.L. Shiffman, R.H. Wiesner (editors)

Chapter 20
Fulminant Hepatic Failure

Paul J. Gaglio, Joshua Aron and Robert S. Brown Jr.

Center for Liver Disease and Transplantation, New York-Presbyterian Hospital, Columbia University College of Physicians and Surgeons, 622 West 168 St, PH 14, New York, NY 10032, USA

1. Introduction 316
   1.1 Definition 316
   1.2 Prevalence and incidence 316
   1.3 Demographics 317
2. Pathophysiology 317
   2.1 Viral hepatitis 317
   2.2 Toxic hepatitis 318
   2.3 Vascular 318
   2.4 Miscellaneous 319
3. Clinical Features 319
   3.1 Neurologic 319
   3.2 Coagulopathy 319
   3.3 Infections 319
   3.4 Renal 319
   3.5 Metabolic 320
   3.6 Cardiovascular 320
4. Diagnosis 320
   4.1 Blood tests 320
   4.2 Imaging studies 320
   4.3 Pathological studies 320
5. Management 321
   5.1 General measures 321
   5.2 Central nervous system 321
      5.2.1 Hepatic encephalopathy 321
      5.2.2 Cerebral edema 322
   5.3 Respiratory 323
   5.4 Cardiovascular 323
   5.5 Nutrition 323
   5.6 Infection 323
   5.7 Renal 324
   5.8 Gastrointestinal 324
   5.9 Hematologic complications 324
   5.10 Specific pharmacologic therapy of FHF 324
      5.10.1 Glucocorticoids 324
      5.10.2 *N*-Acetylcysteine 324
      5.10.3 *S*-Adenosylmethionine 325
      5.10.4 Antiviral agents 325
      5.10.5 Prostaglandin E_1 325
      5.10.6 Insulin–glucagon 325

5.10.7 Liver replacement therapy 325
5.10.8 Orthotopic liver transplantation 325
5.10.9 Living donor liver transplantation 326
5.10.10 Xenograft transplantation 326
5.10.11 Bioartificial liver 326
5.10.12 Hepatocyte transplantation 327
6. Prognosis 327
7. Summary 328
References 328

1. INTRODUCTION

Despite recent advances in medical and surgical therapies, fulminant hepatic failure (FHF) remains the most ominous of all gastroenterologic emergencies. Patients with this rare but devastating form of liver disease have only a 20% chance of survival with medical therapy alone [1]. Early recognition of FHF and anticipation of its potentially fatal complications are essential for successful medical management and appropriate surgical triage of these patients. This chapter will define FHF, identify key prognostic indices that help determine the need for transplantation, and will discuss the pathophysiology and treatment of FHF, including novel treatment options.

1.1 Definition

FHF is defined as the acute onset of profound hepatocellular dysfunction manifested as jaundice accompanied by encephalopathy. This initial description, as proposed by Trey and Davidson in 1970, described patients without a previous history of liver disease [2] but has been expanded to include some patients with pre-existing liver disease. The two most notable exceptions include Wilson's disease and autoimmune hepatitis, which may reflect the initial presentation of an otherwise chronic illness. Further refinement of the definition of FHF has been proposed based on the timing of encephalopathy following the onset of jaundice; hyperacute when encephalopathy occurs within 7 days, acute within 8–28 days, and subacute from 29 to 60 days following jaundice [3]. Although these definitions seem arbitrary, the interval between jaundice and encephalopathy is related to both the etiology and prognosis of the liver disease. For example, patients who develop encephalopathy within 1 week of their jaundice are more likely to have FHF from hepatic ischemia or acetaminophen toxicity when compared to patients who become encephalopathic after a 4-week interval; in these patients a viral or cryptogenic etiology is far more common. In addition, cerebral edema is a more characteristic finding if encephalopathy appears within 1 month of disease onset, while complications of portal hypertension, ascites, and renal failure tend to occur in patients who develop encephalopathy more than 8 weeks from the start of their illness [4]. Finally, survival rates without liver transplantation vary significantly between these subclassifications (Table 1).

1.2 Prevalence and incidence

The true incidence of FHF in the United States is difficult to adequately characterize, as no national acute liver failure database exists. A review

Table 1. Definitions of liver failure.

	Onset of encephalopathy following jaundice (days)	Survival rate (%)
Hyperacute liver failure	7	36
Acute liver failure	8–28	14
Subacute liver failure	2–60	7

Modified from O'Grady, J.G., Schalm, S.W. and Williams, R. (1993) Acute liver failure: redefining the syndromes, *Lancet* **342**, 273–275.

estimated that 2000 patients per year develop FHF in the United States each year [5]. From 1980 to 1988, approximately 7500 deaths were attributed to "hepatic coma" in patients without any prior history of chronic liver disease, alcohol or cancer [6]. These figures may represent underestimates, as under-reporting of FHF likely occurs. Since this is an acute disease from which patients either recover or die, the prevalence of disease is equal to its incidence in the population. Mortality also varies by etiology with Wilson's disease, idiosyncratic drug reactions, and non-A–non-B viral infections associated with a higher mortality than acute liver disease from other causes, with acetaminophen toxicity having the best prognosis [7].

1.3 Demographics

A recently completed review from 13 US centers characterized the demographics and outcomes in 295 patients admitted with FHF over a 2-year period. In this study, 41% of patients ultimately required liver transplantation, 25% recovered with medical therapy and 34% died without undergoing transplantation. Acetaminophen overdose was the most common cause of FHF, followed by cryptogenic/non-A, non-B, non-C hepatitis, idiosyncratic drug reactions, hepatitis B, hepatitis A, Wilson's disease, autoimmune hepatitis, and miscellaneous causes including Budd–Chiari syndrome, herpes simplex, Epstein–Barr, paramyxovirus infection, malignant infiltration, *Amanita* (mushroom) poisoning, ischemia, and acute fatty liver of pregnancy. The mean age of patients was between 35 and 38 years (± 14–17 years), and the female-to-male ratio was 1.17:1 [7].

2. PATHOPHYSIOLOGY

FHF occurs in the setting of massive hepatocellular destruction. The disease processes that induce FHF can be divided into several broad categories: viral infection, metabolic and toxic hepatitis, and ischemia/hypoxia (Table 2). Although the strict definition of FHF implies an acute process in a previously normally functioning liver, there are several conditions associated with histologic and historical evidence of chronic liver disease that may be associated with a fulminant course (Table 3). Several of the etiologic mechanisms leading to FHF deserve further comment.

2.1 Viral hepatitis

Worldwide, viral hepatitis is the most common precipitant of FHF. Hepatitis A virus (HAV) may be associated with FHF, although it accounts for < 0.5% of cases of acute HAV. The risk of liver failure in HAV is higher in patients over age 40 or in patients with pre-existing liver disease such as hepatitis C [8]. Hepatitis B virus (HBV) may induce FHF with or without hepatitis D/delta

Table 2. Precipitating causes of FHF.

Viral infection
Frequent
Hepatitis A, B, D, E
Hepatitis non-A–G
Rare
Hepatitis C
Cytomegalovirus
Epstein–Barr virus
Herpes simplex virus
Metabolic
Acute fatty liver of pregnancy, Reye's SX
Toxin, drugs
Acetaminophen
NSAIDs
CCl_4
Isoniazid
Sodium valproate
Methyl dopa
Tetracycline
Halothane
Amanita phalloides ("mushroom poisoning")
Yellow phosphorus
"Herbal medication"
Drug combinations
Acetaminophen and EtOH
Acetaminophen, barbiturates, isoniazid
Trimethoprim and sulamethoxazole
Amoxicillin and clavulinic acid
Ischemic
Hepatic artery thrombosis
Budd–Chiari syndrome
Right ventricular failure, cardiac tamponade
Shock
Miscellaneous
Hyperthermia
HELPP syndrome

Table 3. "Chronic" liver disease which may be associated with fulminant course.

Wilson's disease
Malignant infiltration of the liver
Post-jejunoileal bypass
Auto-immune hepatitis
Chronic hepatitis B + delta or reactivated hepatitis B
Protoporphyria
Other metabolic diseases (fructose intolerance, tyrosinemia)

Modified from Fingergote, R.F. and Bain, V.G. (1993) Fulminant hepatic failure, *Am. J. Gastroenterol.* **88**(7), 1000–1010.

hepatitis (HDV) co-infection. While HBV accounts for up to 15–20% of all cases of FHF in most retrospective series, the true role of HBV infection is uncertain. In many population-based studies of FHF, HBV prevalence was largely defined by HBsAg seropositivity alone, which may reflect a chronic asymptomatic carrier state. A recently published study analyzing FHF in 377 patients who were hepatitis B surface antigen positive had evidence of acute hepatitis B-related disease based on detectable IgM antibodies to HBV in only 52%. This suggests that half of the patients presenting with HBV and FHF may have an alternative insult in the setting of chronic asymptomatic liver disease, such as toxin exposure or viral co-infection. The contribution of delta virus as a cause of FHF was studied in a recent publication that described 71 HBsAg positive patients with FHF; hepatitis delta virus was found in approximately 33% of patients. This finding is dramatic when it is noted that the prevalence of delta virus co-infection in non-fulminant cases of acute HBV is estimated at 4.4%. As such, delta virus co-infection or superinfection may be underestimated and should be excluded in all cases of HBV and FHF.

Hepatitis E virus (HEV) has been identified in cases of water-borne outbreaks of hepatitis in developing countries, with reports of FHF in some infected patients. Pregnant women are especially vulnerable to FHF following HEV infection [9]. Although a common cause of chronic hepatitis, hepatitis C virus (HCV) rarely induces FHF in the United States [10]. Despite significant improvement in the ability to diagnose viral hepatitis, it is now apparent that in the USA, the majority of cases of FHF due to viral hepatitis are untypable, i.e., non-A through non-E hepatitis. In these cases herpes simplex virus (HSV), cytomegalovirus (CMV), Epstein–Barr virus (EBV) and varicella zoster virus have been commonly implicated.

2.2 Toxic hepatitis

Although almost any medication or chemical can induce hepatitis in an idiosyncratic fashion, various compounds are more common in toxin-induced FHF (Table 2). Toxicity from acetaminophen (and its European cousin paracetamol) is the most common cause of drug-induced FHF. The lethal dose of acetaminophen is between 10 and 20 g. It is the metabolic products of acetaminophen rather than the parent drug that is hepatotoxic. Approximately 5% of acetaminophen is converted to *N*-acetyl-*para*-benzoquinone-imine (NAPQI) by the cytochrome P450 system. This reactive metabolite is rendered non-toxic following conjugation with hepatic glutathione, and then excreted by the kidneys. Following acetaminophen overdosage, excess NAPQI is produced and can deplete hepatic glutathione stores, allowing free NAPQI to induce hepatocellular necrosis. This scenario is enhanced by pre-existing glutathione depletion, which may occur following fasting and chronic alcohol consumption. In addition, alcohol ingestion induces a 5- to 10-fold increase in levels of cytochrome P4502E1, leading to increased NAPQI production. The underappreciated phenomenon of severe hepatotoxicity in chronic alcohol abusers who ingest even small amounts of acetaminophen has been deemed the "therapeutic misadventure" of acetaminophen [11].

Both recreational drugs such as cocaine and ecstasy and prescribed medications such as halothane, sulfonamides, and phenytoin have been implicated in acute liver failure. Mushroom poisoning due to *Amanita phalloides* can occur with very low-level ingestion, with a lethal dose of only three medium-sized mushrooms. Unfortunately, these toxins are heat stable and persist despite cooking.

2.3 Vascular

FHF has been associated with vascular disorders such as Budd–Chiari syndrome, and veno-occlusive disease in patients undergoing chemotherapy or bone marrow transplant. FHF induced by ischemic hepatitis or "shock liver" may occur in the setting of myocardial infarction, cardiomyopathy, hypotension due to any cause, or pulmonary embolism.

2.4 Miscellaneous

Acute fatty liver disease of pregnancy is an uncommon cause of FHF that occurs in the third trimester. Other rare causes of FHF include heat stroke or hyperthermia, rhabdomyolysis, sepsis, jejunoileal bypass, Reye's syndrome, and hepatic infiltration with amyloid, carcinoid, leukemia and oat cell, breast and gastric cancer.

3. CLINICAL FEATURES

The clinical features of FHF are distinct from those of chronic hepatic insufficiency. Spider angiomata, ascites and prominent abdominal venous patterns, which are characteristic of cirrhosis, are usually absent in acute liver failure. Patients typically present with non-specific malaise followed by jaundice and alteration in mental status. The progression may be rapid, occurring over hours to days.

3.1 Neurologic

Upon initial examination, the stage of encephalopathy must be carefully assessed to guide decisions regarding transplantation referral. Mental status changes can be variable and range from agitation, to delusions or hyperkinesis. While exceedingly rare in patients with end stage cirrhosis, cerebral edema with brainstem herniation is the most common cause of death in FHF [12]. It is observed in up to 80% of fatal cases at autopsy and in approximately 75–80% of patients with grade 4 hepatic encephalopathy. The cerebral edema in FHF is most likely a combination of neuronal cell injury, astrocyte hyperplasia, and vasogenic edema due to alterations in the blood–brain barrier. While the risk of cerebral edema increases with the degree of encephalopathy, standard clinical signs of increased intracranial pressure (ICP), such as the Cushing reflex and bradycardia, hypotension, pupillary dilation, posturing and central apnea, have proven unreliable as indicators of elevated ICP [13]. For instance, papilledema, an otherwise classic feature of cerebral edema, is usually absent in FHF. CT scan of the head is also an insensitive marker for cerebral edema but should be performed to exclude intracranial hemorrhage or other causes of altered mentation.

3.2 Coagulopathy

Bleeding is the direct cause of death in up to one-third of patients with FHF. Several factors predispose to bleeding in FHF. The PT and PTT are elevated due to diminished Factor II, V, VII, and IX production, and a bleeding diathesis is exacerbated by low-grade systemic fibrinolysis and disseminated intravascular coagulation. Thrombocytopenia, which may occur due to increased consumption or bone marrow suppression, correlates better with the risk of a gastrointestinal bleed rather than the degree of coagulopathy, which can often be profound.

3.3 Infections

Bacterial and fungal infections occur frequently in patients with FHF. In a recent report, 40 of 50 consecutive patients with FHF developed culture-proven bacterial infection, and 16 of 50 developed fungal infection, which was associated with concomitant bacterial infection in the presence of renal failure [14]. A study at Kings College found that 80% of patients admitted with FHF eventually developed infections, but that only 26.4% of these were identified by bacteremia. Furthermore, fever and leukocytosis were absent in 30% of the cases. Susceptibility to infection is likely multi-factorial, related to polymorphonuclear and Kupffer cell dysfunction, impaired opsonization, and complement deficiency in the setting of liver failure. This is exacerbated by frequent instrumentation for invasive monitoring, use of H2 receptor antagonists or proton pump inhibitors, steroids, and TPN. The most common sources of infection are the lungs, and urine, with Gram-positive cocci (staphylococcus and streptococcus) isolated most often from cultures.

3.4 Renal

Olguria occurs in up to one half of patients with FHF due to hepatorenal syndrome often in combination with acute tubular necrosis (ATN). ATN may be secondary to hemodynamic changes associated with infection or hypovolemia, or due to toxic metabolites resulting from acetaminophen or hydrocarbon ingestion.

3.5 Metabolic

FHF is associated with multiple metabolic complications. Hypoglycemia is an ominous sign that reflects impaired gluconeogenesis and hepatic insulin uptake. Both hypokalemia from respiratory alkalosis or hyperkalemia from renal decompensation may occur. Dilutional hyponatremia and hypophosphatemia occur commonly in FHF, although hypophosphatemia due to rapid hepatocellular phosphate uptake to replenish ATP may portend a good prognosis.

3.6 Cardiovascular

Cardiovascular abnormalities are common in FHF and require careful attention. Hemodynamic parameters in patients with FHF are similar to patients with systemic immune response syndrome, manifested as relative hypotension in the setting of increased cardiac output and decreased systemic vascular resistance. This syndrome may be accompanied by peripheral shunting, abnormal vasomotor tone, and plugging of small vessels by platelet plugs. Decreased tissue extraction of O_2 over a wide range of delivery can lead to hypoxia and resultant lactic acidosis indicating a poor prognosis. In patients who receive overly vigorous volume resuscitation and blood product transfusions, volume overload and adult respiratory distress syndrome can result, especially in the setting of renal dysfunction or multi-organ failure.

4. DIAGNOSIS

In patients who present with jaundice, decreased mentation, and coagulopathy, a prompt, well-orchestrated evaluation is required to identify and potentially treat the conditions responsible for FHF. In general, precipitating factors should be assessed including risk factors for hepatitis, and the use of prescription and non-prescription compounds, especially those recently initiated.

4.1 Blood tests

Blood and urine toxicology screen, including acetaminophen level, should be performed in all patients with suspicion of hepatocellular injury, especially when any suspicion of intentional or unintentional harmful ingestion is present. Serology for hepatotropic viruses should be checked including IgM antibody to HAV, CMV, EBV, HSV, and HDV (when hepatitis B is present). Hepatitis B surface antigen and core antibody IgM and PCR for HCV RNA should be assessed. The evaluation of autoimmune hepatitis requires serum anti-nuclear antibody and anti-smooth muscle antibody. Serum ceruloplasmin levels with ophthalmologic evaluation for Kayser–Fleischer rings should be determined if Wilson's disease is suspected, though these may be absent in the setting of FHF. In preparation for possible liver transplantation, antibody to HIV and ABO blood typing should be determined (Figure 1).

4.2 Imaging studies

In patients who present with FHF, an abdominal ultrasound with Doppler studies should be performed. This test, which can be performed at the patient's bedside, allows prompt evaluation of hepatic parenchyma and patency of the hepatic vasculature including hepatic artery and vein, and portal vein. Computed tomography offers little advantage and requires intravenous contrast which may be associated with significant renal insufficiency in this patient population even when renal function is initially normal.

4.3 Pathological studies

Biopsy is seldom performed in FHF due to coagulopathy. It is rarely informative, as it usually reveals massive hepatocellular necrosis with collapse of lobular architecture and adds little to determining the etiology of FHF if blood testing is inconclusive. However, in the setting of subfulminant liver failure, we have found liver biopsy performed by the transjugular route to be useful to determine

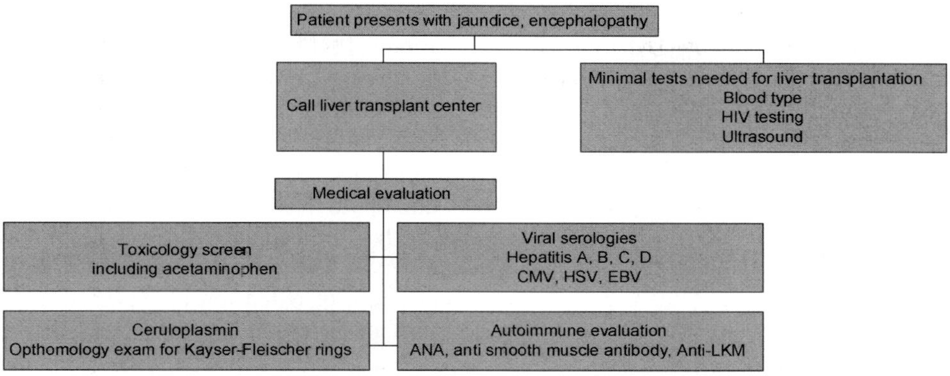

Figure 1. Flowsheet for evaluation of FHF. (*For colored version, see Plate XXX on page 580 at the end of the book.*)

prognosis, as patients with submassive necrosis in this setting will often not improve without liver transplantation. Patients without submassive necrosis will usually improve though cholestasis can be prolonged.

5. MANAGEMENT

5.1 General measures

The most important aspects of management of FHF are recognizing the condition, determining severity, and contacting an institution with the ability to perform liver transplantation or other liver directed therapies (see below). In general, appropriate management of patients with FHF requires ICU care, accurate assessment of central venous pressure, oxygenation, and strict attention to volume status. A specific "organ-system" approach to management with attention toward detecting the manifestations and complications of FHF is essential.

5.2 Central nervous system

5.2.1 Hepatic encephalopathy

As previously stated, the onset of hepatic encephalopathy defines FHF. The treatment of hepatic encephalopathy is controversial; some investigators recommend the use of lactulose, while others decry its usefulness, due to potential negative impact on electrolytes, increased abdominal distension in the presence of ileus, and lack of effect on progressive hepatic coma. In general, lactulose may improve Stage I or II encephalopathy, but should be avoided when patients reach Stage III–IV (see Table 4). In addition, when Stage III encephalopathy is reached, patients should be intubated to manage the airway and prevent aspiration.

During the early stages of FHF, alteration in mentation parallels liver dysfunction and aids in establishing prognosis. Thus, artificially altering mentation with sedating medication should be

Table 4. Stages of hepatic encephalopathy.

Stage	Mental status	Physical exam
I	Euphoria/depression, day–night sleep reversal, poor concentration, mild confusion, slurred speech	Mild asterixis
II	Increased drowsiness, confusion, inability to sustain concentration	Significant asterixis, brisk reflexes
III	Marked confusion, arousable but sleeping continuously	Asterixis, clonus
IV	Minimally responsive to painful stimuli	Patient may "posture" to pain; asterixis absent

avoided. This can often be unintentional, especially with the use of antiemetics with sedating side effects in the setting of acetaminophen ingestion; we prefer the use of serotonin antagonists (e.g., odensetron) for this indication. However, when encephalopathy is associated with agitation, it may be necessary in the interest of effective patient care to provide sedation with a short acting benzodiazepine, especially when agitation is associated with rising ICP.

5.2.2 Cerebral edema

Cerebral edema with elevated ICP is a common finding in patients with FHF who do not spontaneously recover. Sustained elevation in ICP and decreased cerebral perfusion pressures (CPP = mean arterial pressure − ICP) in the peri-operative period are often associated with irreversible neurologic injury following liver transplantation [15]. Though it can be challenging, exquisite attention must be given to diagnosing, monitoring and treating cerebral edema and intracranial hypertension in the setting of FHF. This should be undertaken in an ICU with specific expertise in the management of FHF. Many liver transplantation centers rely on continuous monitoring of ICP/CPP via direct (epidural transducer) or indirect (transcranial Doppler) measurements, thus facilitating proper recognition of diminished CPP, and permitting more prompt treatment as well as avoiding transplantation in those patients who are not likely to recover neurologically. Of additional importance is the ability to treat intra-operative changes in CPP which invariably occur during the liver transplantation procedure itself.

The management of patients with increased ICP and decreased CPP requires an approach directed at minimizing factors that exacerbate ICP elevation, treating diminution of CPP, and recognizing when these efforts are futile. Most importantly, urgent liver transplantation should be performed prior to the development of persistent intracranial hypertension and irreversible neurologic damage, as therapies to effectively control intracranial hypertension in FHF are limited. When patients reach Stage III encephalopathy in the setting of FHF, they should be intubated and cautiously sedated. Patient disturbances and overstimulation should be avoided and auditory disturbances and unnecessary physical contact should be minimized. When ICP changes occur, a sequential approach with a goal to maintain CPP > 40–50 mm Hg and ICP < 30–40 mm Hg should be initiated. The head of the patients' bed should be elevated to 20° above horizontal, in an attempt to decrease ICP. Head elevation greater than 20° has been reported to increase ICP and decrease CPP. In addition, it is important to avoid flexion, rotation, or extension of the head as ICP elevation may occur secondary to decreased cerebral venous return. Of equal importance is maintaining euvolemia as hypovolemia may diminish cerebral perfusion, and hypervolemia with resultant elevation in mean arterial pressure may elevate ICP via the phenomenon of cerebral "luxury-perfusion".

If these measures are unsuccessful, hyperventilation to achieve a pCO_2 of 30 mm Hg is often instituted. Unfortunately, the effect of this intervention is short-lived, but may be useful to transiently decrease ICP. Other modalities which may be used to diminish ICP include the use of intravenous mannitol (0.5–1 g/kg given over 5 min) in patients with normal renal function, with careful attention to avoid increasing the serum osmolarity to greater than 310 mOsm, and, finally, in cases where the above modalities are ineffective, pentobarbitol to induce coma (5 mg/kg iv followed by 1–3 mg/kg/h). Pentobarbitol must be given carefully as it may be associated with a concomitant decrease in systemic blood pressure and ICP, and thus less effect on CPP. Continuous EEG monitoring has been used by many centers as a mechanism to guide pentobarbitol treatment as it may assist in the identification of seizure activity.

Emerging therapies for neurologic complications of FHF are being actively investigated. Some investigators have proposed that benzodiazepine-like substances with GABA-like activity may contribute to cerebral edema in FHF. Support for this hypothesis is obtained from animal studies, which reveal elevated levels of endogenous benzodiazepine in FHF. Human studies in patients treated with the benzodiazepine antagonist flumazenil have revealed transient improvements in coma grade in encephalopathic patients. Most recently, hypothermia has been studied in the treatment of intracranial hypertension.

In an animal model of FHF, mild hypothermia to less than 35°C resulted in decreased CSF lactate, ammonia and glutamate levels, and delayed the onset of encephalopathy and cerebral edema. However, serum ammonia levels were unaffected. This suggests that brain edema may be the consequence of ammonia-induced impairment of cerebral metabolism and hypothermia may inhibit the transfer of ammonia across the blood–brain barrier. In human studies, hypothermia (32°C) induced lowering of ICP by improving cerebral blood flow autoregulation and restored responsiveness to carbon dioxide.

In theory, the above-listed modalities to treat abnormal ICP and CPP in the setting of FHF would appear effective, but in practice, these measures are often ineffective or transiently effective. It is therefore apparent that if not contraindicated, liver transplantation or attempts at liver replacement therapy (see below) should be pursued urgently in patients with FHF and worsening mentation, before the development of changes in ICP and CPP.

5.3 Respiratory

The respiratory support of a patient with FHF requires that the patient be able to protect their airway and handle secretions. When deepening encephalopathy develops, intubation is required to protect the airway, provide pulmonary toilette, and to prevent uncontrolled respiratory failure. Aspiration and pneumonitis with respiratory failure are frequent contraindications to liver transplantation. Maintenance of adequate oxygenation may require positive end expiratory pressure, but should be used judiciously due to associated decreases in cardiac output and hepatic blood flow.

5.4 Cardiovascular

In patients with FHF, attention to hemodynamic parameters and maintenance of a euvolemic state is vital. Reduction in cardiac output, intravascular volume, and tissue oxygen delivery may exacerbate acidosis and diminish cerebral perfusion, while hypervolemia with resultant elevation in mean arterial pressure may elevate ICP via the phenomenon of cerebral "luxury-perfusion". The goal should be to maximize cardiac output while avoiding fluid overload. Inotropic agents may improve cardiac output but decrease peripheral O_2 delivery. In this setting, the prophylactic addition of renal dose dopamine may serve a beneficial role by dilating the microvasculature. The requirement for hemodynamic monitoring must be tempered by the risks of intravascular placement of the monitoring device in a coagulopathic patient. Generally, central venous pressure monitoring is as useful as pulmonary artery pressure monitoring and may suffice in the absence of marked hypotension and oliguria. Increasingly, some transplant centers have utilized non-invasive modalities to monitor and maximize hemodynamic parameters including transcutaneous or transesophageal echocardiography.

5.5 Nutrition

Critically ill patients with liver failure may require significant protein supplementation, ranging from 1.5 to 4.0 g/kg/day. A reasonable approach which balances the requirement to provide adequate calories against the possible risk of exacerbating hepatic encephalopathy would be to give a standard amount of protein (1.0 g/kg/day) initially and modify protein intake depending on the clinical course. The optimal route of nutritional support has not been studied in patients with FHF. However, as in other critically ill patients, enteral nutrition appears to be associated with a better outcome by decreasing the incidence of infectious complications. In patients in coma, airway intubation with transpyloric placement of a nasoduodenal feeding tube may diminish the risk of aspiration.

Hypoglycemia is common in patients with progressive FHF, likely due to the rapid loss of glycogen stores associated with massive liver necrosis. Frequent determinations of blood glucose levels are required, with prompt institution of intravenous dextrose replacement using 5, 10, or 50% dextrose solution intravenously if blood glucose levels are below 150 mg/dl.

5.6 Infection

The serious ramifications of sepsis in the setting of FHF require a vigilant approach with routine chest

X-rays, as well as surveillance urine, blood, sputum and wound cultures. In addition to caring for patients with strict aseptic technique for all urinary catheters and IV lines, many transplant centers institute "prophylactic" antibiotics when patients reach Stage III coma and are intubated. A reasonable approach would be to begin therapy with either an extended penicillin (piperacillin/tazobactam, ampicillin/sulbactam) or a quinolone (or aztreonam if penicillin allergic), and vancomycin for Gram-positive coverage. If bacteremia, renal failure, an unexplained deterioration in liver function, fever or leukocytosis occurs, and/or a patient remains in FHF while on broad spectrum antibiotics for more than 24–48 h, intravenous anti-fungal agents (usually fluconazole or itraconazole due to the lack of nephrotoxicity) should be initiated.

5.7 Renal

The management of renal dysfunction in the setting of FHF requires maintenance of a euvolemic state, optimizing cardiac output, maximizing renal perfusion and avoiding potentially nephrotoxic agents. "Renal dose" dopamine at 2–4 μg/kg/min may increase renal perfusion, natriuresis and water excretion but is generally ineffective as hepatic failure progresses. In this circumstance, renal replacement therapy is mandatory.

"Traditional" hemodialysis is a widely available modality, which has limited efficacy in the setting of renal failure induced by FHF. Both hypotension and refractory elevations of ICP with resultant cerebral edema have been associated with the use of hemodialysis in FHF. Continuous renal replacement therapy using veno-venous hemodialysis minimizes hemodynamic instability, changes in ICP, and cerebral edema when compared to standard hemodialysis and is the preferred modality for fluid removal [16].

5.8 Gastrointestinal

Bleeding from the upper gastrointestinal tract is a common problem in patients with FHF. The coagulopathy inherent to liver failure, exacerbated by thrombocytopenia likely has an additive effect in inducing this phenomenon. An approach designed to maintain intra-gastric contents at a pH > 5 using an H2 receptor antagonist or proton pump inhibitor should be instituted.

5.9 Hematologic complications

Despite the often-profound coagulopathic state in FHF, treatment with FFP should not be instituted unless an invasive procedure is planned or active bleeding is present, as spontaneous changes in prothrombin time (or INR) are helpful in predicting hepatocellular recovery (see Section 6).

5.10 Specific pharmacologic therapy of FHF

5.10.1 Glucocorticoids

Although the use of glucocorticoids in FHF has a historic precedent, their use was not found beneficial in controlled trials and may be potentially deleterious due to the high incidence of sepsis. The use of steroids should be restricted to patients with a high suspicion of autoimmune FHF and should be discontinued promptly in the absence of clear therapeutic benefit.

5.10.2 N-Acetylcysteine

N-Acetylcysteine is an accepted, efficacious therapy in acetaminophen toxicity as it repletes glutathione stores and provides a sulfhydryl group to bind the toxic by-product of acetaminophen metabolism, NAPQI. *N*-Acetylcysteine may be given by mouth or intravenously, although the sterile preparation is presently not FDA approved for intravenous use in the United States. Historically, the determination of toxic acetaminophen levels and need for treatment were based upon the quantity of drug consumed and the timing of the ingestion as charted in the Rumack–Matthew nomogram. However, this approach has not been validated for patients with chronic ingestions or consumption in association with ethanol abuse. As such, many centers recommend therapy with *N*-acetylcysteine irrespective of blood levels of acetaminophen. The recommended dose of *N*-acetylcysteine is the "72 h" regimen based on a 1988 national multicenter study, with a loading dose of 140 mg/kg followed by 17 doses (70 mg/kg) every 4 h by mouth [17]. Any dose that is vomited within 1 h of administration should be repeated.

The accepted timing of administration of *N*-acetylcysteine is within 8 h of acetaminophen ingestion, although benefit may be derived as late as 24 h after ingestion. Benefit has also been reported for patients who developed encephalopathy and other signs of hepatocellular dysfunction more than 24 h following ingestion. Multiple favorable effects from therapy with NAC have been reported, irrespective of the cause of FHF, including improvement in cerebral blood flow, oxygen metabolism and transport, and cardiovascular hemodynamics. These beneficial effects may also accrue in non-acetaminophen induced FHF and is currently under study.

5.10.3 *S*-Adenosylmethionine

S-Adenosylmethionine (SAMe) has been shown in an animal model to increase hepatic glutathione levels and may be theoretically beneficial in the setting of acetaminophen-induced hepatotoxicity. The *in vitro* protective effect of SAMe against the effect of various cytokines may imply that this agent affords "hepatoprotection" in the setting of sepsis as well as FHF.

5.10.4 *Antiviral agents*

The use of antiviral agents in the setting of FHF induced by viral infection makes intuitive sense. There is evidence that herpes simplex hepatitis (Type I or II), which may have a fulminant course during pregnancy, can be successfully treated with acyclovir. In the setting of FHF induced by HBV infection, treatment with lamivudine is often instituted as a mechanism to prevent continued HBV replication, which may diminish rates of post-transplant recurrent HBV. However, antiviral regimens for hepatitis B and C have no established benefit in the setting of FHF.

5.10.5 *Prostaglandin E_1*

Prostaglandin E_1 (PGE_1) is a potent vasodilator, has antiplatelet and fibrinolytic activity, provides cytoprotection in response to injury, inhibits T-cell mediated cytotoxicity, and may improve cerebral oxygen metabolism. Despite reports of 71% survival in patients treated with PGE in the setting of viral-associated FHF, subsequent randomized controlled trials have not demonstrated any overall benefit, although some data suggest a role in the early treatment of drug- or toxin-induced FHF. The use of prostaglandin remains contentious and is generally not recommended pending more conclusive studies.

5.10.6 *Insulin–glucagon*

In animal studies, insulin and glucagon administration was noted to enhance liver regeneration and thus, human trials designed to determine the benefit of this therapy in FHF have been attempted. Unfortunately, no survival benefit was noted in treated patients, and given the concomitant risks of hypoglycemia, insulin–glucagon infusions have been discouraged as a treatment option.

5.10.7 *Liver replacement therapy*

In patients with FHF who do not have spontaneous recovery of hepatocellular function, mortality rates are uniformly high. In this patient population, contemplation must be given to "liver replacement" prior to the development of deleterious complications of FHF. Historically, blood "detoxification" was attempted in individuals suffering from FHF via exchange transfusions, hemo- and peritoneal dialysis, plasmapheresis, and charcoal hemoperfusion. However, direct contact between sorbents and plasma proteins had the undesired effect of removing vital hormones, clotting factors and immunoglobulins, compromising any potential improvement in hepatic function. The lack of success of these modalities initiated a search for a true "liver replacement" technique that would allow blood detoxification and provide products of hepatocellular metabolism.

5.10.8 *Orthotopic liver transplantation*

Orthotopic liver transplantation (OLT) is clearly an effective therapy in patients with FHF who do not spontaneously recover. Carefully selected patients may achieve greater than 90% 1-year survival rate [18]. Clear contraindications to emergency OLT in the setting of FHF include uncontrolled sepsis, uncorrectable metabolic acidosis, multiorgan failure, refractory hypotension, and cerebral perfusion pressure persistently less than 40 mm Hg. Relative contraindications include portal or mesenteric vascular thrombosis, a history of active substance abuse, and a previous psychiatric history, especially in the setting of a suicide attempt.

The major limitation of OLT as a modality in FHF is the constraint of organ availability. Although patients with FHF receive "highest status" and an expedited search for a suitable donor organ occurs, one-third to one-half of patients die or develop contraindications while waiting. Liver transplantation with donors of different ABO blood groups and auxiliary or partial liver transplants have been reported with varying success. However, alternatives to cadaveric liver transplantation or modalities to enhance both spontaneous liver recovery and hepatocellular function while awaiting liver transplantation hold the most promise and are actively being investigated.

5.10.9 Living donor liver transplantation

Living donor liver transplant (LDLT) allows placement of a partial graft "procured" from a living adult donor with a compatible blood type and a significant personal relationship to the recipient. The majority of emergency LDLT in the US has been performed in children with FHF [19]. The theoretic advantage of this technique for adults with FHF includes decreased waiting time for a cadaveric liver and the ability to perform transplantation prior to the onset of complications including sepsis and cerebral edema. The clear limitations to adult-to-adult LDLT include the inability to quickly identify and optimally evaluate an appropriate donor, and the risk to both the donor and recipient; the 60% hepatectomy required to acquire an appropriately sized liver graft may be associated with significant morbidity, and, the potential for graft dysfunction or "small-for-size syndrome" due to an inappropriately sized graft in the recipient. The use of LDLT in adults with FHF is in evolution, and needs to be evaluated in carefully constructed trials.

5.10.10 Xenograft transplantation

The use of organs from non-human species (xenografts) for liver transplantation in the setting of FHF has multiple theoretical advantages. The large reservoir of potential donor organs would obviate the requirement and complications attendant to waiting for an appropriate human donor organ. However, the immunologic barrier to xenotransplantation is significant making it a difficult clinical challenge to realize. Through genetic engineering, it is hoped that "designer" or transgenic animals raised in a germ-free environment with fewer antigens to minimize immunologic recognition by humans will be available in the future, enhancing the success of xenografts as donor organs.

5.10.11 Bioartificial liver

The concept of liver dialysis to provide blood detoxification (non-biologic) and/or hepatocellular synthetic (biologic) support is attractive. Biologic devices that contain either porcine (bioartificial liver or BAL from Circe, Lexington, MA) or transformed human cells, C3A hepatoblastoma cells (extracorporeal liver assist device or ELAD from VitaGen, LaJolla, CA) are in clinical trials. In addition, non-biologic systems, such as the molecular absorbent recirculation system (MARS), which removes protein-bound molecules with countercurrent dialysis against an albumin gradient, are being investigated.

The efficacy and safety of the BAL (Circe, Lexington, MA) was evaluated in a prospective, randomized, controlled multicenter trial of FHF patients in Stages III or IV hepatic encephalopathy. The primary end point was 30-day survival with or without liver transplantation. 146 patients with FHF were included. Overall survival was improved in treated patients vs. controls (73 vs. 59%) but the difference was statistically insignificant ($p = 0.12$). Survival with transplantation was 89 vs. 80%, and 50 vs. 38% without transplantation, when comparing treated to untreated patients. When controlling for the impact of transplantation using a covariate time-dependent proportional hazard model, treatment with the BAL was associated with a 41% reduction in mortality (0.59 RR, $p = 0.068$) particularly in patients with viral infection or chemical/drug toxicity as a precipitant of FHF (0.35 RR, $p = 0.0082$). This has been the largest trial of artificial liver support for FHF to date, and provides preliminary evidence of the efficacy of these devices. This data needs to be confirmed in a second trial, which is in the planning stages.

In a recent Phase I study of the ELAD, 25 patients with acute liver failure and Stage II–IV coma were randomized in a 2:1 ratio to treatment with the ELAD vs. control. Survival was 63% in the ELAD treated group compared to 55% in controls. 81% of treated vs. 56% of untreated patients were successfully "bridged" to transplant or recovery. The ELAD treatments were well tolerated and a larger Phase II trial has been initiated.

Since its first use in 1993, over 800 patients have been treated with MARS. While the majority of treated patients were those with acute exacerbation of chronic liver disease, MARS has been studied in acute liver failure, primary graft dysfunction following liver transplantation, liver trauma and cholestatic syndromes. A preliminary study in 17 patients with acute liver failure has demonstrated a significant reduction of serum ammonia, bilirubin, bile acids, with improvement in hepatic coma grade. Survival in this uncontrolled study was 71% with 24% spontaneous recovery and 8 out of 17 patients went on to undergo liver transplantation. This encouraging data needs to be confirmed in a multi-center controlled trial.

These results are encouraging, but true "liver-replacement" therapy akin to hemodialysis has not yet been achieved using these devices. However, these systems may play a vital role as a bridge to liver transplantation, or support the patient until spontaneous liver recovery is possible.

5.10.12 Hepatocyte transplantation

In recent years, interest in the transplantation of cryopreserved hepatocytes has risen. This technique has multiple theoretical benefits for correcting metabolic deficiencies arising from genetic disorders and both chronic and acute liver disease. Hepatocyte transplantation is achieved by direct implantation into the spleen, liver or other site, or alternatively, by infusion via the splenic or hepatic artery or portal vein. Success with this technique in animals has led to small studies in humans. A recent report cited encouraging results following hepatocyte transplantation in humans with FHF. Following hepatocyte transplantation, metabolic and neurologic improvement was noted, and several patients were successfully bridged to liver transplantation. Various issues regarding hepatocyte transplantation in FHF remain unresolved including the number of cells required, site of implantation, and whether hepatocytes or stem cells should be used. Although this technique is in its infancy, it holds much promise as a potential treatment for both chronic and acute liver disease.

6. PROGNOSIS

The "art" of managing patients with FHF is to predict the outcome of the disease process, and appropriately intervene when it is anticipated that spontaneous recovery is not imminent. Multiple models have been developed to assist in this decision-making process, however, to date, etiology of FHF remains the single most important criterion in assessing prognosis. In a recent report, it was noted that although acetaminophen toxicity was the most common cause of FHF, the majority of these patients recovered spontaneously without the requirement for liver transplantation, while the requirement for liver transplantation was significantly greater in patients with FHF due to Wilson's disease, cryptogenic, also known as non-A, non-B, non-C or sero-negative hepatitis, hepatitis B, or autoimmune hepatitis [7].

In addition to determining the etiology of FHF as a mechanism to predict outcome, other methods to determine prognosis have been adopted. The Kings College Criteria reported by O'Grady and colleagues in 1989 has been found useful as a method to predict which patients with FHF will die without liver transplantation (Table 5) [20]. The strength of this index is that all the measured variables are easily and quickly determined, allowing a rapid decision to be made regarding prognosis. The one caveat of these criteria is that prothrombin time is expressed in British Units. Due to methodological differences in assay performance, prothrombin times are longer in Great Britain than those in the USA. This variance

Table 5. Kings College Criteria for liver transplantation (PT expressed in British units).

Acetaminophen-induced FHF	Non-acetaminophen-induced FHF
pH < 7.3	PT > 100 (INR > 7.7)
Or *all* three below	Or *any* three below
Grade III–IV encephalopathy	Age < 10 or > 40
PT > 100 (INR > 7.7)	Etiology: non-A–B, drug- or halothane-induced, Wilson's disease
Serum creatinine > 3.4 mg/dl	Jaundice to encephalopathy in >7 days
	PT > 50 (INR > 3.85)
	Bilirubin > 17 mg/dl

Adapted from Lee, W.M., Galbraith, R.M., Watt, G.H., Hughes, R.D., McIntire, D.D., Hoffman, B.J., Williams, R. *et al.* (1995) Predicting survival in fulminant hepatic failure using serum Gc protein concentration, *Hepatology* **21**(1), 101–105.

is resolved by using the international normalized ratio in place of PT.

In addition to the importance of etiology of liver failure as a method to predict prognosis, the timing of encephalopathy following the onset of jaundice has been associated with differences in survival without liver transplantation. In patients who develop encephalopathy within 7 days of jaundice, i.e., hyperacute FHF, spontaneous survival was 36%. In patients with acute FHF or encephalopathy within 8–28 days of jaundice, spontaneous survival was 14%. Most ominously, in patients with encephalopathy from 29 to 60 days following jaundice, i.e., subacute FHF, spontaneous survival was <10% (Table 1). The significantly higher survival rate in patients with hyperacute liver failure illustrates the remarkable regenerative capacity of the liver following an acute, massive insult. However, in the setting of continued injury, hepatocyte regeneration may not keep pace with hepatocyte necrosis, resulting in a poor outcome.

In general, patients who survive the acute illness induced by FHF and recover without transplantation will have full recovery of hepatocellular and neurologic function, and a normal life expectancy. A small percentage of patients with acetaminophen-induced FHF develop renal insufficiency for which a limited period of dialysis is required. In patients who develop FHF and do not spontaneously recover and subsequently undergo liver transplantation, 1- and 3-year survival rates closely parallel rates of survival in patients who undergo liver transplantation for other indications.

7. SUMMARY

The management of patients with FHF, a process associated with extensive hepatocellular injury and significant morbidity and mortality, is rapidly evolving. Improvements in understanding the pathophysiology attendant to massive hepatocellular necrosis, prompt recognition of its existence, and system directed therapies have provided improvement in survival. New therapeutic modalities which provide "liver replacement" therapy as a bridge to either liver transplantation or spontaneous recover of hepatocellular function are undergoing evaluation, and will hopefully improve outcomes. Future therapy of FHF including artificial liver support, hepatocyte transplantation, LDLT and xenotransplantation will further enhance our ability to successfully manage these exceptionally ill patients.

REFERENCES

[1] Reigler, J.L. and Lake, J. (1993) Fulminant hepatic failure. *Med. Clin. N. Am.* **77**(5), 1057–1083.

[2] Trey, C. and Davidson, C.S. (1970) The management of fulminant hepatic failure, in *Progress in Liver Diseases*, vol. 3, eds. Popper, H. and Schaffer, F. (Grune & Stratton, New York) pp. 282–298.

[3] Bernuau, J., Rueff, B. and Benhamou, J.P. (1986) Fulminant and subfulminant liver failure: definitions and causes. *Semin. Liver Dis.* **6**(2), 97–106.

[4] Lidofsky, S.D. (1993) Liver transplantation for fulminant hepatic failure. *Gastroenterol. Clin. N. Am.* **22**(2), 257–269.

[5] Lee, W.M. (1993) Medical progress: acute liver failure. *N. Engl. J. Med.* **329**, 1862–1872.

[6] Hoofnagle, J.H., Carithers, R.L., Jr., Shapiro, C., and Ascher, N. (1995) Fulminant hepatic failure: summary of a workshop. *Hepatology* **21**, 240.

[7] Schiodt, F.V., Atillasoy, E., Shakil, A.O., Schiff, E.R., Caldswell, C., Kowdley, K.V., Stribling, R., Crippen, J.S., Flamm, S., Somberg, K.A., Rosen, H., McCashland, T.M., Hay, J.E. and Lee, W.M. (1999) Etiology and outcome for 295 patients with acute liver failure in the United States. *Liver Transplant. Surg.* **5**, 29–34.

[8] Vento, S., Garofano, T., Renzini, C., Cainelli, F., Casali, F., Ghironzi, G., Ferraro, T. and Concia, E. (1998) Fulminant hepatitis associated with hepatitis A virus superinfection in patients with chronic hepatitis C. *N. Engl. J. Med.* **338**(5), 286–290.

[9] Krawczynski, K. (1993) Hepatitis E. *Hepatology* **17**, 932–941.

[10] Gordon, F.D., Anastopoulos, H., Khettry, U., Loda, M., Jenkins, R.L., Lewis, W.D., and Trey, C. (1995) Hepatitis C: a rare cause of fulminant hepatitis failure. *Am. J. Gastroenterol.* **90**(1), 117–120.

[11] Zimmerman, H.J. and Maddrey, W.C. (1995) Acetaminophen (paracetamol) hepatotoxicity with regular intake of alcohol: analysis of instances of therapeutic misadventure. *Hepatology* **22**(3), 767–773.

[12] Almal, T., Schroeder, T. and Ranek, L. (1989) Cerebral blood flow and liver function in patients with encephalopathy due to acute and chronic liver diseases. *Scand. J. Gastroenterol.* **24**, 299–303.

[13] Munoz, S.J., Robinson, M., Northrup, B., Bell, R., Moritz, M., Jarrell, B., Martin, P. and Maddrey, W.C. (1991) Elevated intracranial pressure and computed tomography of the brain in fulminant hepatocellular failure. *Hepatology* **13**, 209–212.

[14] Mutimer, D. and Elias, E. (1992) Liver transplantation for FHF, in *Progress in Liver Disease*, vol. 10, eds. Schaffer, F. and Popper, H. (Grune & Stratton, New York) pp. 349–367.

[15] Schafer, D.F. and Shaw, Jr., B.W. (1989) Fulminant hepatic failure and orthotopic liver transplantation. *Semin. Liver Dis.* **9**(3), 189–194.

[16] Kishimoto, T., Yamagami, S. and Tanaka, H. (1980) Superiority of hemofiltration to hemodialysis for treatment of chronic renal failure: comparative studies between hemofiltration and hemodialysis on dialysis disequilibrium syndrome. *J. Artif. Organs* **4**, 86.

[17] Smilkstein, M.J., Knapp, G.L., Kulig, K.W. and Rumack, B.H. (1988) Efficacy of oral *N*-acetylcysteine in the treatment of acetaminophen overdose; analysis of the national multi-center study. *N. Engl. J. Med.* **319**(24), 1557–1562.

[18] Ascher, N.L., Lake, J.R. and Roberts, J.P. (1993) Liver transplantation for fulminant hepatic failure. *Arch. Surg.* **128**(6), 677–682.

[19] Reding, R., de Goyet Jde, V., Delbeke, I., Sokal, E., Jamart, J., Janssen, M. and Otte, J.B. (1999) Pediatric liver transplantation with cadaveric or living related donors: comparative results in 90 elective recipients of primary grafts. *J. Pediatr.* **143**, 280–286.

[20] O'Grady, J., Alexander, G.J., Hayllar, K.M. and Williams, R. (1989) Early indicators of prognosis in fulminant hepatic failure. *Gastroenterology* **97**, 439–445.

Hepatology: A Practical Approach
B. Al Knawy, M.L. Shiffman, R.H. Wiesner (editors)

Chapter 21
Benign Tumors and Evaluation of Liver Masses

Mindie H. Nguyen and Emmet B. Keeffe

Division of Gastroenterology and Hepatology, Department of Medicine, Stanford University School of Medicine, Stanford, CA, USA

1. Hepatic Adenoma 332
   1.1 Epidemiology and pathogenesis 332
   1.2 Presentation and diagnosis 332
   1.3 Management and prognosis 333
   1.4 Hepatic adenomatosis 335
2. Focal Nodular Hyperplasia 335
   2.1 Epidemiology and pathogenesis 335
   2.2 Presentation and diagnosis 335
   2.3 Management and prognosis 336
   2.4 Multiple focal hyperplasia syndrome 336
3. Nodular Regenerative Hyperplasia 336
   3.1 Epidemiology and pathogenesis 336
   3.2 Presentation and diagnosis 336
   3.3 Management and prognosis 337
4. Macroregenerative Nodules 337
   4.1 Epidemiology and pathogenesis 337
   4.2 Presentation and diagnosis 337
   4.3 Management and prognosis 337
5. Hemangioma 337
   5.1 Epidemiology and pathogenesis 337
   5.2 Presentation and diagnosis 338
   5.3 Management and prognosis 338
6. Other Solid Benign Hepatic Masses 338
   6.1 Lipomatous tumors 338
   6.2 Arteriovenous fistula 339
   6.3 Inflammatory pseudotumor 339
7. Congenital Simple Cysts 339
   7.1 Epidemiology and pathogenesis 339
   7.2 Presentation and diagnosis 339
   7.3 Management and prognosis 339
   7.4 Multiple congenital cysts 339
8. Other Cystic Lesions 339
   8.1 Hydatid cysts 339
   8.2 Caroli's disease 342
   8.3 Peliosis hepatis 342
   8.4 Biliary cystadenoma 342
9. Evaluation of Liver Masses 342
References 342

Benign focal liver lesions are common and increasingly being encountered as incidental findings in patients who undergo ultrasound (US), computed tomography (CT) or magnetic resonance imaging (MRI) for unrelated problems. They may be cystic or solid and arise from a number of different cellular origins. Cystic liver lesions are usually benign while solid hepatic tumors include a variety of benign and malignant neoplasms. It is crucial to correctly classify a hepatic lesion as benign or malignant. It is also important to recognize the different types of benign hepatic tumors, such as hepatic adenoma due to its propensity to rupture leading to life-threatening hemoperitoneum. In addition, certain benign tumors such as hepatic adenoma or macroregenerative nodular hyperplasia (MRN) have the potential to transform into malignant tumors. This chapter will discuss several types of benign hepatic lesions commonly encountered by medical practitioners. Other less important or rare benign hepatic lesions can be found in Table 1 [1–3]. A list of primary and metastatic malignant tumors of the liver provides an important reference for evaluating hepatic masses and is provided in Table 2 [4,5].

1. HEPATIC ADENOMA

1.1 Epidemiology and pathogenesis

Hepatic adenoma or liver cell adenoma is a rare benign condition but one that must be identified and treated promptly due to risk of hemorrhage and malignant transformation. It is most often seen in young women with a history of years of oral contraceptive use [3]. The incidence of hepatic adenoma is about 1 per million in women without a history of oral contraceptive use and was little known prior to 1960 [6]. The incidence increases to 30–40 per million in women who have used oral contraceptive for many years. Hepatic adenomas also occur in men with long-term androgen or anabolic steroid use or in patients with various metabolic disorders such as Type I glycogen storage disease (von Gierke). Sporadic adenomas can also occur but are very rare. One recent case series from Taiwan also reported a higher prevalence of adenoma in men as compared to women, even though there was no history of long-term steroid use in these affected male patients [7].

The pathogenesis of hepatic adenomas is not well understood; however, they seem to be derived from a single clone of proliferative hepatocytes [1]. Alterations in expression of cadherin, a membrane glycoprotein mediating cell–cell adhesion associated with various neoplasia, have been observed in hepatic adenomas.

1.2 Presentation and diagnosis

Patients with hepatic adenomas may be asymptomatic, and tumors are detected on routine physical examination if they are large or as incidental findings on imaging studies [8]. About a quarter of patients

Table 1. Benign lesions of the liver.

Solid lesions	Cystic lesions
Hepatocellular origin	*Cholangiocellular origin*
Hepatocellular adenoma/hepatic adenomatosis[a]	Solitary congenital hepatic cysts[a]
Focal nodular hyperplasia[a]	Congenital hepatic fibrosis/polycystic liver disease/Von
Nodular regenerative hyperplasia[a]	*Meyenburg complexes*[a]
Macroregenerative nodule[a]	Biliary cystadenoma
Mesenchymal origin	Caroli's disease
Hemangioma[a]	*Others*
Lipoma/angiomyolipoma	Peliosis hepatis
Others: hamartoma, fibroma, leiomyoma, lymphagioma	Hydatid cysts
Heterotopic tissue	
Adrenal rests or pancreatic rests	

[a] The more common and/or important benign liver lesions.

Table 2. Malignant neoplasms of the liver.

Primary tumors	Metastatic tumors
Tumors of hepatocellular origin	50% of patients with a primary tumors will eventually have metastases to the liver. Some of the tumors which commonly metastasize to the liver include
Hepatocellular carcinoma[a]	Colorectal carcinoma
Hepatoblastoma	Breast cancer
Tumors of cholangiocellular origin	Lung cancer
Cholangiocarcinoma[a]	Urogenital cancers
Biliary cystadenocarcinoma	Gastrointestinal stromal tumors
Tumors of mesenchymal origin	Other primary gastrointestinal cancers (pancreas, stomach, gallbladder)
Epitheliod hemangioendothelioma	Neuroendocrine tumors
Primary hepatic angiosarcoma	
Primary hepatic lymphoma	
Various other rare types (fibrosarcoma, leiomyosarcoma, etc.)	

[a] The more common and/or important types of primary liver cancers.

have mild and ill-defined epigastric pain. Those with severe pain may have infarction or bleeding into the tumor, or acute hemoperitoneum due to rupture of the tumor. Most hepatic adenomas are fairly large and tend to be subcapsular and spontaneous rupture with catastrophic bleeding is therefore not an uncommon presentation for this disease [1]. The other feared complication of hepatic adenomas is malignant transformation, though this is a rare event [3].

In patients with hepatic adenoma, serum alpha-fetoprotein (AFP) and liver function tests are invariably normal. Diagnosis is made by imaging studies and histologic examination. Macroscopically, most adenomas are round, subcapsular masses without true capsules, range 5–15 cm in diameter, and have large vessels coursing along the outer rim of the tumors [3]. Deeply located and pedunculated adenomas have been described but are uncommon. Microscopically, adenomas consist of sheet-like hepatic cords with compressed sinusoids and normal nuclear:cytoplasmic ratio, an important diagnostic criterion.

On US, adenomas may be hypoechoic or hyperechoic [6,9]. Hemorrhage or calcification associated with necrosis may appear hyperechoic. Though most adenomas are not specifically diagnosed by US, color Doppler US sometimes provides useful clues to help differentiate adenomas from focal nodular hyperplasia (FNH). On color Doppler US, peripheral peritumoral and intratumoral vessels of adenomas typically have a flat continuous or less commonly triphasic waveform which is absent in FNH. Multiphasic CT and MRI allow more specific characterization of adenomas. On unenhanced, portal-venous phase or delayed-phase images, adenomas are nearly isoattenuating relative to surrounding normal liver (hyperattenuating in fatty liver). Hemorrhage can be identified during these phases. During early arterial phase, peripheral enhancement may be seen reflecting the presence of the large subcapsular feeding vessels and centripetal penetrating vessels. On T1-weighted MR images, adenomas are typically bright though they can also be isointense or hypointense. Adenomas are also predominantly hyperintense on T2-weighted images. Comparative features of hepatic adenoma and other common benign hepatic masses are summarized in Table 3.

1.3 Management and prognosis

The natural history and prognosis of hepatic adenomas are not well established. While some adenomas remain stable in size and others regress with discontinuation of estrogen use, the risk of hemorrhage and malignant transformation are the basis for consideration of a more aggressive approach with surgical resection [6,8]. Some have advocated a conservative approach with hormonal withdrawal, serial radiologic examinations and serum AFP to screen for hepatocellular carcinoma (HCC), especially in small isolated adenomas [10]. Laparoscopic surgery offers the alternative of a less invasive

Table 3. Clinical characteristics of more common benign liver lesions and HCC.

Lesions	Prevalence[a]	Gender	Malignant potential	Presentations
Hemangioma	3–20%	F > M	No	Usually asymptomatic Rare complications with large tumors: rupture, hemorrhage, Kasaback–Merritt syndrome
Simple cysts	3.6%	F > M	No	Usually asymptomatic Rare complications with large cysts: hemorrhage, infection
Biliary cystadenoma	Rare	F > M	Yes	Usually asymptomatic
Hepatic adenoma	Rare (<0.001%)	F > M	Yes	Can be asymptomatic Common: rupture and hemorrhage
FNH	Up to 3%	F > M	No or very rare	Usually asymptomatic Rupture and hemorrhage: very rare
NRH[b]	2.6%	–	Yes	Usually asymptomatic Complications: portal hypertension with relatively preserved liver synthetic function
MRN[b]	10.8% (cirrhosis)	–	Yes	Usually asymptomatic Symptoms from underlying liver disease
HCC	Depends on underlying liver disease	M > F	Malignant	Usually asymptomatic in early stages Variable symptoms in later stages (pain, weight loss, liver failure, etc.)

[a] Prevalence from various reports. Exact prevalence is not known for most of these conditions.
[b] Radiographic features of these lesions are nonspecific.

surgical approach to the management of small solid hepatic tumors and favorable results were reported from a few small case series [11,12]. Hepatic arterial embolization can be an effective option in the management of acute hemorrhage in an adenoma [6].

1.4 Hepatic adenomatosis

Hepatic adenomatosis is a rare subset of hepatic adenomas characterized by more than four adenomas within the liver [3]. While the imaging and histopathologic features of the individual adenomas in patients with adenomatosis are similar to those with solitary or only a few adenomas, the prognosis is more ominous and patients may have a more aggressive clinical course with symptomatic, progressive disease that often leads to impaired liver function, hemorrhage, and malignant transformation [13]. Depending on patients' symptoms as well as the size and location of adenomas, treatment options may include surgical resection, liver transplantation or observation [14].

2. FOCAL NODULAR HYPERPLASIA

2.1 Epidemiology and pathogenesis

FNH is the second most common benign lesion of the liver, next to hemangioma [1]. FNH has a prevalence of up to 3% in the general population. As in the case of hepatic adenomas, FNH is often found in young females. However, unlike hepatic adenoma, there is no clear association between oral contraceptive use and the development or progression of FNH.

The pathogenesis of FNH is not clearly understood. It is postulated that FNH may arise as a result of a congenital vascular anomaly. This theory is supported by the finding of abundant arteries in the central scar of FNH and by the high prevalence of other vascular malformation in patients with FNH. On the other hand, some investigators believe FNH may be an inherently proliferative lesion. The presence of cellular clonality as well as growth factors associated with malignancy and hyperproliferation have also been documented in FNH.

2.2 Presentation and diagnosis

FNH cases are usually asymptomatic and are often incidental findings on imaging studies performed for unrelated indications [1]. Some patients may have abdominal pain but spontaneous rupture and hemorrhage are very rare. Malignant transformation in FNH is not clearly documented and unlikely [3].

Macroscopically, FNH is usually subcapsular or exophytic, unencapsulated and usually solitary [3]. Unlike adenoma, most FNH are less than 5 cm in diameter though lesions measuring up to 17 cm have been described. The pathognomonic feature of FNH is the stellate fibrous scar in the center of the FNH nodule that radiates into nodules of hepatic parenchyma. Microscopically, this scar is composed of bile ductules and large muscular arterial vessels with muscular or intimal hyperplasia and capillaries as well as a varying number of chronic inflammatory cells such as lymphocytes, plasma cells, and histiocytes. Radiating from this dense central scar in a stellate fashion are normal-appearing hepatocytes and Kupffer cells.

Noninvasive diagnosis of FNH can be challenging because it is often difficult to differentiate FNH from hepatic adenoma, the other important benign hepatic tumor [1]. US is usually not helpful in the diagnosis of FNH as the normal hepatocytes of the FNH nodule are isodense as the surrounding normal hepatic tissue. As discussed in the last section, color Doppler may be useful in differentiating FNH from adenoma. US may also be useful in 20% of cases when the central scar can be identified. Technetium-99m (99m-Tc) colloid sulfur liver scan may aid in the diagnosis of FNH and is a test that takes advantage of the ability of FNH with its high content of Kupffer cells to take up and concentrate the radioactive-labeled colloid. However, a focal scintigraphic defect could only be observed in approximately 50% of FNH nodules in several small case series while a minority of hepatic adenomas also demonstrated differential uptake of 99m-Tc. Typical features of FNH on multiphase CT and enhanced MRI are similar and most useful diagnostic test for FNH. During arterial phase, FNH becomes hyperdense because of its hypervascularity. During the portal-venous phase, the lesion becomes isodense but the central scar with its particularly rich vasculature (as opposed to an area of necrosis or hemorrhage of hepatic adenoma) may remain enhanced. If there is still any uncertainty about the diagnosis, a tissue diagnosis is warranted.

2.3 Management and prognosis

The most important management issue regarding FNH is to be certain of the diagnosis. Incidental and asymptomatic FNH require no treatment except expectant follow-up and surgical resection when patients develop symptoms or complications such as hemorrhage or rupture [1]. One special case in the management of FNH is during pregnancy due to the concern of progression of FNH at this high-estrogen state. Limited data from small case series, however, reported no increase in tumor size or bleeding. Nevertheless, it is probably prudent to follow pregnant women with FNH with frequent serial US during and after pregnancy.

2.4 Multiple focal hyperplasia syndrome

The multiple FNH syndrome is a variant of FNH [3]. It is defined as two or more FNH lesions in combination with hepatic hemangiomas, tumors of meningeal or astrocytic origin or vascular malformation of the central nervous system. A few patients with multiple FNH nodules have also been reported to have concurrent hepatic adenoma.

3. NODULAR REGENERATIVE HYPERPLASIA

3.1 Epidemiology and pathogenesis

Nodular regenerative hyperplasia (NRH) is another cause of benign hepatic masses on imaging studies [1]. This condition tends to affect older individuals with estimated median age of 53–68 years. It is also known to be associated with several chronic medical conditions commonly found in patients of this age group such as a variety of lymphoproliferative disorders (mastocytosis, bone marrow transplantation); solid organ transplantation (renal and liver transplantation); autoimmune, rheumatologic and collagen vascular diseases (rheumatoid arthritis, Felty's syndrome, polyarteritis nodosa, amyloidosis, primary biliary cirrhosis); chemotherapy; and HCC. NRH has a variable gender distribution with a slight male predominance from one large autopsy series and a 2:1 female predominance from another. In the largest study of 2500 autopsy cases, the prevalence of NRH was 2.6%. However, only one of the 64 NRH nodules (1.5%) found at autopsy had been diagnosed clinically, suggesting that NRH itself probably has a rather benign natural history in most affected patients.

As in the case of most benign hepatic lesions, the pathogenesis of NRH is not well understood. Proposed mechanisms for the formation of NRH include a vascular hypothesis and a generalized proliferative hypothesis. The vascular hypothesis is based on the observation of portal venule phlebosclerosis by some investigators. This vascular aberrancy is hypothesized to lead to ischemia and atrophy of hepatocytes in the central zone, which in turn stimulates proliferation of hepatocytes from the surrounding areas forming NRH. The generalized proliferative hypothesis implies that NRH is composed of hyperplastic hepatocytes, which also indicates that NRH may be a premalignant lesion. There have been case reports of HCC developing in livers with NRH. A high prevalence of liver cell dysplasia (20–42%), a known premalignant condition, has also been described in NRH.

3.2 Presentation and diagnosis

The majority of NRH reported in the literature were diagnosed *postmortem* by autopsies or as incidental findings by imaging studies for unrelated causes. In the minority of patients with NRH who present with symptoms, the most common findings are hepatomegaly and splenomegaly. There may be mild and nonspecific elevated liver function tests or signs and symptoms of portal hypertension. Hepatic failure requiring liver transplantation has occurred but is a rare event. The diagnosis of NRH should therefore be suspected in patients with portal hypertension but with relatively preserved hepatic synthetic function. NRH is also associated with development of HCC.

Macroscopically, a liver with NRH appears similar to a cirrhotic liver and may be entirely replaced by regenerative nodules. Microscopically, NRH is composed of nodules of regenerating hepatocytes and occasional multinucleated cells separated by centrilobular atrophy and not by fibrous band as in the cases of cirrhosis. Radiographic features of NRH are nonspecific. It is isoechoic on US and nonenhancing and hypodense on CT. Histologic examination of NRH nodule is often necessary if definitive diagnosis is warranted. However, liver tissues obtained from needle biopsy may be almost normal in some cases and open biopsy to obtain a larger piece of liver tissue may be indicated if the suspicion for NRH is high.

3.3 Management and prognosis

In most patients, NRH nodules are clinically silent and if discovered incidentally, no specific therapy is necessary. Correct diagnosis is again key to differentiate NRH from malignant tumors or benign lesions with high propensity for complications such as hepatic adenoma. In asymptomatic cases, periodic surveillance is probably warranted due to the low but possible malignant transformation potential of NRH. In patients who present with complications of portal hypertension such as ascites or varices, appropriate therapy for those conditions is indicated. Long-term therapy of portal hypertension with portal caval shunt may be necessary in recurrent or refractory cases. Liver transplantation is an option in patients with liver failure.

4. MACROREGENERATIVE NODULES

4.1 Epidemiology and pathogenesis

MRN, also known as dysplastic nodules (DN) or adenomatous hyperplasia, are benign but premalignant lesions occurring in livers with submassive necrosis or advanced fibrosis or cirrhosis [3]. The reported prevalence of MRN is 10.8% in cases with cirrhosis and 2% in cases with submassive necrosis [5]. The epidemiology of MRN is therefore dependent on the etiology of the underlying liver disease. MRN may result from clonal expansion of neoplastic hepatocytes that are resistant to the necroinflammatory processes leading to fibrosis and cirrhosis of the remaining areas of the affected livers [3]. Clonality of liver cells within MRN and lower proliferation indices of MRN as compared to HCC and unaffected cirrhotic nodules have been described.

4.2 Presentation and diagnosis

MRN are usually discovered by imaging studies during evaluation and surveillance for HCC in patients with cirrhosis or advanced fibrosis. Standard laboratory tests reflect the etiology and severity of underlying liver disease. US and CT features of MRN are generally nonspecific. On T2-weighted MR images, MRN are hypodense and this may be a useful distinguishing feature between MRN and HCC, which typically are hyperintense on T2-weighted images and becomes enhanced during arterial phase of gadolinium injection [1,15]. On histologic examination, hepatocytes within MRN form wide hepatic cords but no greater than three cells in thickness [3]. These hepatocytes may show dysplastic features but do not meet criteria for HCC. Small cell change is a widely recognized premalignant lesion and refers to increased nuclear:cytoplasmic ratio in areas of proliferation. On the other hand, the premalignant potential of large cell change, which refers to the presence of large and hyperchromatic nuclei but with normal nuclear:cytoplasmic ratio, is still controversial. Macroscopically, MRN are usually more green or more pale and distinct from the surrounding cirrhotic liver parenchyma. Hemorrhage and necrosis may occur within larger nodules and these features often herald the development of HCC.

4.3 Management and prognosis

Although some authors may advocate for treating MRN as malignant lesions, many other investigators still recommend close clinical follow-up of patients with MRN [3]. The prognosis and management of MRN remain an area of ongoing investigation and debate.

5. HEMANGIOMA

5.1 Epidemiology and pathogenesis

Hemangioma or cavernous hemangioma is the most common benign liver lesion with a reported prevalence as high as 20% from autopsy series [1]. Prevalence by one ultrasound study is 1.4%. Most hemangiomas are diagnosed in young and middle-aged patients and are more commonly found in women. In addition, women are also more likely to have large and multiple hemangiomas. In addition, hemangioma may have accelerated growth during pregnancy and estrogen supplement.

The pathogenesis of hemangioma is not well understood. Growth of hemangioma is due to ectasia rather than hypertrophy or hyperplasia [5]. Hemangioma should be distinguished from arteriovenous fistula of the liver, which will be discussed later in this chapter.

5.2 Presentation and diagnosis

Most hepatic hemangioma present as incidental findings on imaging studies [1]. Most of these patients are asymptomatic and clinical symptoms such as abdominal pain are very rare in tumors <5 cm. Multiple hemangioma may be found in 5–10% of these patients who may also have hemangioma in other organs such as lungs, brain, or skin. Kasaback–Merritt syndrome is a rare but distinct clinical entity that is associated with giant hemangioma. Patients with this syndrome present with disseminated intravascular coagulation with abdominal pain and bleeding, usually after a surgical or dental procedure. Very rarely, larger hemangioma (usually >5 cm) may also rupture, either spontaneously or as a result of trauma, leading to catastrophic intra-abdominal hemorrhage. Other uncommon but serious clinical sequelae of hemangioma include hemobilia, portal hypertension, cystic degeneration, fluid–fluid levels, pulmonary embolus with caval thrombosis and inflammatory pseudotumors caused by recurrent intratumoral thrombosis.

Hemangiomas are usually diagnosed by characteristic radiographic features. On US, hemangioma is typically a solitary hyperechoic, round or lobular mass with encapsulated appearance and a well-demarcated border. Standard abdominal CT with contrast is unreliable for the diagnosis of hemangioma. Biphasic CT is usually required to establish the diagnosis with the most characteristic finding being globular enhancement due to puddling of contrast in dilated vascular spaces within the tumor. Technetium-labeled red blood cell single photon emission tomographic (SPECT) scanning may be used as a confirmatory test for findings obtained from US or CT. SPECT is an insensitive test and not as specific for small hemangioma as MRI, the best and most expensive imaging study for hemangioma with sensitivity and specificity between 85 and 95%. Cytologic or histologic examination of hemangioma using fine-needle aspiration or biopsy is sometimes necessary for diagnostic confirmation when radiographic features are atypical. No hemorrhage or rupture was reported with fine-needle aspiration of hemangioma from three case series with a total of 64 patients.

5.3 Management and prognosis

Most hemangiomas are asymptomatic and complications are rare with small lesions. Treatment is not indicated for asymptomatic cases though follow-up with annual imaging study is prudent. Asymptomatic patients with giant hemangioma >10 cm should be monitored closely and surgical resection may be advisable, especially in younger patients, due to risks of serious complications. Symptomatic, enlarging or massive hemangioma (>15 cm) should be treated with resection. Transplantation may be necessary in unresectable cases such as in patients with multiple lesions or in those involving the hepatic hilum. Other treatment options include transarterial catheter chemoembolization, ligation of hepatic artery and hepatic irradiation.

6. OTHER SOLID BENIGN HEPATIC MASSES

6.1 Lipomatous tumors

Angiomyolipomas, lipoma and fibrovascular tumors are extremely rare benign hepatic masses. They are usually asymptomatic and diagnosed by identification of intratumoral fat on CT [16]. Fine-needle aspiration may be occasionally required for definitive diagnosis of lipomatous tumors and reveals epitheliod smooth muscle cells, fat cells and blood vessels.

Bile duct hamartomas are usually asymptomatic benign liver lesions without risk of malignant transformation [1]. They are usually discovered incidentally and should be distinguished from more serious lesions such as cholangiocarcinoma to avoid unnecessary invasive surgical treatment. Von Meyenburg's complexes are biliary microhamartomas and are usually associated with underlying polycystic liver disease, congenital hepatic fibrosis and Caroli's disease.

6.2 Arteriovenous fistula

Arteriovenous (AV) fistula of the liver usually occurs as a result of prior trauma such as surgery or liver biopsy or in association with intrahepatic malignancy [17]. They may be diagnosed by imaging studies such as enhanced CT or MRI; however, AV fistula is best examined by angiography. Although most patients with arterioportal venous fistula may be asymptomatic, abdominal pain, abdominal bruit, and serious portal hypertension can occur. Other systemic complications of large AV fistula such as high-output cardiac failure and renal failure are other possible presentations. Hepatic AV fistula may be treated by transcatheter arterial embolization of the feeding artery.

6.3 Inflammatory pseudotumor

Inflammatory pseudotumor is another extremely rare benign lesion of the liver that merits a brief discussion. It is diagnosed primarily in middle-aged men who present with fever, weight loss, and malaise. The etiology of this condition is unknown and may resolve spontaneously without surgery or any other interventions.

7. CONGENITAL SIMPLE CYSTS

7.1 Epidemiology and pathogenesis

Hepatic cysts are one of the more common benign liver masses [1]. The reported ultrasound prevalence from one large multicenter study is 3.6% and increases with age. The prevalence increased from 0.83% in young persons below 40 years of age to 7.8% in patients older than 60 years. There is also a strong female predominance with benign hepatic cysts.

7.2 Presentation and diagnosis

Simple hepatic cysts are usually discovered incidentally, asymptomatic, and have no malignant potential. Symptoms such as abdominal pain are uncommon for lesions less than 5 cm. Rare complications include intracystic hemorrhage and infection. On CT, a simple cyst has water attenuation, with imperceptible wall, without septations, and does not enhance with intravenous contrast [16]. Hepatic cysts can usually be diagnosed by ultrasound. Pathologically, simple cysts are lined by simple cuboidal epithelium.

7.3 Management and prognosis

The majority of solitary simple cysts of the liver have excellent prognosis and should be managed conservatively. Symptomatic cases can be treated effectively by percutaneous cyst aspiration and sclerotherapy (with alcohol or doxycycline). Surgical cyst fenestration may be necessary in a minority of cases. Laparoscopic unroofing of simple cysts has been described to safe and as effective as open surgical unroofing by cases series with long-term follow-up [18].

7.4 Multiple congenital cysts

Patients with multiple hepatic cysts often have concurrent renal cysts are more likely to be symptomatic [18]. Besides abdominal pain, other presenting signs and symptoms may be abdominal mass, early satiety, and obstructive hepatopathy.

8. OTHER CYSTIC LESIONS

8.1 Hydatid cysts

Hydatid cysts or echinococcosis is caused by the tapeworms *Echinococcus granulosus* or *Echinococcus multilocularis*, both of which have a world-wide distribution and live in sheep, cats, dogs, cattle, humans and a variety of other wild animals as their intermediate and/or definitive hosts [5]. Most patients with hydatid cysts are asymptomatic. Patients with large cysts or subcapsular cysts may present with abdominal pain, cholangitis, or portal hypertension. Anaphylactic shock may occur

Table 4. Typical histologic and radiographic features of selected benign liver lesions.

Diagnostic studies	Hemangioma	Adenoma	FNH
Histology	Endothelium-lined fibrous septa	Sheet-like hepatic cords with normal nuclear:cytoplasmic ratio	Dense central fibrovascular scar
US	Hyperechoic	Variable	Hypervascularity with Doppler Central scar in 20%
CT			
Arterial phase	Lobular peripheral "puddling" enhancement	Peripheral/centripetal enhancement	Early peripheral enhancement
Portal phase	Hypoattenuating	Nearly isoattenuating enhanced if hemorrhage	Isoattenuating with delayed enhancement of central scar
MRI			
T1-weighted	Hypointense	Variable	Hypointense scar
T2-weighted	Very hyperintense ("light-bulb")	Hyperintense	Hyperintense scar
Arterial phase	Same enhancement pattern as CT	Early enhancement	Early enhancement
99m-Tc	Radionuclide pools in delayed phase	Usually normal uptake but also variable	Increased uptake but variable
Angiography	Early, persistent irregular areas ("lakes") without abnormal or neovascularization	"Spoke-wheel" pattern from centripetal vessels	Hypervascular with tortuous intratumoral vessels

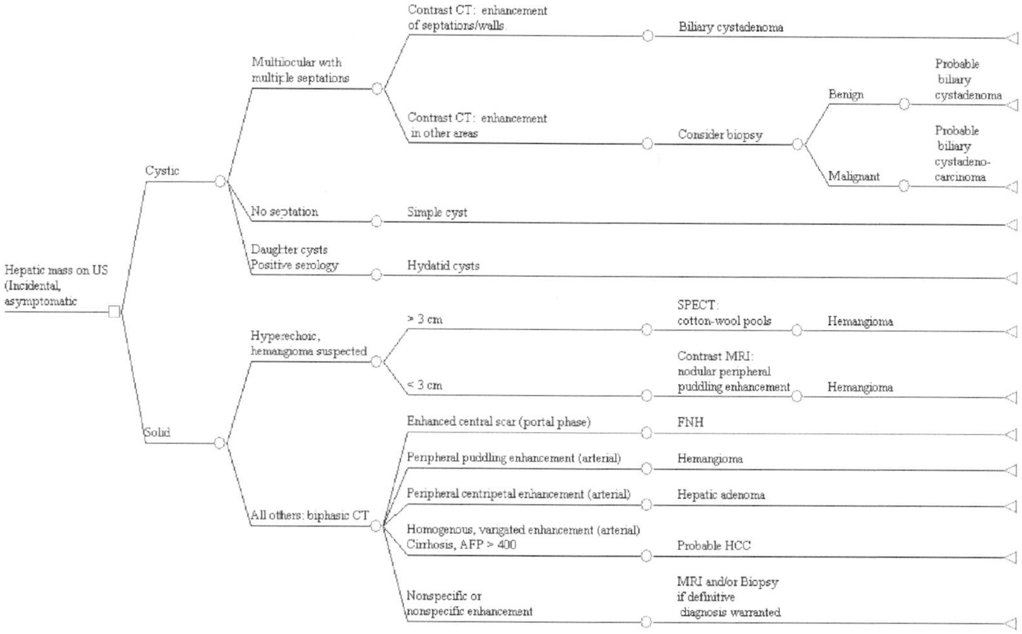

Figure 1. Evaluation for asymptomatic liver masses. (*For colored version, see Plate XXXI on page 580 at the end of the book.*)

due to rupture of cysts into the peritoneal cavity. Helpful diagnostic features include eosinophilia, positive serologic tests, and the presence of intracystic septations, calcified cystic rims and daughter cysts on US or CT. Medical treatment of hydatid cysts with mebendazole or albendazole is usually disappointing, while safe and successful laparoscopic unroofing of these cysts have been reported [5,18].

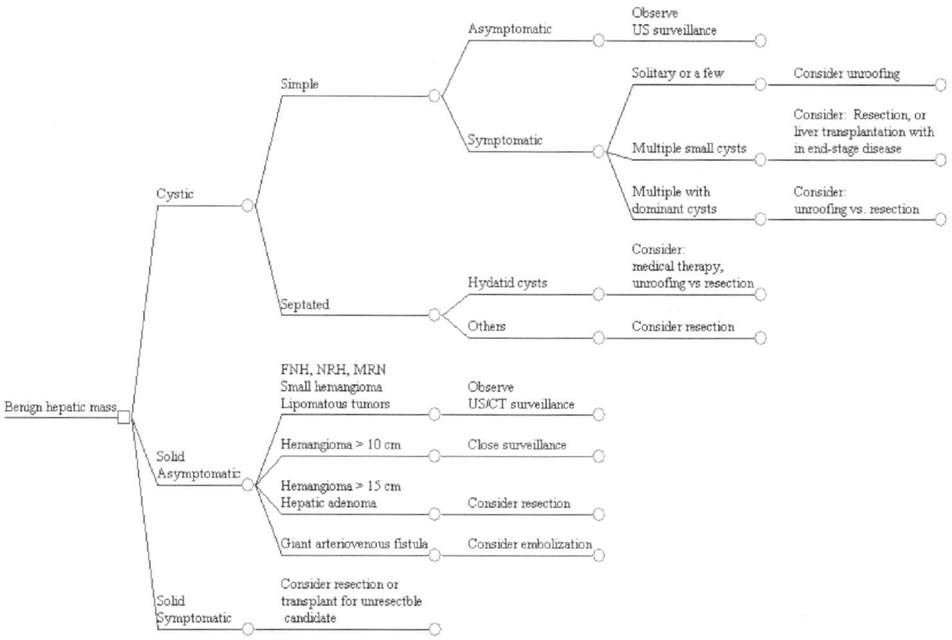

Figure 2. Follow-up and management of benign liver masses. (*For colored version, see Plate XXXII on page 581 at the end of the book.*)

8.2 Caroli's disease

Patients with Caroli's disease have grossly ectatic bile ducts [5]. It is an autosomal-recessive disease and is associated with polycystic kidney disease and choledochal cysts. Cholelithiasis and cholangitis are the most common complications of this disease. Irregular intrahepatic biliary dilation is the typical radiographic feature of Caroli's disease.

8.3 Peliosis hepatis

Peliosis hepatis is characterized by blood-filled cavities within the liver [5]. It usually occurs in association with malnutrition, tuberculosis, malignancies, androgenic steroid use and has also been described in patients with acquired immunodeficiency syndrome (AIDS).

8.4 Biliary cystadenoma

Biliary adenoma is a rare hepatic tumor that occurs primarily in middle-aged women without underlying chronic biliary or liver disease [3]. Biliary cystadenoma can be differentiated from simple hepatic cysts by the presence of multiple septations and multilocular appearance on US or CT. On CT with intravenous contrast, the tumor is typically hypovascular with enhancement of the cystic walls and septations only [16]. Enhancement of the center of the tumor should raise suspicion for a diagnosis of biliary cystadenocarcinoma since malignant transformation of biliary cystadenoma to biliary cystadenocarcinoma is not uncommon [19].

9. EVALUATION OF LIVER MASSES

Appropriate evaluation of liver masses depends on clinical, pathological, and radiographic characteristics of the lesions under investigation, many of which were discussed earlier in this chapter and are now summarized in Tables 3 and 4. Typical features of malignant tumors such as HCC are included for comparison. Metastatic tumors to the liver usually have ring enhancement with a complete ring while the enhancement pattern in HCC is more often homogenous or variegated with abnormal internal vessels [20]. As with evaluation of many other clinical entities, the differentiation between benign and malignant disease is paramount, classifying liver lesions into cystic or solid lesions appears a logical starting point since this task can usually be accomplished by less expensive noninvasive testings such as US and most cystic lesions are benign lesions. Based on this starting point, an algorithmic approach to the evaluation of hepatic masses is proposed in Figure 1. In addition, because definitive diagnosis of a number of hepatic lesions may require long-term follow-up, suggestions for follow-up and management of both solid and cystic hepatic masses are also included in Figure 2.

REFERENCES

[1] Trotter, J.F. and Everson, G.T. (2001) Benign focal lesions of the liver. *Clin. Liver Dis.* **5**, 17–42.

[2] Mergo, P.J. and Ros, P.R. (1998) Benign lesions of the liver. *Radiol. Clin. N. Am.* **36**, 319–331.

[3] Brunt, E.M. (2001) Benign tumors of the liver. *Clin. Liver Dis.* **5**, 1–15.

[4] Mani, H. and Van Thiel, D.H. (2001) Mesenchymal tumors of the liver. *Clin. Liver Dis.* **5**, 219–257.

[5] Di Bisceglie Adrian, M. (1999) Malignant neoplasm of the liver, in *Schiff's Diseases of the Liver*, eds. Schiff, E.R., Sorrell, M.F. and Maddrey, W.C., 8th edition (Lippincott Williams & Wilkins, Philadelphia, PA).

[6] Grazioli, L., Federle, M.P., Brancatelli, G., Ichikawa, T., Olivetti, L. and Blachar, A. (2001) Hepatic adenoma: imaging and pathologic findings. *Radiographics* **21**, 877–892.

[7] Wu, N.H., Wang, C.C., Huang, G.T., Yang, P.M., Sheu, J.C. and Chen, D.S. (1999) A different experience of hepatic adenoma in Taiwan with emphasis on clinical manifestation and ultrasonographic features. *Hepatogastroenterology* **46**, 3197–3200.

[8] Kew, M.C. (1998) Hepatic tumors and cysts, in *Sleisneger & Fodtran's Gastrointestinal and Liver Disease*, eds. Feldman, M., Scharschmidt, B.F. and Sleisenger, M.H., 6th edition (W.B. Saunders, Philadelphia, PA).

[9] Hung, C.H., Changchien, C.S., Lu, S.N., Eng, H.L., Wang, J.H., Lee, C.M., Hsu, C.C. and Tung, H.D. (2001) Sonographic features of hepatic adenomas with pathologic correlation. *Abdom. Imaging* **26**, 500–506.

[10] Terkivatan, T., de Wilt, J.H., de Man, R.A., van Rijn, R.R., Zondervan, P.E., Tilanus, H.W. and Ijermans, J.N. (2001) Indications and long-term outcome of

treatment for benign hepatic tumors: a critical appraisal. *Arch. Surg.* **136**, 1033–1038.

[11] Descottes, B., Lachachi, F., Sodji, M., Valleix,, Durand-Fontanier, S., Pech de Laclause, B. and Grousseau, D. (2000) Early experience with laparoscopic approach for solid liver tumors: initial 16 cases. *Ann. Surg.* **232**, 641–645.

[12] Katkhouda, N. and Mavor, E. (2000) Laparoscopic management of benign liver disease. *Surg. Clin. N. Am.* **80**, 1203–1211.

[13] Grazioli, L., Federle, M.P., Ichikawa, T., Balzano, E., Nalesnik, M. and Madariaga, J. (2000) Liver adenomatosis: clinical, histopathologic, and imaging findings in 15 patients. *Radiology* **21**, 395–402.

[14] Yoshidome, H., McMasters, K.M. and Edwards, M.J. (1999) Management issues regarding hepatic adenomatosis. *Am. Surg.* **65**, 1070–1076.

[15] Peterson, M.S. and Baron, R.L. (2001) Radiologic diagnosis of hepatocellular carcinoma. *Clin. Liver Dis.* **5**, 123–144.

[16] Horton, K.M., Bluemke, D.A., Hruban, R.H., Soyer, P. and Fishman, E.K. (1999) CT and MR imaging of benign hepatic and biliary tumors. *Radiographics* **19**, 431–451.

[17] Choi, B.I., Lee, K.H., Han, J.K. and Lee, J.M. (2002) Hepatic arterioportal shunts: dynamic CT and MR features. *Korean J. Radiol.* **3**, 1–15.

[18] Hansman, M.F., Ryan, Jr., J.A., Holmes, IV, J.H., Hogan, S., Lee, F.T., Kramer, D. and Biehl, T. (2001) Management and long-term follow-up of hepatic cysts. *Am. J. Surg.* **181**, 404–410.

[19] Kinoshita, H., Tanimura, H., Osishi, H., Kasano, Y., Uchiyama, K. and Yamaue, H. (2001) Clinical features and imaging diagnosis of biliary cystadenocarcinoma of the liver. *Hepatogastroenterology* **48**, 250–252.

[20] Nino-Murcia, M., Olcott, E.W., Jeffrey, R.B., Lamm, R.L., Beaulieu, C.F. and Jain, K.A. (2000) Focal liver lesions: pattern-based classification scheme for enhancement at arterial phase CT. *Radiology* **215**, 746.

Section III
Complications of End-Stage Liver Disease

Section Editor – B. Al Knawy

Hepatology: A Practical Approach
B. Al Knawy, M.L. Shiffman, R.H. Wiesner (editors)

Chapter 1
Ascites

Andrés Cárdenas[a] *and Vicente Arroyo*[b]

[a]Division of Gastroenterology and Hepatology, Beth Israel Deaconess Medical Center, Harvard Medical School, Boston, MA, USA

[b]Liver Unit, Institut de Malalties Digestives, Hospital Clinic, IDIBAPS, University of Barcelona, Barcelona, Spain

1. Introduction 347
2. Pathophysiology of Ascites 348
   2.1 Splanchnic and systemic hemodynamics 348
   2.2 Renal functional abnormalities 348
3. Theories of Ascites Formation 349
4. Evaluation of Cirrhotic Patients with Ascites 350
   4.1 History 350
   4.2 Examination 351
   4.3 Diagnostic tests 351
5. Therapeutic Methods 352
   5.1 Sodium restriction 352
   5.2 Diuretic therapy 353
   5.3 Therapeutic paracentesis 353
6. Practical Approach of the Patient with Ascites 353
   6.1 Mild or moderate ascites 354
   6.2 Large ascites 355
   6.3 Refractory ascites 355
   6.4 Dilutional hyponatremia 356
   6.5 Spontaneous bacterial peritonitis 356
   6.6 Hepatic hydrothorax 357
References 358

1. INTRODUCTION

Ascites is the pathological accumulation of free fluid in the peritoneal cavity. It is a manifestation of an underlying pathological process; most often advanced liver disease. Cirrhosis due to alcohol abuse and hepatitis C is the most common cause of ascites and accounts for 80% of the cases in United States and Europe. Malignancy, congestive heart failure, and tuberculosis are the cause of ascites in a minority of patients. This condition is an outstanding complication of cirrhosis associated with a poor quality of life, increased risk for infections, renal failure, and decreased survival. Nearly 60% of patients with compensated cirrhosis develop ascites within 10 years of disease. The development of ascites in cirrhosis is an important prognostic feature, as 50% of these patients will die in approximately 2 years. The presence of ascites in a cirrhotic patient is an indication for liver transplantation. Most patients with cirrhosis and ascites respond to low-sodium diet and diuretic treatment, whereas patients with non-cirrhotic ascites respond to therapy of the underlying disease. This chapter will focus on the pathophysiology, clinical features, diagnostic methods, and current therapy of ascites in cirrhosis.

2. PATHOPHYSIOLOGY OF ASCITES

Although sinusoidal portal hypertension is required for the accumulation of ascites, it alone cannot account for its development. Increased lymph formation (due to elevated portal blood inflow) with leakage into the peritoneal cavity is a self-limited process. Ongoing replenishment of the intravascular space by means of sodium and water retention is what perpetuates this pathological state. The formation of ascites in cirrhosis is the final consequence of a combination of abnormalities in the splanchnic and systemic circulation as well as renal function abnormalities that bring about the accumulation of fluid in the peritoneal cavity [1].

2.1 Splanchnic and systemic hemodynamics

Cirrhosis causes marked structural abnormalities in the liver that lead to a severe disturbance of the hepatic and splanchnic circulation. Liver fibrosis and nodule formation alter the hepatic vasculature with resulting increase of portal flow. Elevated resistance to blood flow causes significant effects not only in the portal venous system but also in the splanchnic arterial bed. In the venous side, there is development of portal hypertension with collateral formation and shunting of blood from the portal to the systemic circulation. In the arterial side, marked vasodilation contributes to portal hypertension by increasing portal venous inflow and inducing changes in the microcirculation that predispose to increased filtration of plasma. Several vasodilator factors, including nitric oxide (NO), glucagon, and substance P are responsible for this vasodilation. Most of the available data suggest that NO, a potent arterial vasodilator, is the main factor involved [2].

Aside from changes in splanchnic hemodynamics, cirrhotic patients with ascites develop a hyperdynamic state characterized by reduced systemic vascular resistance and arterial pressure, increased cardiac output, and activation of vasoconstrictor and antinatriuretic systems (renin–angiotensin and sympathetic nervous systems and antidiuretic hormone or arginine vasopressin). Splanchnic vasodilation by decreasing the effective arterial blood volume unloads the central baroreceptors thereby triggering the activation of these systems, which play a fundamental role in the development of ascites.

2.2 Renal functional abnormalities

Patients with cirrhosis develop three renal functional abnormalities; sodium retention, water retention, and renal vasoconstriction [3]. Impairment in the renal ability to excrete sodium is the earliest renal dysfunction in cirrhosis and occurs before water retention and renal vasoconstriction (Figure 1). Patients without the development of any of the major complications of cirrhosis such as ascites, variceal hemorrhage, or hepatic encephalopathy have subtle abnormalities in renal sodium metabolism. For example they may be unable to excrete a sodium overload, as occurs in hospitalized patients with cirrhosis that receive intravenous saline infusions. With time cirrhotic patients develop an inability to excrete their regular sodium intake and develop sodium retention. This derangement precedes the onset of ascites indicating that it is a cause and not a consequence of fluid retention. In advanced cirrhosis sodium retention further leads to the expansion of extracellular fluid volume and an increased amount of fluid in the interstitial tissue. The pathogenesis is due to an abnormally increased reabsorption of sodium in the renal tubules (proximal and distal) because it occurs in the setting of a normal filtered sodium load [4]. The three major hormones acting on the renal tubules to retain sodium are aldosterone, angiotensin, and norepinephrine.

Water retention is common in advanced cirrhosis and occurs several months after the onset of sodium retention. The major clinical consequence is the development of dilutional hyponatremia (serum sodium concentration less than 130 mEq/l), which occurs despite avid sodium retention because water is retained in excess of sodium. The prevalence of spontaneous hyponatremia in hospitalized patients with cirrhosis and ascites is near 35% [5]. The intensity of this disorder is not uniform in all patients. Some patients have normal serum sodium levels but

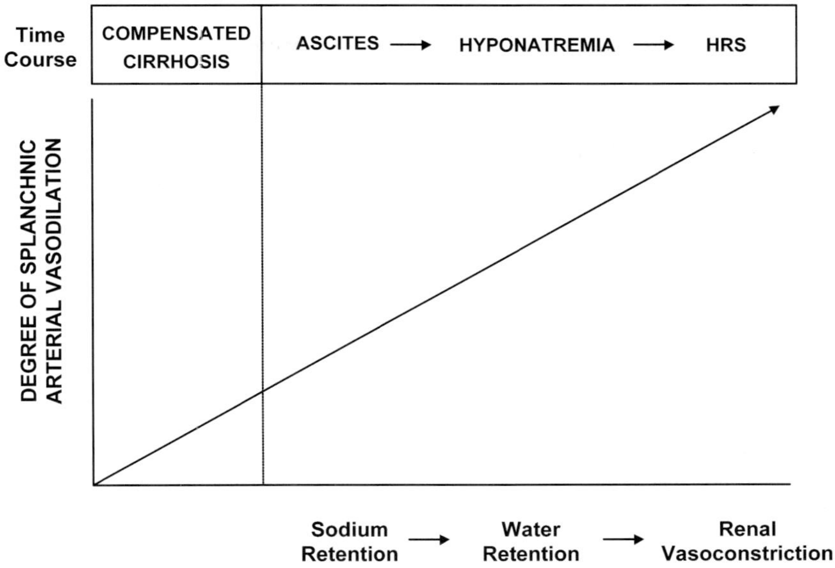

Figure 1. Time course of functional renal abnormalities in relation to splanchnic arterial vasodilation in cirrhosis. There is a progressive worsening of renal function as liver disease advances. HRS: Hepatorenal syndrome.

can become hyponatremic when they drink large amounts of water, whereas others can develop hyponatremia spontaneously and become symptomatic. The pathogenesis of water retention in cirrhosis is complex and involves three factors, including a reduced delivery of filtrate to the ascending limb of the loop of Henle, reduced renal synthesis of prostaglandins, and most importantly increased non-osmotic secretion of antidiuretic hormone.

Renal vasoconstriction is the renal functional abnormality that develops latest in patients with cirrhosis and ascites. The clinical consequence is the development of hepatorenal syndrome, which occurs in the late stages of cirrhosis. Increased activity of vasoconstrictor factors and reduced activity of renal vasodilator factors acting on the renal circulation play a crucial role because renal vasoconstriction in cirrhosis occurs in the absence of morphological or histological changes in the kidney [6]. The degree of renal dysfunction may range from a modest renal impairment with serum creatinine levels ranging between 1.2 and 1.4 mg/dl to severe renal failure with elevation of serum creatinine above 1.5 mg/dl and oligoanuria. Renal vasoconstriction is the consequence of extreme underfilling of the arterial circulation.

3. THEORIES OF ASCITES FORMATION

All theories involve sodium and water retention either as a primary event or due to changes in systemic hemodynamics. The *overfill theory* suggests that in advanced cirrhosis a "sodium-retaining signal" is produced with subsequent sodium and water retention in the renal tubules [7]. The existence of this "sodium-retaining signal" has been suggested by two mechanisms; one is the presence of a "hepatorenal reflex" arising from intrahepatic baroreceptors and the other is the decreased clearance of a sodium-retaining substance. To date, there is no clear evidence to fully support this concept. Another argument against this theory relies on the fact that these patients have an underfilled arterial vascular bed as opposed to it being overfilled.

The *forward theory* considers that the first event in ascites formation is sinusoidal portal hypertension, which causes splanchnic arteriolar vasodilation (Figure 2) [1]. Vasodilation in the splanchnic circulation simultaneously produces systemic arterial vascular underfilling and a "forward" increase in

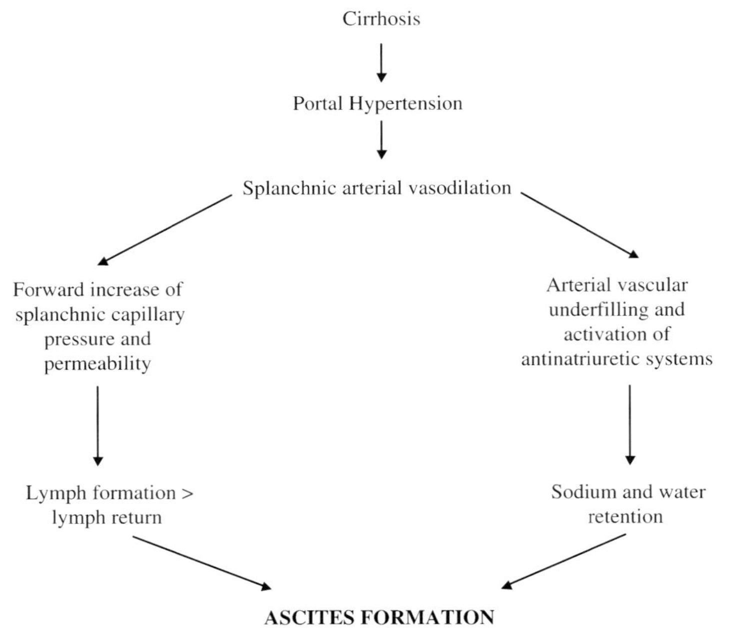

Figure 2. The forward theory of ascites formation. Antinatriuretic systems include the renin–angiotensin–aldosterone system and the sympathetic nervous system.

the splanchnic capillary pressure and filtration coefficient. In patients with compensated cirrhosis, the degree of portal hypertension and splanchnic arterial vasodilation is moderate. Arterial underfilling is compensated by an increase in plasma volume and cardiac output. In these patients the lymphatic system is able to return the moderate increase in lymph produced to the systemic circulation, thus preventing leakage of fluid into the abdominal cavity. As cirrhosis progresses, portal hypertension and decreased splanchnic vascular resistance turn progressively worse and a critical point is reached in which the consequences of this intense splanchnic arterial vasodilation cannot be compensated for by increasing lymph return, plasma volume, and cardiac output. The maintenance of arterial pressure then requires persistent activation of the renin–angiotensin–aldosterone system, the sympathetic nervous system, and the antidiuretic hormone, which produce continuous sodium and water retention. The retained fluid is, however, ineffective in refilling the dilated arterial vascular bed because it escapes from the intravascular compartment, due to an imbalance between the excessive lymph production and the ability of the lymphatic system to return it to the systemic circulation. The final consequence of both disorders is persistent renal sodium and water retention with ongoing leakage of fluid into the abdominal cavity and the formation of ascites.

4. EVALUATION OF CIRRHOTIC PATIENTS WITH ASCITES

4.1 History

Patients should be questioned about precipitating events such as excessive salt intake, alcohol consumption, infections, medications such as non-steroidal anti-inflammatory drugs, and non-compliance of diuretic therapy (Table 1). Worsening liver disease, portal vein thrombosis, and development of hepatocellular carcinoma also precipitate the development of ascites. In the setting of acute liver failure, such as in alcoholic hepatitis, ascites forms rapidly but there is resolution following therapy and abstinence. More commonly, ascites develops

Table 1. Evaluation of patients with cirrhosis and ascites.

General evaluation
Complete history and physical examination
Standard hematology, coagulation, and liver tests
Abdominal ultrasonography and Doppler flow (including the kidneys)
Upper gastrointestinal endoscopy
Liver biopsy
Diagnostic paracentesis
Total protein and albumin measurement
Cell count
Culture in blood culture bottles
Optional tests (see text)
Evaluation of renal function
24 h urine sodium
Serum electrolytes and serum creatinine
Urine sediment and protein excretion
Evaluation of circulatory function
Arterial pressure and heart rate
Plasma renin activity and plasma norepinephrine concentration (see text)

Renal and circulatory function should be assessed under low-sodium diet and without diuretic therapy.

insidiously over the course of weeks to months. The main symptoms are an increase in abdominal girth often accompanied by lower extremity edema. In patients with a large amount of ascites, the respiratory function and physical activity may be impaired. Dyspnea occurs as a consequence of increasing abdominal distention or due to pleural effusions. Patients with spontaneous bacterial peritonitis (SBP) can present with fever, chills, abdominal pain, encephalopathy, and rebound abdominal tenderness. However, often they are asymptomatic and the diagnosis relies on the examination of peritoneal fluid. Other common manifestations of patients with ascites include dull abdominal pain, anorexia, malaise, weakness, difficulty in sleeping, and muscle cramps. Finally, questions regarding nutritional intake and complete evaluation of nutritional status should be performed.

4.2 Examination

The hyperdynamic state of advanced cirrhotic patients is associated with resting tachycardia, low arterial blood pressure, and bounding peripheral pulses. Most patients are malnourished and have signs of muscle wasting, palmar erythema, spider angiomata, and lower extremity edema. Patients either have mild to moderate or large (tense or not) ascites. The abdomen is distended with bulging flanks; dullness to percussion in these areas indicates ascites. When free fluid is present in the abdominal cavity, it moves to the flanks and the intestines float upward when the patient is supine. The air–fluid level is higher than that normally found on the lateral aspect of the abdomen, if the patient is turned on his/her side the dullness will shift and percussion over the uppermost part becomes tympanic, because that area is occupied by intestines as fluid shifts to the other side. This maneuver is called shifting dullness and is very sensitive for detecting ascites [8]. Other maneuvers to detect ascites such as fluid wave and puddle sign are less reliable. In some patients with previous abdominal surgery increased intra-abdominal pressure favors the development of umbilical, femoral, and inguinal hernias. Mild or moderate pleural effusions are common in patients with ascites. Large pleural effusions, usually greater than 500 ml, in cirrhotic patients without cardiopulmonary disease are known as hepatic hydrothorax (see below).

4.3 Diagnostic tests

Standard electrolyte, renal, hematology, and coagulation tests should be performed. Hyponatremia and hyper- or hypokalemia are common, especially in patients taking diuretics. Liver tests required include aminotransferases, bilirubin, albumin, total protein, alkaline phosphatase, prothrombin time, and alpha-fetoprotein. All cirrhotic patients with ascites need an abdominal ultrasound to rule out hepatocellular carcinoma, evaluate the patency of portal and hepatic flow and in some cases confirm its presence. An upper gastrointestinal endoscopy, to assess the presence and characteristics of esophageal or gastric varices or portal hypertensive gastropathy should be done. In patients with previously unknown liver disease, the diagnosis of cirrhosis can be confirmed either histologically or by a combination of exploratory, ultrasonographical, and endoscopic findings. A percutaneous liver biopsy should only be performed after resolution of ascites, because its presence increases the risk of complications. In patients with coagulopathy and large ascites the liver biopsy may be performed through a transjugular approach [9]. Finally, a 24 h urine collection on a low-salt diet and off diuretics for at least 4 days for determination of volume and urinary sodium excretion is helpful in determining prognosis and how patients will respond to therapy.

Diagnostic paracentesis is required in all patients presenting with ascites *de novo*. The technique for performing an adequate diagnostic paracentesis is explained elsewhere [10]. The ascitic fluid in cirrhotics is transparent and yellow/amber in color. Basic parameters to be determined in ascitic fluid are cell count, culture in blood culture bottles, albumin, and total protein. Glucose, lactate dehydrogenase, amylase, triglyceride, tuberculosis smear, and cytological analysis of the fluid are optional and provide important information in differential diagnosis of ascites. The cell count is the most helpful test in determining bacterial infection. The ascitic fluid white blood cell count is less than 500 mm^{-3} in most cases, with predominance of mononuclear cells (>75%) and very low number of polymorphonuclear (PMN) cells. An elevated white blood cell count with predominance of PMN cells is indicative of a peritoneal infection. The diagnosis of SBP is made when the fluid sample has a PMN count greater than 250 mm^{-3} [11]. Cultures are positive in approximately 50% of patients if blood culture bottles are used [12]. Bloody ascites may lead to a higher PMN count in the absence of infection. A low proportion of patients may have a positive ascitic fluid culture without increased PMN cell count. This condition is known as bacterascites. Conversely, as indicated above many patients with high PMN count suggestive of peritoneal infection may have a negative ascitic fluid culture. This condition is known as culture-negative SBP or neutrocytic ascites. Both are managed as a culture-positive SBP [11] (see below).

The difference between serum albumin concentration and ascites albumin concentration (serum–ascites albumin gradient) in patients with cirrhosis and ascites is usually greater than 1.1 g/dl [13]. Values lower than 1.1 g/dl suggest a cause of ascites other than cirrhosis (Table 2). Most patients with cirrhosis

Table 2. Classification of ascites by the serum–ascites albumin gradient.

High gradient (≥ 1.1 g/dl)	Low gradient (< 1.1 g/dl)
Cirrhosis	Peritoneal carcinomatosis
Congestive heart failure	Tuberculosis (without cirrhosis)
Fulminant hepatic failure	Pancreatitis (without cirrhosis)
Portal vein thrombosis	Biliary (without cirrhosis)
Liver metastasis	Nephrotic syndrome
Alcoholic hepatitis	Connective tissue diseases
Budd–Chiari syndrome	Chlamydia/gonococccal infection
Veno-occlusive disease	
Myxedema	

Serum–ascites albumin gradient = Ascites albumin concentration − serum albumin concentration.

have a total ascitic fluid protein concentration less than 1.0 g/dl. However, values greater than 1.0 g/dl are not uncommon. Patients with protein concentration in ascitic fluid lower than 1.0 g/l have a greater risk of developing SBP. The mobilization of ascites with diuretics may also increase the concentration of proteins in the ascitic fluid. The red blood cell (RBC) count in ascitic fluid is usually low in patients with cirrhosis (below 1000 cells/mm^3). Bloody ascites (more than 50,000 RBC/mm^3) may be observed in patients with a traumatic tap or hepatocellular carcinoma; in these cases a correction factor of 1 PMN per 250 RBC is recommended [11].

5. THERAPEUTIC METHODS

5.1 Sodium restriction

This is the first and most important step in treating cirrhotic patients with ascites. A low-sodium diet of 70–90 mmol/day (1.5–2 g of salt) is required and in general is well tolerated. This restriction causes a negative sodium balance and loss of ascites and edema in those patients with a urinary sodium excretion greater than 100 mEq/day as measured by a 24 h urine collection. In patients with marked sodium retention (urinary sodium excretion less than 10 mEq/day) such sodium restriction is not sufficient by itself to achieve negative sodium balance, but it may slow the accumulation of fluid. These patients need diuretic therapy.

5.2 Diuretic therapy

Diuretic therapy in cirrhosis is based on the administration of spironolactone, a drug that competes with aldosterone for the binding to the mineralocorticoid receptor in the collecting tubular epithelial cells, alone or in combination with a loop diuretic, furosemide, which acts by inhibiting the $Na^+-K^+-2Cl^-$ cotransporter in the loop of Henle. The response to diuretic therapy in cirrhotic patients should be evaluated by measuring body weight, urine volume, and sodium excretion (spot sample) on a regular basis. Patients may fail to respond to diuretics when they do not comply with a low-sodium diet. This should be suspected when body weight and ascites do not decrease despite a high urine volume and natriuresis. Approximately 10–15% of patients with ascites either do not respond to diuretic therapy or develop diuretic-induced complications that prevent the use of high doses of these drugs [14]. This condition is known as refractory ascites (see below). Common complications of diuretic therapy in patients with cirrhosis include electrolyte disturbances (hyponatremia and hypo/hyperkalemia), hepatic encephalopathy, renal impairment, gynecomastia, and muscle cramps. Patients receiving diuretics need to be followed closely with frequent visits and have electrolytes, serum creatinine, and urinary sodium monitored regularly in order to prevent and treat these complications.

5.3 Therapeutic paracentesis

Therapeutic paracentesis is the treatment of choice in the management of large ascites in patients with cirrhosis. We recommend total paracentesis with complete removal of ascites in one tap or repeated taps of 4–6 l/day associated with intravenous albumin (6–8 g/l tapped) [15]. Paracentesis is quick, effective and associated with lower number of complications than conventional diuretic therapy. Post-paracentesis circulatory dysfunction is a circulatory derangement with marked activation of the renin–angiotensin system that occurs in most patients treated with large taps [16]. This disorder is clinically silent, not spontaneously reversible, and is associated with renal impairment and decreased survival. This complication is prevented either with the administration of plasma expanders like albumin, dextran-70 and polygeline or with terlipressin [17,18]. Among the plasma expanders, albumin is the most effective and improves survival when more than 5 l are removed [17].

Therapeutic paracentesis should be performed in sterile conditions using specially designed large gauge needles with side holes and with aid of a suction pump, to facilitate a rapid removal of ascites (100–200 ml/h). With this technique the rate of local complications is considerably reduced. In general, the duration of the treatment ranges between 30 and 90 min depending on the amount of fluid removed. Albumin is infused immediately after the procedure and patients may be discharged from the hospital the same day if done as an outpatient procedure. Coagulopathy should not preclude a paracentesis unless there is disseminated intravascular coagulation. Hemorrhage into the ascitic fluid or hematoma of the abdominal wall is uncommon (less than 2%) and usually mild.

6. PRACTICAL APPROACH OF THE PATIENT WITH ASCITES

The first and most important aspect in the management of all patients with cirrhosis and ascites is an evaluation for liver transplant (Figure 3). A number of predictive factors of survival described in patients with cirrhosis and ascites are helpful in identifying candidates for liver transplantation [19]. The most valuable factors associated with a poor prognosis in these patients are the following:

1. An impaired ability to excrete a water load (urine volume of <8 ml/min after a water load of 20 mg/kg with intravenous dextrose).
2. Dilutional hyponatremia (serum sodium <130 mEq/l).
3. Arterial hypotension (mean arterial pressure <80 mm Hg).
4. Serum creatinine >1.2 mg/dl.
5. Marked sodium retention (urine sodium <10 mEq/day).
6. Increased plasma renin activity and norepinephrine concentration.

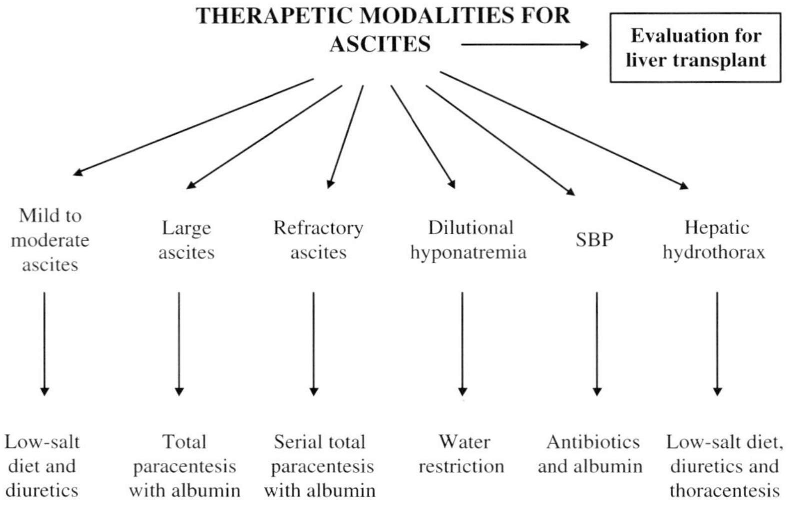

Figure 3. Therapeutic modalities for patients with cirrhosis and ascites. The first and most important step is referring the patient for evaluation for liver transplantation. SBP: spontaneous bacterial peritonitis.

Interestingly, in patients with ascites these parameters are better predictors of prognosis than liver tests, such as albumin, bilirubin, and prothrombin time.

6.1 Mild or moderate ascites

These patients usually have less than 5 l of ascitic fluid and are treated with a low-sodium diet and diuretics (Table 3). There is no need for hospitalization. Patients are started on spironolactone 100 mg/day. If there is no response, the dose is increased progressively to 200 mg/day up to 400 mg/day. Furosemide is added at increasing doses (40, 80, and 160 mg/day) in patients not responding to 400 mg/day of spironolactone. Alternatively they can be treated with simultaneous administration of spironolactone and furosemide starting with 100 and 40 mg/day, respectively. If there is no response with this approach, one must check compliance with diet and medications, and afterwards diuretics may be increased in a stepwise fashion every 7 days, spironolactone up to 400 mg/day and furosemide up to 160 mg/day. There is a general agreement that these are the highest doses of diuretics to be used in cirrhotics. Higher doses will not increase the rate of response. The goal of treatment is to achieve a weight loss of 300–500 g/day in patients without peripheral edema and 800–1000 g/day in patients with peripheral edema. Greater weight losses should not be attempted, at least in the outpatient setting, because of there is a higher risk of intravascular

Table 3. Treatment strategy for patients with cirrhosis and mild or moderate ascites.

Initial therapy

Begin with low-sodium diet (70–90 mmol/day) and spironolactone (100–200 mg/day as single dose). Monitor body weight daily and spot urine sodium weekly. Ideal weight loss should be between 300 and 500 g/day in patients without peripheral edema and 800–1000 g/day in patients with peripheral edema. Outpatients should be instructed to reduce the diuretic dosage in case of greater weight loss

Furosemide 20–40 mg/day may be used in combination with spironolactone to increase the natriuretic effect

If there is no response, check compliance with treatment and low-sodium diet. Increase the dose of diuretics in stepwise fashion every 7 days up to 400 mg/day of spironolactone and 160 mg/day of furosemide

Maintenance therapy

Maintain sodium restriction and reduce diuretic dosage if possible

If ascites or edema does not recur, increase sodium intake progressively and maintain a low dose of diuretics volume depletion and renal failure. Once ascites has been reduced, sodium restriction should be maintained while the dose of diuretics can be cut in half.

6.2 Large ascites

The preferred treatment for patients with large ascites is total or repeated paracentesis plus intravenous albumin (6–8 g/l tapped), followed by diuretics (Table 4). Patients with a known history of cirrhosis and without any complications can be managed as outpatients. However, patients in whom large ascites is the first manifestation of cirrhosis or those with associated hepatic encephalopathy, gastrointestinal bleeding, SBP, or hepatocellular carcinoma require hospitalization. Since these patients usually have marked sodium retention they need to be started or continued on relatively high doses of diuretics (i.e., spironolactone 200 mg/day and furosemide 40 mg/day) after paracentesis together with a low-sodium diet. Diuretics are then adjusted according to individual responses.

Table 4. Treatment strategy for patients with cirrhosis and large ascites.

Initial therapy

Total paracentesis plus intravenous albumin (8 g/l of ascites removed)

Maintenance therapy

Low-sodium diet (70–90 mmol/day) associated with diuretic therapy

If the patient was not on diuretics before the development of arge ascites, start with spironolactone (200 mg/day as single dose) and furosemide 40 mg/day and adjust the dose to maintain the patient with mild or no ascites or edema. Check body weight daily and spot urine sodium weekly. Monitor the patient closely during the first 3–4 weeks of therapy

If the patient was on diuretics before the development of severe ascites, start with a dose higher than the dose taken before paracentesis

If ascites and edema increase, check compliance with treatment and low-sodium diet. Increase the dose of diuretics in stepwise fashion every 7 days up to 400 mg/day of spironolactone and 160 mg/day of furosemide

6.3 Refractory ascites

As discussed above between 10 and 15% of patients are refractory to treatment with diuretics. This situation is known as refractory ascites, the definition and diagnostic criteria are described in Table 5 [14]. These patients have a very poor prognosis, survival is near 50% at 6 months and 25% at 1 year. Patients with refractory ascites have marked sodium retention (less than 10 mEq/day), dilutional hyponatremia, and frequently have type 2 hepatorenal syndrome (see Chapter 4, Section III). In refractory ascites, sodium excretion cannot be achieved with drugs either because patients do not respond to high doses of diuretics or because they develop side effects that preclude the use of an effective diuretic dose.

There are three ways of treating patients with refractory ascites; peritoneovenous shunt, repeated total paracentesis plus intravenous albumin, and transjugular intrahepatic portosystemic shunts (TIPS). Surgical shunts, although very effective, were abandoned due to significant complications

Table 5. Definition and diagnostic criteria of refractory ascites in cirrhosis.

Diuretic-resistant ascites

Ascites that cannot be mobilized or the early recurrence of which cannot be prevented due to a lack of response to sodium restriction and diuretic treatment (mean loss of weight less than 200 g/day during the last 4 days of intensive diuretic therapy – spironolactone 400 mg/day and furosemide 160 mg/day – and urinary sodium excretion less than 50 mEq/day)

Diuretic-intractable ascites

Ascites that cannot be mobilized or the early recurrence of which cannot be prevented due to the development of diuretic-induced complications[a] that preclude the use of an effective diuretic dosage

[a] *Diuretic-induced hepatic encephalopathy*: development of hepatic encephalopathy in the absence of other precipitating factors.
Diuretic-induced renal failure: increase in serum creatinine by greater than 100% to a value above 2 mg/dl in patients with ascites responding to diuretic treatment.
Diuretic-induced hyponatremia: decrease in serum sodium concentration by greater than 10 mEq/l to a level lower than 125 mEq/l.
Diuretic induced hypo or hyperkalemia: decrease of serum potassium concentration to less than 3 mEq/l or increase to more than 6.0 mEq/l despite appropriate measures to normalize potassium levels.

that caused increased mortality when compared to paracentesis. Total paracentesis is the most accepted therapy for refractory ascites. Patients, on average, require a therapeutic tap every 2 weeks. They can get tapped as outpatients, making this option very safe and easy to perform. TIPS, a non-surgical method of portal decompression that acts as a side-to-side portocaval shunt, by reducing portal pressure improves sodium excretion, ascites volume, and diuretic requirements in patients with refractory ascites. The main disadvantage is frequent obstruction of the prosthesis, which precipitates rapid reaccumulation of ascites in some patients. Side effects include hepatic encephalopathy, congestive heart failure, and impairment in liver function due to the shunting of blood from the liver to the systemic circulation.

Three comparative studies of TIPS vs. repeated paracentesis show that TIPS is associated with a lower rate of ascites recurrence when compared with paracentesis. However, side effects such as hepatic encephalopathy and impaired liver function are more common with TIPS. The studies illustrate discrepant findings with respect to survival; one showed improved survival with paracentesis, the other showed a benefit with TIPS, and the third showed no difference [20–22]. In our opinion patients with poor hepatic function and hepatic encephalopathy should not be offered a TIPS. The recommendation to perform TIPS should be individualized and reserved for patients with preserved hepatic function, no hepatic encephalopathy, compartmentalized fluid, and those unwilling to have repeated paracentesis every 2 weeks. The recommendations for treating refractory ascites are listed in Table 6.

Table 6. Treatment strategy for patients with refractory ascites.

Initial therapy

- Total paracentesis plus intravenous albumin (8 g/l of ascites removed)

Maintenance therapy

- Maintain a low-sodium diet (70–90 mmol/day) constantly
- In patients taking the highest doses of diuretics, check urinary sodium. If less than 10 mEq/l, stop diuretic therapy
- Total paracentesis plus intravenous albumin when necessary (approximately every 2–3 weeks)
- Consider use of TIPS in patients with preserved hepatic function, no hepatic encephalopathy, compartmentalized fluid, and those unwilling to have repeated paracentesis every 2 weeks

6.4 Dilutional hyponatremia

In most patients, dilutional hyponatremia (serum sodium <130 mEq/l) is asymptomatic, but in some it may associated with symptoms such as anorexia, headache, poor concentration, lethargy, nausea, vomiting, and occasionally seizures. Presently there is no pharmacological therapy for dilutional hyponatremia and the only therapeutic measure that improves or stops the progressive decrease in serum sodium concentration is water restriction. We recommend strict fluid restriction to 1 l/day. The administration of hypertonic saline solutions is not recommended because it invariably leads to further expansion of extracellular fluid volume and accumulation of ascites and edema. Preliminary studies show that two types of drugs selectively increase water excretion in hyponatremic patients with congestive heart failure and cirrhosis. The first are antagonists of the V2 receptor of antidiuretic hormone and the second are selective kappa opioid agonists. The former group of drugs antagonize selectively the water-retaining effect of antidiuretic hormone in the cortical collecting duct whereas the latter inhibit antidiuretic hormone release from the neurohypophysis [23]. These compounds when available for use in clinical practice would offer a novel therapeutic approach for the treatment of water retention and dilutional hyponatremia in cirrhotic patients with ascites.

6.5 Spontaneous bacterial peritonitis

This is a common and severe complication of cirrhotic patients with ascites characterized by infection of ascitic fluid in the absence of other contiguous sources of infection, such as abdominal abscess or intestinal perforation (Table 7). The prevalence of SBP in hospitalized cirrhotic patients ranges between 20 and 30%. Aerobic Gram-negative bacteria are responsible for nearly 80% of cases and *Escherichia coli* accounts for most of them. Aerobic Gram-positive bacteria, mostly *Streptococcus*

Table 7. Treatment strategy for patients with cirrhosis and spontaneous bacterial peritonitis.

Begin empiric antibiotic therapy with an intravenous third-generation cephalosporin, preferably cefotaxime (2 g every 8–12 h) for at least 5 days, after diagnosis is confirmed
Infuse albumin at a dose of 1.5 g/kg at diagnosis of the infection and 1 g/kg 48 h later
Repeat diagnostic paracentesis 2 days after beginning antibiotics. In case of treatment failure (worsening infection or no decrease in PMN count), antibiotic therapy should be revised and appropriately changed
Treat until the complete disappearance of all signs of infection (fever, abdominal pain, normalization of blood PMN count) and decrease of PMN count in ascitic fluid below 250 mm^{-3}
After resolution of infection, start long-term prophylaxis norfloxacin 400 mg/day orally

viridans, *Staphylococcus aureus*, and *Enterococcus fecalis* are isolated in approximately 20% of cases [12]. Patients with hepatic hydrothorax that develop a spontaneous infection of pleural fluid are treated as SBP. Anaerobic and microaerophilic organisms, although very abundant in gut flora, rarely cause SBP. The pathogenesis of SBP involves passage of bacteria from the intestinal lumen to the systemic circulation, bacteremia secondary to the impairment of the reticuloendothelial system phagocytic activity, and infection due to poor opsonization and defective bactericidal activity of ascitic fluid [24].

Empiric antibiotic therapy with an intravenous third-generation cephalosporin, preferably cefotaxime (2 g every 8–12 h) for at least 5 days, is required after diagnosis is confirmed [11]. Therapy modification depends on results from cultures. Responses to therapy include frequent clinical evaluation and repeat diagnostic paracentesis 2 days after beginning antibiotics. In case of treatment failure (worsening infection or no decrease in PMN count), antibiotic therapy should be revised and appropriately changed. We recommend treating until the complete disappearance of all signs of infection (fever, abdominal pain, normalization of blood PMN count) and decrease of PMN count in ascitic fluid below 250 mm^{-3}.

SBP improves in approximately 90% of cases if treated with the above regimens. However, hospital mortality remains near 30%, because most of these patients have advanced liver failure and complications like gastrointestinal bleeding, renal failure, and hepatic encephalopathy. The most important predictor of survival in patients with SBP is the development of renal failure during the infection. Renal failure is triggered by an impairment of circulatory function with activation of the vasoconstrictor systems. The administration of albumin at a dose of 1.5 g/kg at the diagnosis of the infection and 1 g/kg 48 h later prevents renal failure and improves survival in patients with SBP. Unfortunately life expectancy after an episode of SBP is short, with a 1-year probability of survival of 30–50% if antibiotic prophylaxis. Recurrence is very common, nearly 70% in 1 year, and constitutes a major cause of death in these patients.

Two groups of cirrhotic patients benefit from prophylaxis [11]. These are patients with a prior episode of SBP and cirrhotics with gastrointestinal bleeding. In the first group, long-term norfloxacin therapy (400 mg/day orally) is recommended. In patients with gastrointestinal hemorrhage, administration of norfloxacin (400 mg/12 h orally or per gastric tube) for 7 days is also recommended. Antibiotic prophylaxis may be also effective in the prevention of the first SBP episode in patients with low ascitic fluid protein (<1 g/dl), but this indication requires further evaluation.

6.6 Hepatic hydrothorax

Hepatic hydrothorax is an infrequent complication of cirrhosis. It occurs due to small diaphragmatic defects, which favor the passage of fluid from the peritoneal to the pleural cavity [25]. The effusion is usually right sided, although it can be present on the left side. Negative pressure in the pleural space favors the transfer of fluid across these defects. Patients with hepatic hydrothorax are treated similarly to those with ascites. The first step is starting the patient on a low-sodium diet and diuretics as described above. Therapeutic thoracentesis is reserved for patients with large effusions and dyspnea or those refractory to diuretic therapy. Pleurodesis is in general unsuccessful because rapid reaccumulation of fluid does not allow the visceral and parietal pleural surfaces to adhere. Chest tube placement should always be avoided, as it is a set up for infections and massive fluid losses. Repair of diaphragmatic defects using videothoracoscopy may be considered in patients with large defects. In patients with refractory hepatic hydrothorax requiring a thoracentesis for symptomatic relief more often than every 2 weeks, TIPS may be beneficial as a bridge to transplantation in those with preserved hepatic function. This is particularly true if the patient is a candidate for liver transplantation, the only long-term solution in patients with refractory hepatic hydrothorax.

REFERENCES

[1] Cardenas, A., Bataller, R. and Arroyo, V. (2000) Mechanisms of ascites formation. *Clin. Liver Dis.* **4**, 447–465.

[2] Martin, P.Y., Ginès, P. and Schrier, R.W. (1998) Nitric oxide as a mediator of hemodynamic abnormalities and sodium and water retention in cirrhosis. *N. Engl. J. Med.* **339**, 533–541.

[3] Gines, P., Cardenas, A. and Schrier, R. (2001) Liver disease and the kidney, in *Diseases of the Kidney and Urinary Tract*, ed. Schrier, R. 7th edition (Lippincott Williams & Wilkins, Philadelphia, PA) pp. 2167–2203.

[4] Ginès, P. and Rodés, J. (1999) Clinical disorders of renal function in cirrhosis with ascites, in *Ascites and Renal Dysfunction in Liver Disease*, eds. Arroyo, V., Ginès, P., Rodés, J. and Schrier, R.W. (Blackwell Science, Malden) p. 36.

[5] Arroyo, V., Rodés, J., Gutiérrez-Lizarraga, M.A. and Revert, L. (1976) Prognostic value of spontaneous hyponatremia in cirrhosis with ascites. *Am. J. Dig. Dis.* **21**, 249–256.

[6] Dagher, L. and Moore, K. (2001) The hepatorenal syndrome. *Gut* **49**, 729–737.

[7] Lieberman, F.L., Denison, E.K. and Reynolds, T.B. (1970) The relationship of plasma volume, portal hypertension, ascites, and renal sodium retention in cirrhosis: the overflow theory of ascites formation. *Ann. N.Y. Acad. Sci.* **170**, 202.

[8] Williams, Jr., J.W. and Simel, D.L. (1992) Does this patient have ascites? How to divine fluid in the abdomen. *J. Am. Med. Assoc.* **267**, 2645–2648.

[9] Bravo, A.A., Sheth, S.G. and Chopra, S. (2001) Liver biopsy. *N. Engl. J. Med.* **344**, 495–500.

[10] Runyon, B. (1999) Approach to the patient with ascites, in *Textbook of Gastroenterology*, ed. Yamada, T. 3rd edition (Lippincott Williams & Wilkins, Philadelphia, PA) p. 966.

[11] Rimola, A., Garcia-Tsao, G., Navasa, M., Piddock, L.J., Planas, R., Bernard, B. and Inadomi, J.M. (2000) Diagnosis, treatment and prophylaxis of spontaneous bacterial peritonitis: a consensus document. International Ascites Club. *J. Hepatol.* **32**, 142–153.

[12] Fernandez, J., Navasa, M., Gomez, J., Colmenerom, J., Vila, J., Arroyo, V. and Rodes, J. (2002) Bacterial infections in cirrhosis: epidemiological changes with invasive procedures and norfloxacin prophylaxis. *Hepatology* **35**, 140–148.

[13] Runyon, B.A., Montano, A.A., Akriviadis, E.A., Antillon, M.R., Irving, M.A. and McHutchison, J.G. (1992) The serum–ascites albumin gradient is superior to the exudate-transudate concept in the differential diagnosis of ascites. *Ann. Intern. Med.* **117**, 215–220.

[14] Arroyo, V., Ginès, P., Gerbes, A., Dudley, F.J., Gentilini, P., Laff, G., Reynolds, T.B., Ring-Larsen, H. and Scholmerich, J. (1996) Definition and diagnostic criteria of refractory ascites and hepatorenal syndrome in cirrhosis. *Hepatology* **23**, 164–176.

[15] Ginès, P., Arroyo, V., Quintero, E., Planas, R., Bory, F., Cabrera, J., Rimola, A., Viver, J., Camps, J. and Jiménez, W. (1987) Comparison of paracentesis and diuretics in the treatment of cirrhotics with tense ascites. Results of a randomized study. *Gastroenterology* **93**, 234–241.

[16] Ruiz-del-Arbol, L., Monescillo, A., Jimenez, W., Garcia-Plaza, A., Arroyo, V. and Rodes, J. (1997) Paracentesis-induced circulatory dysfunction: mechanism and effect on hepatic hemodynamics in cirrhosis. *Gastroenterology* **113**(2), 579–586.

[17] Ginès, A., Arroyo, V., Monescillo, A., Vila, C., Doménech Abecasis, R., Angeli, P., Ruiz del Árbol, L., Planas, R., Sola, R., Gines, P., Terg, R., Inglada, L., Vaque, P., Salemo, F., Vargas, V., Clemente, G., Quer, J.C., Jiménez, W., Arroyo, V. and Rodes, J. (1996) Randomized trial comparing albumin, dextran-70 and polygelin in cirrhotic patients with ascites treated by paracentesis. *Gastroenterology* **111**, 1002–1010.

[18] Moreau, R., Asselah, T., Condat, B., de Kerguenec, C., Pessione, F., Bernard, B., Poynard, T., Binn, M., Grange, J.D., Valla, D. and Lebrec, D. (2002) Comparison of the effect of terlipressin and albumin on arterial blood volume in patients with cirrhosis and

tense ascites treated by paracentesis: a randomised pilot study. *Gut* **50**, 90–94.

[19] Llach, J., Ginès, P., Arroyo, V., Rimola, A., Tito, L., Badalamenti, S., Jimenez, W., Gaya, J., Rivera, F. and Rodes, J. (1988) Prognostic value of arterial pressure, endogenous vasoactive systems, and renal function in cirrhotic patients admitted to the hospital for the treatment of ascites. *Gastroenterology* **94**, 482–487.

[20] Lebrec, D., Giuily, N., Hadengue, A., Vilgrain, V., Moreau, R., Poynard, T., Gadano, A., Lassen, C., Benhamou, J.P. and Erlinger, S. (1996) Transjugular intrahepatic portosystemic shunts: comparison with paracentesis in patients with cirrhosis and refractory ascites: a randomized trial. *J. Hepatol.* **25**, 135–144.

[21] Rossle, M., Ochs, A., Gulberg, V., Siegerstetter, V., Holl, J., Deibert, P., Olschewski, M., Reiser, M. and Gerbes, A.L. (2000) A comparison of paracentesis and transjugular intrahepatic portosystemic shunting in patients with ascites. *N. Engl. J. Med.* **342**, 1701–1707.

[22] Gines, P., Uriz, J., Calahorra, B., Garcia-Tsao, G., Kamath, P.S., Del Arbol, L.R., Planas, R., Bosch, J., Arroyo, V. and Rodes, J. (2002) Transjugular intrahepatic portosystemic shunting versus paracentesis plus albumin for refractory ascites in cirrhosis. *Gastroenterology* **123**, 1839–1847.

[23] Cárdenas, A. and Ginès, P. (1999) Treatment of water retention and dilutional hyponatremia in cirrhosis, in *Treatment of Liver Diseases*, eds. Arroyo, V., Bosch, J., Brugera, M., Rodés, J. and Sánchez-Tapias, J.M. (Masson, Barcelona) p. 61.

[24] Such, J. and Runyon, B.A. (1998) Spontaneous bacterial peritonitis. *Clin. Infect. Dis.* **27**, 669–674.

[25] Lazaridis, K.N., Frank, J.W., Krowka, M.J. and Kamath, P.S. (1999) Hepatic hydrothorax: pathogenesis, diagnosis, and management. *Am. J. Med.* **107**, 262–267.

Hepatology: A Practical Approach
B. Al Knawy, M.L. Shiffman, R.H. Wiesner (editors)

Chapter 2
Management of Variceal Hemorrhage

Arun J. Sanyal

Division of Gastroenterology, Department of Internal Medicine, Medical College of Virginia Campus of the Virginia Commonwealth University, Richmond, VA, USA

1. Gastro-esophageal Varices: Anatomy and Classification 362
2. Pathophysiology of Portal Hypertension 363
3. Natural History of Gastric and Esophageal Varices 364
   3.1 Esophageal varices 364
   3.2 Gastric varices 365
4. Primary Prophylaxis of Variceal Hemorrhage 365
   4.1 Pharmacologic treatment 366
      4.1.1 Non-selective beta-blockers 366
      4.1.2 Nitrates 367
      4.1.3 Combination of beta-blockers and nitrates 368
   4.2 Mechanical portal decompression (surgery and transjugular intrahepatic portasystemic shunts) 368
   4.3 Endoscopic sclerotherapy and band ligation 368
   4.4 Clinical recommendations for primary prevention of variceal hemorrhage 369
5. Management of Active Hemorrhage 369
   5.1 Pharmacologic treatment 370
      5.1.1 Vasopressin and its analogs 370
      5.1.2 Somatostatin and its analogs 371
   5.2 Endoscopic treatment 371
   5.3 What to do when endoscopic and pharmacologic treatment fails? 372
   5.4 An algorithm for the management of active variceal hemorrhage 373
6. Prevention of Recurrent Variceal Hemorrhage 373
   6.1 Endoscopic treatment 374
   6.2 Pharmacologic treatment 374
   6.3 Transjugular intrahepatic portasystemic shunts 375
   6.4 Surgery and orthotopic liver transplant 377
      6.4.1 An algorithm for the prevention of recurrent variceal hemorrhage 377
References 378

Portal hypertension is defined as an increase in portal venous pressure over 5 mmHg. Portal hypertension is causally related to the development of ascites and variceal hemorrhage, the two major complications of cirrhosis. Of these, variceal hemorrhage represents an immediate threat to life and must be treated as a medical emergency. The optimal management of gastro-esophageal varices requires a clear understanding of the anatomy of the varices, their pathophysiology and natural history and the relative efficacy and safety of various therapeutic modalities at different stages in the natural history of variceal hemorrhage. These are discussed below.

1. GASTRO-ESOPHAGEAL VARICES: ANATOMY AND CLASSIFICATION

The portal vein is formed by the confluence of the superior mesenteric vein and splenic vein. The tributaries of these veins also communicate with veins, which drain into the superior or inferior vena cava. Such communications exist mainly (1) at the cardia via the intrinsic and extrinsic veins of the region, (2) in the anal canal via anastomoses between the superior and middle hemorrhoidal veins, (3) in the falciform ligament via recanalization of the paraumbilical veins and direction of flow to the veins draining the abdominal wall, (4) in the splenic venous bed and the left renal vein and (5) in the retroperitoneum. When portal pressures rise, these communications provide a mechanism for decompression of the portal vein. In the process, they dilate and form varicosities; of the various sites, varices in the gastro-esophageal region are most likely to bleed and come to clinical attention.

The extrinsic veins of the gastro-esophageal region communicate with the intrinsic veins of the region. The intrinsic veins in this region are organized in four specific zones (Figure 1) [1]. (1) Gastric: a 2–3 cm zone of radially arranged veins in the submucosa and lamina propria. (2) Palisade zone: this extends cranially for 2–3 cm from the top of the gastric zone and is a direct extension of the veins of the gastric zone the area of which is arranged longitudinally in the lamina propria. (3) Perforating zone: this extends for 2–3 cm cranially from the top of the palisade zone and involves veins which curve around and penetrate the wall of the esophagus to communicate with the periesophageal plexus of veins. These perforating veins normally only allow flow from the intrinsic to the extrinsic veins due to the presence of valves in the veins. (4) Truncal zone: a 8–10 cm zone extending upwards from the perforating zone. The intrinsic veins are composed of 3–4 large venous trunks in the submucosa which communicate with an irregular polygonal venous plexus in the submucosa. Blood in these veins flow from a cranial to caudal direction and drain via the perforating veins into the extrinsic veins.

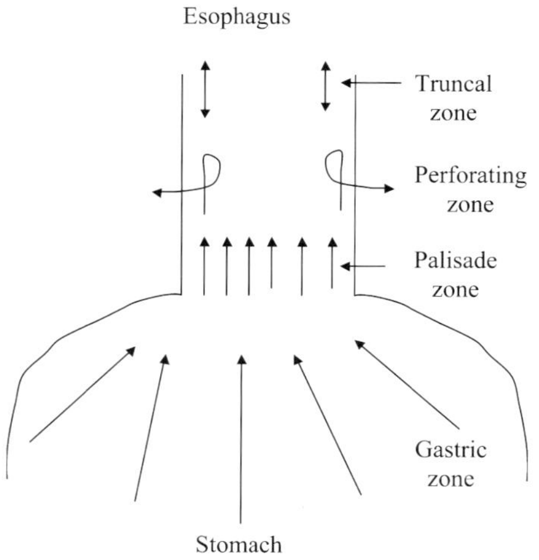

Figure 1. The intrinsic venous drainage of the gastro-esophageal junction. The region may be subdivided in to four zones: (1) gastric, where radially arranged veins drain towards the gastro-esophageal junction, (2) palisade, where parallel rows of superficial veins drain cranially towards the perforating zone, (3) perforating, where the veins perforate the esophageal wall and communicate with the extrinsic venous plexus around the esophagus, and (4) truncal, where blood can flow in a bidirectional manner. Based on the descriptions of Vianna [1].

When portal hypertension occurs, the intrinsic veins around the GE junction dilate and become tortuous forming varicose veins. In contrast to normal individuals, the valves in the perforating veins become incompetent thereby permitting reverse flow into the intrinsic plexus from the extrinsic veins.

Clinically, varices are classified by their location into esophageal and gastric varices. Esophageal varices are graded by their size [2]:

F1: small straight varices
F2: enlarged, tortuous, occupy less than 1/3 of lumen
F3: large, coil-shaped, occupy more than 1/3 of lumen

In contrast, gastric varices are classified primarily by their location (Figure 2) [3]:

A: *Gastro-esophageal varices (GOV)*: gastric varices in continuity with esophageal varices
 Type I (GOV1): along the lesser curve (usually 2–5 cm in length)
 Type II (GOV2): along the greater curve extending towards the fundus of the stomach

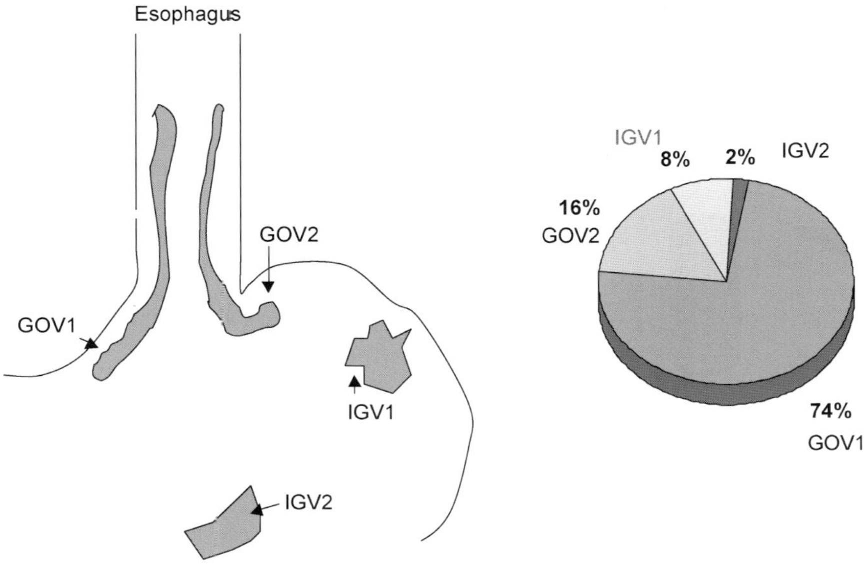

Figure 2. Types and prevalence of gastric varices. Gastro-oesophageal varices (GOV) are varices in continuity with esophageal varices along the lesser curve (Type 1) or greater curve (Type 2). Isolated gastric varices (IGV) are present in the fundus (Type 1) or elsewhere in the stomach (Type 2). Based on the descriptions of Sarin *et al.* (1992) *Hepatology* **16**, 1342. (*For colored version, see Plate XXXIII on page 581 at the end of the book.*)

B: *Isolated gastric varices (IGV)*:
Type I (IGV1): isolated cluster of varices in the fundus of the stomach
Type II (IGV2): isolated gastric varices in other parts of the stomach.

2. PATHOPHYSIOLOGY OF PORTAL HYPERTENSION

The portal pressure is directly related to portal inflow and outflow resistance (Figure 3):

$$\text{portal pressure} = \text{portal venous inflow} \times \text{outflow resistance} \quad (2.1)$$

Portal pressure is usually determined by hepatic venous catheterization and measurement of the free hepatic venous (FHV) and wedged hepatic venous pressures (WHVP) and calculation of the hepatic venous pressure gradient (HVPG):

$$\text{HVPG} = \text{WHVP} - \text{FHV} \quad (2.2)$$

Wedged hepatic pressures reflect sinusoidal pressures while the free hepatic venous pressure corrects for the effects of intra-abdominal pressures. Ideally, the hepatic vein is cannulated with a 7 Fr balloon catheter using a transjugular or transfemoral approach. Once the hepatic vein is cannulated, the catheter is advanced by 2–3 cm and the balloon inflated. Next, 2–3 cc of radiocontrast is injected to document the position of the catheter and complete occlusion of the hepatic vein. The balloon is then deflated and the catheter flushed. The balloon is again reinflated and pressure measurements obtained over a 30–45 s period. It is critically important to measure the zero point of the pressure tracing and calibrate the tracing prior to each measurement. An average of three measurements each with the balloon inflated (wedged pressure) and also with the balloon deflated (free hepatic venous pressure) are taken. A review of the pressure tracing should be done to ensure that there are no respiratory or motion artifacts. Reading the pressure off a digital counter is misleading and should be avoided.

Portal hypertension is initiated by an increase in outflow resistance from the portal venous bed. Table 1 lists the sites and common causes of portal hypertension. Once portal hypertension occurs, a collateral circulation develops to return

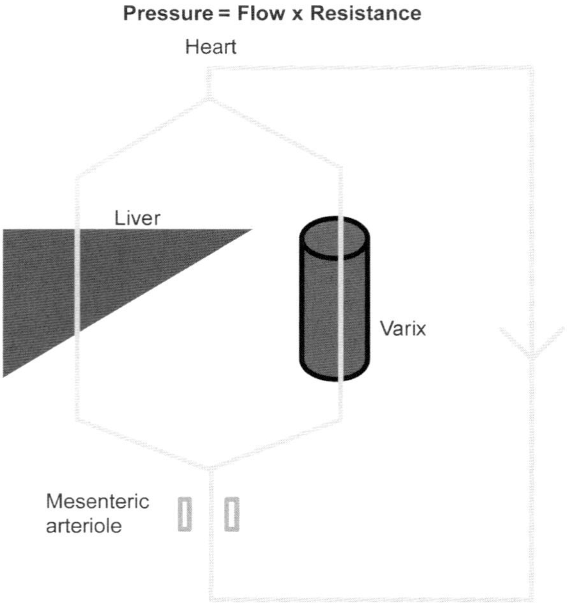

Figure 3. A cartoon showing the functional anatomy of the splanchnic circulation and variceal circulation. Published with permission from Sanyal *et al.* (2001) *Clin. Liver Dis.* (*For colored version, see Plate XXXIV on page 582 at the end of the book.*)

blood to the systemic circulation. For a given varix, the transmural pressure gradient is the product of flow and resistance

$$P_1 - P_2 = QR \tag{2.3}$$

where P_1 and P_2 are the pressures within and outside the varix, respectively; Q the blood flow per unit time and R the resistance to flow through the varix. The resistance to flow can also be expressed as a function of the blood viscosity (n) and the vessel radius (r) as:

$$R = nl/\pi r^4 \tag{2.4}$$

Variceal wall tension determines its probability of rupture. Variceal wall tension is determined by the transmural pressure, radius, and its wall thickness (w) (Laplace's law):

$$\text{Wall tension} = [Q(nl/\pi r^4)](r/w) \tag{2.5}$$

Thus, long, large varices with high flow rates and a thin wall are most likely to rupture and bleed. On the other hand, decreasing collateral flow, resistance to flow or increasing wall thickness should decrease the risk of variceal rupture.

Table 1. Causes of portal hypertension.

Causes
Presinusoidal portal hypertension
Prehepatic
Portal vein thrombosis
Tumor encasement of portal vein
Intrahepatic
Non-cirrhotic portal hypertension (idiopathic portal hypertension)
Schistosomiasis
Some cases of primary biliary cirrhosis
Sarcoidosis
Sinusoidal portal hypertension
Cirrhosis
Vitamin A toxicity
Post-sinusoidal portal hypertension
Veno-occlusive disease
Budd–Chiari syndrome
Constrictive pericarditis

Most pharmacologic treatments are directed at decreasing collateral flow which is usually achieved by decreasing portal pressure and/or increasing collateral resistance.

3. NATURAL HISTORY OF GASTRIC AND ESOPHAGEAL VARICES

3.1 Esophageal varices

Approximately 2–5% of patients with cirrhosis without varices develop varices *de novo* each year. Approximately a third of all patients with esophageal varices experience variceal hemorrhage. Considering the approximately 20–30% mortality from each episode of variceal hemorrhage, it is important to be able to target those at greatest risk of bleeding. Several factors predict the risk of bleeding from esophageal varices. These include:

1. *Portal pressures*: When the HVPG is less than 12 mmHg, varices do not form and therefore can not bleed [4]. At HVPG values over 12 mmHg, varices both form and bleed; however, the precise degree of elevation of HVPG does not correlate with the risk of bleeding. It has also been noted that, amongst those who bleed, those with higher levels of HVPG have a greater risk of severe bleeding and failure of medical treatment.

2. *Varix size and location*: The likelihood of variceal rupture is directly related to its diameter due to the effects of the radius on wall tension (see above). Varices at the GE junction and palisade zone lie in the lamina propria and thus have a thinner coat and are most likely to bleed.
3. *Variceal features on endoscopy*: Several endoscopic features of esophageal varices have been shown to predict the risk of hemorrhage. Together, these are often referred to as "red signs" due to their color [5]. Such findings include:
   a. *red wale marks*: these are longitudinal red streaks on varices which resemble red corduroy wales
   b. *cherry red spots*: these are discrete red cherry-colored spots which are flat and overlie varices
   c. *hematocystic spots*: these are raised discrete red spots overlying varices and resemble "blood blisters"
   d. *diffuse erythema*: as self-evident, this denotes a diffuse red color of the varix
4. *Degree of liver failure*: There is a direct relationship between the severity of liver failure and the risk of variceal hemorrahge.
5. *Presence of ascites*: Tense ascites is also an important risk factor for variceal hemorrhage.

All these risk factors have been used to estimate the probability of variceal hemorrhage with relative precision [2] (Table 2). The risk of bleeding is greatest in the first 2 years after varices are detected and decreases after that time.

Table 2. Prediction of the risk of variceal hemorrhage from DeFranchis *et al.* (1998) *New Engl. J. Med.* **319**(5), 983–989 (published with permission).

Red Wale Marks	Child Class								
	A			B			C		
	F1	F2	F3	F1	F2	F3	F1	F2	F3
−	6	10	15	10	16	26	20	30	42
+	8	12	19	15	23	33	28	38	54
+ + +	16	23	34	28	40	52	44	60	76

F1, F2, F3 are progressively larger varices.

In contrast to GI bleeding from other sources, variceal hemorrahge only stops spontaneously in 50% of cases. Advanced liver failure and actively spurting varices at the time of endoscopy are risk factors for exsanguination. Once active bleeding stops, bleeding often recurs within the first 48–72 h [6,7]. Subsequently, the risk of rebleeding declines to baseline values by 6 weeks. Large varices, age >60 years, renal failure, and severe initial bleeding as defined by a hemoglobin <8 g/dl at admission are risk factors for early rebleeding. Aggressive volume replacement may also cause rebound portal hypertension and precipitate early rebleeding. Survival during this acute phase depends not only on the control of active hemorrhage but also on the recurrence of bleeding.

In the absence of specific treatment, 70% of those who survive a variceal bleed will bleed again and approximately 70% of such survivors die in the first year after the index bleed [6]. The risk of recurrent bleeding is related to the degree of liver failure, continued alcoholism, variceal size, renal failure and the presence of a hepatoma.

3.2 Gastric varices

The likelihood of bleeding from gastric varices depends on their location [8]. Although GOV1 constitute over 70% of gastric varices, only 11% of GOV1 will ever bleed. In contrast, about 80% of IGV1 experience hemorrhage even though they comprise only 8% of all gastric varices. Bleeding from IGV often occurs at relatively low portal pressures and is often severe and associated with crippling encephalopathy. This is due to their association with spontaneous large spleno-renal collaterals, which feed these varices and function as large portasystemic shunt collaterals (Figure 4). Recently, the risk of bleeding from IGV1 was shown to correlate with the size of the varices (>10 mm), Child class and the presence of a red spot on the varices.

4. PRIMARY PROPHYLAXIS OF VARICEAL HEMORRHAGE

A key objective of management of the cirrhotic subject is the primary prevention of variceal

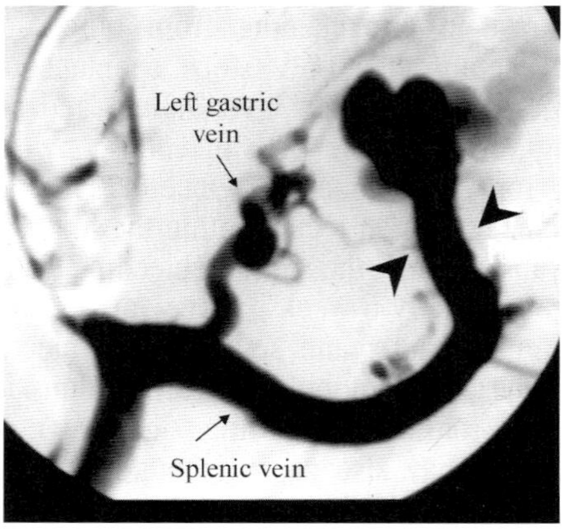

Figure 4. An angiogram demonstrating an isolated gastric varix (Type 1) associated with a large spontaneous spleno-renal collateral.

hemorrhage. The importance of primary prevention is underscored by the continuing high mortality from active hemorrhage as well as the progressive decline in survival following the index bleed.

4.1 Pharmacologic treatment

4.1.1. Non-selective beta-blockers

Pharmacodynamic considerations: Portal pressure is critically dependent on portal venous inflow which, in turn, is dependent on the mesenteric arteriolar tone. Non-selective beta-blockers block β-adrenergic receptor-mediated vasodilatory effects and allow unopposed α-adrenergic receptor-mediated vasoconstriction in the mesenteric arterioles. At high doses, they produce a drop in cardiac output that further contributes to the decrease in mesenteric arterial flow. Both effects decrease portal venous inflow and thereby decrease portal pressure. Thus, the principal hemodynamic effect of such agents is a decrease in hepatic venous pressure gradient due to a decrease in wedged hepatic venous pressure.

Propranolol and nadolol are the two most-studied non-selective β-blockers for the management of portal hypertension. Following either an oral or intravenous dose of propranolol, the hepatic venous pressure gradient decreases by 9–31%. However, up to 50% of patients fail to maintain the initial portal hypotensive effect over time. This is due to an increase in collateral venous resistance and/or an increase in hepatic arterial flow.

Pharmacokinetic considerations: Propranolol is highly lipophilic and is almost completely absorbed after oral administration. It undergoes first-pass elimination to a variable degree causing plasma levels to vary by up to 20-fold. A sustained-release form of propranolol has also been developed which allows once daily dosing. The clinical effects often do not correlate well with the plasma levels because of the formation of active metabolites, especially the (−) enantiomers, which are taken up by sympathetic nerve endings and then released slowly.

In contrast, nadolol is water soluble and only incompletely absorbed orally. Also, the interindividual pharmacokinetic variability is much less than propranolol. Due to its hydrophilic nature, it does not cross the blood–brain barrier well. However, clinical trials have not shown a significant decrease in the incidence of CNS side effects compared to propranolol. It is excreted via the kidney and its dose has to be modified in response to renal insufficiency.

Clinical trials of beta-blockers for primary prevention of variceal hemorrhage: Numerous clinical trials have evaluated the utility of propranolol or nadolol for primary prophylaxis of variceal hemorrhage (Figure 5). Alcoholic liver disease was the most common etiology of cirrhosis across all trials. Analysis of the data is, however, complicated by the considerable heterogeneity among the patients studied and the treatment regimen used. The majority of patients studied had relatively preserved liver function. The dose was titrated in these studies to achieve a decrease in the heart rate by 25% or to 55–60 beats/min.

Beta-blockers are associated with a lower risk of variceal hemorrhage than placebo (0–18 vs 12–30%) [9]. Although four studies showed a significant decrease in bleeding risk, only one found a survival advantage for those treated with beta-blockers. However, variceal hemorrhage-related deaths were less likely among those receiving beta-blockers. Meta-analyses of the data suggest that non-selective beta-blockade reduces the risks of initial variceal hemorrhage by 45% and bleeding-related

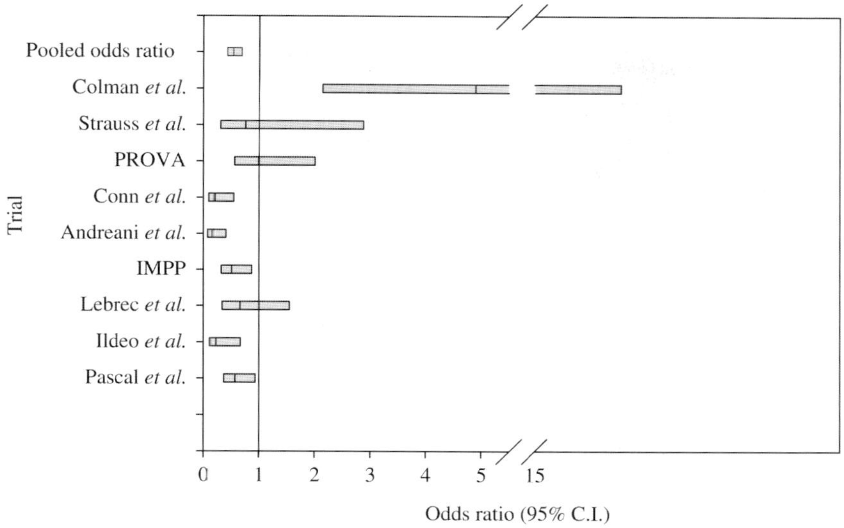

Figure 5. A meta-analysis of β-blockers for primary prophylaxis of variceal hemorrhage. The bleeding risk was decreased in 7 of 9 published studies. Overall, there was a significant decrease in bleeding risk with beta-blockers (Odds ratio = 0.54; 95% C.I.: 0.39–0.74). Based on data from Ref. [22].

deaths by 50% (Figure 5) [9]. Compliance with treatment was an important predictor of a good outcome while failure of therapy was associated with younger age, large variceal size, advanced liver failure and lower propranolol doses.

Adverse effects: β-Blockers are associated with numerous side effects and multiple drug interactions. The most clinically important side effects involve bronchoconstriction, development of heart failure, and impotence in cirrhotics. Despite the increase in renin activity and decrease in renal blood flow, renal dysfunction is rare. The administration of β-blockers has not been shown to impair the hemodynamic response to acute blood loss.

4.1.2. Nitrates

Pharmacodynamics: Nitric oxide (NO) is a potent vasodilator and is an important mediator of the vasodilated state seen in cirrhosis. The "nitrosovasodilator" group of drugs act via nitric oxide pathway producing vasodilation in their target vascular beds. At usual pharmacologic doses, these agents are primarily venodilators and decrease the hepatic venous pressure gradient by decreasing post-sinusoidal resistance to flow. At high doses, arterial dilation and systemic hypotension occur causing reflex splanchnic vasoconstriction and further decrease in portal pressures. Splanchnic vasoconstriction can also result from a nitrate-mediated baroreceptor reflex, which originates from the pulmonary vascular bed. Plasma norepinephrine and renin activity increase during chronic nitrate therapy indicating increased sympathetic activity and enhanced tendency to retain Na. In the long term, the degree of portal decompression is variable and the systemic hemodynamic effects become less pronounced. The effects of isosorbide dinitrate (ISDN) are less predictable than isosorbide mononitrate (ISMN) presumably due to their variable hepatic extraction in cirrhotic subjects. Therefore, ISMN is the long-acting nitrate of choice for the treatment of portal hypertension.

Clinical trials of nitrates for primary prevention of variceal hemorrhage: An important study [10] prospectively randomized 118 patients to receive either ISMN (20 mg tid) or propranolol (to maximum tolerated dose). After a median follow-up of 29 months, no significant differences were noted in either bleeding rates (18 vs 14%) or mortality (18 vs 15%). However, after 7 years [10], an increased mortality especially in those >51 years of age (72 vs 48%) was noted in those receiving ISMN.

It is unclear whether the above findings reflect a beneficial effect of propranolol or an adverse effect of nitrates. Interpretation of the data is further confounded by the fact that about 50% of patients enrolled in either arm withdrew from the study. Nitrates are known to increase Na retention, and cause tissue hypoxia and increased lactate levels in cirrhotic individuals. At this time, the data do not support a role for nitrates as monotherapy for the primary prophylaxis of variceal hemorrhage.

4.1.3. Combination of beta-blockers and nitrates

It has been shown that combination of beta-blockers and nitrates have a synergistic effect in terms of decreasing portal pressures. This synergism is maintained over time. Clinically, a long-term trial demonstrated that combination therapy was superior to beta-blocker therapy alone for primary prophylaxis of variceal hemorrhage (Figure 6) [11]. It was also found that those who had a decrease in hepatic venous pressure gradient by 20% or to values less than 12 mmHg and were able to maintain this drop were essentially free of bleeding. These data provide strong evidence to support the use of combination therapy for primary prophylaxis of variceal hemorrhage. However, it must be remembered that the majority of patients in this trial had Child class A cirrhosis and that 20–30% of subjects were intolerant to this combination of drugs. The increased mortality seen in those over 51 years of age treated with nitrates alone is also worrisome. While there is no consensus on when to use combination therapy, this author restricts their use to those with early-stage cirrhosis (Child class A or B) with high-risk varices who have normal systemic hemodynamics and are under 50 years of age.

4.2 Mechanical portal decompression (surgery and transjugular intrahepatic portasystemic shunts)

Four prospective randomized trials comparing surgical portacaval shunts to medical therapy were carried out over 25 years ago [12]. They demonstrated that while surgery could effectively prevent variceal hemorrhage, the benefit was offset by severe encephalopathy which ensued in 30–60% of patients. Moreover, medically treated patients survived longer. Thus, this modality has been eliminated as an option for the primary prevention of variceal hemorrhage. Similarly, there is no role for transjugular intrahepatic portasystemic shunts (TIPS) for primary prophylaxis of variceal hemorrhage.

4.3 Endoscopic sclerotherapy and band ligation

Injection of sclerosant substances into varices may be used to obliterate varices and treat

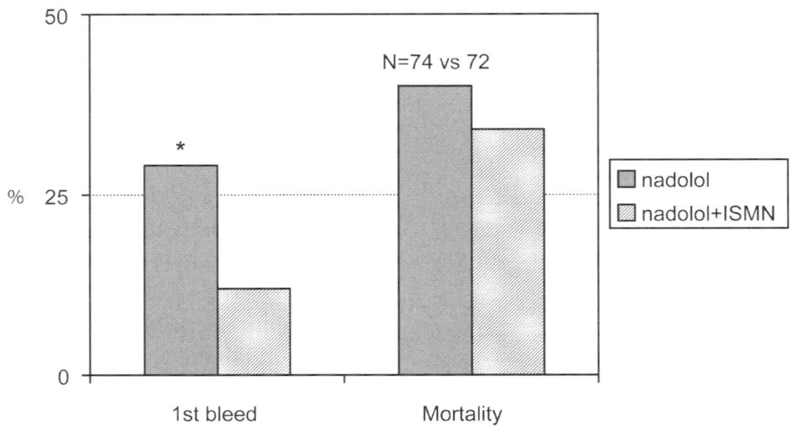

Figure 6. Nadolol vs nadolol + isosorbide mononitrate (ISMN) for primary prophylaxis of variceal hemorrhage. Combination therapy was associated with a significantly superior bleeding rate, i.e., less bleeding although the mortality data were comparable. Data from Ref. [11]. *(For colored version, see Plate XXXV on page 582 at the end of the book.)*

variceal hemorrhage. Endoscopic sclerotherapy was found to be associated with increased mortality despite a decrease in bleeding in a large multicenter study. Also, beta-blockers alone are superior to sclerotherapy and equivalent to beta-blocker and sclerotherapy for this indication. Thus, sclerotherapy should not be used either alone or with beta-blockers for the primary prevention of variceal hemorrhage.

In contrast, several clinical trials have shown that the endoscopic variceal band ligation is superior to no therapy for primary prophylaxis of variceal hemorrhage. It has also been found to be superior to propranolol in one trial [13]. This study has, however, been criticized because of the low dose of propranolol used and a very high rate of bleeding in the propranolol arm. Studies are currently in progress to determine the relative utility of band ligation vs pharmacologic treatment for primary prophylaxis of variceal hemorrhage.

4.4 Clinical recommendations for primary prevention of variceal hemorrhage

Non-selective beta-blockers remain the first-line therapy for the primary prevention of variceal hemorrhage in cirrhotic patients. All patients with cirrhosis should undergo an endoscopic examination as part of their evaluation. Patients with Child class B or C cirrhosis with esophageal varices of any grade and those with Child class A cirrhosis and large varices, especially with red signs, should be targeted for treatment with propranolol or nadolol. In selected cases, combination pharmacologic therapy may be used. In those where varices are not present, endoscopy should be repeated at 2–3 year intervals. No evaluable data currently exist for the clinical utility of beta-blockers for the various types of gastric varices although it appears to make intuitive sense to treat those especially at high risk for bleeding. Endoscopic band ligation may be used in cases where the patients are intolerant to pharmacologic therapy.

It has been shown that those who experience a 20% or greater drop in HVPG or HVPG values <12 mmHg and maintain these changes over time are most likely to remain free of bleeding [14]. It has therefore been recommended that the HVPG be measured prior to initiation of therapy and after 1–3 months of treatment and the dosage of the drug changed appropriately to achieve the desired endpoints. However, the cost-effectiveness of this approach remains to be demonstrated. Moreover, HVPG measurement is not possible at many medical centers. Where such facilities are unavailable, the dose should be titrated to achieve a decrease in resting heart rate to values of 55–60 beats/min.

5. MANAGEMENT OF ACTIVE HEMORRHAGE

Active variceal hemorrhage accounts for about a third of all deaths related to cirrhosis of the liver. There are three primary goals of management during the active bleeding episode. These include hemodynamic resuscitation, prevention and treatment of complications and treatment of bleeding (Table 3). All three need to be pursued simultaneously and often require the coordinated care of a hepatologist, critical care physician, critical care nurse, surgeon and interventional radiologist.

Hemodynamic resuscitation: This should be aggressively managed with large bore peripheral i.v. lines or a central line. Blood loss should be replaced by packed cells and clotting factors should be replaced as needed. In those requiring large amounts of blood, attention to development of hypocalcemia and thrombocytopenia should also be given. The hemoglobin should be brought to the 9–10 g/dl range and over transfusion should be avoided due to the risks of rebound portal hypertension and rebleeding.

Prevention and management of complications: Complications related to bleeding as well as the treatment of bleeding contribute substantially to mortality from active hemorrhage. Pulmonary aspiration is often fatal and careful attention to protection of the airway is very important. The renal function must be monitored and fluid administered to maintain a urine output of at least 50 cc/h. If renal failure develops, it must be evaluated quickly and managed appropriately. Lactulose should be given orally once

Table 3. Management of acute variceal hemorrhage.

Hemodynamic resuscitation
Keep Hgb ~9–10 g/dl
Fluids to maintain urine output >50 ml/h
Correct severe coagulopathy with fresh frozen plasma
Correct severe thrombocytopenia (platelets <50,000 mm^{-3})

Prevent and treat complications
Airway-related
  Protect airway if compromised
  Monitor and treat aspiration aggressively

Sepsis
  Diagnostic paracentesis and blood cultures upon admission
  Empiric treatment of sepsis until culture and paracentesis results back
  Prophylaxis for spontaneous bacterial peritonitis after i.v. antibiotics stopped
  Monitor periodically for sepsis (urine, chest X-ray, blood cultures)

Renal failure
  Maintain euvolemia (judicious use of colloids along with crystalloids)
  Avoid NSAIDS, aminoglycosides
  Avoid sepsis or treat aggressively
  Monitor for development of hepatorenal syndrome

Hepatic encephalopathy
  Lactulose via NG tube once bleeding is controlled
  Look for sepsis, medications, renal failure, electrolyte and acid–base disturbances as reversible causes of worsening mental status

Nutrition and metabolic disturbances
  Start enteral feeds as soon as bleeding is controlled
  Consider TPN for prolonged ileus
  Monitor glucose, electrolytes, Ca^{2+}, Mg^{2+}, phosphates

Related to blood transfusions
  Check platelets [Ca^{2+}] if large amounts of blood transfused

Achieve and maintain hemostasis
First-line therapy: pharmacologic treatment (somatostatin, terlipressin or octreotide) + endoscopic sclerotherapy or band ligation
Salvage therapy: TIPS or surgery

bleeding is controlled to wash out the blood from the GI tract and also to prevent encephalopathy.

Approximately 20% of patients with cirrhosis have subclinical evidence of infection at the time of hospitalization for a variety of indications. It has been shown that such infections are associated with continued hemorrhage and failure of medical therapy. Also, patients with ascites may develop spontaneous bacterial peritonitis, which further adds to bleeding-related mortality. All patients with variceal hemorrhage should therefore have blood cultures and a diagnostic paracentesis soon after admission. They should also receive a dose of a third generation antibiotic, e.g., cefotaxime whose cultures are awaited. If all cultures are negative, those at risk for spontaneous bacterial peritonitis should be given norfloxacin 400 mg p.o. daily for 7–14 days. Aminoglycosides should be avoided due to their high incidence of nephrotoxicity in patients with advanced cirrhosis unless documented sepsis with bacteria only sensitive to aminoglycosides are found.

Treatment of active hemorrhage: All the modalities discussed above for primary prevention are also available for active bleeding. The choice of treatment depends on its relative efficacy and safety, the expediency with which it can be implemented and cost considerations. These are discussed below.

5.1 Pharmacologic treatment

5.1.1. Vasopressin and its analogs

Vasopressin is a non-specific vasoconstrictor and produces mesenteric arteriolar vasoconstriction. Although vasopressin can achieve initial hemostasis in 60–80% of cases, rebleeding often occurs and overall mortality is not improved. It has also been associated with increased fibrinolysis and failure to produce additional decreases in hepatic venous pressure gradient in those who are already bleeding. It also produces coronary vasoconstriction and should always be given along with nitrates either intravenously or percutaneously to prevent this complication. The concomitant use of nitrates is also associated with a synergistic effect on portal pressures.

Terlipressin is an analog of vasopressin where a triglycyl group is attached to the n-terminal of lysine-vasopressin. Cleavage of this residue releases the drug in a slow and sustained manner at the vascular smooth muscle. Several clinical trials have shown equivalence to somatostatin and greater efficacy than placebo (Figure 7). This is the only drug that has been found to be associated with an improvement in

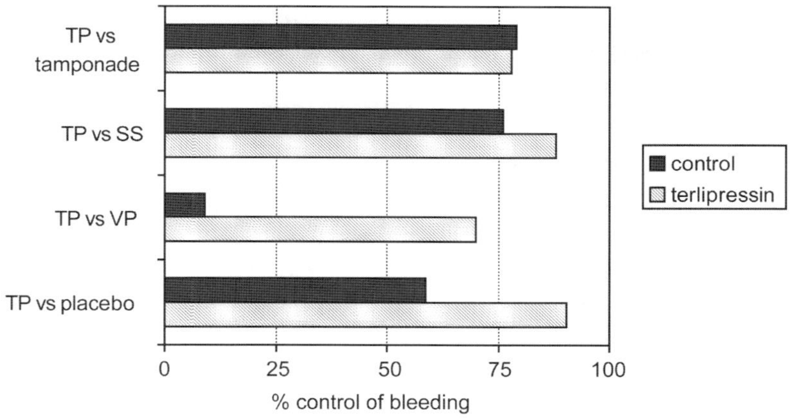

Figure 7. Comparison of terlipressin (TP) vs placebo, vasopressin (VP), somatostatin (SS) or tamponade in the management of acute variceal hemorrhage. (*For colored version, see Plate XXXVI on page 583 at the end of the book.*)

survival in cases of active variceal hemorrhage. It is not available in the US.

5.1.2. Somatostatin and its analogs

Somatostatin is a 14 amino acid peptide, named for its growth-hormone inhibiting properties. Somatostatin inhibits release of vasodilator hormones, e.g., glucagon and thereby indirectly causes splanchnic vasoconstriction and decreased portal inflow. Somatostatin has a very short half-life and disappears within minutes of a bolus infusion. Octreotide is a long-acting analog of somatostatin.

Following a bolus injection of either agent, portal venous inflow, portal pressures, azygous flow and intravariceal pressures decrease within seconds. Of these effects, the changes in portal pressures, as measured by wedged hepatic pressures, are most variable and the decreases in collateral flow (azygous flow) are those most consistently observed. Bolus doses are more likely to decrease cardiac output than continuous infusions. The overall effects of a 250 μg of somatostatin followed by an infusion at 250 μg/h has the same effects as a 500 μg bolus. Tachyphylaxis occurs after repeated bolus injections or during infusion of octreotide. Given their modest direct effects on portal hemodynamics, it is likely that the principal mechanism of action of these agents is to decrease the reflex increase in mesenteric blood flow which occurs in response to blood in the GI tract, a phenomenon mediated by glucagon and other gut-related hormones. Neither drug causes clinically significant toxicity in clinical trials of variceal hemorrhage.

Clinical trials: Somatostatin is significantly superior to placebo with respect to achievement of hemostasis as well as prevention of early rebleeding. It is also superior to vasopressin and balloon tamponade due to the virtual absence of side effects associated with somatostatin or octreotide therapy (Figure 8). Somatostatin is equivalent to endoscopic sclerotherapy. Also, the use of either somatostatin or octreotide infusion for 5 days in addition to sclerotherapy has been shown, in one study each, to be superior to sclerotherapy alone for prevention of early rebleeding and improving survival. Similar data have been shown with octreotide and endoscopic band ligation. Thus, these agents are principally used as adjunctive therapy along with endoscopic treatment.

5.2 Endoscopic treatment

Endoscopic treatment is currently the definitive treatment of choice for active variceal hemorrhage. It can be performed at the same time as diagnostic endoscopy at the bedside by virtually all trained gastro-enterologists. Two forms of endoscopic treatment are available: endoscopic sclerotherapy and endoscopic variceal band ligation.

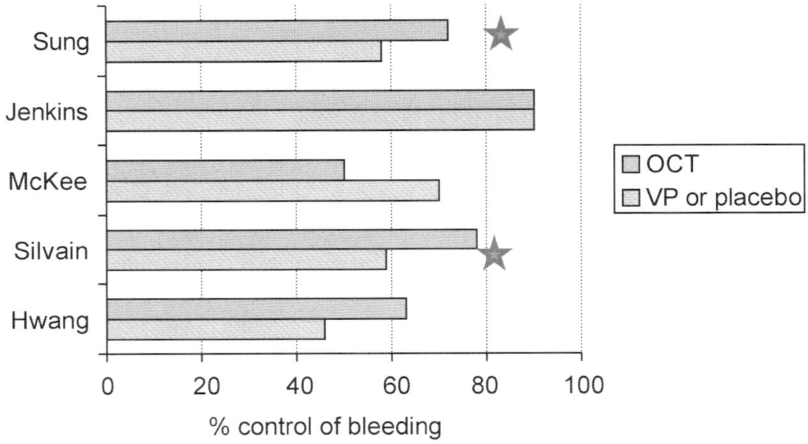

Figure 8. Clinical trials demonstrating the relative efficacy of octreotide vs either vasopressin or placebo in the control of variceal hemorrhage. (*For colored version, see Plate XXXVII on page 583 at the end of the book.*)

Clinical trials: Both esophageal as well as GOV Types I and II are amenable to treatment by sclerotherapy or band ligation. However, IGV do not lend themselves to these modalities of treatment. Sclerotherapy is superior to balloon tamponade alone, vasopressin alone as well as a combination of vasopressin and balloon tamponade for control of active hemorrhage, prevention of early rebleeding, complication rates and survival (Figure 9). Both intravariceal and paravariceal injections are effective. Band ligation is equally effective as sclerotherapy for achieving hemostasis and prevention of early rebleeding. It is therefore reasonable to use either modality in the setting of active hemorrhage.

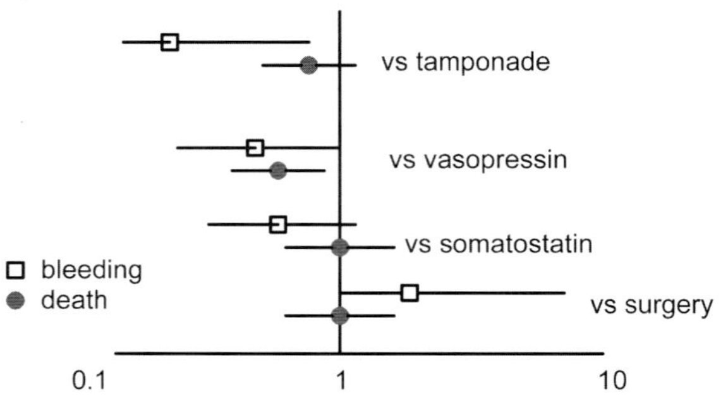

Figure 9. The relative efficacy of endoscopic sclerotherapy vs other modalities of treatment for the management of acute variceal hemorrhage. Sclerotherapy was superior to tamponade, vasopressin for prevention of bleeding. Although it appeared superior to somatostatin, this did not reach significance. Surgery was more effective than sclerotherapy for the control of bleeding but was not associated with an improvement in survival. Based on data from Ref. [22]. (*For colored version, see Plate XXXVIII on page 584 at the end of the book.*)

Complications: Local complications (Table 4) include ulceration, bleeding, dysmotility, stricture formation while regional complications include esophageal perforation and mediastinitis. Systemic complications include sepsis, aspiration and ventilation perfusion mismatch with hypoxemia. All these complications occur more frequently when endoscopy is performed emergently rather than electively.

5.3 What to do when endoscopic and pharmacologic treatment fails?

Emergent endoscopic treatment fails to control bleeding in 10–20% of patients. These patients are at high risk for both exsanguination as well as all the complications related to active bleeding. In such patients, a second attempt at endoscopic hemostasis may be made. However, if bleeding is not quickly and effectively stopped, more definitive therapy must be instituted immediately.

Balloon tamponade: This is an effective way to achieve short-term hemostasis. The use of balloon tamponade compromises the airway and it must be

Table 4. Complications of endoscopic therapy of varices.

Complication
Local
Pain
Ulceration
Strictures
Regional
Mediatinitis
Mediastinal abscess
Systemic
Sepsis
Pleural effusion
Ventilation–perfusion mismatch

These are mainly associated with sclerotherapy although local complications can also occur with band ligation.

protected before such a tube is placed. It is also associated with a risk of pressure necrosis of the mucosa when used for long periods of time (>72 h) and a high risk of rebleeding when the balloon is deflated. Its use is therefore restricted to the temporary stabilization of the patient until definitive treatment can be instituted.

Surgery: Both portal decompressive surgery as well as esophageal transection have been shown to be highly effective in achieving hemostasis. The use of surgery as first-line treatment has declined because sclerotherapy has been shown to be as effective as surgical portacaval shunt in those with advanced cirrhosis and variceal hemorrhage [15]. Also, portacaval shunts have been associated with an approximately 40–50% incidence of encephalopathy. These considerations have led to a decline in the use of surgery as first-line treatment of variceal hemorrhage. Nevertheless, surgical portal decompression or esophageal transection remains an effective way to arrest variceal hemorrhage and prevent rebleeding. The ideal patient for surgical therapy is one with well-preserved liver function who fails emergent endoscopic treatment and has no complications from the bleeding or endoscopy. The choice of surgery is usually dependent on the training and expertise of the surgeon.

TIPS: It functions like side-to-side surgical portacaval shunts without exposing the patient to the risks of general anesthesia or major surgery. This has led to a resurgence of interest in portal decompression as a treatment of variceal hemorrhage. Two important studies have shown that TIPS can be placed in practically all patients with severe active variceal hemorrhage refractory to endoscopic therapy [16,17] who had advanced liver failure. While one study focused on those with esophageal bleeding, the other focused on gastric variceal hemorrhage. In both studies, hemostasis was achieved in over 90% of individuals and the 30 day survival approached 50–60%. These data are far superior to those obtained with conventional treatment, i.e., surgery for this subset where a 10–20% survival would have been expected. Thus, TIPS is the procedure of choice in patients with active hemorrhage despite endoscopic treatment who are high-risk for surgery. The utility of TIPS vs surgery in those with variceal hemorrhage and good liver functions remains under investigation.

5.4 An algorithm for the management of active variceal hemorrhage

The initial treatment of active hemorrhage must include hemodynamic resuscitation, prevention of complications and early endoscopy to establish the diagnosis and initiate specific treatment (Figure 10). Somatostatin or octreotide (50 μg bolus followed by 50 μg/h by i.v. infusion) may be started in the emergency room in those having a high index of suspicion for variceal hemorrhage. At endoscopy, bleeding esophageal varices are treated by either sclerotherapy or band ligation. If active bleeding persists or recurs within 48 h, bleeding may be controlled by a definitive procedure, e.g., surgery or TIPS performed. The choice of the definitive procedure depends on the clinical condition of the patient and the expertise available. When bleeding occurs over 48 h after initial endoscopic treatment, a second attempt at controlling hemorrhage by endoscopy is reasonable before proceeding to salvage therapy.

6. PREVENTION OF RECURRENT VARICEAL HEMORRHAGE

The natural history of the untreated patient who has survived an episode of variceal hemorrhage is characterized by recurrent hemorrhage with consequent liver failure, hepatic encephalopathy and eventually death [6]. It is therefore imperative

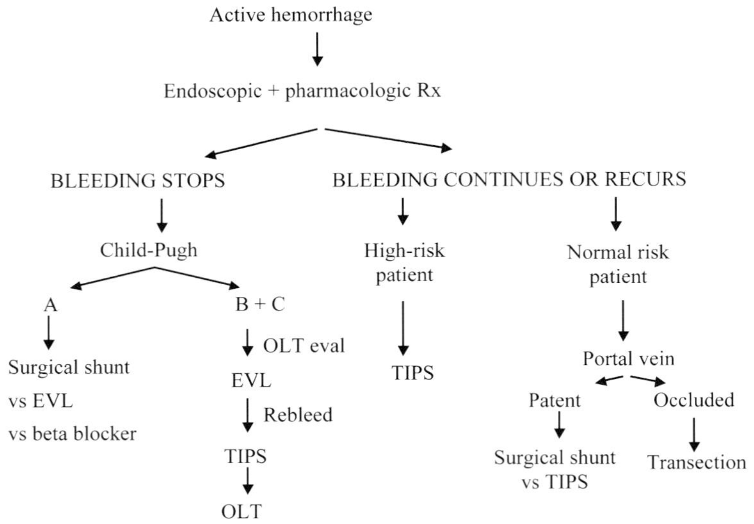

Figure 10. An algorithm for the management of variceal hemorrhage. Published with permission from Garcia and Sanyal (2001) *Clin. Liver Dis.* **5**, 509–540.

to prevent such rebleeding. All the modalities discussed above are also available for prevention for recurrent variceal hemorrhage.

6.1 Endoscopic treatment

Endoscopic sclerotherapy decreases both the risk of rebleeding (40–50% vs 70%) and death (30–60% vs 50–75%) compared to placebo. There is controversy about whether this represents the beneficial effects of sclerotherapy performed during episodes of active bleeding or the ability of sclerotherapy to obliterate esophageal varices. The nature of the sclerosant, frequency of sclerotherapy (weekly vs 2–3 week intervals), site of injection (intravariceal vs paravariceal) and volume of sclerosant do not affect the outcome of the treatment. Breakthrough hemorrhage usually occurs before varices are obliterated. There is an approximately 20% recurrence rate for varices over time after they have been obliterated. Therefore, surveillance endoscopy is usually performed at 6-month intervals in most cases. In the absence of hard evidence, this author reduces the frequency of surveillance endoscopy to annual intervals, once a year has gone by without evidence of variceal recurrence. All the side effects of sclerotherapy described above during emergent sclerotherapy may also occur during repeated sessions.

Endoscopic band ligation has now replaced sclerotherapy as first-line treatment for the prevention of recurrent variceal hemorrhage (Figure 11). It is associated with earlier variceal obliteration, less complications and less rebleeding as well as improved survival compared to sclerotherapy [18]. Band ligation is associated with a greater risk of variceal recurrence compared to sclerotherapy. Those with paraesophageal varices >5 mm in diameter have the greatest risk of variceal recurrence. The role of endoscopic ultrasound in predicting variceal recurrence is currently under study.

6.2 Pharmacologic treatment

A large number of controlled clinical trials have examined the role of β-blockers for prevention of recurrent variceal hemorrhage [19]. As in studies of primary prophylaxis, most trials of secondary prophylaxis have also included subjects with relatively preserved liver function. The principal source of heterogeneity between studies stem from the varying times of entry into studies (1 day–1 month). β-Blocker doses were titrated to achieve a 25% decrease in resting heart rates. An improvement in rebleeding rates was noted in most studies although a survival advantage was shown only in a single trial

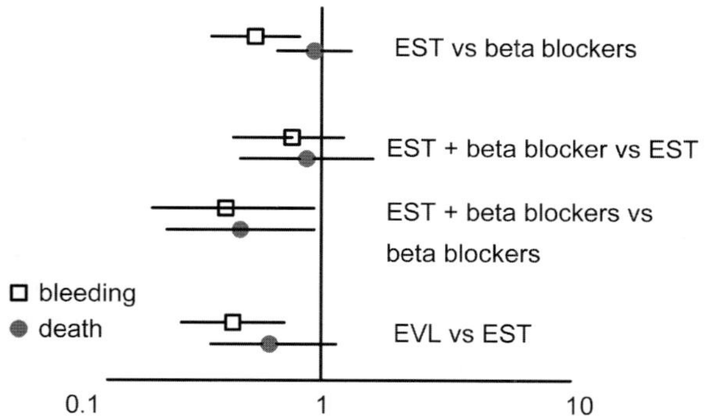

Figure 11. The relative efficacy of endoscopic therapies for the prevention of recurrent variceal hemorrhage. Endoscopic sclerotherapy (EST) was associated with improved rebleeding rates compared to β-blockers but the survival data were unchanged. Endoscopic band ligation (EVL) was superior to EST for prevention of rebleeding. There was also a trend towards improved survival. Based on data from Ref. [22]. *(For colored version, see Plate XXXIX on page 584 at the end of the book.)*

[20]. Meta-analyses of these data have also been performed and suggest that the risk of bleeding is decreased by approximately 40% while the risk of death is decreased by 20% [21].

The utility of β-blockers vs other modalities of treatment have been extensively studied and the data subjected to meta-analyses [22]. β-Blockers are inferior to sclerotherapy with respect to prevention of recurrent bleeding although the two treatments are similar with respect to effect on mortality. Also, β-blockers and sclerotherapy is equi-efficaceous to sclerotherapy alone while the combination is superior to β-blockers alone. Two studies have found combination pharmacologic treatment with β-blockers and nitrates to be more effective in preventing recurrent bleeding than sclerotherapy and band ligation, respectively. However, this did not translate into a survival advantage. Combination pharmacologic treatment or β-blockers alone are used for secondary prophylaxis mainly in those with relatively preserved liver functions (Figure 12).

6.3 Transjugular intrahepatic portasystemic shunts

Several clinical trials have evaluated the efficacy of TIPS vs endoscopic treatment for the prevention of recurrent variceal hemorrhage (Figure 13). These studies show that TIPS is substantially superior to endoscopic treatment for prevention of recurrent bleeding. However, this was offset by a higher likelihood of encephalopathy and a lack of effect on mortality. TIPS is therefore used primarily as a salvage therapy for those with recurrent bleeding despite an adequate trial of endoscopic treatment.

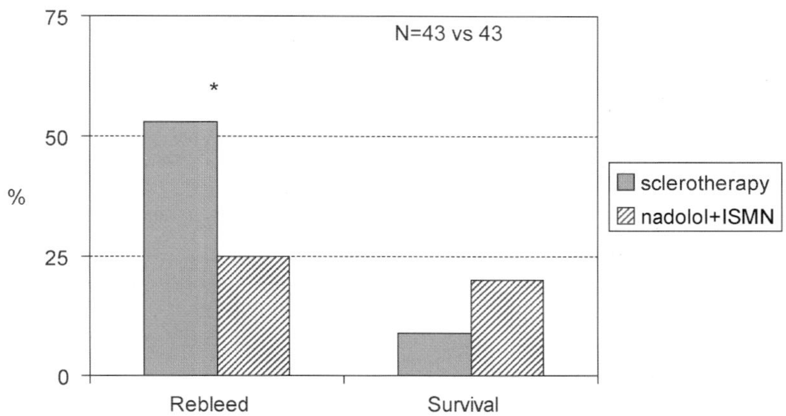

Figure 12. The effects of sclerotherapy vs nadolol and isosorbide mononitrate (ISMN) on prevention of recurrent variceal hemorrhage. Combination therapy was associated with a lower rebleed rate although the survival data were not significantly different. Based on data from Villanueva *et al.* (1996) *N. Engl. J. Med.* **334**, 1624–1629. (*For colored version, see Plate XL on page 584 at the end of the book.*)

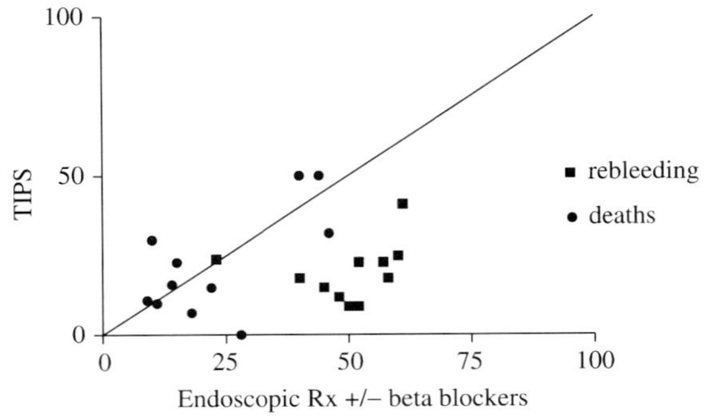

Figure 13. A L'Abbe plot comparing the results of studies of TIPS vs endoscopic therapy with or without additional pharmacologic therapy for the prevention of recurrent variceal hemorrhage. The unit line represents the theoretical region where the data would be expected if the treatments were similar. TIPS was associated with significantly less rebleeding. However, the mortality data fall around the unit line indicating that TIPS did not improve survival. Published with permission from Garcia and Sanyal (2001) *Clin. Liver Dis.* **5**, 509–540.

The principal cause of rebleeding after TIPS is the recurrence of portal hypertension (Table 5). This may result from TIPS thrombosis, stent retraction and kinking, stent stenosis and development of right heart failure [23]. TIPS thrombosis usually occurs early and its development has been associated with the presence of a biliary-TIPS fistula. Although anticoagulation is routinely used in many European centers, this is rarely used in North America. There are no hard data to clearly demonstrate either the need or value of routine anticoagulation for the prevention of stent thrombosis.

The most common cause of recurrent portal hypertension is the ingrowth of tissue from the surrounding liver into the stent lumen eventually occluding it [24]. Such pseudointimal hyperplasia results from the proliferation and migration of mesenchymal cells of smooth muscle phenotype into the lumen where they synthesize and secrete collagen. Virtually all long-term survivors after TIPS experience TIPS stenosis within the first 2 years necessitating surveillance by either Doppler sonography or angiography [23]. Doppler sonography is specific but somewhat insensitive depending on the specific cutoffs used for the diagnosis of stent stenosis (Table 6). Angiography is the gold standard for the detection of stent stenosis and is required for its treatment. The propensity for development of stent stenosis decreases after 4 years [23]. There is no established standard of care for the long-term monitoring of stent patency once a TIPS is placed.

The adverse effects of TIPS [24] are listed in Table 7. Hepatic encephalopathy occurs in about 30% of individuals after TIPS. It manifests as altered mental status and usually manifests about 2–3 weeks after TIPS placement. It is often precipitated with dietary indiscretion, constipation, urinary tract infections or electrolyte imbalances. Six weeks after TIPS, most episodes are related to recurrent GI bleeding. Advanced age (>60 years), Child class C and prior history of encephalopathy are risk factors for encephalopathy in addition to shunt diameter. Occasionally, progressive liver failure develops following TIPS placement. Those with advanced liver failure are at the greatest risk of such progression. This usually culminates in death unless a liver transplant is performed.

Hemolytic anemia (Sanyal's syndrome) occurs in about 10% of patients after TIPS. It is usually asymptomatic although it may occasionally be severe enough to cause high-output heart failure. It is diagnosed by an increase in unconjugated bilirubin and reticulocytosis after TIPS. Hemolysis usually

Table 5. Causes of rebleeding after TIPS placement.

TIPS thrombosis
Technical problems
Kinking of stent
Stent retraction
Hemobilia
Development of severe right heart failure
Pseudointimal hyperplasia

Table 6. Specificity and sensitivity of sonographic criteria for TIPS stenosis.

Parameter (cm/s)	Sensitivity	Specificity
<50	78	99
<70	89	83
<80	92	60
<100	98	4

Data from Feldstein *et al.* (1996) *Radiology* **202**, 141.

Table 7. Complications of TIPS.

Technical
Shunt displacement
Inadequately deployed shunt
Cardiac arrythmias during placement
Rupture of the liver or inferior vena cava
Extrahepatic puncture of the portal vein with hemoperitoneum
TIPS-biliary fistula
TIPS-arterial fistula
Infarction of the liver
Related to portasystemic shunting
Hepatic encephalopathy
Increased susceptibility to sepsis
Specific complications
Progressive liver failure
Hemolytic anemia
Infective endotipsitis

subsides within 8 weeks although rarely it may be unremitting and require liver transplant or shunt occlusion.

6.4 Surgery and orthotopic liver transplant

A vast body of literature about the value of surgical treatment for prevention of recurrent variceal hemorrhage exists. Surgical therapy either decompresses the portal vein or disconnects the varices in the esophagus. Portal decompression is achieved by connecting the portal circulation to the systemic venous circulation thereby bypassing the area of increased resistance to flow within the liver. Such shunts may be either total, e.g., end-to-side or side-to-side portacaval shunt, which diverts all the portal flow to the systemic circulation, or partial which diverts only part of the portal flow and maintains some antegrade flow to the liver, e.g., a small diameter H graft between the portal vein and inferior vena cava. Shunts are also classified as non-selective or selective. The latter, e.g., the distal spleno-renal shunt preserves some sinusoidal perfusion while decompressing the portal veins. Each particular operation has its proponents and their data are not easily generalizable due the failure of others to obtain similar data. Virtually all the operations described are effective in arresting hemorrhage and preventing rebleeding. However, they often do not provide any survival advantage over endoscopic treatment. They are therefore primarily used as salvage treatment for those who have failed endoscopic treatment (Figure 14). Theoretically, a patient with Child class A cirrhosis may benefit from surgery (compared to TIPS) if they fail endoscopic treatment. The non-decompressive operations do not treat the portal hypertension and are generally not recommended.

Orthotopic liver transplant is the only treatment which not only effectively corrects the portal hypertension but also removes the cirrhotic liver and corrects liver failure [25]. It is the only treatment that substantially improves the long-term outcome after variceal hemorrhage and must be considered in all patients who have survived an episode of variceal bleeding unless a contraindication exists.

6.4.1. An algorithm for the prevention of recurrent variceal hemorrhage

The goal of long-term treatment is prevention of rebleeding, hepatic decompensation and death (Figure 10). Orthotopic liver transplantation is

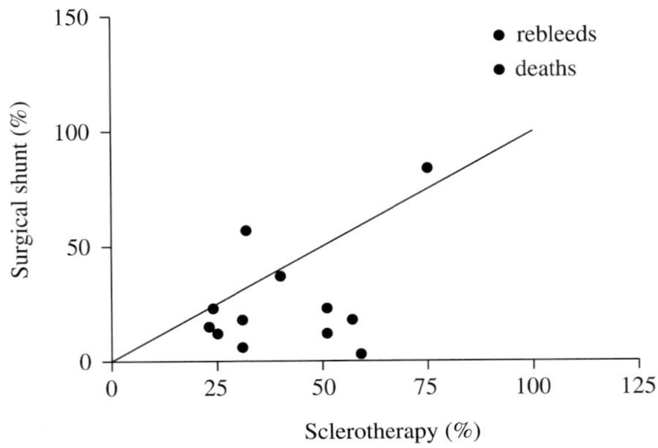

Figure 14. A L'Abbe plot of surgical therapy vs sclerotherapy for the prevention of recurrent variceal hemorrhage. Surgery was associated with less rebleeding but this did not translate in to a survival advantage. Published with permission from Garcia and Sanyal (2001) *Clin. Liver Dis.* **5**, 509–540.

the only treatment that reliably achieves all three objectives. Thus, all survivors of a variceal bleed should be evaluated for liver transplant. While waiting for transplant, endoscopic band ligation is the initial treatment of choice in most individuals. Some patients with Child class A cirrhosis who are compliant with therapy may be treated with pharmacologic treament. Selected patients with Child class A cirrhosis may benefit from surgical portal decompression.

If bleeding recurs, the acute bleeding is managed by endoscopic treatment. Those who continue to bleed or those who have bled despite adequate endoscopic treatment should be considered for salvage treatment with either TIPS or surgery. The choice of procedure should be individualized based on the patients' condition and operator expertise. Bleeding occurring after surgery or TIPS should lead to a work up for shunt thrombosis or stenosis. Angiography is the procedure of choice in such a patient because a patent Doppler sonogram does not exclude the possibility of TIPS stenosis.

REFERENCES

[1] Vianna, A., Hayes, P.C. and Moscoso, G. (1987) Normal venous circulation of the gastroesophageal junction. A route to understanding varices. *Gastroenterology* **93**, 876–889.

[2] deFranchis, R. (1988) Prediction of the first variceal hemorrhage in patients with cirrhosis of the liver and esophageal varices. *N. Engl. J. Med.* **319**, 983–989.

[3] Sarin, S.K., Lahoti, D., Saxena, S.P., Murthi, N.S. and Makwane, U.K. (1992) Prevalence, classification and natural history of gastric varices: long-term follow up study in 568 patients with portal hypertension. *Hepatology* **95**, 434–440.

[4] Garcia-Tsao, G., Groszmann, R., Fisher, R.L., Conn, H.O., Atterbury, C.E. and Glickman, M. (1985) Portal pressures, presence of gastroesophageal varices and variceal bleeding. *Hepatology* **5**, 419–424.

[5] Beppu, K., Inokuchi, K., Koyanagi, N., Nakayama, S., Sakata, H., Kitano, S. and Kobayashi, M. (1981) Prediction of variceal hemorrhage by esophageal endoscopy. *Gastrointest. Endosc.* **27**, 213–218.

[6] Graham, D.Y. and Smith, J.L. (1981) The course of patients after variceal hemorrhage. *Gastroenterology* **80**, 800–809.

[7] Smith, J.L. and Graham, D.Y. (1982) Variceal hemorrhage. A critical evaluation of survival analysis. *Gastroenterology* **82**, 968–973.

[8] Sarin, S.K. (1996) Diagnostic issues: portal hypertensive gastropathy and gastric varices, in *Portal Hypertension II. Proceedings of the Second Baveno International Consensus Workshop on Definitions, Methodology and Therapeutic Strategies*, ed. DeFranchis, R. (Blackwell Science, Oxford) pp. 30–55.

[9] Poynard, T., Cales, P., Pasta, L., Ideo, G., Pascal, J.P., Pagliaro, L. and Lebrec, D. (1991) Beta-adrenergic antagonist drugs in the prevention of gastrointestinal bleeding in patients with cirrhosis and esophageal varices, an analysis of data and prognostic factors in 589 patients from four randomized clinical trials. *N. Engl. J. Med.* **324**, 1532–1538.

[10] Angelico, M., Carli, L., Piat, C., Gentile, S. and Capocaccia, L. (1997) Effects of isosorbide 5 mononitrate compared to propranolol on first bleeding and long-term survival in cirrhosis. *Gastroenterology* **113**, 1632–1639.

[11] Merkel, C., Marin, R., Sacerdoti, D., Donada, C., Cavallarin, G., Torboli, P., Amodio, P., Sebastianelli, G., Bolognesi, M., Felder, M., Felder, M., Mazzaro, C. and Gatta, A. (2000) Long-term results of a clinical trial of nadolol with or without isosorbide mononitrate for primary prophylaxis of variceal bleeding in cirrhosis. *Hepatology* **31**, 324–329.

[12] Grace, N.D. (1992) Prevention of initial variceal hemorrhage. *Gastroenterol. Clin. N. Am.* **21**, 149–161.

[13] Sarin, S.K., Lamba, G.S., Kumar, M., Misra, A. and Murthy, N.S. (1999) Comparison of endoscopic ligation and propranolol for the primary prevention of variceal bleeding. *N. Engl. J. Med.* **340**, 988–993.

[14] Groszmann, R.J., Bosch, J., Grace, N.D., Conn, H.O., Garcia-Tsao, G., Navasa, M., Alberts, J., Rodes, J., Fischer, R. and Bermann, M. (1990) Hemodynamic events in a prospective randomized trial of propranolol versus placebo in the prevention of a first variceal hemorrhage. *Gastroenterology* **99**, 1401–1407.

[15] Cello, J.P., Grendell, J.H., Crass, R.A., Trunkey, D.D., Cobb, E.E. and Heilbron, D.C. (1984) Endoscopic sclerotherapy versus portacaval shunt in patients with severe cirrhosis and variceal hemorrhage. *N. Engl. J. Med.* **311**, 1589–1594.

[16] Sanyal, A.J., Freedman, A.M., Luketic, V.A., Purdum, P.P., Shiffman, M.L., Tisnado, J. and Cole, P.E. (1996)

Transjugular intrahepatic portosystemic shunts for patients with active variceal hemorrhage unresponsive to sclerotherapy. *Gastroenterology* **111**, 138–146.
[17] Chau, T.N., Patch, D., Chan, Y.W., Nagral, A., Dick, R. and Burroughs, A.K. (1998) "Salvage" transjugular intrahepatic portasystemic shunts: gastric fundal compared with esophageal variceal bleeding. *Gastroenterology* **114**, 981–987.
[18] Laine, L. and Cook, D.J. (1995) Endoscopic ligation compared with sclerotherapy for treatment of esophageal variceal bleeding. *Ann. Intern. Med.* **123**, 280–287.
[19] Sanyal, A.J. and Shiffman, M.L. (1997) The pharmacologic treatment of portal hypertension. *Curr. Clin. Top. Gastrointest. Pharmacol.* **1**, 242–275.
[20] Lebrec, D., Poynard, T., Bernuau, J., Bercoff, E., Nouel, O., Capron, J.P., Poupon, R., Bouvry, M., Rueff, B. and Behamou, J.P. (1984) A randomized controlled study of propranolol for prevention of recurrent gastrointestinal bleeding in patients with cirrhosis: a final report. *Hepatology* **4**, 355–358.
[21] Hayes, P.C., Davis, J.M., Lewis, J.A. and Bouchier, I.A.D. (1990) Meta-analysis of value of propranolol in prevention of variceal hemorrhage. *Lancet* **336**, 153–156.
[22] D'Amico, G., Pagliaro, L. and Bosch, J. (1995) The treatment of portal hypertension: a meta-analytic review. *Hepatology* **22**, 332–354.
[23] Sanyal, A.J., Freedman, A.M., Luketic, V.A., Purdum, P.P., III, Shiffman, M.L., DeMeo, J., Cole, P.E. and Tisnado, J. (1997) The natural history of portal hypertension after transjugular intrahepatic portosystemic shunts (comment). *Gastroenterology* **112**, 889–898.
[24] Freedman, A.M. and Sanyal, A.J. (1994) The spectrum of complications following transjugular intrahepatic portasystemic shunts (TIPS). *Semin. Interventional Radiol.* **11**, 161–177.
[25] Garrett, K.O., Reilly, J.J., Schade, R.R. and Van Thiel, D.H. (1988) Bleeding esophageal varices: treatment with sclerotherapy and liver transplant. *Surgery* **104**, 819–823.

Hepatology: A Practical Approach
B. Al Knawy, M.L. Shiffman, R.H. Wiesner (editors)

Chapter 3
Hepatic Encephalopathy

Bandar Al Knawy

Section of Gastroenterology/Hepatology, King Abdulaziz Medical City, P.O. Box 22490, Riyadh 11425, Saudi Arabia

1. Introduction 381
   1.1 Pathophysiology 381
      1.1.1 Ammonia 382
      1.1.2 Gamma-aminobutyric acid–benzodiazepine receptor complex 382
      1.1.3 Manganese 382
   1.2 Types of hepatic encephalopathy 383
   1.3 Precipitating factors 383
2. Clinical Features 383
   2.1 Investigation 385
   2.2 Management 385
References 386

1. INTRODUCTION

Hepatic encephalopathy (HE) is a potentially reversible, severe, neuropsychiatric syndrome [1,2]. It occurs in patients with acute and chronic hepatic failure and usually reflects the severity of hepatic dysfunction. Therefore, the development of HE carries an important prognostic implication. In acute hepatic failure, it indicates the development of cerebral edema, which may lead to intracranial hypertension, brainstem herniation and mortality; whereas in cirrhosis, the clinical stage of HE is one of the five components used in the Child–Pugh's score [3]. This score is a reliable predictor of liver disease progression and is used as an essential criterion for liver transplant listing. HE associated with cirrhosis is frequently referred to as portosystemic encephalopathy (PSE) due to the influence of portosystemic shunts in the development of mental state changes. HE associated with acute liver failure is addressed in Chapter 20 of Section II.

1.1 Pathophysiology

Neuropathological changes in cirrhotic patients who died following hepatic coma have revealed astrocytic changes known as Alzheimer type II astrocytosis [4]. They are found in the gray matter of the cerebrum, cerebellum, putamen, and globus pallidus. Morphologically, the astrocytes are enlarged with prominent nucleoli, margination of chromatin, and large pale nuclei.

The precise mechanism involved in the development of HE is not fully understood. However, it is generally assumed that it is due to portosystemic shunting of intestinal nitrogenous substances from the portal to the systemic circulation.

Ammonia, neurotoxicity, endogenous benzodiazapines, aromatic/branched chain amino acid imbalance, increased neuroinhibition mediated by gamma-aminobutyric acid (GABA), manganese, false neurotransmitters, and alteration in the blood–brain barrier permeability are potential mechanisms involved in the pathogenesis of HE. The pathogenesis of HE syndrome appears to be multifactoral with an interplay between the different mechanisms. In brief, the role of ammonia, gamma-aminobutyric acid–benzodiazepine receptor complex and manganese will be discussed.

1.1.1 Ammonia

Abnormalities of ammonia metabolism are most frequently incriminated in the pathophysiology of HE [5–9]. The bacteria in the normal gut flora produce urease that enzymatically cleaves ammonia from protein in the intestinal lumen, which is then absorbed into the portal circulation. In the liver, ammonia is metabolized (detoxified) into urea and then excreted through the kidneys and the colon. In cirrhosis, ammonia reaches the systemic circulation because of portosystemic shunts and the presence of poor hepatocellular function. The role of ammonia as the principal toxin can be deduced from (1) elevated serum and cerebrospinal fluid ammonia levels in the majority of patients with HE, (2) reversal of clinical features following medical therapy directed toward reduction of blood ammonia (dietary protein restriction, non-absorbable disaccharides and antibodies), (3) presence of HE in children with hyperammonemia secondary to genetic abnormalities of urea cycle synthesis, (4) Eck fistula, end-to-side portocaval shunt, surgically created shunt in dogs where they developed coma after eating meat, (5) increased cerebral metabolism of ammonia as detected by positron emission tomography (PET), and (6) astrocytes, the cells in the brain responsible for ammonia metabolism.

The mechanism of ammonia neurotoxicity is still unknown. However, recent evidence suggests that mitochondrial dysfunction plays an important role in the pathogenesis of ammonia neurotoxicity [10] (Figure 1).

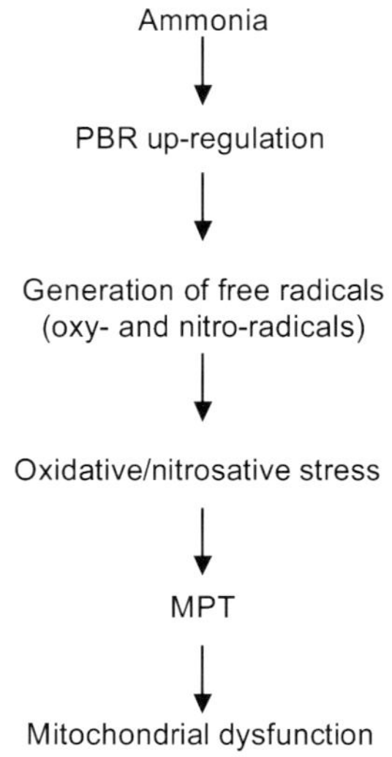

Figure 1. Ammonia neurotoxicity. PBR, peripheral benzodiazepine receptor; MPT, mitochondrial permeability transition.

1.1.2 Gamma-aminobutyric acid–benzodiazepine receptor complex

HE is a neuroinhibition state. GABA is the principal neurotransmitter inhibitor [11,12]. The plasma level of GABA is increased in cirrhotic patients with HE. The major source of the increased plasma GABA levels is the gut. GABA crosses the blood–brain barrier to reach the GABA receptors and augment GABA-ergic neurotransmission. It is stored in the presynaptic neurons. The postsynaptic membrane contains a receptor complex that binds benzodiazepines (BZs). The GABA–BZ receptor complex is the principal neuroinhibitory network in the brain. Benzodiazepine antagonists, flumazinel, caused transient improvement of the HE symptoms. The importance of increased GABA levels, and GABA-B_2 receptors is still unclear.

1.1.3 Manganese

The potential role of manganese in the pathophysiology of HE is based on the following observations [13–16]:

(1) Increased blood manganese in cirrhotic patients with HE, since the liver is important for the excretion of manganese; (2) manganese intoxication in non-human primates results in Alzheimer type II astrocytosis; (3) bilateral T_1-weighted magnetic resonance imaging (MRI) signal hyperintensity in basal ganglia of cirrhotic patients. Similar MRI findings are seen in patients receiving manganese on

long-term total parenteral nutrition; (4) Deposition of manganese in the globus pallidus and other basal ganglia is found in autopsy samples of patients with chronic HE.

1.2 Types of hepatic encephalopathy

The working party at the 11th World Congress of Gastroenterology, Vienna, 1998, proposed a consensus terminology for the different clinical presentations of HE [17] (Table 1). This classification should standardize the definitions of the different clinical subtypes of HE.

Type C HE is relevant to this chapter and will be discussed here. It is further categorized into episodic, persistent and minimal HE.

Episodic HE is subdivided into: (i) *precipitated*, where the symptoms are induced by precipitating factors (Table 2), (ii) *spontaneous*, without recognized precipitating factors and usually occurring with the terminal stage of cirrhosis and carrying a serious prognostic state, (iii) *recurrent*: when two episodes of episodic HE occur within 1 year. *Persistent HE* can be either mild (Grade I), severe (Grades 2–4) or dependent on medical therapy. *Minimal HE* is sometimes referred to as "subclinical" or stage O. These patients have no recognizable clinical features of brain dysfunction, have normal neurological examination but have impaired psychometric tests such as digit-symbol, block-design or number connection tests. Minimal HE is diagnosed in 30–80% of patients with liver cirrhosis. Impaired performance of cirrhotic patients by psychometric tests indicates neurological deficit secondary to basal ganglia involvement. Mild–moderate degrees of extrapyramidal signs are found in 52.4% of cirrhotic patients with minimal HE [18]. This is supported by T_1-weighted MRI signal hyperintensity, observed in basal ganglia of cirrhotic patients. The clinical significance of minimal HE is that it affects a patient's cognitive ability at work, at home and whilst driving [19].

1.3 Precipitating factors

The majority of hepatic encephalopathies are secondary to precipitating factors (Table 2). Spontaneous HE is uncommon and reflects a profound deterioration of hepatic function. Clinically, hepatic encephalopathies are precipitated by either nitrogenous or non-nitrogenous causes. The nitrogenous causes are azotemia, gastrointestinal hemorrhage, hypokalemia, bacterial infections, constipation and excess dietary protein. Non-nitrogenous causes are drugs (tranquilizers, sedatives and analgesics), hypoxia, hypoglycemia and progressive hepatic damage. Classically, blood ammonia level is elevated in nitrogenous causes and normal in non-nitrogenous. Azotemia, tranquilizers, sedative, analgesia and gastrointestinal hemorrhage account for 75% of hospital admissions in patients diagnosed with HE.

2. CLINICAL FEATURES

In the presence of advanced liver disease, HE is characterized by disturbance in cognition, consciousness, personality, behavior and neurological function.

Table 1. Proposed nomenclature of HE.

HE type	Nomenclature	Subcategory	Subdivisions
A	Encephalopathy associated with *acute* liver failure		
B	Encephalopathy associated with portal-systemic *bypass* and no intrinsic hepatocellular disease		
C	Encephalopathy associated with *cirrhosis* and portal hypertension, hypertension/or portal-systemic shunts	Episodic HE	Precipitated, spontaneous[a], recurrent
		Persistent HE	Mild, severe, treatment-dependent
		Minimal HE	

[a]Without recognized precipitating factors.

Table 2. Precipitating factors.

Gastrointestinal bleeding
Impaired renal function
Excess dietary protein
Infection (especially spontaneous bacterial peritonitis)
Constipation
Drugs (sedative, antihistamine, narcotics, etc.)
Dehydration
Hypokalemia
Hypoglycemia
Hypoxia
Surgical procedures

The onset of encephalopathy is either abrupt or insidious. The earliest features of HE are changes in personality, hypersomnia and minor behavioral changes, which can only be noticed by the patient's family. Later features are progressive deterioration in the level of consciousness, impairment of intellectual function and symmetrical neurological deficits. On physical examination, characteristic stigmata of advanced liver disease, such as ascites, shrunken liver, splenomegaly and jaundice, are always present. Fetor hepaticus is a sulfur, musty or rotten-egg odor. It is often present in patients with HE and has no correlation to the grade of HE. It is probably related to the presence of mercaptans in the patient's breath. Detailed neurological examination of the motor system is very difficult in stuporous or comatose patients. Various neurological signs are present according to the grade of HE. Apraxia, coordination and impaired handwriting in Grade 1, ataxia and hyporeflexia in Grade 2, hyperreflexia, Babinski's sign and muscle rigidity in Grade 3 while decerebrate posture is elicited in Grade 4. While focal neurological signs have been reported [20], alternative diagnoses should always be excluded. Asterixis or flapping tremor is best demonstrated in cooperative patients with the arms outstretched, the hands dorsiflexed and fingers spread. This posture should be maintained for at least 20 s. It can be demonstrated in patients with Grades 2 and 3 HE. In comatose patients, the examiner can elicit asterixis by dorsiflexing the patient's fingers. Asterixis is not specific for HE, and can also be found in renal failure, congestive heart failure, pulmonary insufficiency and drug overdosage. These neurological manifestations are generally reversible and, rarely, HE has progressive, debilitating symptoms including dementia, spastic paraparesis, cerebellar degeneration and extrapyramidal movement disorders. The West Haven Criteria for Grading Hepatic Encephalopathy summarizes the spectrum of the neuropsychiatric features according to the clinical presentation and physical findings [21].

Grade 0
lack of detectable changes in personality or behavior; asterixis absent
Grade 1
trivial lack of awareness; shortened attention span; impaired addition or subtraction; hypersomnia, insomnia, or inversion of sleep pattern; euphoria or depression; asterixis can be detected
Grade 2
lethargy or apathy; disorientation; inappropriate behavior; slurred speech; obvious asterixis
Grade 3
gross disorientation; bizarre behavior; semi-stupor to stupor; asterixis generally absent
Grade 4
coma

Grading of HE is very beneficial, as it helps to determine the aggressiveness of clinical care, the appropriate place for admission (intensive care unit or hospital ward) and sequences the steps of therapeutic interventions. Furthermore, it is very useful in monitoring the improvement or deterioration of the patient's condition.

HE is a diagnosis of exclusion. Therefore, during the evaluation of patients presenting with HE, it is essential to consider the differential diagnosis (Table 3).

Table 3. Differential diagnosis for HE.

Metabolic encephalopathies
Toxic or drug encephalopathies (alcohol, psychoactive drugs, heavy metals)
Encephalitis and meningitis
Intracranial lesions (subdural, intracerebral or subarachnoid hemorrhage; cerebral infarction; cerebral abscess and cerebral tumor)

2.1 Investigation

The diagnosis of HE is entirely clinical; there are no specific laboratory tests that confirm the diagnosis. Laboratory blood tests indicate hepatic dysfunction like abnormal serum transaminases, albumin, bilirubin, and prothrombin time. The serum ammonia is frequently elevated in patients presenting with HE. Arterial ammonia levels correlate better with the grade of HE. Normal values do not exclude the diagnosis. It should be obtained on a fasting state. Cerebrospinal fluid is normal, without increase in intracerebral pressure. Changes in the electroencephalogram (EEG) are predominantly over the frontal regions in patients with clinical features of Grade II HE onwards. Slow (5 cycles/s), triphasic waves are seen in Grades II and III HE while very slow (2–3 cycles/s), and delta waves are seen in Grade IV HE. These findings are clear with the progressive clinical improvement of mental status. They are non-specific and have limited application in clinical practice. Other metabolic disorders can have similar EEG findings.

Computed tomography (CT) of the brain may show mild cerebral atrophy, especially in patients with ethanol-induced cirrhosis. It is an essential diagnostic tool to rule out structural brain lesions (e.g., subdural hematoma). CT should be obtained in patients with focal neurological signs, lack of clinical correlation between the grade of HE and the severity of hepatic dysfunction and delayed clinical improvement in spite of aggressive medical therapy. Non-structural, neurophysiological or neurobiochemical imaging techniques such as magnetic resonance spectroscopy or PET may prove useful in the diagnosis of HE. Labeled neurotransmitters are used to study the metabolic and physiological changes during the different stages of HE. At the present time, they have limited clinical use.

2.2 Management

There are four essential therapeutic measures in the management of patients with HE: (i) meticulous care of confused and comatose patients; (ii) prompt identification and correction of precipitating factors; (iii) exclusion of alternative diagnoses; (iv) reduction of intestinal ammonia.

Special and immediate attention should be directed towards airway management, hemodynamic and metabolic status in order to support the confused and comatose patients. A systematic approach to look for potential precipitating factors is essential, as the majority of HE episodes have an underlying cause. Impairment of renal function, drugs (sedatives, antihistamines and tranquilizers), gastrointestinal bleeding, infection (like spontaneous bacterial peritonitis, pneumonia, urinary tract infection, etc.) and hypokalemia are the most common precipitating factors. Appropriate initial workup should include renal function, liver profile, K^+ level, blood culture, ascitic fluid analysis, hemoglobin level, white blood count, and, in addition, careful history taking with regards to new medication(s), high protein intake and constipation. Therapeutic measures such as urgent endoscopic therapy to control gastrointestinal hemorrhage, antibiotic coverage for SBP or other infectious process, fluid and electrolytes management, etc. should be implemented immediately.

HE may mimic other causes of altered mental state such as primary neurological disorders or metabolic encephalopathies. Such diagnoses once suspected, should be excluded (Table 3).

Reduction of intestinal ammonia can be achieved by either reduction of its production or its absorption. The intestinal production of ammonia can be lowered by dietary protein restriction while its absorption can be lowered by non-absorbable synthetic disaccharides and antibiotics. The degree of protein restriction depends on the stage of HE. In an advanced stage of HE, dietary protein should be eliminated and once improvement occurs, reinstituted gradually, ideally 10 g increments every 3–5 days, until clinical protein tolerance is established. Vegetable protein is preferred because of its lower rate of ammonia production. Additionally, the higher content of fiber in a vegetable diet accelerates the intestinal transit time of food. The daily protein intake should be equally divided between the meals.

The non-absorbable synthetic disaccharides such as *lactulose* (β-galactoside fructose) and lactitol (β-galactosidosorbitol) are the main therapeutic agents for HE [22]. The colonic bacteria metabolize lactulose to various organic acids, which lower the colonic pH to produce colonic acidification and osmotic diarrhea. These agents impair the absorption of ammonia. It is administered orally with an adult dose up to 160 g/day (240 ml). The starting dose, orally or via nasogastric tube, is 30–45 ml, followed by dosing every hour until diarrhea occurs. The dose is then titrated to give 2–4 soft stools per day and stool pH <6. The average maintenance dose is approximately 45–60 ml/day. In comatose patients, lactulose is given either by nasogastric tube or as retention enema. Lactulose enema dose is 300 ml in 700 ml of water. Lactulose is generally well tolerated with few side effects. Abdominal cramping, diarrhea, flatulence, dehydration and hypernatemia may occur as a result of severe diarrhea. *Lactitol* is equally effective, more palatable and associated with fewer side effects such as flatulence [23].

Antibiotics act by reducing ammonia absorption through the reduction of colonic bacteria and a concomitant decrease in bacterial urease, the main enzyme responsible for ammonia generation. *Neomycin* (2–4 g/day) and *metronidazole* (250 mg twice/day) are effective either alone, as an alternative to lactulose or in addition to lactulose in refractory HE. Despite its minimal absorption, chronic use of neomycin can cause ototoxicity, malabsorption, bacterial overgrowth and renal tubular toxicity. Theoretically, antibiotics and synthetic disaccharides should have an antagonistic action because the former eliminates the gut flora required for the pharmacological action of lactulose or lactitol. The combination of both agents proves to be beneficial in a subset of patients with intractable encephalopathy.

Branched-chain amino acids are metabolized by skeletal muscle and the aromatic amino acids are metabolized by the liver. Patients with cirrhosis have an altered ratio of branched-chain amino acids (valine, leucine, isoleucine) to aromatic amino acids (phenylalanine, tyrosine, tryptophan) from normal 3:1 to about 1:1 [24]. The increase of aromatic amino acids in serum indicates a corresponding elevation in their level in the central nervous system. Their accumulation within the central nervous system produces false neurotransmitters and promotes HE. Parenteral infusion and oral administration of formulas enriched in branched-chain amino acids showed no clinical benefit [25]. Enteral administration of branched-chain amino acids (Hepatic-Aid®) improves the nitrogen balance in malnourished cirrhotic patients who are intolerant to dietary protein without precipitating HE. This is especially useful for malnourished patients prior to liver transplantation.

Ornithine–aspartate are both important substrates in the metabolic conversion of ammonia to urea, glutamine–urea formation and glutamine synthesis, which are the major hepatic pathways for ammonia detoxification (clearance). In cirrhosis, these pathways are impaired, resulting in hyperammonemia. Administration of ornithine–aspartate may increase ammonia removal by stimulation of glutamine synthesis and ureagenesis. Clinical trails showed significant reduction of ammonia level and clinical improvement [25,26]. It is only available in Europe.

Zinc is a co-enzyme in the metabolism of ammonia to urea. It is commonly deficient in patients with cirrhosis due to increased urinary loss and malnutrition. Zinc sulfate 600 mg/day is useful when given over a long period (3 months) and in patients with documented zinc deficiency [27].

Flumazenil is a benzodiazepine receptor antagonist which has showed unimpressive therapeutic benefit. It should not be used unless there is a suspicion of benzodiazepine intake [26].

REFERENCES

[1] Blei, A.T., Cordoba, J. and Practice Parameters Committee of the American College of Gastroenterology. (2001) Hepatic encephalopathy. *Am. J. Gastroenterol.* **96**, 1968–1975.

[2] Butterworth, R.F. (2000) Complications of cirrhosis III. Hepatic encephalopathy. *J. Hepatol.* **32**(Suppl. 1), 171–180.

[3] Bustamante, J., Rimola, A., Ventura, P.J., Navasa, M., Cirera, I., Reggiardo, V. and Rodes, J. (1999) Prognostic significance of hepatic encephalopathy in patients with cirrhosis. *J. Hepatol.* **30**, 890–895.

[4] Weissenborn, K., Ehrenheim, C.H., Hori, A., Kubicka, S. and Manns, M.P. (1995) Pallidal lesions in patients with liver cirrhosis: clinical and MRI evaluation. *Metab. Brain Dis.* **10**, 219–231.

[5] Ferenci, P., Puspok, A. and Steindl, P. (1992) Current concepts in the pathophysiology of hepatic encephalopathy. *Eur. J. Clin. Invest.* **22**, 573.

[6] Lockwood, A.H., McDonald, J.M., Reiman, R.E. *et al.* (1979) The dynamics of ammonia metabolism in man: effects of liver disease and hyperammonia. *J. Clin. Invest.* **63**, 449.

[7] Matthews, S.A. (1992) Ammonia, a causative factor in meat poisoning in Eck fistula dogs. *Am. J. Physiol.* **59**, 459.

[8] Lockwood, A.H., Yap, E.W.H. and Wong, W.-H. (1991) Cerebral ammonia metabolism in patients with severe liver disease and minimal hepatic encephalopathy. *J. Cereb. Blood Flow Metab.* **11**, 337–341.

[9] Norenberg, M.D. (1996) Astrocytic–ammonia interactions in hepatic encephalopathy. *Semin. Liver Dis.* **16**, 245–253.

[10] Norenberg, M.D. (2003) Oxidative and nitrosative stress in ammonia neurotoxicity. *Hepatology* **37**, 245–248.

[11] Schafer, D.F. and Jones, E.A. (1982) Hepatic encephalopathy and the amino butyric acid neurotransmitter system. *Lancet* **ii**, 18.

[12] Jones, A., Skolnick, P., Gammal, S.H., Basile, A.S. and Mullen, K.D. (1989) The γ-aminobutyric acid a (GABA) receptor complex and hepatic encephalopathy: some recent advances. *Ann. Intern. Med.* **110**, 532.

[13] Spahr, L., Butterworth, R.F., Fontaine, S., Bui, L., Therrien, G., Milette, P.C., Hebrun, L.H., Zayed, J., Leblanc, A. and Layrargues, G.P. (1996) Increased blood manganese in cirrhotic patients: relationship to pallidal magnetic resonance signal hyperintensity and neurological symptoms. *Hepatology* **24**, 1116–1120.

[14] Krieger, D., Krieger, S., Jansen, O., Gass, P., Theilmann, L. and Lichtnecker, H. (1995) Manganese and chronic encephalopathy. *Lancet* **346**, 270–274.

[15] Kulisevsky, J., Pujol, J., Balanzo, J., Junque, C., Deus, J., Capdevilla, A. and Villanueva, C. (1992) Pallidal hyperintensity on magnetic resonance imaging in cirrhotic patients: clinical correlations. *Hepatology* **16**, 1382–1388.

[16] Pomier Layrargues, G., Sphar, L. and Butterworth, R.F. (1995) Increased manganese concentrations in pallidum of cirrhotic patients. *Lancet* **345**, 735.

[17] Ferenci, P., Lockwood, A., Mullen, K., Tarter, R., Weissenborn, K., Blei, A.T. and the Members of the Working Party (2002) Hepatic encephalopathy – definition, nomenclature, diagnosis, and quantification: Final Report of the Working Party at the 11th World Congresses of Gastroenterology, Vienna, 1998. Special Article. *Hepatology* **35**, 716–719.

[18] Jover, R., Company, L., Gutierrez, A., Zapater, P., Perez-Serra, J., Girona, E., Aparicio, J.R. and Perez-Mateo, M. (2003) Minimal hepatic encephalopathy and extrapyramidal signs in patients with cirrhosis. *Am. J. Gastroenterol.* **98**(7), 1599–1604.

[19] Groenewag, M., Quero, J.C., De Bruijn, I., Hartmann, I.J., Essink-bor, M.L., Hop, W.C. and Schalm, S.W. (1998) Subclinical hepatic encephalopathy impairs daily functioning. *Hepatology* **28**, 45–49.

[20] Cadranel, J.F., Lebiez, E., Martino, V.D., Bernard, B., El Koury, S., Tourbah, A., Pidoux, B., Valla, D. and Opolon, P. (2001) Focal neurological signs in hepatic encephalopathy in cirrhotic patients: an underestimated entity? *Am. J. Gastroenterol.* **96**, 515–518.

[21] Atterbury, C.E., Maddrey, W.C. and Conn, H.O. (1978) Neomycin–sorbitol and lactulose in the treatment of acute portal-systemic encephalopathy: a controlled, double-blind clinical trial. *Am. J. Dig. Dis.* **23**, 398–406.

[22] Cordoba, J. and Blei, A.T. (1997) Treatment of hepatic encephalopathy. *Am. J. Gastroenterol.* **92**, 1429–1439.

[23] Camma, C., Fiorello, F., Tine, F., Marchesini, G., Fabbri, A. and Pagliaro, L. (1993) Lactitol in treatment of chronic hepatic encephalopathy: a meta-analysis. *Dig. Dis. Sci.* **38**, 916–922.

[24] Rosen, H.M., Yoshimura, N., Hodgman, J.M. and Fischer, J.E. (1977) Plasma amino acid patterns in hepatic encephalopathy of differing etiology. *Gastroenterology* **72**, 483–487.

[25] Riordan, S.M. and Williams, R. (1997) Treatment of hepatic encephalopathy. *N. Engl. J. Med.* **337**, 473–479.

[26] Grimm, G., Ferenci, P., Katzenschlager, R., Schneeweiss, B., Lenz, K., Madl, C., Laggner, A.N. and Gangl, A. (1988) Improvement of hepatic encephalopathy treatment with flumazenil. *Lancet* **2**, 1392–1394.

[27] Rading, P., Duchateau, J. and Bataille, C. (1984) Oral zinc supplementation improves hepatic encephalopathy: results of a randomized controlled trial. *Lancet* **2**, 493–495.

Hepatology: A Practical Approach
B. Al Knawy, M.L. Shiffman, R.H. Wiesner (editors)

Chapter 4
Hepatorenal Syndrome

Andrés Cárdenas[a] *and Pere Ginès*[b]

[a]Division of Gastroenterology and Hepatology, Beth Israel Deaconess Medical Center, Harvard Medical School, Boston, MA, USA

[b]Liver Unit, Institut de Malalties Digestives, Hospital Clinic, IDIBAPS, University of Barcelona, Villaroel 170, Barcelona 08036, Spain

1. Introduction 389
2. Pathophysiology 390
   2.1 Extrarenal factors 390
   2.2 Intrarenal factors 390
   2.3 The arterial vasodilation theory 391
3. Clinical and Laboratory Findings 391
4. Diagnosis 393
5. Management 394
   5.1 General measures 394
   5.2 Pharmacologic therapy 394
   5.3 Transjugular intrahepatic portosystemic shunt 395
   5.4 Dialysis 395
   5.5 Liver transplantation 396
   5.6 Prevention 396
6. Summary 396
References 397

1. INTRODUCTION

Hepatorenal syndrome (HRS) is the development of functional renal failure in patients with advanced chronic liver disease, liver failure, and portal hypertension in the absence of any identifiable renal pathology. Patients with HRS show a severe disturbance in their systemic hemodynamics with low arterial pressure and high cardiac output. The splanchnic circulation in patients with HRS is subjected to the effects of circulating vasodilators arising from the endothelium that cause significant arterial vasodilation in this vascular bed with resulting activation of endogenous vasoconstrictor systems. In all non-splanchnic vascular beds there is marked vasoconstriction, which in the kidney results in low glomerular filtration rate (GFR). Although HRS occurs predominantly in advanced cirrhosis, it may also develop in other chronic liver diseases associated with severe liver failure and portal hypertension, such as alcoholic hepatitis, or in acute liver failure [1].

This entity is a relatively common complication of patients with cirrhosis with a reported incidence of about 10% among hospitalized patients with ascites. The probability of developing HRS in patients with cirrhosis and ascites is near 20% at 1 year and increases to 40% at 5 years [2]. Patients with ascites and marked sodium and water retention as well as those with marked arterial hypotension have the highest risk of developing HRS. Two types of HRS are observed in the clinical setting. Type 1 HRS is an acute form that has a very poor prognosis. Type 2 HRS develops slowly over the course of weeks; these patients have diuretic-resistant ascites and have a slightly better prognosis compared with those that have type 1 HRS.

There are several mechanisms that play a contributory role in pathogenesis of HRS which include extrarenal and intrarenal factors, abnormalities in systemic hemodynamics, and the diseased liver causing portal hypertension and hepatic failure. The present chapter will describe the pathogenesis, clinical features, diagnostic approach and treatment of HRS in cirrhosis.

2. PATHOPHYSIOLOGY

The pathophysiologic hallmark of HRS is vasoconstriction of the renal circulation. The mechanisms underlying renal vasoconstriction are multifactorial and include changes in systemic arterial circulation, portal hypertension, activation of vasoconstrictor factors, and suppression of vasodilator factors acting on the renal circulation (Table 1). Nonetheless, a common pathway for these derangements seems to be the development of an intense splanchnic arterial vasodilation which triggers an important compensatory response accounting for the sodium and water retention as well as renal vasoconstriction [3] (Figure 1).

2.1 Extrarenal factors

The renin–angiotensin–aldosterone system (RAAS) and the sympathetic nervous system (SNS) are overactivated in most cirrhotic patients with ascites in response to a reduced effective arterial blood volume, which is due to marked splanchnic arterial vasodilation [4,5]. In patients with HRS this activation is particularly intense suggesting that they play an important role in producing vasoconstriction of the renal circulation. Another important vasoconstrictor factor that is frequently increased in cirrhosis with ascites is arginine vasopressin (AVP) [6]. This hormone is mainly responsible for increased water reabsorption in the renal tubules and the subsequent development of dilutional hyponatremia. The circulating levels of endothelin-1, an endothelial-derived peptide with potent vasoconstrictor effect, are also increased in patients with HRS [7]. Increased levels are due to an enhanced release of the peptide from the hepatic and splanchnic circulation. Endothelin also induces vasoconstriction of the renal circulation and may play a role in the pathogenesis of HRS.

Table 1. Vasoactive factors likely involved in regulation of renal perfusion in cirrhosis and the pathogenesis of hepatorenal syndrome.

Vasodilators
Prostacyclin
Prostaglandin E2
Nitric oxide
Atrial natriuretic peptide
Kallikrein–kinin system
Vasoconstrictors
Angiotensin II
Norepinephrine
Neuropeptide Y
Endothelin-1
Adenosine
Thromboxane A2
Cysteinyl leukotrienes
F2-isoprostanes

The major natriuretic hormones, namely, atrial natriuretic peptide and brain natriuretic peptide, are increased in patients with cirrhosis and ascites [8]. These peptides by inducing renal vasodilation and natriuresis may act as a homeostatic response to counteract the effects of RAAS and SNS on the renal circulation.

2.2 Intrarenal factors

Metabolites of arachidonic acid are the intrarenal system most widely studied in cirrhosis. Arachidonic acid is metabolized in the kidney through three separate pathways. The most important of these three pathways is dependent on cyclooxygenases and gives rise to prostaglandins (PGs). Patients with cirrhosis and ascites without HRS have an increased renal production of PGs when compared with controls and cirrhotics without ascites [9]. The renal PGs cause renal vasodilation and by doing so protect the kidney from the effects of the above-mentioned vasoconstrictors. This is demonstrated by the fact that PGs synthesis inhibition by non-steroidal anti-inflammatory agents causes renal vasoconstriction and subsequent renal failure in cirrhotics with ascites [10]. With disease progression and development of HRS, renal production of PGs is reduced. Therefore, an imbalance between the vasoconstrictor systems and PGs may result in severe renal vasoconstriction.

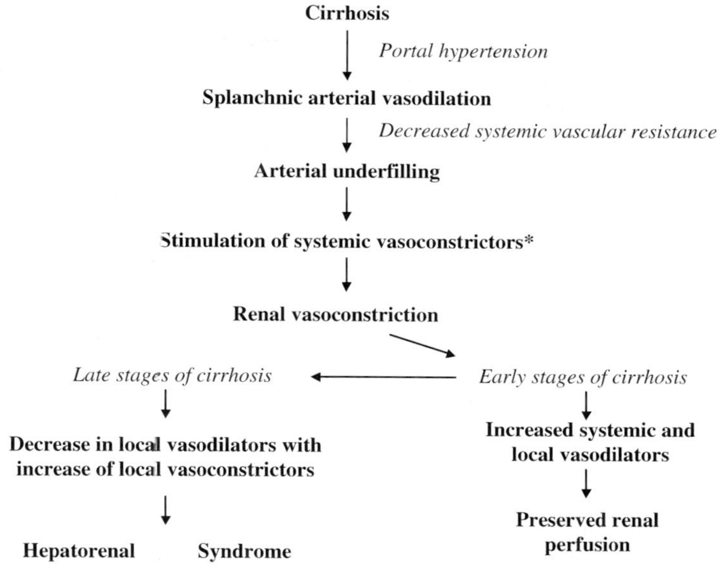

Figure 1. Pathogenesis of hepatorenal syndrome as proposed by the peripheral arterial vasodilation theory. *Vasoconstrictors: renin–angiotensin–aldosterone system (RAAS), sympathetic nervous system (SNS), endothelin and arginine vasopressin.

Other intrarenal factors that may play a role in the regulation of renal perfusion in cirrhosis and pathogenesis of HRS are nitric oxide (a potent vasodilator), intrarenal kallikrein–kinin and renin–angiotensin systems and adenosine.

2.3 The arterial vasodilation theory

The theory that better explains the relationship between changes in the renal circulation, activation of vasoconstrictor mechanisms, and presence of marked disturbances in systemic hemodynamics is the arterial vasodilation theory [3] (Figure 1). This theory proposes that renal hypoperfusion represents the extreme manifestation of underfilling of the arterial circulation secondary to a marked vasodilation of the splanchnic vascular bed. Arterial underfilling by causing a baroreceptor-mediated activation of vasoconstrictor systems (RAAS and SNS) would lead to vasoconstriction not only in the renal circulation but also in other vascular beds. In consequence, the splanchnic area would escape the effect of vasoconstrictors due to an enhanced local production of vasodilator factors, mainly nitric oxide. In the early stages of cirrhosis and portal hypertension, renal perfusion initially would be maintained within normal limits despite the high levels of RAAS and SNS due to increased levels of renal vasodilators. However, with progression of disease, renal perfusion could not be maintained because of extreme arterial underfilling causing maximal activation of vasoconstrictor systems and decreased activity of renal vasodilators. At this critical point HRS would ensue.

3. CLINICAL AND LABORATORY FINDINGS

There are no specific clinical findings in HRS. The majority of patients have features of advanced liver disease (hyperbilirubinemia, elevated prothrombin time, and hepatic encephalopathy), impairment of circulatory function and ascites (see Chapter 1 of Section III). Renal failure in HRS is often associated with oliguria, urinary sodium retention, and spontaneous dilutional hyponatremia. There are two types of HRS [1,11] (Table 2). Type 1 HRS is characterized by a rapid and progressive impairment of renal function as defined by a doubling of the initial serum creatinine to a level higher than 2.5 mg/dl or a 50% reduction of the initial 24-h creatinine clearance to a level lower than 20 ml/min in less than 2 weeks. Serum creatinine levels in patients with HRS are

Table 2. Clinical types of hepatorenal syndrome.

Type 1. Rapid and progressive impairment of renal function as defined by a doubling of the initial serum creatinine to a level higher than 2.5 mg/dl or a 50% reduction of the initial 24-h creatinine clearance to a level lower than 20 ml/min in less than 2 weeks
Type 2. Impairment in renal function (serum creatinine >1.5 mg/dl) that does not meet the criteria of type 1

usually lower than values observed in patients with acute renal failure without liver disease probably due to a reduced muscle mass and low endogenous production of creatinine. In some patients, this type of HRS develops spontaneously without any identifiable precipitating factor, whereas in others it can occur in close association with systemic bacterial infections specially spontaneous bacterial peritonitis (SBP) or acute alcoholic hepatitis. SBP is the most common precipitating cause of type 1 HRS [12]. It occurs in approximately one-third of cases with SBP despite a rapid resolution of the infection with intravenous antibiotics. In addition, large-volume paracentesis without plasma expansion may precipitate type 1 HRS. Although gastrointestinal bleeding is considered to be a major precipitating factor of HRS, the development of renal failure after this complication is uncommon in patients with cirrhosis and occurs almost exclusively in patients who develop hypovolemic shock, and in most cases is associated with ischemic hepatitis, which suggests that renal failure in patients with gastrointestinal bleeding is probably related to the development of acute tubular necrosis [13]. Nevertheless, a small percentage of patients with gastrointestinal bleeding may develop renal failure which fulfills criteria for HRS [13]. Without treatment, the median survival time of patients with type 1 HRS is less than 2 weeks and practically all patients die within 8–10 weeks after the onset of renal failure (Figure 2).

In contrast to type 1 HRS, type 2 HRS is characterized by a less severe course with serum creatinine levels below 2.0 mg/dl in most cases. The main clinical consequence of type 2 HRS is diuretic-resistant ascites. As expected, survival is longer in this group of patients than in those with type 1 HRS (median survival of 5 months), but is shorter than that of cirrhotic patients with ascites without renal failure.

Predictive factors associated with a greater risk of developing HRS in cirrhotic patients with ascites are listed in Table 3. The most easily recognized are severe urinary sodium retention (<10 mEq/day), spontaneous dilutional hyponatremia (serum sodium <130 mEq/l), and low mean arterial blood pressure

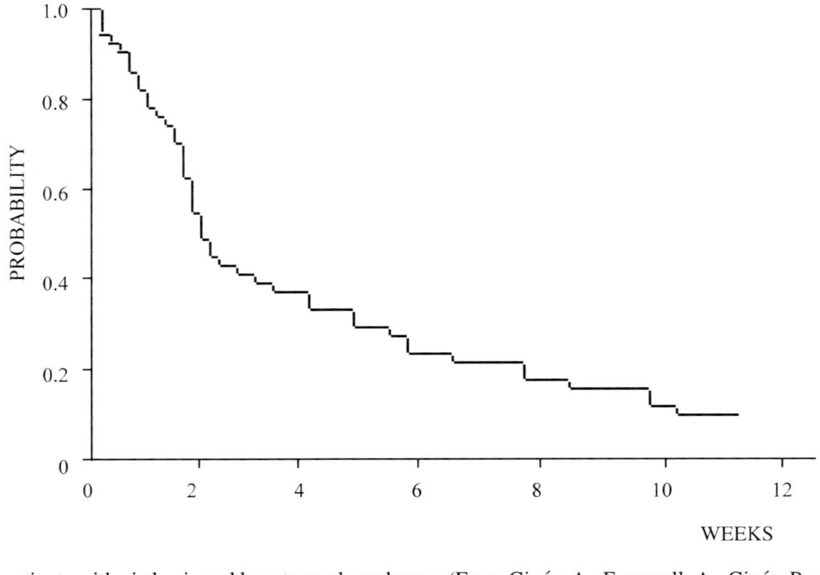

Figure 2. Survival of patients with cirrhosis and hepatorenal syndrome. (From Ginés, A., Escorsell, A., Ginés, P. *et al.* (1993) Incidence, predictive factors, and prognosis of the hepatorenal syndrome in cirrhosis with ascites. *Gastroenterology* **105**, 229–236, with permission.)

Table 3. Parameters associated with a higher risk of hepatorenal syndrome development in nonazotemic cirrhotic patients with ascites.

Slightly increased BUN and/or serum creatinine levels[a]
Dilutional hyponatremia
Reduced free water excretion after water load
Low urinary sodium excretion
Arterial hypotension
High plasma renin activity
High plasma norepinephrine concentration
Previous episodes of ascites
Absence of hepatomegaly
Poor nutritional status
Moderately increased renal vascular resistive index

[a]Blood urea nitrogen (BUN) and serum creatinine lower than 30 and 1.5 mg/dl, respectively.

(<80 mmHg) [2]. Interestingly, neither the degree of liver failure, as assessed by classic parameters of liver function (serum bilirubin, albumin, and prothrombin time), nor the Child–Pugh classification correlates with the risk of developing HRS.

4. DIAGNOSIS

Due to the lack of specific diagnostic tests to distinguish between HRS and other causes of renal failure that may occur in cirrhosis, the diagnosis of HRS is based on several diagnostic criteria described in Table 4 [1]. Low GFR is defined as serum creatinine greater than 1.5 mg/dl or 24-h creatinine clearance lower than 40 ml/min, without diuretic therapy. Other criteria include the absence of clinical conditions that predispose to the development of acute renal failure, no improvement of renal function following diuretic withdrawal and plasma expansion, no proteinuria, and a normal renal ultrasound. Most cases of HRS have urine sodium below 10 mEq/l and urine osmolality above plasma osmolality because of a preserved tubular function. Nevertheless, a minority of patients may have higher urine sodium and low urine osmolality, similar to values found in acute tubular necrosis. Conversely, some cirrhotic patients with acute tubular necrosis may have low urine sodium and high urine osmolality. For these reasons, urinary indices are not considered major criteria for the diagnosis of HRS [1].

Table 4. Diagnostic criteria of hepatorenal syndrome.

Criteria
Major criteria[a]
Low glomerular filtration rate, as indicated by serum creatinine greater than 1.5 mg/dl or 24-h creatinine clearance lower than 40 ml/min
Absence of shock, ongoing bacterial infection, fluid losses and current treatment with nephrotoxic drugs
No sustained improvement in renal function (decrease in serum creatinine to 1.5 mg/dl or less or increase in creatinine clearance to 40 ml/min or more) following diuretic withdrawal and expansion of plasma volume with 1.5 l of a plasma expander
Proteinuria lower than 500 mg/day and no ultrasonographic evidence of obstructive uropathy or parenchymal renal disease
Additional criteria
Urine volume lower than 500 ml/day
Urine sodium lower than 10 mEq/l
Urine osmolality greater than plasma osmolality
Urine red blood cells less than 50 per high power field
Serum sodium concentration lower than 130 mEq/l

[a]Only major criteria are necessary for the diagnosis of hepatorenal syndrome.

Other causes of renal failure, particularly prerenal failure secondary to volume depletion, acute tubular necrosis, drug-induced nephrotoxicity, and glomerulonephritis should be excluded before the diagnosis of HRS is made. Causes that may predispose to prerenal failure such as volume depletion due to vomiting or diarrhea, or renal fluid losses due to excessive diuretic therapy are common in cirrhotic patients and should be sought after. In prerenal failure due to volume depletion, renal function improves rapidly after the intravenous administration of fluids, whereas no improvement occurs in patients with HRS. Shock before the development of renal failure in a cirrhotic patient precludes the diagnosis of HRS, and usually indicates acute tubular necrosis. Likewise, the diagnosis of HRS should not be made in patients with recent or current treatment with nephrotoxic drugs, mainly non-steroidal anti-inflammatory drugs or aminoglycosides. Proteinuria (>500 mg/day) and/or ultrasonographic abnormalities in the kidneys indicate organic renal disease, mainly glomerulonephritis, which is commonly associated with alcoholic cirrhosis or hepatitis B or C associated cirrhosis. In these patients, a renal biopsy should be performed in selected cases.

5. MANAGEMENT

5.1 General measures

In the majority of patients HRS develops in the setting of advanced liver disease and in some others in the setting of acute liver failure. In either case these patients are unstable and require hospitalization, preferably in an intensive care unit for those with type 1 HRS. Continuous monitorization of vital signs, fluid intake, daily weights and urinary output should be performed. Central line access with central venous pressure measurement is helpful in assessing volume status, particularly when intravenous fluid challenge of a plasma expander is administered to rule out renal failure due to intravascular volume depletion (Table 4). Adequate measures to ensure proper nutrition with a low salt diet are extremely important as these patients are frequently malnourished. Since the majority of patients have ascites, diagnostic paracentesis must be performed to rule out SBP (see Chapter 1 of Section III). In patients with tense ascites, a therapeutic tap of 5 l associated with albumin infusion may aid in providing comfort.

The most accepted therapies for HRS include the use splanchnic vasoconstrictors, portosystemic shunts, and liver transplantation, which are described below (Figure 3).

5.2 Pharmacologic therapy

A variety of pharmacologic interventions have been used over the years to treat HRS. Although the use of renal vasodilator drugs such as dopamine and prostaglandin analogues to treat HRS was adopted by many groups, their use over the course of the last 2 decades has been progressively abandoned due to lack of substantial data confirming adequate benefit [14]. Other approaches such as the use of endothelin blockers (BQ123) and *N*-acetylcysteine seem to be promising, but larger uncontrolled as well as controlled studies are needed to confirm their role in the therapy of HRS [14]. The use of systemic vasoconstrictors with plasma expansion seems to be the most promising approach to therapy now that several uncontrolled studies have confirmed their beneficial role in HRS. Although using vasoconstrictors in a condition characterized by renal vasoconstriction seems paradoxical, the rationale is based on the fact that the initial event in the pathogenesis of HRS is an arterial splanchnic vasodilation causing activation of endogenous vasoconstrictors systems.

The vasoconstrictors used include vasopressin analogues (ornipressin and terlipressin), somatostatin analogues (octreotide), and catecholamines (midodrine and noradrenaline). Vasopressin analogues have a marked vasoconstrictor effect in the splanchnic circulation and have been used for many years in

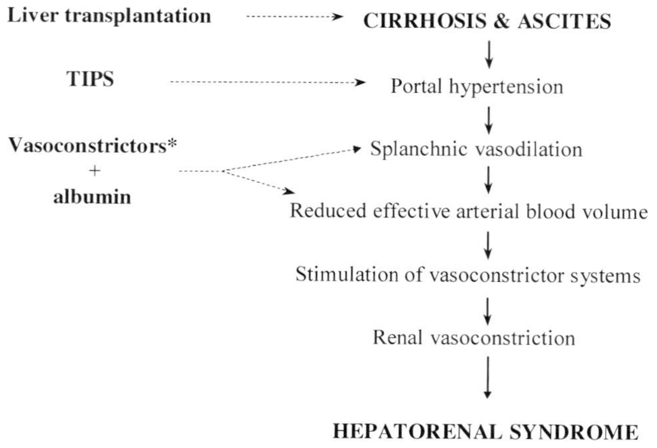

Figure 3. Proposed therapies for hepatorenal syndrome in relation to the pathophysiological events leading to its development. TIPS: transjugular intrahepatic portosystemic shunt. *Vasoconstrictors: terlipressin, midodrine, octreotide and noradrenaline.

the management of acute variceal bleeding in cirrhotic patients. The most studied vasopressin analogue in HRS is terlipressin. The administration of terlipressin and albumin is associated with a significant improvement of GFR and normalization of serum creatinine in approximately two-thirds of patients with cirrhosis and HRS [15–17]. One of the initial concerns about terlipressin was the development of ischemia, however, this has not been the case. There is a low incidence of ischemic side effects (approximately 5%) as demonstrated by several studies that now pool more than 120 patients [15–17]. The administration of midodrine, an alpha-adrenergic agonist in association with octreotide, an inhibitor of the release of glucagon and other vasodilator peptides, and albumin also improves renal function in cirrhotic patients with HRS although information about this therapeutic approach is still very limited [18]. Finally, the administration of noradrenaline in association with intravenous albumin resulted in a significant improvement of renal function in a small group of cirrhotic patients with type 1 HRS [19]. In all the studies recurrence of HRS after discontinuation of therapy in patients showing a normalization of serum creatinine was uncommon. Because of limited information and the possibility of side effects, treatment with vasoconstrictors should probably be restricted at present to patients with type 1 HRS. One of the primary goals of pharmacological therapy is that of successfully reversing renal failure so that suitable liver transplant candidates can undergo transplantation with less morbidity and mortality. Non-transplant candidates may also benefit from such therapy by reducing morbidity and mortality. In two studies, patients that responded to therapy of HRS (decrease of creatinine to <1.5 mg/dl) with terlipressin and albumin had an increased survival compared to those that did not respond to this therapy [16,17]. The recommended doses and duration of vasoconstrictor therapy are summarized in Table 5.

Table 5. Recommendations for using vasoconstrictors in hepatorenal syndrome.

Duration of therapy should be anywhere between 5 and 15 days, because improvement of renal function usually occurs slowly
Therapy should be aimed at reducing serum creatinine below 1.5 mg/dl
The recommended doses are
Terlipressin 0.5 mg intravenously every 4 h with an increase of the dose in a stepwise fashion (i.e., every 2–3 days) to 1 mg/4 h and then up to 2 mg/4 h in cases showing no response to therapy
Midodrine 7.5 mg orally three times daily with an increase to 12.5 mg three times daily if needed and octreotide 100 ug subcutaneously three times daily with an increase to 200 ug three times daily if needed
Noradrenaline 0.5–3 mg/h continuous intravenous infusion
Concomitant intravenous albumin infusion (1 g/kg on the first day, followed by 20–40 g/day) should be administered to all patients
These drugs should be avoided in patients with cardiac diseases, peripheral vascular disease, and/or cerebrovascular disease, dueto a likely high risk of ischemic events

5.3 Transjugular intrahepatic portosystemic shunt

Transjugular intrahepatic portosystemic shunt (TIPS) is a non-surgical method of portal decompression used as an alternative therapy for cirrhotic patients bleeding from esophageal or gastric varices that are refractory to endoscopic and medical treatment. From a pathophysiological point of view, TIPS by reducing portal pressure returns some of the volume of blood pooled in the splanchnic circulation to the systemic circulation. This event suppresses RAAS and SNS activity and ameliorates their vasoconstrictor effect on the renal circulation. Small studies indicate that TIPS may improve renal function and GFR as well as reduce the activity of RAAS and SNS in cirrhotics with type 1 HRS. However, the effects on renal function and the clinical course of patients after TIPS insertion are variable; some have a delayed response and others actually do worse. Experience from series of cirrhotic patients undergoing TIPS for refractory ascites indicates that those with hepatic encephalopathy and severe coagulopathy are prone to more complications and decreased survival. Although uncontrolled studies suggest that TIPS improves prognosis in patients with type 1 and 2 HRS [20], the impact of this therapy on patient survival remains to be assessed.

5.4 Dialysis

Small and uncontrolled studies using hemodialysis and peritoneal dialysis suggest that both are ineffective because of a high incidence severe side effects, including arterial hypotension, coagulopathy and gastrointestinal bleeding and increased mortality. In some centers, hemodialysis is used to treat patients with HRS awaiting liver transplantation. The effectiveness of dialysis in this setting has not been appropriately studied. Continuous arterio-venous or veno-venous hemofiltration have also been used but their efficacy remains to be determined. The beneficial effect of an extracorporeal albumin dialysis system (MARS), which consists of a modified dialysis method that enables the selective removal of albumin-bound substances that accumulate in liver failure by the use of an albumin containing dialysate has been recently reported in patients with HRS [21]. Although promising, these results require further evaluation in order to consider dialysis as a therapy, or more importantly as a bridge to liver transplantation in patients with HRS.

5.5 Liver transplantation

Liver transplantation is the best treatment for selected patients with HRS, as it offers a cure to both the diseased liver and the circulatory and renal dysfunction. The long-term outcome of cirrhotic patients with HRS treated by liver transplantation is usually good, although the presence of HRS is associated with increased morbidity and early mortality after transplantation [22]. After transplantation, a further impairment in renal function may be observed in some patients that will require hemodialysis during their postoperative stage. Nonetheless, only 5% will need long-term hemodialysis. Because cyclosporine and FK506 treatment may contribute to this degree of renal impairment postoperatively, other drugs such as azathioprine, steroids, IL-2 receptor antagonists or anti-lymphocyte agents should preferably be used until diuresis and improvement of renal function is observed, usually in 48–72 h after transplantation. After this initial impairment, GFR starts to improve and reaches an average of 40–50 ml/min by the sixth week after the surgery. Aside from renal impairment, patients develop more complications, spend more days in the intensive care unit and in the hospital, and have a higher in-hospital mortality rate than patients without HRS. Therefore, successful pharmacological therapy of HRS before transplantation may prevent and decrease the high incidence of complications these patients experience after the surgery. Despite this increased morbidity, long-term survival of transplanted patients with HRS is not markedly different from that of cirrhotic patients without HRS; the probability of survival after 2–3 years of transplantation is approximately 60% [23].

5.6 Prevention

HRS can be prevented in two clinical settings. First, in patients with SBP the administration of albumin (1.5 g/kg at diagnosis of infection and 1 g/kg 48 h later) prevents the circulatory dysfunction and subsequent development of HRS [24]. The incidence of HRS in patients with SBP receiving albumin together with antibiotic therapy is of 10%, compared with an incidence of 30% in patients not receiving albumin. Most importantly, the administration of albumin improves survival in these patients. Second, in patients with acute alcoholic hepatitis the administration of pentoxifylline, an inhibitor of tumor necrosis factor (400 mg tid orally for 28 days), also prevents the development of HRS and improves survival in this setting [25].

6. SUMMARY

HRS is a common complication of advanced cirrhosis characterized by renal failure, changes in systemic blood pressure, and increased activity of endogenous vasoactive systems. Renal failure is due to severe renal vasoconstriction developing in the late stages of cirrhosis. The pathogenesis of HRS is the result of an extreme underfilling of the arterial circulation secondary to an arterial vasodilation located in the splanchnic circulation. This underfilling triggers a compensatory response with activation of vasoconstrictor systems. Aside from the renal circulation, other extrasplanchnic vascular beds appear also to be vasoconstricted. The diagnosis of HRS is based on established diagnostic criteria aimed at excluding nonfunctional causes of renal failure. The prognosis of patients with HRS is very poor. Liver transplantation is the best option in selected patients, but it is not always applicable due to the short survival expectancy and donor shortage. Pharmacological therapies based on the use of vasoconstrictor drugs (terlipressin, midodrine, octreotide or noradrenaline) are the most promising in aims of successfully offering a bridge to liver transplantation. Prevention of HRS with albumin infusion is recommended in patients with SBP and with pentoxifylline in patients with acute alcoholic hepatitis.

REFERENCES

[1] Arroyo, V., Ginès, P., Gerbes, A., Dudley, F.J., Gentilini, P., Laffi, G., Reynolds, T.B., Ring-Larsen, H. and Scholmerich, J. (1996) Definition and diagnostic criteria of refractory ascites and hepatorenal syndrome in cirrhosis. *Hepatology* **23**, 164–176.

[2] Ginès, A., Escorsell, A., Ginès, P., Salo, J., Jimenez, W., Inglada, L., Navasa, M., Claria, J., Rimola, A. and Arroya, V. (1993) Incidence, predictive factors, and prognosis of hepatorenal syndrome in cirrhosis. *Gastroenterology* **105**, 229–236.

[3] Schrier, R.W., Arroyo, V., Bernardi, M., Epstein, M., Henriksen, J.H. and Rodes, J. (1988) Peripheral arterial vasodilation hypothesis: a proposal for the initiation of renal sodium and water retention in cirrhosis. *Hepatology* **8**, 1151–1157.

[4] Moller, S., Bendtsen, F. and Henriksen, J.H. (2001) Vasoactive substances in the circulatory dysfunction of cirrhosis. *Scand. J. Clin. Lab. Invest.* **61**, 421–429.

[5] Dudley, F.J. and Esler, M.D. (1999) The sympathetic nervous system in cirrhosis, in *Ascites and Renal Dysfunction in Liver Disease*, eds. Arroyo, V., Ginès, P., Rodés, J. and Schrier, R.W. (Blackwell Science, Malden) pp. 198–219.

[6] Arroyo, V., Clària, J., Saló, J. and Jimenez, W. (1994) Antidiuretic hormone and the pathogenesis of water retention in cirrhosis with ascites. *Semin. Liv. Dis.* **14**, 44–58.

[7] Moore, K., Wendon, J., Frazer, M., Karani, J., Williams, R. and Badr, K. (1992) Plasma endothelin immunoreactivity in liver disease and the hepatorenal syndrome. *N. Engl. J. Med.* **327**, 1774–1778.

[8] Gines, P., Jimenez, W., Arroyo, V., Navasa, M., Lopez, C., Tito, L., Serra, A., Bosch, J., Sanz, G. and Rivera, F. (1988) Atrial natriuretic factor in cirrhosis with ascites: plasma levels, cardiac release and splanchnic extraction. *Hepatology* **8**, 636–642.

[9] Moore, K. (1999) Arachidonic acid Metabolites and the kidney in cirrhosis, in *Ascites and Renal Dysfunction in Liver Disease*, eds. Arroyo, V., Ginès, P., Rodés, J. and Schrier, R.W. (Blackwell Science, Malden) pp. 249–272.

[10] Boyer, T.D., Zia, P. and Reynolds, T.B. (1979) Effect of indomethacin and prostaglandin A1 on renal function and plasma renin activity in alcoholic liver disease. *Gastroenterology* **77**, 215–222.

[11] Arroyo, V., Guevara, M. and Gines, P. (2002) Hepatorenal syndrome in cirrhosis: pathogenesis and treatment. *Gastroenterology* **122**, 1658–1676.

[12] Folio, A., Llovet, J.M., Navasa, M., Planas, R., Forns, X., Francitorra, A., Rimola, A., Gassull, M.A., Arroyo, V. and Rodes, J. (1994) Renal impairment after spontaneous bacterial peritonitis in cirrhosis: incidence, clinical course, predictive factors and prognosis. *Hepatology* **20**, 1495–1501.

[13] Cárdenas, A., Ginés, P., Uriz, J., Bessa, X., Salmeron, J.M., Mas, A., Ortega, R., Calahorra, B., De Las Heras, D., Bosch, J., Arroyo, V. and Rodes, J. (2001) Renal failure after upper gastrointestinal bleeding in cirrhosis. Incidence, clinical course, predictive factors and short-term prognosis. *Hepatology* **34**, 671–676.

[14] Wong, F. and Blendis, L. (2001) New challenge of hepatorenal syndrome: prevention and treatment. *Hepatology* **34**, 1242–1251.

[15] Uriz, J., Gines, P., Cardenas, A., Sort, P., Jimenez, W., Salmeron, J.M., Bataller, R., Mas, A., Navasa, M., Arroyo, V. and Rodes, J. (2000) Terlipressin plus albumin infusion: an effective and safe therapy of hepatorenal syndrome. *J. Hepatol.* **33**, 43–48.

[16] Moreau, R., Durand, F., Poynard, T., Duhamel, C., Cervoni, J.P., Ichai, P., Abergel, A., Halimi, C., Pauwels, M., Bronowicki, J.P., Giostra, E., Fleurot, C., Gurnot, D., Nouel, O., Renard, P., Rivoal, M., Blanc, P., Coumaros, D., Ducloux, S., Levy, S., Pariente, A., Perarnau, J.M., Roche, J., Scribe-Outtas, M., Valla, D., Bernard, B., Samuel, D., Butel, J., Hadengue, A., Platek, A., Lebrec, D. and Cadranel, J.F. (2002) Terlipressin in patients with cirrhosis and type 1 hepatorenal syndrome: a retrospective multicenter study. *Gastroenterology* **122**, 923–930.

[17] Ortega, R., Ginés, P., Uriz, J., Cardenas, A., Calahorra, B., De Las Heras, D., Guevara, M., Bataller, R., Jimenez, W., Arroyo, V. and Rodes, J. (2002) Terlipressin therapy with and without albumin for patients with hepatorenal syndrome. Results of a prospective, non-randomized study. *Hepatology* **36**, 941–948.

[18] Angell, P., Volpin, R., Gerunda, G., Craighero, R., Roner, P., Merenda, R., Amodio, P., Sticca, A., Caregaro, L., Maffei-Faccioli, A. and Gatta, A. (1999) Reversal of type 1 hepatorenal syndrome with

the administration of midodrine and octreotide. *Hepatology* **29**, 1690–1697.

[19] Duvoux, C., Zanditenas, D., Hezode, C., Chauvat, A., Monin, J.L., Roudot-Thoraval, F., Mallat, A. and Dhumeaux, D. (2002) Effects of noradrenalin and albumin in patients with type 1 hepatorenal syndrome: a pilot study. *Hepatology* **36**(2), 374–380.

[20] Brensing, K.A., Textor, J., Perz, J., Schiedermaier, P., Raab, P., Strunk, H., Klehr, H.U., Kramer, H.J., Spengler, U., Schild, H. and Sauerbruch, T. (2000) Long term outcome after transjugular intrahepatic portosystemic stent-shunt in non-transplant cirrhotics with hepatorenal syndrome: a phase II study. *Gut* **47**, 288–295.

[21] Mitzner, S.R., Stange, J., Klammt, S., Risler, T., Erley, C.M., Bader, B.D., Berger, E.D., Lauchart, W., Peszynski, P., Freytag, J., Hickstein, H., Loock, J., Lohr, J.M., Liebe, S., Emmrich, J., Korten, G. and Schmidt, R. (2000) Improvement of hepatorenal syndrome with extracorporeal albumin dialysis MARS: results of a prospective, randomized, controlled clinical trial. *Liver Transpl.* **6**, 277–286.

[22] Gonwa, T.A., Morris, C.A., Goldstein, R.M., Husberg, B.S. and Klintmalm, G.B. (1991) Long-term survival and renal function following liver transplantation in patients with and without hepatorenal syndrome-experience in 300 patients. *Transplantation* **51**, 428–430.

[23] Gonwa, T.A., Klintmalm, G.B., Levy, M., Jennings, L.S., Goldstein, R.M. and Husberg, B.S. (1995) Impact of pretransplant renal function on survival after liver transplantation. *Transplantation* **59**, 361–365.

[24] Sort, P., Navasa, M., Arroyo, V., Aldeguer, X., Planas, R., Ruiz-del-Arbol, L., Castells, L., Vargas, V., Soriano, G., Guevara, M., Gines, P. and Rodes, J. (1999) Effect of intravenous albumin on renal impairment and mortality in patients with cirrhosis and spontaneous bacterial peritonitis. *N. Eng. J. Med.* **5**, 403–409.

[25] Akriviadis, E., Botla, R., Briggs, W., Han, S., Reynolds, T. and Shakil, O. (2000) Pentoxifylline improves short-term survival in severe acute alcoholic hepatitis: a double-blind, placebo-controlled trial. *Gastroenterology* **119**, 1637–1648.

Hepatology: A Practical Approach
B. Al Knawy, M.L. Shiffman, R.H. Wiesner (editors)

Chapter 5
Hepatopulmonary Syndrome

Karen L. Swanson and Michael J. Krowka

Division of Pulmonary and Critical Care, Mayo Clinic College of Medicine, Mayo Clinic, 200 First Street SW, Rochester, MN 55905, USA

1. Introduction 399
2. Pathophysiology 400
3. Clinical Features 402
4. Diagnosis 402
5. Management 404
6. Prognosis 406
7. Summary 406
References 407

---

1. INTRODUCTION

A spectrum of pulmonary vascular pathologies can occur in the setting of chronic liver disease. At one end of the spectrum, pulmonary vasoproliferation characterized by medial hypertrophy, intimal hyperplasia and plexogenic pulmonary arteriopathy results in obstruction to pulmonary blood flow and "portopulmonary hypertension" [1]. At the other end, intrapulmonary vascular dilatations develop and result in arterial hypoxemia with normal or low pulmonary vascular resistance leading to the "hepatopulmonary syndrome" (HPS) [1].

The clinical triad of chronic liver disease, arterial hypoxemia and intrapulmonary vascular dilatations characterizes the HPS [2]. The chronic liver disease generally involves cirrhotic or non-cirrhotic portal hypertension. Arterial hypoxemia is defined as an arterial PaO_2 of less than 70 mmHg or an alveolar–arterial oxygen gradient greater than 20 mmHg while breathing room air [1]. Some authors advocate using the age-corrected alveolar–arterial oxygen gradient rather than a standard value of 20 mmHg. Intrapulmonary vascular dilatations are documented with either transthoracic contrast echocardiography or brain imaging following lung perfusion scanning using technetium-labeled macroaggregated albumin particles (^{99m}TcMAA).

Prevalence rates for HPS in the literature have ranged from 5 to 29% in patients with end-stage liver disease undergoing liver transplantation evaluation [2]. The true prevalence of HPS in patients with various stages of liver disease is unknown. In the largest prospective study to date of 80 patients with cirrhosis undergoing liver transplant evaluation, the prevalence rate of HPS was 17.5% [3].

Positive contrast echocardiography with *normal* gas exchange has been documented in patients with cirrhosis. Table 1 compares several studies of patients with cirrhosis evaluated using both contrast echocardiography and arterial oxygenation assessment. Positive contrast echocardiography documenting intrapulmonary vascular dilatation ranged from 3.0 to 20.0% [3–6]. Arterial hypoxemia ranged from 0.0 to 17.5%. Do patients with positive contrast echocardiography, but normal gas exchange, have a higher incidence of developing HPS or an early form of HPS? The answers to these questions currently are not known and can only be answered through future prospective studies.

HPS occurs with equal frequency in men and women, as well as in the pediatric population. Portal hypertension appears to be the necessary factor for the development of HPS [1]. The incidence of HPS is not related to any specific

Table 1. The prevalence of positive transthoracic echocardiography in patients with portal hypertension in relation to abnormal oxygenation (true HPS).

	N	+CE − hypoxemia	+CE + hypoxemia	DLCO < 80%
Martinez *et al.* [3]	80	2 (3)	14 (17.5)	14 (18)
Mimidis *et al.* [4]	75	8 (10.7)	0	8 (11)
Gupta *et al.* [5]	54	4 (7.4)	6 (11.1)	5 (9)
Abrams *et al.* [6]	40	8 (20)	7 (17.5)	11 (14)

N: total number; CE: transthoracic contrast echocardiography, number (percent); DLCO: diffusion capacity for carbon monoxide in pulmonary function testing.

etiology of liver disease [1,2,6,7]. Oxygenation abnormalities have not correlated with the severity of portal hypertension as measured by portal pressure or the severity of liver disease as measured by the Child–Pugh score [6,7]. Severity of hepatic dysfunction associated with portal hypertension does not predict the presence or severity of HPS. HPS has been documented in patients with mild degrees of hepatic dysfunction (Child–Pugh "A"), and hypoxemia has progressed in the setting of stable hepatic dysfunction [6,7].

2. PATHOPHYSIOLOGY

The primary problem in HPS is a gas exchange abnormality resulting in hypoxemia caused by changes in the arterial pulmonary vascular bed [2]. An imbalance between vasodilating and vasoconstricting vascular mediators has been proposed as a probable cause for the pathological changes that are seen at autopsy. Normal capillary diameter in the pulmonary vascular system ranges from 8 to 10 μm [1]. Autopsy studies and pulmonary angiography have demonstrated two different types of vascular dilatations that exist in HPS (see Figure 1A–C). Remarkably, physiologic studies suggest that these changes can reverse following liver transplantation in most cases [8].

Type I dilatations (Figure 1B) consist of diffuse precapillary and capillary vascular dilatations between 15 and 500 μm in diameter [2,9]. These types of dilatations lead to ventilation–perfusion mismatching caused by excessive perfusion for a given unit of normal ventilation. Type II dilatations (Figure 1C) involve distinct arteriovenous communications resulting in the *absence* of ventilation with increased perfusion and the presence of true anatomic shunting. The response to 100% oxygen varies with both the degree and type of intrapulmonary vascular dilatations present [7]. With type I lesions, the response to 100% oxygen may be near normal, while in a pure shunt (type II lesions), there will be minimal or no response to 100% oxygen. Dilated pleural vessels similar to spider angiomata in liver disease can also be found in HPS, but they do not appear to participate in gas exchange [9].

The mechanism of hypoxemia in HPS is likely multi-factorial and, in a given patient, may include the co-existence of other non-vascular reasons for hypoxemia [3,7]. Patients with advanced liver disease often have pre-existing gas exchange abnormalities due to the presence of pleural effusions ("hepatic hydrothorax"), ascites, interstitial lung diseases and/or obstructive lung disease (emphysema, bronchitis or asthma) [3,7]. In the absence of these co-existing, "intrinsic" pulmonary abnormalities, at least three mechanisms of hypoxemia exist in HPS and are described in Table 2 [1,2,9]. These mechanisms have been documented through the use of the multiple inert gas elimination technique [2,9]. First, due to the hyperdynamic circulation associated with advanced liver disease, the increased cardiac output probably increases the transit time through the pulmonary circulation, thus decreasing the time for capillary oxygenation to occur resulting in ventilation–perfusion mismatch (normal ventilation with increased perfusion).

A second mechanism of hypoxemia is caused by a diffusion–perfusion limitation due to the presence of Type I diffuse intrapulmonary vascular dilatations. As the degree of dilatation increases, there is more distance from the alveoli to the center of the capillary

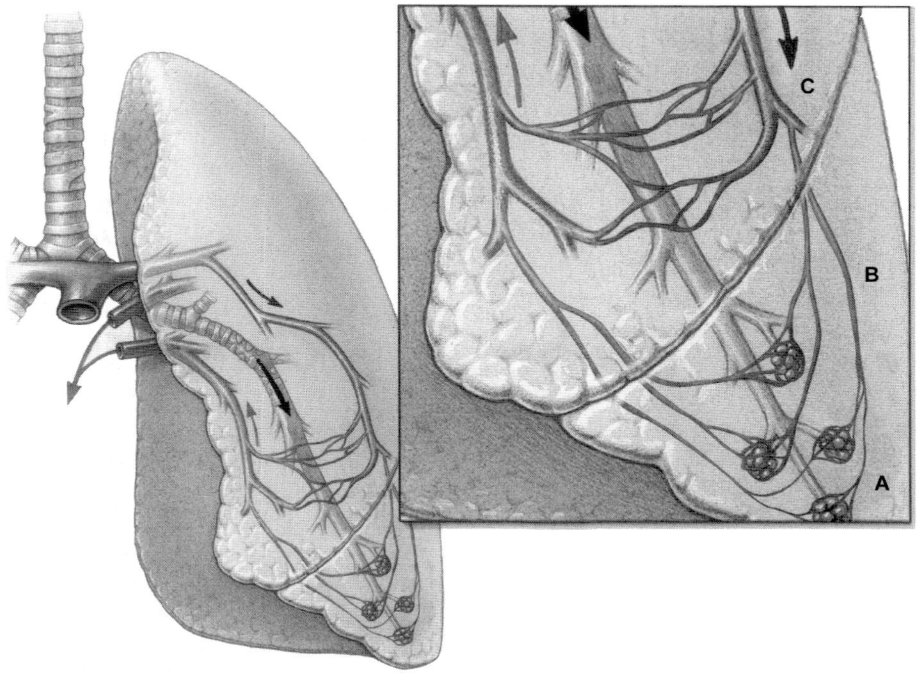

Figure 1. (A) Normal intrapulmonary arterial–capillary–venule interface. (B) Type I intrapulmonary vascular dilatations showing the diffuse pre-capillary and capillary vascular dilatations. (C) Type II intrapulmonary vascular dilatations showing distinct arteriovenous communications that result in a true right to left shunt.

and thus, a limitation to the passive diffusion of oxygen molecules to the center of the unoxygenated venous blood flow. With a higher partial pressure of alveolar oxygen (obtained while breathing 100% oxygen), there is an increased driving force for oxygen to diffuse into the capillaries, resulting in a dramatic increase in PaO_2 despite severe hypoxemia when breathing room air [7]. Such diffusion limitation in combination with the possible increased blood transit time due to the hyperdynamic circulation seen in liver disease can result in severe arterial hypoxemia at rest ($PaO_2 < 50$ mmHg).

Table 2. Mechanisms of hypoxemia in hepatopulmonary syndrome are shown.

Abnormality	Mechanism
Hyperdynamic circulation	Ventilation–perfusion mismatch
↑ cardiac output = ↑ transit time in capillary bed	Normal V/↑ Q
↓ time for gas exchange (oxygenation)	
Diffusion–perfusion limitation	Ventilation–perfusion mismatch
(Type I intrapulmonary vascular dilatations)	Normal V/↑ Q
↑ distance to center of capillary = limitation to diffusion	Diffusion abnormality
True right to left shunt	Ventilation–perfusion mismatch
(Type II intrapulmonary vascular dilatations)	Shunt = absent V/↑ Q
Intrinsic cardiopulmonary disease if present	

Any combination of the four abnormalities may be present in patients with HPS resulting in both varying severities of hypoxemia and responses to oxygen therapy. V: ventilation; Q: perfusion.

The third mechanism of hypoxemia is the presence of right to left anatomic intrapulmonary shunting. This appears to be uncommon as demonstrated by pulmonary angiography or contrast-enhanced CT scanning of the chest. Unoxygenated venous blood simply bypasses gas exchange units via direct arteriovenous communications of varying size and configuration (see Figure 1C). If macroscopic in size (>3 mm in diameter), they may be amenable to coil embolotherapy. These abnormalities may result in severe hypoxemia with very poor response to 100% inspired oxygen ($PaO_2 < 300$ mmHg) [7].

Recently, much interest has developed regarding the interaction of vascular mediators between the liver and the lung. Is the diseased liver tilting the balance between vasodilating and vasoconstricting substances so that there is an unopposed action of vasodilators? Does the pulmonary vascular bed require vasomodulating factors produced by the liver to maintain control of the pulmonary circulation? An intriguing response to this question may be found in the pediatric congenital heart disease literature. Pulmonary vascular dilatation with severe hypoxemia developed *after* the creation of cavopulmonary shunts as a treatment approach to tricuspid atresia (and its associated vascular abnormalities) [10]. In some patients who had aberrant hepatic venous drainage (emptying into the left atrium), arterial hypoxemia and intrapulmonary vascular dilatations resolved with redirection of the hepatic venous effluent into the pulmonary arterial circulation. This well-documented experience provides evidence for a probable vasomodulating mediator arising from the liver that affects the structure and vasomotor tone of the pulmonary arterial circulation.

In a bile duct ligation rat model of HPS, pulmonary vascular endothelial nitric oxide synthase levels are increased and the increased nitric oxide levels have been found to correlate with the development of pulmonary vasodilatation [11]. Nitric oxide is a potent vasodilator in the vascular system. In a subsequent study by the same investigators, both hepatic and plasma endothelin-1 levels were increased after bile duct ligation in the rat with subsequent portal hypertension [12]. In this situation, endothelin-1 likely acts on the endothelin-B receptors on the endothelial cell to stimulate nitric oxide production. The plasma endothelin-1 levels positively correlated with pulmonary endothelial nitric oxide synthase levels and alveolar–arterial oxygen gradients. No human studies have addressed the endothelin-B hypothesis to date. Indeed, increased levels of exhaled nitric oxide have been documented in HPS at levels (ppb) which appear to be greater than those measured in cirrhotic patients without hypoxemia [2,9].

3. CLINICAL FEATURES

The clinical features seen in HPS are those typically seen in underlying liver disease [13]. On physical examination these include spider angiomata, palmar erythema, gynecomastia, splenomegaly and jaundice. As the severity of HPS increases, other physical findings may evolve, including cyanosis, tachypnea, clubbing and orthodeoxia. Orthodeoxia is defined as a decrease in arterial PaO_2 greater than 3 mmHg in the upright versus the supine position [9,13]. Patients frequently present with the insidious onset of dyspnea and platypnea (dyspnea exaggerated in the upright position). Orthodeoxia and platypnea, although uncommon, are two of the cardinal manifestations of HPS although not specific for HPS. Hypoxemia that is worse in the upright position is due to the increased presence of intrapulmonary vascular dilatations in the mid and basal portions of the lungs. In the upright position, there is increased perfusion to these dependent areas with worsening ventilation–perfusion mismatching and resultant hypoxemia. When compared to patients with cirrhosis alone, HPS patients have higher incidences of finger clubbing, spider angiomas and dyspnea [2]. Progressive hypoxemia may occur in the setting of apparently stable hepatic dysfunction [14].

4. DIAGNOSIS

The diagnosis of HPS relies on the documentation of arterial hypoxemia and intrapulmonary vascular dilatation in the setting of chronic liver disease [1]. The hypoxemia in HPS is defined as an arterial PaO_2 of less than 70 mmHg or an alveolar–arterial oxygen gradient of greater than 20 mmHg (some authors use 15 mmHg) [1,2]. Arterial blood gases obtained in both the supine and upright positions will document the presence and severity of orthodeoxia. Similarly arterial blood gases in room air and 100% oxygen will document the presence or absence of a true shunt by the response to oxygen. The shunt fraction can be estimated by the 100% oxygen technique, but unless used correctly, the hyperdynamic state generally present in chronic liver disease can result in the shunt equation underestimating the true shunt [15].

Two-dimensional transthoracic contrast echocardiography is the most sensitive study to detect the presence of intrapulmonary vascular dilatation [6]. It is not able to differentiate between the two different types of intrapulmonary vascular dilatations; however, it can differentiate between intrapulmonary and intracardiac sources of right to left shunt. Contrast echocardiography detects vascular dilatation via micro-bubbles (diameter 10–60 microns) created by hand-agitated saline that is injected into a peripheral arm vein. Normally these micro-bubbles are absorbed at the capillary–alveolar level through the first pass into the pulmonary circulation. If vascular dilatations exist, the micro-bubbles pass through the pulmonary vascular bed into the left atrium where they can be seen 3–6 cardiac cycles after their appearance in the right ventricle. If micro-bubbles are seen in the left heart within three cardiac cycles, then an intracardiac shunt may exist (atrial or ventricular septal defect).

If the contrast echocardiogram is positive, the degree of intrapulmonary vascular dilatation can be quantified by lung–brain perfusion scanning with technetium-99-labeled macroaggregated albumin (^{99m}TcMAA) [7,16]. Technically, we measure the degree of dilatation with this method, although many authors have loosely used the term "shunt". It should be remembered that although the vascular dilatations may include true anatomic shunts, the ^{99m}TcMAA method (or contrast echocardiogram) does not distinguish between the types of vasodilatation. Figure 2 shows a positive lung–brain perfusion scan with the intrapulmonary right to left shunt quantified at 27.47%. Normal shunt fractions are less than 6%. This radionuclide scan is specific for the diagnosis of HPS in the setting of chronic liver disease and hypoxemia if the shunt fraction is greater than or equal to 6% [16].

The perfusion scan is very helpful in quantifying the oxygenation abnormality in HPS, since it is specific for vascular dilatation and is not affected by other non-vascular reasons for hypoxemia [7,16]. The macroaggregated albumin, with diameters between 20 and 90 microns, passes through the dilated pulmonary vascular bed and can be detected by imaging over the brain and kidneys. Abrams *et al.* [16] studied the role of macroaggregated albumin lung perfusion scans in the diagnosis of HPS given that many cirrhotics may have positive contrast echocardiography in the absence of hypoxemia. They found that the lung perfusion scans were positive in 21 of 25 patients with HPS (84% sensitivity) and *negative in all controls* (cirrhotic patients with normal contrast echocardiograms). All patients with positive lung perfusion scans were hypoxemic with PaO_2 values of less then 60 mmHg. They concluded that a positive lung perfusion scan in cirrhosis was specific for the presence of HPS. They also found a strong inverse correlation between the quantitated shunt fraction and room air arterial PaO_2 and a strong direct correlation between the shunt fraction and the alveolar–arterial oxygen gradient. Mayo Clinic investigators have reported very similar relationships between lung perfusion scanning and oxygenation in patients with HPS [7].

In patients with a large shunt by ^{99m}TcMAA lung scanning and a poor response to 100% oxygen ($PaO_2 < 300$ mmHg; normal > 500 mmHg), pulmonary angiography may be indicated to determine if discrete arteriovenous communications are present [7]. These vascular lesions are often amendable to vascular intervention with coil embolotherapy and elimination of shunting. More frequently in HPS, however, the intrapulmonary vascular dilatations are small and diffuse with normal pulmonary angiograms when performed. One potential algorithm (currently followed at Mayo Clinic) for evaluating patients with suspected HPS can be seen in Figure 3.

Finally, a reduction in the single breath diffusing capacity for carbon monoxide (DLCO) is the most common abnormality observed in pulmonary function tests in patients with any type of chronic liver disease; it is not specific for HPS [2,9]. An abnormal diffusing capacity may correlate quite closely with the severity of hypoxemia due to HPS, at least prior

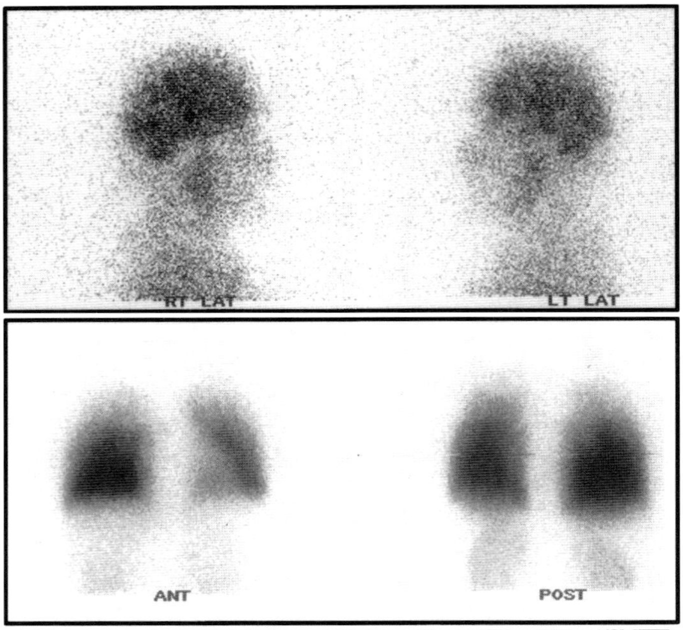

Geometric mean counts			
	Ant	Post	Geometric Mean
Lung	255244	368446	306665
	Left Lat	Rt Lat	
Brain	15333	14876	15103
	Shunt Index %	=	27.47
	Normal shunt index < 5%		

Figure 2. Lung perfusion scanning with brain imaging using technetium-99-labeled macroaggregated albumin (assumes 13% cardiac output to brain).

to liver transplantation [2]. There are no patterns in expiratory flow or the flow volume loop that are specific for HPS. There are no specific findings in chest roentgenogram for the diagnosis of HPS. Chest radiographs can show basal shadowing, specific arteriovenous malformations (uncommon), pleural effusions, or may be normal. In conventional computed tomography scanning of the chest, peripheral pulmonary vascular dilatations can be seen with normal central pulmonary artery diameter [17].

5. MANAGEMENT

The treatment of HPS can be focused on three areas as seen in Table 3. The first intervention involves the treatment of hypoxemia with oxygen. Some patients will respond quite well simply to the administration of oxygen. However, as the severity of the intrapulmonary vascular dilatations progresses, oxygen alone will be less effective. A second focus of therapy is in the treatment of the pulmonary vascular dilatations. Presently, there is no consistently effective treatment for the type I dilatations. Several agents discussed below have been used with various degrees of success. Treatment for the type II dilatations causing right to left shunting involves coil embolotherapy. The type I dilatations are more commonly seen, however. Treatment of the underlying liver disease is the third aim of treatment, although HPS can progress even with stable hepatic dysfunction.

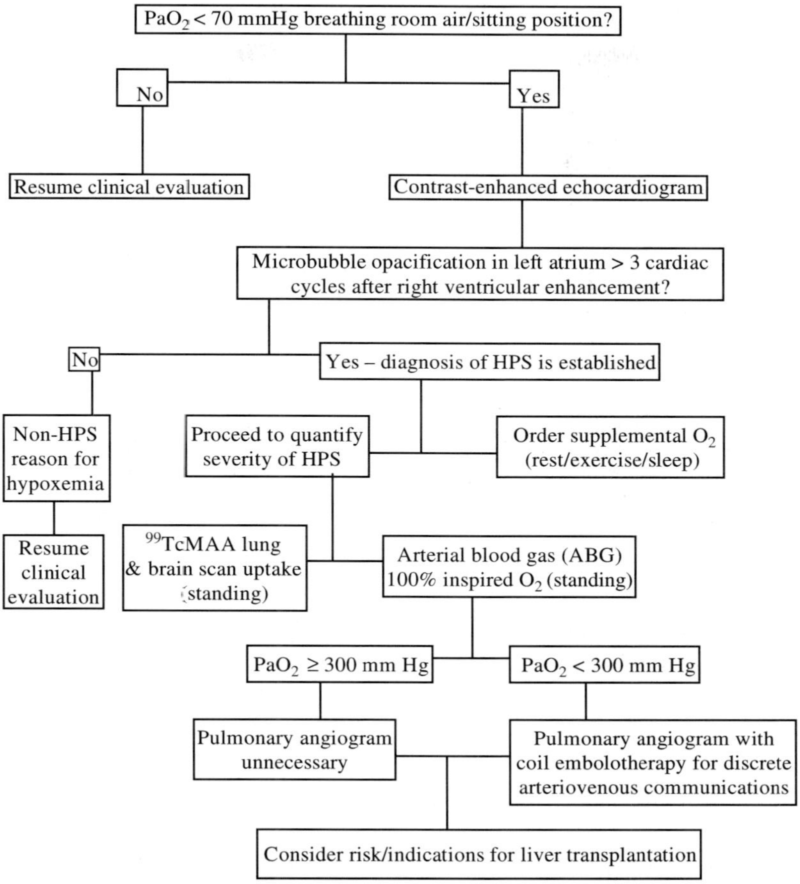

Figure 3. Diagnostic algorithm for hepatopulmonary syndrome screening and diagnosis.

Rarely, HPS can spontaneously resolve [9,15]. Pharmacologic treatment in the management of HPS has been disappointing thus far. Many agents have been tried without much benefit including almitrine, antimicrobial agents, prednisone, indomethacin and octreotide [9,15]. Recently, methylene blue administered intravenously to seven patients with moderate to severe HPS was found to improve oxygenation with a maximum effect seen at 5 h and continued improvement at 10 h following a single infusion [18]. This supports the idea of nitric oxide induced pulmonary vasodilatation. *Allium sativum* (garlic) has also been shown to improve oxygenation in 6 of 15 patients with HPS in a prospective, pilot

Table 3. Hepatopulmonary syndrome treatment options.

	Pharmacology	Interventional	Surgery
Hypoxemia	Oxygen		
Pulmonary vascular dilatation	Multiple agents attempted (see text)	Coil embolotherapy (type II)	
Hepatic dysfunction		TIPS, cavoplasty	OLT

OLT: orthotopic liver transplantation.

study to determine if a standardized garlic powder improved oxygenation and dyspnea in HPS [19]. Transjugular intrahepatic portosystemic shunting (TIPS) and cavoplasty (for portal hypertension caused by inferior vena cava obstruction due to chronic Budd–Chiari syndrome) via interventional radiology techniques are additional interventions with variable results in HPS [20,21].

There is no question that HPS can resolve following orthotopic liver transplantation (OLT) [8,14]. Recurrence of HPS after OLT is rare. Many institutions currently consider HPS to be an indication for OLT even in the setting of stable hepatic dysfunction as long as transplant-listing criteria are met [2,14]. In a review of 81 total patients undergoing OLT as treatment for HPS, Krowka *et al.* [14] found an overall mortality of 16% within 3 months after OLT. No intraoperative deaths occurred. In this literature review, 82% of patients undergoing OLT for HPS experienced an improvement in or normalization of hypoxemia within 15 months following OLT. Unfortunately, recent case reports have described the resolution of HPS following OLT with the subsequent development of pulmonary hypertension [22]. This is an uncommon occurrence and presently patients who may develop this phenomenon cannot be identified before transplant. Genetic abnormalities that may affect vascular mediators and the development of pulmonary hypertension are currently being sought.

An active area of interest is the optimal timing of when the OLT should be performed in patients with HPS. The United Network for Organ Sharing (UNOS) is a non-profit charitable organization that maintains the nation's organ transplant waiting list [23]. Recently, the UNOS policy regarding liver transplantation adopted the Model for End-Stage Liver Disease (MELD) scale to assess a patient's risk of 3-month mortality on the waiting list so that patients could be better prioritized based on the severity of their illness, using objective, verifiable medical criteria. The MELD scale is a continuous disease severity scale (based upon levels of bilirubin, creatinine and INR) that is highly predictive of the risk of dying from liver disease for patients waiting on the transplant list [24].

Patients with HPS may have stable hepatic dysfunction so that their MELD score may not reflect their need for urgent liver transplantation. Because of this, UNOS and the Liver Disease Severity Scale Committee developed guidelines for adjusting the MELD score for this group of patients. The current policy now states that "patients with clinical evidence of portal hypertension, evidence of a shunt and a $PaO_2 < 60$ mmHg on room air may be referred to the Regional Review Board for consideration of a MELD score that would provide them a reasonable probability of being transplanted with 3 months".

6. PROGNOSIS

The natural history of HPS is as yet unknown. Most patients with HPS will continue to deteriorate with worsening hypoxemia and dyspnea despite stable hepatic dysfunction unless transplanted. Nonetheless, some prognostic factors have been defined by reviewing the literature. In the review by Krowka *et al.* [14], transplanted patients who died had significantly lower mean PaO_2 values compared with patients who survived (44.7 mmHg versus 54.2 mmHg; $p < 0.03$). Also 30% of patients with severe hypoxemia, defined as a $PaO_2 < 50$ mmHg, died after OLT compared with those with a $PaO_2 > 50$ mmHg ($p < 0.02$). Unpublished data from Mayo Clinic, studying the clinical course of 37 patients with HPS who did not undergo liver transplantation, demonstrated a 30% 5-year survival. Only by gaining an understanding of the natural history and prognostic factors involved in HPS, will investigators be able to determine the optimal timing of OLT in these patients.

7. SUMMARY

HPS is an uncommon condition generally resulting in progressive hypoxemia caused by increasing intrapulmonary vascular dilatations in patients with chronic liver disease. The degree of hypoxemia caused by HPS does not appear to be related to the severity of the liver disease. Many patients with end-stage liver disease may complain of dyspnea, however, a high degree of suspicion in patients with liver disease and hypoxemia will enable clinicians to diagnose HPS. The evaluation of these patients is focused on the documentation and severity of hypoxemia and intrapulmonary vascular dilatations with arterial blood gases, contrast echocardiography and lung perfusion–brain scanning. Treatment of the underlying liver disease and alleviating hypoxemia with the use of oxygen is appropriate. OLT currently is the mainstay of therapy for the treatment of HPS. As further insight emerges regarding the vascular mediators involved, future drug therapy may involve manipulation of the various mediators.

REFERENCES

[1] Krowka, M.J. (2000) Hepatopulmonary syndromes. *Gut* **40**, 1–4.

[2] Rodriguez-Roisin, R. and Roca, J. (1997) Hepatopulmonary syndrome: the paradigm of liver-induced hypoxaemia. *Baillieres Clin. Gastroenterol.* **11**, 387–406.

[3] Martinez, G.P., Barbera, J.A., Visa, J., Rimola, A., Parc, J.G., Roca, J., Navasa, M., Rodes, J. and Rodriguez-Roisin, R. (2001) Hepatopulmonary syndrome in candidates for liver transplantation. *J. Hepatol.* **34**, 651–657.

[4] Mimidis, K.P., Karatza, C., Spiropoulos, K.V., Toulgaridis, T., Charokopos, N., Thomopoulos, K.C., Margaritis, V.G. and Nikolopoulou, V.N. (1998) Prevalence of intrapulmonary vascular dilatations in normoxaemic patients with early liver cirrhosis. *Scand J. Gastroenterol.* **33**, 988–992.

[5] Gupta, D., Vijaya, D.R., Gupta, R., Dhiman, R.K., Bhargava, M., Verma, J. and Chawla, Y.K. (2001) Prevalence of hepatopulmonary syndrome in cirrhosis and extrahepatic portal venous obstruction. *Am. J. Gastroenterol.* **96**, 3395–3399.

[6] Abrams, G.A., Jaffe, C.C., Hoffer, P.B., Binder, H.J. and Fallon, M.B. (1995) Diagnostic utility of contrast echocardiography and lung perfusion scan in patients with hepatopulmonary syndrome. *Gastroenterology* **109**, 1283–1288.

[7] Krowka, M.J., Wiseman, G.A., Burnett, O.L., Spivey, J.R., Therneau, T.M., Porayko, M.K. and Wiesner, R.H. (2000) Hepatopulmonary syndrome: a prospective study of relationships between severity of liver disease, PaO_2 response to 100% oxygen, and brain uptake after 99mTcMaa lung scanning. *Chest* **118**, 615–624.

[8] Krowka, M.J. (2000) Hepatopulmonary syndrome: recent literature (1997 to 1999) and implications for liver transplantation. *Liver Transpl.* **6**, S31–S35.

[9] Herve, P., Lebrec, D., Brenot, F., Simonneau, G., Humbert, M., Sitbon, O. and Duroux, P. (1998) Pulmonary vascular disorders in portal hypertension. *Eur. Respir. J.* **11**, 1153–1166.

[10] Vettukattil, J.J., Slavik, Z., Lamb, R.K., Monro, J.L., Keeton, B.R., Tsang, V.T., Aldous, A.J., Zivanovic, A., Johns, S., Lewington, V. and Salmon, A.P. (2000) Intrapulmonary arteriovenous shunting may be a universal phenomenon in patients with the superior cavopulmonary anastomosis: a radionuclide study. *Heart* **83**, 425–428.

[11] Fallon, M.B., Abrams, G.A., Lua, B., Hou, Z., Dai, J. and Ku, D.D. (1997) The role of endothelial nitric oxide synthase in the pathogenesis of a rat model of hepatopulmonary syndrome. *Gastroenterology* **113**, 606–614.

[12] Luo, B., Abrams, G.A. and Fallon, M.B. (1998) Endothelin-1 in the rat bile duct ligation model of hepatopulmonary syndrome: correlation with pulmonary dysfunction. *J. Hepatol.* **29**, 571–578.

[13] Castro, M. and Krowka, M.J. (1996) Hepatopulmonary syndrome: a pulmonary vascular complication of liver disease. *Clin. Chest Med.* **17**, 35–48.

[14] Krowka, M.J., Porayko, M.K., Plevak, D.J., Pappas, C., Steers, J.L., Krom, R.A. and Wiesner, R.H. (1997) Hepatopulmonary syndrome with progressive hypoxemia as an indication for liver transplantation: case reports and literature review. *Mayo Clin. Proc.* **72**, 44–53.

[15] Aboussouan, L.S. and Stoller, J.K. (2000) The hepatopulmonary syndrome. *Ballieres Clin. Gastroenterol.* **14**, 1033–1048.

[16] Abrams, G.A., Nanda, N.C., Dubovsky, E.V., Krowka, M.J. and Fallon, M.B. (1998) Use of macroaggregated albumin lung perfusion scan to diagnose hepatopulmonary syndrome: a new approach. *Gastroenterology* **114**, 305–310.

[17] Lee, K.N., Lee, H.J., Shin, W.W. and Web, W.R. (1999) Hypoxemia and liver cirrhosis (hepatopulmonary syndrome) in eight patients: comparison of the central and peripheral pulmonary vasculature. *Radiology* **211**, 549–553.

[18] Schenk, P., Madl, C., Majd-Rezaie, S., Rezaie-Majd, S., Lehr, S. and Muller, C. (2000) Methylene blue improves the hepatopulmonary syndrome. *Ann. Intern. Med.* **133**, 701–706.

[19] Abrams, G.A. and Fallon, M.B. (1998) Treatment of hepatopulmonary syndrome with *Allium sativum* L

(garlic): a pilot trial. *J. Clin. Gastroenterol.* **27**, 232–235.

[20] Lasch, H.M., Fried, M.W., Zacks, S.L., Odell, P., Johnson, M.W., Gerber, D.A., Sandu, F.S., Fait, J.H. and Shrestha, R. (2001) Use of transjugular intrahepatic portosystemic shunt as a bridge to liver transplantation in a patient with severe hepatopulmonary syndrome. *Liver Transpl.* **17**, 147–149.

[21] De, B.K., Sen, S., Biswas, P.K., Mandel, S.K., Das, D., Das, U., Guru, S. and Bandyopadhyay, K. (2002) Occurrence of hepatopulmonary syndrome in Budd-Chiari syndrome and the role of venous decompression. *Gastroenterology* **122**, 897–903.

[22] Martinez-Palli, G., Barbera, J.A., Taura, P., Cirera, I., Visa, J. and Rodriguez-Raisin, R. (1999) Severe portopulmonary hypertension after liver transplantation in a patient with pre-existing hepatopulmonary syndrome. *J. Hepatol.* **31**, 1075–1079.

[23] United Network for Organ Sharing (UNOS). Online: http://www.unos.org

[24] Kamath, P.S., Wiesner, R.H., Malinchoc, M., Kremers, W., Therneau, T.M., Kosberg, C.L., D'Amico, G., Dickson, E.R. and Kim, W.R. (2001) A model to predict survival in patients with end-stage liver disease. *Hepatology* **33**, 464–470.

Hepatology: A Practical Approach
B. Al Knawy, M.L. Shiffman, R.H. Wiesner (editors)

Chapter 6
Hepatocellular Carcinoma

Hashem B. El-Serag

Gastroenterology and Health Services Research Sections, Baylor College of Medicine, The Houston VA Medical Center, Houston, TX, USA

1. Epidemiology 409
2. Risk Factors 411
   2.1 Hepatitis C virus 411
      2.1.1 Alcohol 411
      2.1.2 Human immunodeficiency virus 411
      2.1.3 Antiviral therapy and HCC 412
   2.2 Hepatitis B virus 412
   2.3 Diabetes 412
   2.4 Idiopathic HCC 412
3. Clinical Features 412
4. Pathology 413
5. Prevention 413
6. Diagnosis 414
   6.1 Imaging 414
   6.2 Biopsy 415
7. Staging 415
8. Treatment 415
   8.1 Surgical resection 416
   8.2 Liver transplantation 417
   8.3 Non-surgical ablative therapies 417
9. Prognosis 418
References 418

1. EPIDEMIOLOGY

Hepatocellular carcinoma (HCC) affects approximately half a million persons each year worldwide making it the fifth most common malignancy in men and the ninth most common in women. HCC is a rapidly fatal cancer that mostly affects persons in developing countries (Southeast Asia and sub-Saharan Africa) where hepatitis B virus (HBV) is endemic. However, the incidence of HCC has been increasing rapidly in several developed countries in Europe and North America.

HCC is rarely seen during the first 4 decades of life except in populations where HBV infection is hyperendemic. The incidence of HCC increases progressively with older age, reaching a peak between the ages of 70 and 75 years. In general, patients with HCC are younger in high-incidence areas than those in low-incidence area. In high-incidence areas, HBV is the major risk factor for HCC and is acquired early in life. However, in areas with low HCC incidence, the main risk factors, hepatitis C virus (HCV) and alcoholic cirrhosis, are acquired relatively late in life. With the exception of areas in the world where HBV is endemic, it is uncommon to find HCC in the absence of cirrhosis (Figure 1). Once cirrhosis is established, the annual rate of HCC is between 1 and 6% [1].

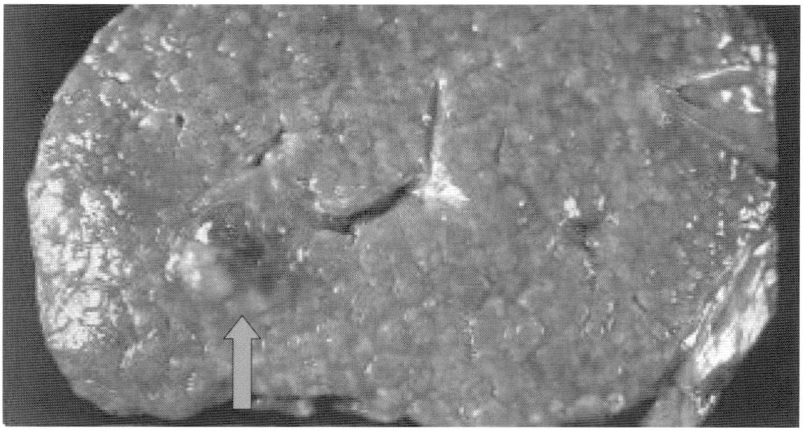

Figure 1. Nodular HCC in a liver with cirrhosis (most common form of HCC in the most common setting). (*For colored version, see Plate XLI on page 585 at the end of the book.*)

In countries with multi-ethnic groups such as the United States, Caucasians are 2–3 times less affected than African-Americans, who, in turn, are 2–3 times less affected than Asians, Pacific Islanders or Native Americans. In all ethnic groups, men are 2–3 times more affected than women. The magnitude of these marked ethnic and gender differences in HCC has remained largely constant even when the overall rates of HCC have risen significantly. The reason(s) for these ethnic differences probably relates to the prevalence and acquisition time of the major HCC risk factors (HCV, HBV, and alcoholic liver disease). Higher levels of testosterone or bigger body mass index have been suggested as possible explanations for the higher risk in men.

Recently, a trend of rising incidence rates of HCC has been reported from several developed countries in North America, Europe, and Asia. For example, the age-adjusted incidence rate of HCC increased from 1.4 per 100,000 during 1976–1980 to 3.0 per 100,000 during 1996–1998, representing a twofold increase (Figure 2) [2]. Due to the essential role of cirrhosis in the development of HCC in most patients, an increase in the number of persons living with cirrhosis is the likely explanation for the rising incidence of HCC (Table 3). This has resulted from a combination of rising incidence of cirrhosis as well as general improvement in the survival of patients with cirrhosis. The prolonged survival of patients with cirrhosis, related to better clinical management

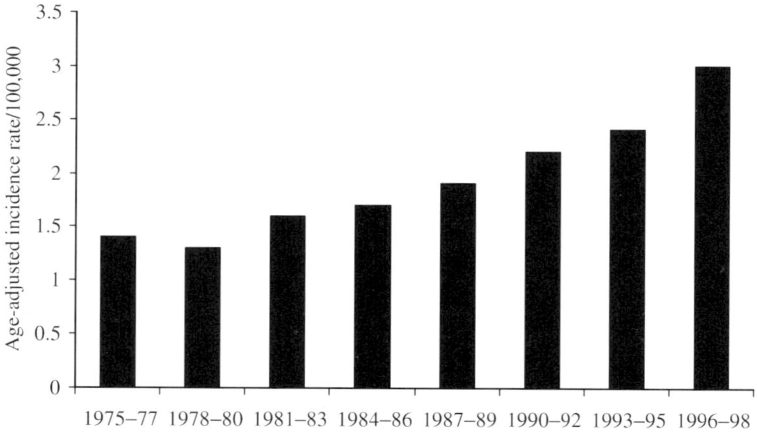

Figure 2. The age-adjusted incidence rates of hepatocellular carcinoma in the United States.

(e.g., esophageal variceal hemorrhage) may allow enough time for some patients to develop symptomatic HCC. In the US, HCV-related HCC accounts for at least half of the recent increase in HCC. Importantly, Caucasian men between the ages of 45 and 65 represent the group most affected by the rising rates of HCC.

2. RISK FACTORS

A list of risk factors is shown in Table 1.

2.1 Hepatitis C virus

Several lines of evidence indicate a strong causal association between HCV and HCC. HCV-RNA can be found in the serum, liver, and tumor tissues of patients with HCC, but unlike HBV it does not integrate into the host genome. Markers of HCV infection are found in HCC cases depending on the geographic regions; for example, 30% in the US, and more than 80% of HCC cases in Japan [3].

Table 1. Causes and risk factors for hepatocellular carcinoma.

Causes and risk factors
Cirrhosis from any cause (including alcohol)[a]
Chronic viral hepatitis
Hepatitis C[a]
Hepatitis B[a]
Hepatitis D
Diabetes mellitus
Non-alcoholic fatty liver disease
Hemochromatosis
Other rare metabolic disorders:
Alpha-1 antitrypsin deficiency
Tyrosinemia
Porphyrias: cutanea tarda and intermittent
Wilson's disease
Glycogen storage disease types 1 and 2
Toxins
Aflatoxins
Thorium dioxide
Possible carcinogens
Anabolic steroids
Estrogens
Not proven
Oral contraceptives
Smoking

[a]Most common causes.

HCV increases the risk of HCC by promoting fibrosis and cirrhosis; virtually all HCV-related HCC cases occur among patients with cirrhosis or advanced fibrosis. The duration of HCV infection is especially relevant to HCC development, most cases of HCC occurring after 2–3 decades of chronic infection. HCV infection increases the relative risk of HCC several-fold (up to 25 times) as compared to non-infected people.

In HCV-infected patients, there are several host-related factors that increase the progression of HCV infection to cirrhosis and HCC. These include older age at the time of acquisition of infection, male gender, heavy alcohol intake (more than 50 g daily), co-infection with HBV or HIV, and possibly a transfusion mode of HCV acquisition. Viral factors seem to be less important in determining the progression of HCV. There is no evidence that either viral load, genotype, or viral quasispecies are important in determining the risk of HCV progression to cirrhosis or HCC [4].

2.1.1 Alcohol

HCV and alcohol increase the risk of HCC by more actively promoting the development of cirrhosis. Among alcohol drinkers, the risk of HCC increases with a daily intake greater than 40–60 g, and that the presence of HCV had a positive synergistic action with an additional twofold increase in the risk over that caused by alcohol alone. The effect of occasional or "social" alcohol drinking on the progression of HCV infection is less well understood. Excessive alcohol drinking increases the risk of HCC through the formation of cirrhosis, even in the absence of viral hepatitis, but to a much lesser degree.

2.1.2 Human immunodeficiency virus

Higher HCV-RNA counts have been reported in patients with dual HCV/HIV infection as compared to patients with HCV monoinfection. Several studies have indicated that co-infection with HCV and HIV is associated with an increased risk of chronic liver disease especially in patients with low CD-4 cell count; however, the clinical importance of these lesions and whether they lead to a subsequent increase in HCC is related in no small part to the overall mortality of HIV-infected patients. As the overall mortality is increased due to wider implementation of highly active anti-retroviral therapy and the reduction in opportunistic infections, insidious infections such as HCV or HBV might become a more important cause of morbidity and mortality [4].

2.1.3 Antiviral therapy and HCC

There was only one prospective, randomized, controlled trial that examined the effects of therapy on HCC, a trial from Japan in which 100 patients were randomized to receive either 6 million units of interferon-α thrice weekly for 3–6 months or were followed without treatment. After a 2- to 7-year period of follow-up, HCC was significantly reduced in the treated group (4%) as compared to the non-treated controls (38%), a 93% reduction in the adjusted risk ratio. However, a large degree of this risk reduction was a result of the unusually high rate of HCC in the control group. Several retrospective, non-randomized studies suggested a moderate decrease in the risk of HCC among HCV-infected patients treated with interferon. The benefit was better appreciated in younger patients, those with sustained biochemical and or virological response than non-responders. Patients with cirrhosis are more likely to have contraindications to treatment (e.g., low platelets) or be discontinued due to side effects. However, the lack of randomization requires caution in interpreting these studies. In non-randomized trials, an exaggerated treatment benefits are likely as healthier patients tend to get treated more frequently than those with advanced liver disease.

2.2 Hepatitis B virus

During the course of HBV infection, it becomes integrated with the host chromosomal DNA. However, chronic hepatitis leading to cirrhosis is the most important precancerous etiological factor in HBV-infected patients. In places where HBV is acquired at birth through vertical transmission (mother to infant) or during early childhood, up to half of HBV infections follow a chronic course, and the risk of HBV-related HCC is high.

2.3 Diabetes

Several reports have suggested that persons with diabetes mellitus are at an increased risk (approximately double) of developing HCC, while others have found either a weak association or no association between HCC and diabetes. Diabetes predisposes to non-alcoholic steatohepatitis, which may progress to cirrhosis in up to 5% of cases. Diabetes is also associated with increased levels of insulin-like factors that are potential carcinogenic factors. Obesity, which frequently accompanies diabetes, has also been reported to increase the risk of hepatic steatosis and fibrosis in HCV-infected patients [5].

2.4 Idiopathic HCC

Between 15 and 40% of patients with HCC in the US have none of the etiologic factors listed in Table 1. More than half of "idiopathic" cases have evidence of advanced liver damage usually cirrhosis or advanced fibrosis. "Cryptic" viral hepatitis may be found in some patients where viral nucleic acids is found within hepatocytes despite the absence of conventional virological markers in the serum. Some of these cases may also represent "burnt out" non-alcoholic steatohepatitis (with or without diabetes) or autoimmune hepatitis [4].

3. CLINICAL FEATURES

Patients with HCC present with one or more of several clinical features including right upper quadrant pain, weight loss, worsening liver enzymes in a patient known to have cirrhosis. Rare presenting features include acute abdominal catastrophe from rupture of HCC with intra-abdominal bleeding or extra-hepatic manifestations (e.g., hypercalcemia, hyperglycemia, thyrotoxicosis). Anemia is present in more than half of cases, although rarely erythrocytosis can be seen due to extra-renal synthesis of erythropoietin. In addition to signs of cirrhosis (e.g., jaundice, palmar erythema, gynecomastia) and portal hypertension (e.g., ascites, varices), a hepatic bruit could be detected in 10–20% of patients with HCC. More patients are being diagnosed with HCC at an asymptomatic stage as a result of widespread imaging studies [6].

4. PATHOLOGY

There are three main types of HCC based on gross appearance: nodular (75%), massive (25%), and diffuse (<1%). The massive variety is prone to rupture and hemorrhage. The diffuse variety notoriously escapes detection by ultrasound examination. Histologically, despite the poor prognosis, most HCC is well differentiated. Both trabecular and acinar forms are seen, and bile production is the cardinal feature of HCC. The portal vein or its branches are invaded by HCC in the majority of cases. Extra-hepatic spread, primarily to the lungs and lymph nodes, is present in more than half of the cases at autopsy. Bone or skin metastasis is rare.

5. PREVENTION

(1) *HBV immunization*: Immunization for HBV has been proven to reduce the incidence of HCC in countries where HBV is endemic. A safe and effective HBV vaccine is currently available. It is especially important for those with liver disease due to any cause to receive such immunization.

(2) *Counseling for alcohol ingestion*: Epidemiological studies have found that ingesting alcohol in daily amounts that exceed 40–60 g to be significantly associated with the risk of alcoholic liver disease (including cirrhosis and HCC). The amounts of alcohol in common beverages are provided in Table 2. HCV or HBV infected persons should have special counseling. Treatment for alcohol dependence associated with relapse rate is very high; however, joining a support group has been shown to decrease this rate.

(3) *Screening/surveillance for HCC*: *Screening* refers to the process of identifying a condition in average risk healthy persons, while *surveillance* aims at identifying a condition among persons with a high risk. Although frequently interchangeable, strictly speaking, screening for HCC is not indicated due to its relative infrequent occurrence in the general population. The majority of hepatologists employ some sort of HCC surveillance. However, the efficacy of HCC surveillance programs has not been examined in randomized controlled trials. Studies that used mathematical modeling have suggested a small benefit for HCC surveillance, which may be cost-effective in high-risk patients. There are several tests that have been used for HCC surveillance [7].

Table 2. The amount of alcohol (ethanol) contained in common beverages.

	Serving (oz)	Ethanol, % (ml/100 ml)	Ethanol/ serving (g)
Beer (average can)	12	5	14.2
Wine (glass)	5	12	14.2
Whiskey shot (80 proof)	1.5	40	14.2

α-Fetoprotein (AFP): AFP is a fetal protein whose serum levels become undetectable soon after birth. The normal AFP level in adults is <10 ng/l. Modest elevation of AFP levels (10–100 ng/ml) can be seen in some patients with chronic viral hepatitis, especially those with HCV, and cirrhosis, whereas normal levels have been reported in patients with small HCC. AFP levels may also increase >20 ng/ml with pregnancy and gonadal germ cell tumors; however, in the latter two conditions there is a concomitant rise in serum levels of β-HCG. As a surveillance test for HCC, AFP level >20 ng/ml has an average sensitivity of 50% and a specificity of 80%. Due to low sensitivity the use of AFP alone in HCC surveillance is not recommended. On the other hand, in the presence of a liver mass, a diagnostic test of an AFP level >400 ng/ml is highly specific and almost diagnostic of HCC. Measurement of various isoforms of AFP has been investigated to improve sensitivity and specificity. The best studied is Lens culinaris agglutinin A-reactive α-fetoprotein, which improves specificity but still has relatively low sensitivity.

Des-gamma-carboxy prothrombin (DCP): DCP is a form of prothrombin that is deficient in carboxyglutamic acid residues making the molecule inactive as a prothrombin. DCP is elevated in patients deficient in vitamin K (including those taking coumadin), as well as patients with viral hepatitis, cirrhosis, and HCC. Normal values vary among the available assays. In general, DCP has low sensitivity for small HCC and is not widely used.

Ultrasound (US): US is a non-invasive, painless procedure with no known side effects. The use of US examination of the liver in HCC surveillance has a sensitivity and specificity of up to 80 and 90%, respectively. The diagnostic accuracy of ultrasound depends partly on the operator's experience, the size of the patient (i.e., significant obesity) and the texture of the liver (the presence of coarse liver can hinder correct identification of HCC). US has poor sensitivity in detecting HCC lesions < 3 cm, multifocal or diffuse HCC.

Helical computed tomography (CT) scans and magnetic resonance imaging (MRI) are commonly used to diagnose HCC as follow-up test for AFP or US; however, these tests are expensive and their benefit in HCC surveillance has not yet been proven.

On average, the tumor mean doubling time of HCC is approximately 4–6 months and therefore a suggested surveillance strategy is to perform an ultrasound combined with measuring serum levels of AFP every 6 months (Figure 3). Patients with an elevated AFP or a mass on ultrasound should receive CT scan and or MRI to confirm HCC, and to determine its stage (Table 3). These tests have greater accuracy for detecting HCC, however, their utility as surveillance tests is unknown, and because these are expensive tests, they are usually reserved as confirmatory or diagnostic tests.

6. DIAGNOSIS

The requirements for HCC diagnosis are listed in Table 4 [8,9].

6.1 Imaging

On ultrasound examination, HCC is typically hypoechoic and a capsule may be noted. However, CT scan and MRI are the main diagnostic modalities. HCC derives its blood supply predominantly from the hepatic artery whereas the remainder of the liver receives both arterial and portal blood. HCCs therefore enhance early or during the infusion of contrast, in the arterial phase of the triphasic CT scan or dual-contrast MRI of liver (negative contrast medium chondroitin sulfate iron colloid and positive contrast medium gadopentate dimeglumine) is highly accurate in detecting HCC. In MRI, HCC appears hypointense on T-1-weighted images and hyperintense on T-2-weighted images. The sensitivity and specificity of contrast-enhanced spiral CT is 68 and 81%, respectively. These figures are

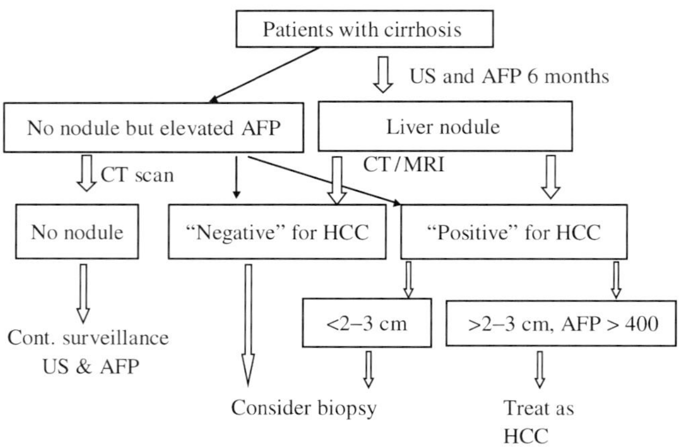

Figure 3. A suggested algorithm for surveillance in hepatocellular carcinoma.

Table 3. Recommendations for hepatocellular carcinoma (HCC) surveillance.

Surveillance for HCC is recommended for the following groups
Cirrhosis due to any reason
Adult persons with chronic hepatitis B especially if acquired early in life
Adult patients with hereditary hemochromatosis
Previously resected HCC
Surveillance for HCC is *not* recommended for the following groups
Healthy individuals with no liver disease (i.e., screening)
Patients with HCV infection and no cirrhosis
Patients who are not candidates for surgical resection, liver transplantation, or ablative therapy

slightly higher for MRI. Although CT scan and MRI detect lesions as small as 0.5–1 cm, their sensitivity for HCC decreases with small tumors and is the lowest in tumors less than 2 cm in diameter. Radioisotope scans of the liver lack both sensitivity and specificity, and should not be used. Angiography use is limited nowadays to the administration of chemoembolization.

6.2 Biopsy

The routine use of needle biopsy under radiologic guidance of HCC is controversial, particularly in patients with HCC who may be potentially cured by surgical resection or liver transplantation. One possible but small risk (1%) of percutaneous needle biopsy is local spread of HCC along the needle track. Open surgical biopsy procedures may sometimes be performed, if HCC is suspected but the tumor cannot be located with precision by radiographic methods. In general, biopsy is not required if the diagnosis of HCC can be made accurately by non-invasion tests (Table 5).

Table 4. Diagnosis of hepatocellular carcinoma.

Cyto-histological criteria (biopsy whether percutaneous, laparoscopic, or open)
Non-invasive criteria
Radiological criteria
Two coincident imaging techniques
c/w a focal lesion >2 cm with arterial hypervascularization
Combined criteria: one imaging technique associated with AFP
Focal lesion >2 cm with arterial hypervascularization
AFP levels >400 ng/ml

Table 5. Recommendation on the use of needle biopsy for HCC diagnosis.

Not required in the presence of a mass >3 cm with characteristic features of HCC on CT/MRI/angiography, and AFP > 400–500 ng/ml
Usually required for small lesions <2 cm; or lesions difficult to distinguish on imaging studies

7. STAGING

Survival is based on the extent of the tumor, as well as on underlying hepatic function. The currently available staging systems for HCC include: pathologic tumor-node metastasis (PTNM), Okuda, Cancer of the Liver Italian Program (CLIP), and Barcelona Clinic Liver Cancer (BCLC).

PTNM staging system similar to that for other solid tumors is limited by not accounting for the severity of underlying hepatic function, and therefore does not accurately predict survival in patients undergoing hepatic resection for HCC.

The Okuda system (Table 6) incorporates the underlying liver disease, in addition to the spread of the tumor. Patients with Okuda stage 3 HCC have a very poor prognosis and should receive supportive care only. The CLIP score (Table 7) better explains variability in survival especially within Okuda stage 1 and 2. Okuda, CLIP, and BCLC are all effective at selecting patients with extremely poor prognosis who should only receive supportive care.

8. TREATMENT

In general, no treatment modality has been shown in randomized controlled trials to decrease the mortality related to HCC. Lack of randomized control trials makes it difficult to avoid "lead-time bias" in interpreting the available literature. Lead-time bias

Table 6. Okuda staging system.

Clinical parameters	Cut-off values	Points
Tumor size (cross-sectional area on imaging)	>50%	1
	<50%	0
Ascites	Present	1
	Absent	0
Serum albumin (mg/dl)	>3	0
	<3	1
Serum total bilirubin	<3	0
	>3	1
Number of points	**Stage**	**Median survival (years)**
0	1	8.3
1–2	2	2
3–4	3	6.7

is the apparent improvement in survival that is exclusively caused by early detection, and it occurs when studies compare different treatments in groups of patients with different degrees of severity of liver disease, or with different sizes of tumor. Potentially curative therapies (resection, liver transplantation, percutaneous ablation) are recommended for patients with early HCC; again, there are no RCT comparing these therapies.

The algorithm for HCC management is outlined in Figure 4 [8,9].

8.1 Surgical resection

Resection of HCC should be considered for all non-cirrhotic patients who lack extra-hepatic spread. Unfortunately, the great majority of patients with HCC are not suitable candidates for surgical resection. Because most HCCs occur in patients with advanced cirrhosis and concomitant portal hypertension, these patients are at high risk of decompensation if surgical resection is attempted (Figure 4). Optimal candidates include patients with Child–Pugh class A cirrhosis with normal serum total bilirubin values, absence of clinically relevant portal hypertension, and small asymptomatic tumors and no evidence of distant spread. Liver resection has the disadvantage of not eliminating remaining portions of the liver at risk for malignant transformation. The post-resection residual liver, often cirrhotic, has the same high potential for HCC. Therefore, even following "complete" resection, recurrence rate/new cancer is high and the 3-year recurrence free survival is 30–40%. Further refinement of Child A by ruling out significant portal hypertension (bilirubin <1–2) may improve the 5-year survival even further (60–70%), however, it further limits the number of suitable candidates (<5% of all patients).

Table 7. CLIP staging system.

Variables	0	1	2
Child–Pugh class	A	B	C
Tumor morphology	Single nodule and <50% area	Multiple nodules and <50% area	Massive or >50% area
AFP (ng/ml)	<400	>400	
Portal vein thrombosis	No	Yes	

	HCC prognosis using the CLIP staging system		
CLIP score	Median survival (Months)	One-year survival (%)	Two-year survival (%)
0	36	84	65
1	22	66	45
2	9	45	17
3	7	36	12
4–6	3	9	0

The score ranges between 0 and 6. *Cross-sectional area on imaging.

8.2 Liver transplantation

Orthotopic liver transplantation (OLT) is theoretically the best treatment for HCC because it removes the cancer and the surrounding tissue, removes the remaining liver tissue that is at risk for the development of *de novo* cancer, and restores hepatic function. Unfortunately, the limited availability of donor organs with the resulting delay to transplantation makes OLT impractical. The 5-year survival rate after OLT is 75% for solitary HCCs less than 5 cm in diameter or two tumors of smaller size. As median waiting time for transplantation is currently greater than 1 year, the development of contra-indications to transplantation increases development in up to 70% of the patients usually because of progression of HCC. Patients are often treated with chemoembolization while waiting transplantation, although with unproven benefit. There are only limited but promising data on survival after living donor liver transplantation but most series show comparable short-term patient survival with that in cadaveric transplants.

8.3 Non-surgical ablative therapies

Ablation may be accomplished by either chemical means (e.g., absolute ethanol) or physical means (e.g., cryoablation, radiofrequency ablation, or microwave coagulation. Ultrasound or CT-guided percutaneous ethanol injection is considered the standard ablative technique for <3 lesions that are <5 cm, in patients with no significant coagulopathy, and no ascites. The most frequent side effect is local pain, however, serious complications are rare. Almost all tumors smaller than 2 cm in diameter can be completely ablated in a single session for patients with a single small (<3 cm) HCC recurrence free survival similar to that of surgical resection. Recently, the use of radiofrequency ablation has become an established mode of therapy for HCC because of its ability to destroy HCC (up to 5 cm in size) at one sitting. However, one early study reported that 12.5% of patients treated with radiofrequency ablation had biopsy-proven needle-track seeding 4–18 months later. More recent studies have failed to corroborate these results. In tumors larger than 3 cm, alcohol diffusion is often incomplete, thus leaving viable neoplastic tissue after treatment.

Chemoembolization is performed by injecting chemotherapeutic agents intra-arterially into the hepatic artery, which is then occluded by injection of particulate materials such as Gelfoam to obstruct flow. Extensive tumor necrosis can be achieved in more than 80% of patients. However, the side effects of chemoembolization can be severe and include severe pain, liver failure, and formation of liver abscess. Chemoembolization is relatively contra-indicated when the tumor is diffuse throughout the liver, in the presence of liver failure (Child–Pugh class C), and in the presence of portal vein

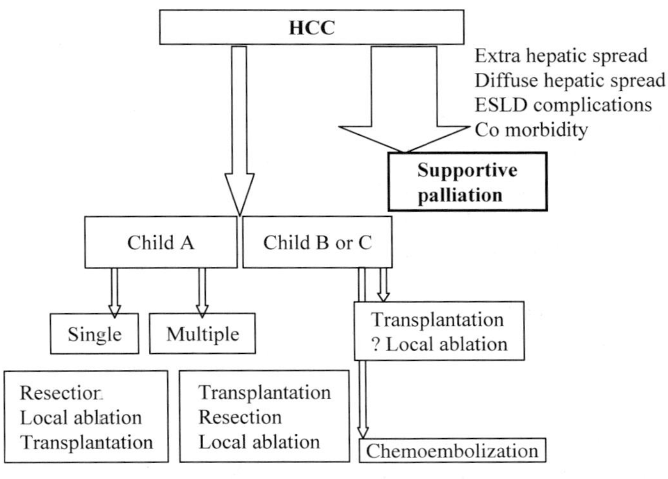

Figure 4. Management algorithm for hepatocellular carcinoma.

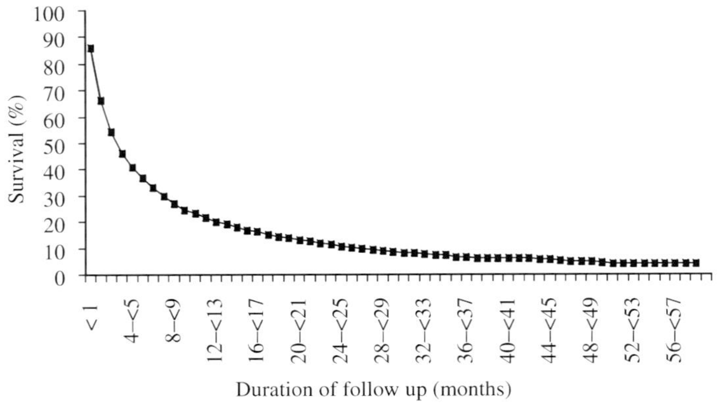

Figure 5. The overall survival of patients with HCC who are examined in population-based studies.

thrombosis. A recent meta-analysis of seven randomized controlled trials indicated a small survival benefit with arterial chemoembolization in patients with compensated (Child A or B) cirrhosis [10].

9. PROGNOSIS

Overall the 5-year survival of patients with HCC remains at a dismal rate of 6% (median of 7–8 months) (Figure 5). Both Okuda (Table 6) and CLIP staging (Table 7) allows for individualized prognosis data. Survival of patients with HCC is strongly dependent on the stage of cancer at the time of diagnosis, the underlying severity of liver disease and whether potentially curative therapy is applied. If an HCC lesion is smaller than 2 cm at the time of diagnosis in a patient with Child A cirrhosis and is successfully resected, the 5-year survival rate approaches 70–85%. Unfortunately, HCC is commonly diagnosed at an advanced stage in patients with decompensated liver disease, making curative therapy unlikely. Less than 10% of patients diagnosed with HCC in the US undergo potentially curative therapy. Caution has to be exercised in extrapolating the occasionally optimistic results often reported in small non-randomized studies of patients with HCC treated at referral centers. The multiple sources of bias that affect these studies tend to exaggerate the actual benefit. The overall survival of patients in HCC population-based studies has changed very little indicating that either therapy is not as effective as reported or it has not been applied on a large scale. Selection bias in which patients with no major comorbidity are included in the studies [11].

REFERENCES

[1] El-Serag, H.B. (2001) Global epidemiology of hepatocellular carcinoma. *Clin. Liver Dis.* **5**, 87–107. vi.

[2] El-Serag, H.B. and Mason, A.C. (1999) Rising incidence of hepatocellular carcinoma in the United States. *N. Engl. J. Med.* **340**, 745–750.

[3] Colombo, M. (2000) Hepatocellular carcinoma in patients with HCV. *Baillieres Best Pract. Res. Clin. Gastroenterol.* **14**, 327–339.

[4] El-Serag, H.B. (2002) Hepatocellular carcinoma and hepatitis C in the United States. *Hepatology* **36**, S74–S83.

[5] El-Serag, H.B., Richardson, P. and Everhart, J.E. (2001) The role of diabetes in hepatocellular carcinoma among veterans: a case-control study. *Am. J. Gastroenterol.* **96**, 2462–2467.

[6] Befeler, A.S. and Di Bisceglie, A.M. (2002) Hepatocellular carcinoma: diagnosis and treatment. *Gastroenterology* **122**, 1609–1619.

[7] Sherman, M. (2001) Surveillance for hepatocellular carcinoma. *Semin. Oncol.* **28**, 450–459.

[8] Bruix, J. and Llovet, J.M. (2002) Prognostic prediction and treatment strategy in hepatocellular carcinoma. *Hepatology* **35**, 519–524.

[9] Bruix, J., Sherman, M., Llovet, J.M., Beaugrand, M., Lencioni, R., Burroughs, A.K., Christensen, E., Pagliaro, L., Colombo, M., Rodes, J. and EASL Panel of Experts on HCC (2001) Clinical management of

hepatocellular carcinoma. Conclusions of the Barcelona-2000 EASL conference. European Association for the Study of the Liver. *J. Hepatol.* **35**, 421–430.

[10] Llovet, J.M. and Bruix, J. (2003) Systematic review of randomized trials for unresectable hepatocellular carcinoma: chemoembolization improves survival. *Hepatology* **37**, 429–442.

[11] El-Serag, H.B., Mason, A.C. and Key, C.R. (2001) Temporal trends in survival of patients with hepatocellular carcinoma in the US. *Hepatology* **33**, 62–65.

Section IV

Systemic Effect of Liver Diseases

Section Editor – B. Al Knawy

Hepatology: A Practical Approach
B. Al Knawy, M.L. Shiffman, R.H. Wiesner (editors)

Chapter 1
Nutrition in Liver Disease

Wael I. Youssef and Arthur J. McCullough

MetroHealth Medical Center, Case Western Reserve University, 2500, MetroHealth Drive, Cleveland, OH 44109, USA

1. Introduction 424
   1.1 Definition 424
   1.2 Prevalence 425
   1.3 General demographics 425
      1.3.1 Protein energy 425
      1.3.2 Obesity 426
2. Pathophysiology of Malnutrition 426
   2.1 Nutrient intake 426
   2.2 Absorption and metabolism 427
      2.2.1 Malabsorption 427
   2.3 Alcohol 427
   2.4 Protein and energy 427
      2.4.1 Protein 427
      2.4.2 Energy 428
3. Clinical Features 429
   3.1 Medical history 429
   3.2 Physical examination 430
4. Diagnosis 430
5. Management 431
   5.1 Nutritional requirements 431
      5.1.1 Protein requirements 431
      5.1.2 Energy 432
      5.1.3 Vitamins 432
   5.2 Specific alterations in liver disease 433
      5.2.1 Accelerated starvation 433
      5.2.2 Protein imbalance 433
         5.2.2.1 Hepatic encephalopathy 433
         5.2.2.2 Protein restriction 434
         5.2.2.3 Non-essential amino acids 434
      5.2.3 Salt restriction 434
      5.2.4 Alcohol-related alterations 434
         5.2.4.1 Alcohol toxicity 434
         5.2.4.2 Alcohol as empty calories 434
   5.3 Nutritional therapy 435
      5.3.1 Goals 435
      5.3.2 Specific patient populations 435
         5.3.2.1 Cirrhosis 435
         5.3.2.2 Alcoholic hepatitis 435
         5.3.2.3 Fulminant hepatic failure 435
         5.3.2.4 Perioperative 436

5.3.3 Liver transplant 436
5.3.3.1 Pre-transplant 436
5.3.3.2 Post-transplant 436
5.3.3.3 Long-term 437
5.3.4 Principles and practical implementation 437
5.3.4.1 Glucose requirement 437
5.3.4.2 Route of nutrient administration 437
5.3.4.3 Protein restriction 438
5.3.5 Prognosis 439
5.3.5.1 PEM 439
5.3.5.2 Obesity 439
6. Summary 440
References 440

1. INTRODUCTION

The liver is primarily a metabolic organ that orchestrates a complex array of physiological and biochemical processes, including the regulation of protein and energy metabolism (PEM). Consequently, it is not surprising that patients with advanced liver disease commonly have malnutrition. Increasing information suggests that PEM itself may accelerate deteriorating liver function and adversely affects clinical outcome.

The importance of this concept has led to the development of guidelines for the nutritional management of patients with liver disease [1,2]. The rationale for aggressive nutritional therapy in these patients is based on promising, but nascent clinical information and a number of nutritional axioms relative to chronic liver disease. First, malnutrition is common, but often underdiagnosed. Second, these patients have alterations in energy metabolism and nutritional status that mimic starvation. Third, many of the complications associated with chronic liver disease (such as hepatic encephalopathy, ascites and sepsis) occur *pari passu* with a negative nitrogen state, such as that before and immediately after liver transplantation. Finally, there is the expectation that correction of malnutrition may improve the clinical outcome of these patients.

This review will focus on the management of malnutrition in liver disease patients with the realization that the specific logistics of identifying patients most in need of nutritional therapy, as well as, choosing the type, duration and quantity of nutritional supplementation is a phase of clinical care that remains in evolution.

1.1 Definition

Protein energy malnutrition can be defined as the loss of protein stores (both visceral and muscle/somatic) and fat mass. Two forms are described: marasmus (combined protein energy malnutrition) and kwashiorkor (hypoalbuminemic) malnutrition. The former is an insufficient amount of both protein and calories resulting in the loss of muscle and fat mass with relative sparing of visceral proteins, such as albumin and fibrinogen. The latter is an insufficient amount of predominantly protein that results in diminished protein stores that occurs to a greater extent in visceral proteins as compared to muscle proteins.

In addition to these more classical forms of malnutrition it is also important to realize that over nutrition in the form of obesity is occurring more frequently in patients with liver disease. Obesity – defined as a body mass index (BMI) ≥ 30 – when present in liver disease poses specific and important issues regarding the nutritional management of these patients, as well as a potential etiologic factor for the development of advanced liver disease [3].

1.2 Prevalence

PEM is uncommon in the pre-cirrhotic stages of liver disease, except in the setting of extra-hepatic biliary obstruction. However, the prevalence of protein energy malnutrition in cirrhosis has been reported to range between 10 and 100% and may correlate with the severity of disease defined by the Child–Pugh–Turcotte score [4]. In one study, PEM was reported to be present in 20% of patients with compensated cirrhosis (Child's A) and in 50–60% of patients with decompensated cirrhosis (Child's C). The large range in reported prevalence rate may depend on how nutritional assessment is performed. For example, a large study of hospitalized patients with acute alcoholic hepatitis initially report a 100% prevalence of malnutrition based on at least one abnormal marker of malnutrition. However, the prevalence dropped to approximately 50% when a more complete pattern of marasmus or kwashiorkor was required [4].

1.3 General demographics

1.3.1. Protein energy

Although most of the earlier studies have concentrated on patients with alcoholic liver disease, the prevalence of PEM is high in all forms of cirrhosis [5]. Figure 1 shows four studies that have measured nutritional status in both alcoholic and non-alcoholic cirrhosis. These studies show that the prevalence of PEM is high and almost identical in

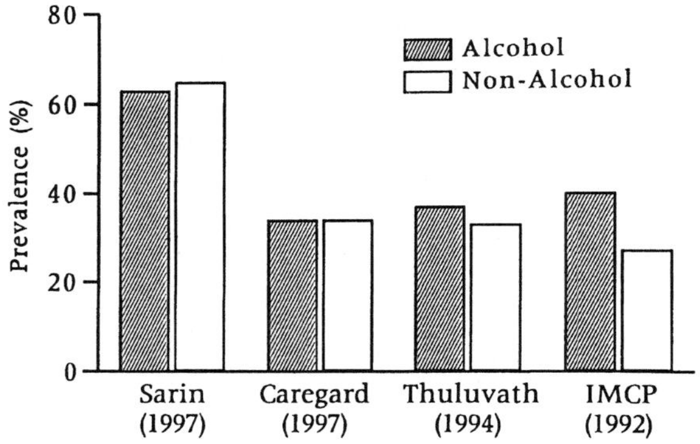

Fig. 1. The prevalence of PEM in alcoholic and non-alcoholic cirrhosis is shown for the only four available studies.

these two different types of cirrhosis. Based on anthropometric measurements of the lowest fifth percentile of a control population, the prevalence of PEM varied between 34 and 62, and 27 and 67% in these studies for alcoholic and non-alcoholic cirrhosis, respectively. There is also a high prevalence of PEM in patients awaiting liver transplantation with estimates ranging between 18 and 100% [6]. Data from the two most detailed studies of transplant patients are shown in Figure 2, which shows the moderate or severe PEM found in 70–80% of these patients. As listed in Table 1, disease-specific patterns of PEM have also been shown in patients with cirrhosis awaiting liver transplantation. Therefore, clinicians need to be aware that PEM is very common in these patients, especially because it has prognostic significance.

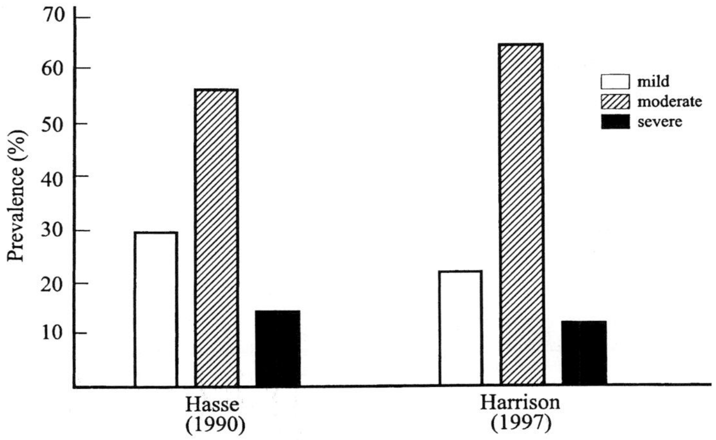

Fig. 2. The prevalence of PEM in patients awaiting liver transplantation.

Table 1. Pattern of malnutrition in chronic liver disease.

	Muscle wasting	Loss of fat stores	Synthetic function
Alcohol	+++	+	++
Viral	++	++	+
Primary biliary cirrhosis	+++	+++	+
Primary sclerosing cholangitis	++	+	+

(+) mild, (++) moderate, and (+++) severe abnormalities.

1.3.2. Obesity

The prevalence of obesity is approximately 30% of the adult population in the US and its prevalence increases at an alarming rate worldwide [7]. Obesity has also been reported as a risk factor for the development of cirrhosis in alcoholic, viral and non-alcoholic fatty liver disease [3].

Although the prevalence of obesity is unknown in patients with liver disease, obesity has been evaluated in patients awaiting transplantation. Although the definition of obesity differed among the studies, it appears that moderate or severe obesity is present in 6.5–31.5% of patients at the time of transplantation. Notably, the prevalence of different degrees of obesity is uniform among the different types of liver disease with the exception of cryptogenic cirrhosis, which accounts for an increasing proportion of liver transplants as the severity of obesity increases (Figure 3).

2. PATHOPHYSIOLOGY OF MALNUTRITION

There are multiple factors (as listed in Table 2) involved in the etiology of malnutrition which accelerates significantly after the development of cirrhosis and portosystemic shunting. As noted in Table 2, many of the factors can be treated successfully when nutritional status is recognized and treated as a priority.

2.1 Nutrient intake

Many studies have demonstrated inadequate dietary intake in a large percentage of patients with chronic liver disease prior to hospitalization [2]. Such poor intake is prevalent (27–87%) in patients with both alcoholic and non-alcoholic liver disease and has been attributed to anorexia, nausea, early satiety (especially in the presence of ascites) dysgeusia (possibly related to zinc deficiency) and unpalatable sodium- and protein-restricted diets. Inadequate dietary intake also continues after hospitalization with these patients ingesting approximately only 50%

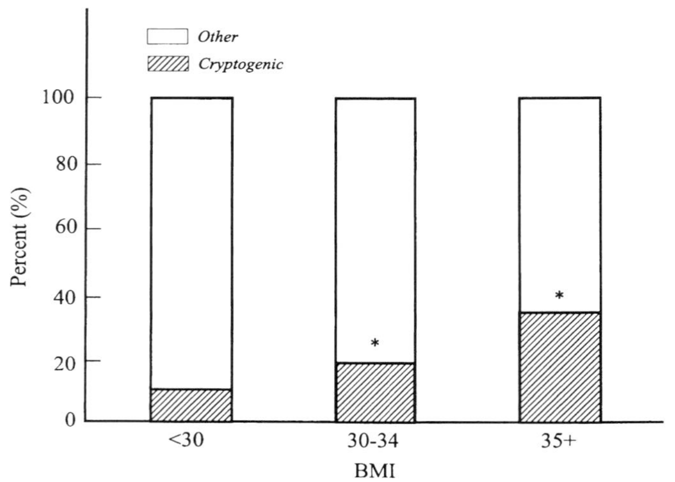

Fig. 3. The proportion of cryptogenic cirrhosis as the cause of liver disease in patients undergoing liver transplantation increases as the degree of obesity increases.

Table 2. Protein energy malnutrition in cirrhosis: etiologic factors.

Non-hospitalized patients
Inadequate diet[a]
Quantitative
Iatrogenic
(protein, fluid/salt restriction)
Malabsorption[a]
Pancreatic and bile salt deficiency
Enteropathy
Anorexia, nausea and vomiting.
Alcohol toxicity on energy and protein.
Altered protein and energy metabolism
Amino acid oxidation
Increased protein breakdown
Accelerated fat oxidation and gluconeogenesis
Hospitalized patients
Fasting status[a]
Diagnostic testing
Gastrointestinal bleeding
Altered neurologic status
Purgation and neomycin toxicity
Unpalatable diets[a]
Stressful complications[a]

[a]Factors that can be currently altered or treated.

of their calculated protein and caloric needs during their first 10 days of hospitalization. In hospitalized patients, the deficient intake is often iatrogenic and related to diagnostic and therapeutic procedures. The importance of these observations are emphasized by recent work, which demonstrated that a regular oral diet can improve PEM in cirrhotic patients [8].

2.2 Absorption and metabolism

Some studies have also demonstrated PEM in cirrhotics despite normal dietary intake. Therefore, other factors (such as those listed in Table 2 as altered PEM) must be involved.

2.2.1. Malabsorption

Although malabsorption is not usually considered a major cause of PEM in cirrhosis, moderate steatorrhea (< 12 g daily) occurs in both cholestatic and non-cholestatic liver disease. It has been reported to occur in as many as 40% of cirrhotic patients and may exceed 30 g daily in 10% of cirrhotic patients. This malabsorption has been attributed to decreased intestinal bile acids, pancreatic insufficiency and a diminished capacity for long-chain fatty acid absorption. These abnormalities are more severe in cholestatic liver disease [9]. In patients with extrahepatic biliary obstruction, the absence of bile acids in the duodenum induce anorexic factors – cholecystokinin and leptin appear to be particularly important. In addition, celiac sprue occurs more frequently in primary biliary cirrhosis, while inflammatory bowel disease and exocrine pancreatic abnormalities are more common in primary sclerosing cholangitis.

Although evidence for malabsorption should be sought in cirrhotic patients, malabsorption is not usually considered a major cause of PEM in these patients, with the exception of patients with cholestatic liver disease. The use of oral lactulose or neomycin for hepatic encephalopathy may also exacerbate nutrient malabsorption in all forms of liver disease.

2.3 Alcohol

Although alcohol is recognized as a direct hepatotoxin, it also has profound effects on PEM as recently reviewed elsewhere [10]. From a practical approach, these adverse effects can be avoided by abstinence from alcohol use.

2.4 Protein and energy

2.4.1. Protein

Underlying pathophysiological factors cause loss in both fat and protein stores. After an overnight fast, cirrhotics have an increased rate of protein breakdown that is not suppressed normally in response to feeding. Additionally, because of alterations in energy metabolism, due to glucagon resistance and diminished glycogenolysis (Figure 4), amino acids are oxidized for energy, especially the ketogenic amino acid leucine. This irreversible loss of

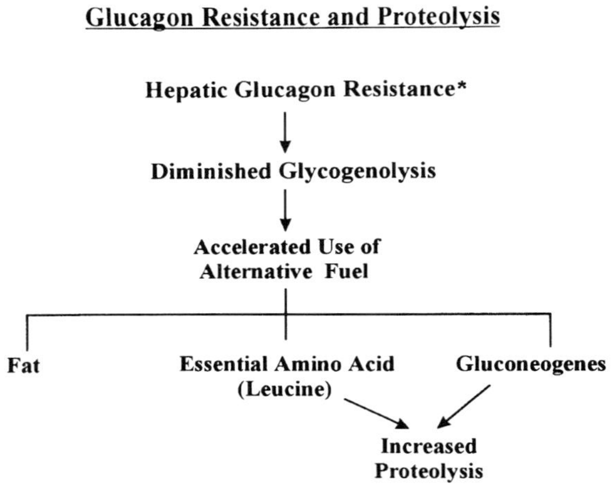

Fig. 4. The hypothesis: decreased hepatic glucose production caused by hepatic glucagon resistance leads to the use of alternative fuels and increased proteolysis in cirrhosis.

nitrogen is also associated with an increased rate of gluconeogenesis.

Gastroesophageal bleeding may also contribute to protein loss. Because hemoglobin lacks the essential amino acid isoleucine, it is relatively a low-quality protein source. Digestion of hemoglobin causes an increased rate of protein breakdown and urea synthesis. Clinical trials have shown that the administration of exogenous isoleucine in patients with gastrointestinal bleeding decreases protein breakdown and urea synthesis while improving protein synthesis. Large-volume paracentesis may also increase protein loss.

2.4.2. Energy

Although highly variable, when corrected for lean body mass, resting energy expenditure has been shown to be increased in cirrhotics [11]. When measured energy expenditure is compared with predicted energy expenditure, −30, 20 and 50 of cirrhotics have high, low, or normal metabolic rates [12]. Patients with hypermetabolism have increased rates (as shown in Table 3) of morbidity and mortality after liver transplantation. Therefore, a clinician can tailor specific energy requirements for individual patients using simple calculations.

Regardless of the rate of energy expenditure, the preferred fuel substrate is clearly altered in cirrhosis [5,11] Cirrhotics have a decrease in the respiratory quotient, which is the rate of carbon dioxide production divided by the rate of oxygen consumption after an overnight fast. Cirrhotics obtain 75% of their calories from fat after an overnight fast compared with 35% for controls, who would take 48–72 h of starvation to obtain the low respiratory quotient levels that cirrhotics obtain after only 12–18 h (Figure 5). In addition, amino acids are oxidized for energy and converted to glucose *via* gluconeogenesis in cirrhosis, therefore this is a disease of accelerated starvation with early recruitment of alternative fuels. Consequently, food should not be withheld from cirrhotic patients for any extended period, and frequent feedings need to be encouraged. Cirrhotic patients given an evening snack to supply energy

Table 3. Percentage of cirrhotic patient populations.

Study and year	Patients (%)		
	Hypometabolic	Normometabolic	Hypermetabolic
Müller *et al.* (1999) ($n = 473$)[a]	3	63	34
Müller *et al.* (1992) ($n = 123$)[b]	30	55	17
Bossari *et al.* (1984) ($n = 30$)[c]	24	60	16

Resting energy expenditure (REE) based on the comparison of measured (indirect calorimetry) which predicted (Harris–Benedict equation) REE.
[a]Hypometabolic, <80% of predicted, hypometabolic >120% of predicted.
[b]Hypometabolic <80% of predicted; hypermetabolic >130% of predicted; hypometabolic <40 kcal kg FFM^{-1} d^{-1} (to convert kilocalories to kilojoules, multiply by 4.184). (FFM^{-1}, d^{-1} = per fat free mass (g) per day).
[c]Hypometabolic; <75% of predicted; hypermetabolic >125% of predicted.

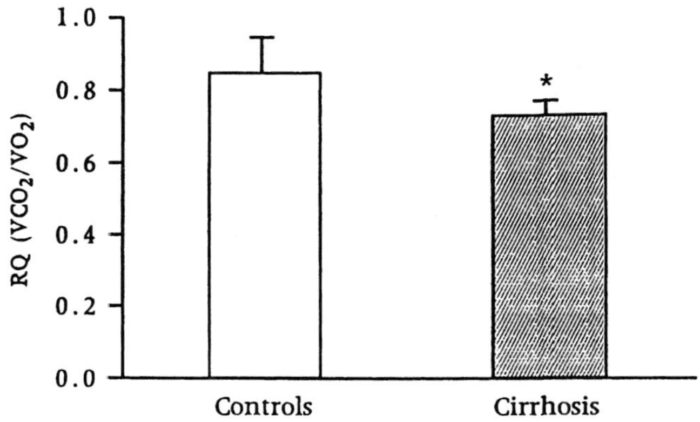

Fig. 5. The respiratory exchange ratio (referred to as the respiratory quotient) is shown as the aggregated data from 7 published trials for controls and patients with cirrhosis.

during the sleeping hours have been shown to maintain a greater positive nitrogen balance than those who were given less frequent interval feedings (Figure 6).

The metabolic profile in advanced liver disease resembles that of the stressed state (such as septicemia) superimposed on that of chronic starvation or prolonged fasting [13]. The similarities between cirrhosis and starvation include decreased glycogen stores and a low respiratory quotient. Features consistent with stress include carbohydrate intolerance, increased lipolysis, negative nitrogen balance, decreased plasma concentrations of branched-chain amino acids, increased energy expenditure, and increased protein breakdown.

3. CLINICAL FEATURES

3.1 Medical history

The duration, severity, and etiology of liver disease are pertinent to PEM in patients with liver disease [14] (Table 4). Other disease processes, such as renal failure, cardiac and pancreatic disease in alcoholism, and diabetes and cardiac disease in hemochromatosis, should also be evaluated. Factors that may limit nutrient ingestion and absorption, such as anorexia, early satiety, vomiting, and diarrhea should be identified. If possible, dietary recall should estimate macronutrient and micronutrient intake and the consumption of alcoholic beverages. Because cirrhotic patients often self-select a higher proportion

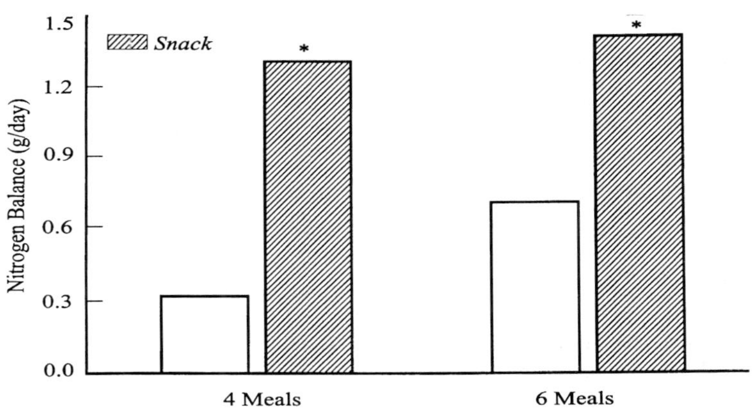

Fig. 6. The effect of a night-time snack with frequent feedings on nitrogen balance.

Table 4. Nutrition assessment in advanced liver disease.

History	Physical examination	Laboratory tests
Weight loss >10% of usual weight	Wasting of skeletal muscle mass (temporal muscles)	Visceral proteins albumin, pre-albumin and retinol-binding protein
Loss of appetite	Skin/hairs	Vitamin and mineral levels; assess micronutrient deficiencies
Decrease energy level	Flashing point (zinc deficiency)	Total lymphocyte count
Vomiting and/or diarrhea	Dry rash (vitamin A deficiency)	
	Oral mucosa (vitamin B deficiency)	
	Peripheral neuropathy (thiamine deficiency)	
	Hyper-reflexia (magnesium deficiency)	

of their dietary intake at breakfast, a full day's calorie count is required to obtain an accurate assessment.

3.2 Physical examination

During physical examination one should look for signs of decompensation, such as mental status changes, asterixis, jaundice, ascites, leg edema, and bruising [14]. Weight should be recorded with specific attention to fluid overload. Signs of specific nutritional deficiency, such as acrodermatitis from zinc deficiency or pellagra from niacin deficiency, should be sought. Patients with cholestatic liver disease and steatorrhea may have skin excoriations related to pruritus, xanthomas due to hyperlipidemia, or dermatitis from essential fatty acid deficiency.

Evaluation of the oral mucosa, skin and hair are particularly important [14]. In the oral mucosa, glossitis (raw tongue), atrophic tongue (slick tongue) and angular stomatitis are common findings and result from deficiencies in the B vitamins, iron, folate and vitamin B_{12}. Less common are gingivitis (vitamin C deficiency) and altered taste/smell (zinc deficiency).

On the skin, petechiae (vitamin C deficiency) purpura (vitamin A and zinc deficiency) may be present. Hair may demonstrate sparseness (protein, zinc and biotin deficiencies), follicular hyperkeratosis (vitamins A and C deficiency) or be corkscrewed and coiled (vitamin C deficiency).

4. DIAGNOSIS

Nutritional assessment can be difficult in patients with chronic liver disease [15]. Parameters of common use in clinical practice should diagnose protein (kwashiorkor or hypoalbuminemic) or combined protein calorie (marasmic) forms of malnutrition (Table 5). Fluid excess is universal in end-stage liver disease and may be present even in earlier stages of disease. This excess in fluid causes weight-to-height parameters (such as percentage of ideal body weight or BMI) to underestimate the prevalence of chronic liver disease as it may also cause alterations in visceral protein synthesis, cellular immunity, and total lymphocyte count independent of PEM. This causes an overestimation of the degree but not necessarily the prevalence of PEM. In contrast, markers of muscle mass (creatinine height index and midarm muscle circumference) and fat mass (triceps skinfold thickness) are less influenced by either alcohol or chronic liver disease. When performing a creatinine height index estimation, creatinine clearance should be measured to confirm the precision of the creatinine height index.

In addition to these anthropometric and laboratory parameter, bioelectrical impedance analysis has been used to estimate total lean body mass rather than just skeletal mass and is logistically convenient and relatively inexpensive. Because this method is inaccurate in cirrhotic patients with ascites or edema and has some imprecision even in those without ascites or edema, it may be best used to serially monitor the response to nutritional feeding.

Table 5. Factors affecting nutritional assessment.

Measurements used to assess nutritional status	Malnutrition		Alcohol toxicity	Liver disease	Renal function
	Protein	Protein/calorie			
Visceral proteins	×		×	×	
Lymphocyte count	×		×	×	×
Cellular immunity	×		×	×	×
% Ideal body weight		×		×	×
Anthropometry		×		(?)	(?)
Creatinine height index		×		(?)	×
SGA[a]		×		×	(?)
BIA[b]		×		×	
DEXA[c]		×		×	

[a]SGA, subjective global assessment.
[b]BIA, bioelectrical impedance analysis.
[c]DEXA, dual energy X-ray absorptiometry.

Dual-energy X-ray absorptiometry (DEXA) is a non-invasive method with minimal radiation that provides accurate measurements of total body bone mineral, fat, and fat-free soft tissue mass. The accuracy of this method is also influenced by fluid retention as with BIA.

Subjective global assessment is an evaluation of PEM based predominantly on the following clinical findings: the presence of edema, muscle wasting, subcutaneous fat loss, glossitis, and cheilosis. As a practical method for estimating PEM it compares favorably with standard measures in patients without liver disease. Subjective global assessment in cirrhotic patients especially helps evaluate patients prior to liver transplantation [6].

Despite limitations, nutritional assessment is useful in all types of cirrhosis, especially when a composite score emphasizing anthropometry and creatinine height index is performed and combined with overall clinical judgment.

5. MANAGEMENT

Goals: Although early studies used survival as the primary outcome measure for determining the efficacy of nutritional therapy, more recently improvement in nutritional status, infection rates, immune function, nitrogen balance, and perioperative morbidity have been shown with nutritional therapy in cirrhotic patients. It is most effective when used for longer periods or in certain subgroups such as in those with severe malnutrition, chronic hepatic encephalopathy, and decompensated liver disease. No reliable information is available regarding the cost-effectiveness of nutritional therapy or its effect on the quality of life of cirrhotic patients.

5.1 Nutritional requirements

5.1.1. Protein requirements

In stable cirrhotics, the average protein requirement to maintain positive nitrogen balance is $0.8\ g\ kg^{-1}\ day^{-1}$, which is similar to that required in the normal population. Because the range of protein required is larger in cirrhotics than in controls, compensated cirrhotics should receive at least $1.2\ g\ kg^{-1}\ day^{-1}$. Although nitrogen balance is achieved at this amount, nitrogen retention continues to improve up $1.8\ g\ kg^{-1}\ day^{-1}$ [16]. Even stable cirrhotics are protein deficient and this is an important management consideration. Cirrhotic patients undergoing surgery should receive protein doses between 1.2 and $1.5\ g\ kg^{-1}\ day^{-1}$ (Table 6).

Table 6. Guidelines for nutritional therapy liver disease.

	Protein ($g\ kg^{-1}\ day^{-1}$)	Energy ($kcal\ kg^{-1}\ day^{-1}$)	Energy substrate		Nutritional goal
			%CHO	%Fat	
Hepatitis (acute or chronic)[a]	1.0–1.5	30–40	67–80	20–33	Prevent malnutrition, enhance regeneration
Cirrhosis (uncomplicated)	1.0–1.2	30–40	67–80	20–33	
Cirrhosis (complicated)[b]	1.2–1.8	40–50	72	28	Restore normal nutritional status
Malnutrition					Prevent malnutrition, enhance regeneration
Cholestasis	1.0–1.5	30–40	73–80	20–27	Prevent malnutrition Treat fat malabsorption[c]
Encephalopathy[d]					
Grade 1 or 2	0.5–1.2	25–40	75	25	
Grade 3 or 4	0.5	25–40	75	25	Provide nutritional needs without precipitating encephalopathy
Liver transplant					
Peri-transplant	1.2–1.8	30–50	70–80	20–30	Restore normal nutritional status
Post-transplant	1.0	30–35	>70	≤30	Retain and maintain ideal body weight

[a]There are no convincing data indicating any extraordinary vitamin or trace metal requirements in liver disease. A typical substitution solution for parenteral feeding is provided. Vitamins: ($10\ cm^3\ l^{-1}$) – ascorbic acid ($20\ mg\ ml^{-1}$), Vitamin A ($660\ IU\ ml^{-1}$), Vitamin D ($40\ IU\ ml^{-1}$), thiamine HCL ($0.6\ mg\ ml^{-1}$), riboflavin phosphate ($0.72\ mg\ ml^{-1}$), pyridoxine HCI ($0.8\ mg\ ml^{-1}$) niacinamide ($8\ mg\ ml^{-1}$), D-pantothenic acid ($3\ mg\ ml^{-1}$), Vitamin E ($2\ IU\ ml^{-1}$), Biotin ($12\ mcq\ ml^{-1}$), folic acid ($0.08\ mg\ 5\ ml^{-1}$), Vitamin B_{12} ($1\ mcq\ 5\ ml^{-1}$). Trace Metals ($1\ ml\ l^{-1}$): zinc chloride ($10.42\ mq\ 5\ ml^{-1}$, copper chloride ($2.68\ mq\ 5\ ml^{-1}$), manganese ($1.44\ mq\ 5\ ml^{-1}$), chromium chloride ($0.012\ mq\ 5\ ml^{-1}$).

[b]Ascites and sepsis are two complications which are not listed but which should be treated aggressively as part of nutritional therapy (see text).

[c]Medium chain triglycerides may be necessary if fat malabsorption is present. Pancreatic enzymes are necessary if pancreatic insufficiency is present; especially in alcoholic cirrhosis and primary sclerosing cholangitis.

[d]Branched-chain amino acid (BCAA) formulations may be necessary. Available hepatic enteral formulations are 45% BCAA enriched and parenteral formulations are 36% BCAA enriched. This compares to standard for preparations which contain 26% BCAA. For outpatients, diets high in vegetable protein or casein hydrolysates may be better tolerated than standard dietary protein in the protein intolerant patient with cirrhosis.

5.1.2. Energy

Abnormalities in extracellular fluid levels and in fat and non-fat body compartments, portosystemic shunting, and variability in energy expenditure between different body compartments make the prediction of energy compartments quantitatively unreliable in cirrhosis. Therefore, with knowledge that hypermetabolism may have adverse clinical sequelae energy expenditure should be measured with indirect calorimetry, especially in hospitalized patients undergoing liver transplantation. If indirect calorimetry is not available, the daily resting energy expenditure for cirrhosis should be assumed as 25–30 $kcal\ kg^{-1}$ body weight (based on ideal body weight if ascites and/or edema is present) for decisions regarding restorative or maintenance needs.

Energy is proportionally provided by carbohydrates and fat (Table 6). Two points are important: (1) insulin resistance is universal in cirrhosis irrespective of the type of severity of the disease. Glucose intolerance is not typically an important management issue, except hypoglycemia, which develops in up to 50% of cirrhotic patients during sepsis. (2) Lipid formulations are very useful in cirrhosis because of their low water content and high caloric density. Initial concerns that lipids might precipitate encephalopathy have not been confirmed.

5.1.3. Vitamins

Approximately 40% of patients with non-alcoholic liver disease have fat soluble vitamin deficiencies (Vitamin A and E); 8–10% have deficiencies in the B complex vitamins (nicotinic acid, thiamine,

Table 7. Vitamins in liver disease.

Many complications associated with liver disease are manifestations of vitamin deficiencies. These include macrocytic anemia (folate and Vitamin B_{12} deficiency); neuropathy (pyridoxine, thiamine or Vitamin B_{12}); confusion, ataxia and ocular disturbances (thiamine) and impaired adaptation to dark (Vitamin A)
Pyridoxine phosphate (the major active form of pyridoxine) rather than pyridoxine itself may be required to correct pyridoxine deficiency; especially in alcoholics
The clinical response to thiamine is usually rapid and effective. However, the neuropathy may be irreversible and abnormalities in red cell transketolase may not improve
Deficiencies in Vitamin B_{12} and folic acid may develop faster in cirrhotic patients due to diminished hepatic storage
In the presence of active hepatic inflammation, fatty liver or hepatocellular cancer, normal or elevated levels of Vitamin B_{12} levels do not exclude a deficiency of this vitamin
Decreased serum levels of Vitamin A do not necessarily reflect Vitamin A deficiency. Zinc deficiency may be causing decreased transport out of the liver
In non-cholestatic liver disease, abnormal serum levels of fat-soluble vitamins should not be sought or treated in the absence of clinical or laboratory abnormalities, which indicate a functional vitamin deficiency. In cholestatic liver diseases, abnormal serum levels of the fat-soluble vitamins may be treated even in the absence of clinical symptoms or laboratory abnormalities
Suggestions for us of vitamin supplements: (A) Water-soluble vitamins may be supplied with a multivitamin preparation; (B) fat-soluble vitamins should be used in a water-soluble form whenever possible. Vitamin A, Aquasol 1 capsule daily (50,000 IU), Vitamin K, Synkayvite, 1 tablet daily (15 mg). Vitamin D treatment should be individualized by monitoring plasma 25-hydroxy vitamin D levels and serum and urinary calcium levels. Vitamin D_2 (ergocalciferol), 1.25 mg (50,000) U, 1 tablet 3–4 times a day, may be adequate. Vitamin E (D-α-tocopheryl polyethelene glycol 1000 succinate (TPGS) 23 IU kg^{-1} day^{-1})

Vitamin B_{12}, riboflavin and pyridoxine) and 17% have folate deficiency. These abnormalities are related more to disordered hepatic function and diminished reserve rather than deficient dietary intake or malabsorption. However, in severe advanced cirrhosis, malabsorption may play a role in both fat-soluble vitamins and the B complex vitamins. These vitamin deficiencies are more prevalent and severe in alcoholic than non-alcoholic liver disease. Specific issues regarding vitamins in liver disease are provided in Table 7.

5.2 Specific alterations in liver disease

5.2.1. Accelerated starvation

The preferred fuel substrate is altered in cirrhosis. After an overnight fast, cirrhotics have a decreased respiratory exchange ratio or respiratory quotient indicating that approximately 75% of their calories are derived from fat as compared to 35% for normal controls. This metabolic profile after an overnight fast in cirrhotics is similar to normal individuals undergoing more prolonged (48–72 h) starvation. Hepatic glucose production from glycogen is reduced; gluconeogenesis is increased and peripheral glucose utilization is decreased.

Therefore, cirrhosis should be considered a disease of accelerated starvation with early recruitment of alternative fuels. Cirrhotic patients should avoid any extended period of time without feeding. The advantage of a frequent feeding approach has been confirmed by nitrogen balance and indirect calorimetry measurements in cirrhotic patients.

5.2.2. Protein imbalance

5.2.2.1 Hepatic encephalopathy. Advanced acute or chronic liber failure often presents with a constellation of neuropsychiatric abnormalities known as hepatic encephalopathy. These mental status alterations may range from mild behavioral changes to deep coma. Subclinical hepatic encephalopathy is present in 70% of patients with cirrhosis and currently does not require any specific nutritional therapy. However, liver failure associated with hepatic encephalopathy is the third most common cause of death in cirrhosis and is responsible for approximately 20% of the deaths from this disease. Although the pathogenesis of hepatic encephalopathy remains ill-defined, all the proposed toxins (ammonia, mercaptans, fatty acids, gamma-amino-butyric acid, an altered plasmino acid profile and an endogenous benzodiazepines), appear to be related in part to protein feeding. Overt encephalopathy is almost always associated with some precipitating event such as gastrointestinal bleeding, infection/sepsis, fluid and electrolyte imbalances constipation, acid-base abnormalities or the inappropriate use of sedating drugs. In a minority of cirrhotic patients, hepatic encephalopathy may be precipitated by protein intake (especially animal protein) without any other precipitating factor. These patients are considered protein intolerant. More than 95% of cirrhotic patients can tolerate diets containing as much as 1.5 gm kg^{-1} day^{-1} of mixed proteins. Therefore, true protein intolerance is rare except for fulminant hepatic failure, or the occasional patient with 'endogenous' chronic encephalopathy or fulminant hepatic failure.

In those few cirrhotic patients with endogenous protein intolerance, it has been demonstrated that branched-chain amino acid formulations are better tolerated than standard amino acid supplements and can achieve positive nitrogen balance. It should be emphasized, however, that there is no clearly proven benefit that branched-chain amino acids are standard amino acids for the majority of patients with chronic liver disease.

5.2.2.2 Protein restriction. There is no justification for the routine use of protein restriction as prophylaxis against precipitating hepatic encephalopathy [2]. Available data indicate that the vast majority of cirrhotic patients and even patients with severe alcoholic hepatitis can tolerate large quantities of protein feeding (up to 1.75 g kg^{-1} day^{-1}).

If the amount of protein cannot be provided without precipitating hepatic encephalopathy, specialized formulations enriched with branched-chain amino acids should be substituted for standard formulations.

5.2.2.3 Non-essential amino acids. Precautions are required with amino acid preparations (especially branched-chain amino acid enriched preparations) used for nutritional purposes in patients with liver disease to insure that the deficiencies of other amino acids do not develop [13]. Administration of standard or specialized total parenteral nutrition solutions devoid of the non-essential amino acids tyrosine and cysteine may not achieve positive nitrogen balance in cirrhosis despite provisions of adequate amounts of essential amino acids. This observation emphasized that certain intrinsic liver functions may be rate limiting in cirrhosis such as the ability to synthesize cysteine from methionine and tyrosine from phenylalanine.

5.2.3. Salt restriction

Abnormalities in salt and water retention may necessitate sodium restriction in the cirrhotic patient with fluid overload. However, sodium and consequently salt restriction significantly decreases the palatability of the diet and consequently may diminish food intake. In the hospitalized patient, very low (250–500 mg) sodium (0.63–1.3 g salt) diets may be appropriate. In the non-hospitalized patient, every effort should be made to avoid salt restriction. In those patients with fluid overload who otherwise cannot be managed effectively, the least sodium restriction that is effective should be employed. A 2.5-g sodium (6.3 g salt) intake approximates a no added salt diet. This mild restriction can be tolerated by the compliant patient and is usually effective for fluid management in most patients, but does not significantly limit calorie or protein intake.

5.2.4. Alcohol-related alterations

Alcoholic liver disease has specific nutritional features that are direct effects of alcohol toxicity and are not related to liver disease *per se* [10].

5.2.4.1 Alcohol toxicity. Alcohol has deleterious effects on muscle protein status independent of associated liver injury. Alcohol is known to inhibit meal stimulated hepatic protein production, which is an important contributor to skeletal muscle and whole body protein synthesis in humans. In addition alcohol increases intestinal permeability, which in turn initiates endotoxin/cytokine-induced muscle proteolysis. Recent work also suggests that alcohol induced cirrhosis may be associated with a greater decrease in muscle mass but a relative sparing of fat stores as compared to non-alcoholic cirrhosis.

5.2.4.2 Alcohol as empty calories. Alcohol has a caloric density of seven but produces less efficient energy per gram of nutrient than both carbohydrates and lipids. In addition, it often replaces other more beneficial calorie sources.

5.3 Nutritional therapy

5.3.1. Goals

The general goals of nutritional support of patients with acute or chronic liver are similar to those of other patients. In the stressed patient, nutritional substrates should be given to (1) prevent the catabolic breakdown of body protein and provide sufficient amino acids for the acute phase response and (2) provide adequate fuel to sustain energy balance [16].

Regarding goals specific to liver disease, nutritional therapy needs to correct pre-existing PEM while simultaneously providing sufficient amino acids to encourage hepatic regeneration and normalization of function without precipitating encephalopathy. Although attempts have been made to treat hepatic encephalopathy with modified amino acid formulations or using nutritional supplements as a primary therapy for the liver disease itself, the clinical emphasis should be placed on supplying the basic requirements of nitrogen and calories. Specialized formulations and nutritional supplements should be withheld for those select cases when standard nitrogen sources cannot provide the necessary requirements without precipitating encephalopathy, for severely malnourished patients.

Contrary to past studies which used survival as the primary outcome measure of nutritional therapy, recent investigations using more realistic outcomes such as improvement in nutritional status, immune function, infection rates, length of hospital stay and perioperative morbidity have demonstrated the efficacy of nutritional therapy. In addition, nutritional therapy may be used most effectively when used for longer time periods or in certain subgroups of liver disease patients. It should be emphasized that there is no reliable information available regarding the cost effectiveness of nutritional therapy or its impact of nutritional therapy on the quality of life of these patients.

5.3.2. Specific patient populations

5.3.2.1 Cirrhosis. Two studies indicate that enteral feeding improves liver function, encephalopathy and perhaps survival in severely malnourished cirrhotics and in patients with decompensated alcoholic liver disease. The significance and reason for these benefits remain a much discussed area of clinical nutrition. However, nutrient intake is increased by enteral nutrition in all published studies to date and may in part be responsible for these benefits.

Another study provided nutritional supplements (1000 cal and 34 g of protein–casein based) for 1 year to patients with complicated alcoholic cirrhosis. These supplements resulted in higher protein and caloric intake to levels, which simply met their required needs.

5.3.2.2 Alcoholic hepatitis. There have been eight published trials on the use of standard intravenous amino acid formulations as primary therapy for alcoholic hepatitis. The results are conflicting, but six of the eight studies showed improvement in either liver histology or function. One of these studies additionally showed a strong trend toward an improvement in mortality. Two of the studies concluded that supplemental amino acids were of no benefit. In one of these negative studies, the mortality was 3.3% in the 30 patients in whom positive nitrogen balance was achieved, but 58% in those patients who remained in negative nitrogen balance despite nutritional therapy.

These combined data emphasized that there is no reason to routinely restrict protein in these patients and that positive nitrogen balance should be a goal.

5.3.2.3 Fulminant hepatic failure. Fulminant hepatic failure defined as the development of hepatic encephalopathy within 8 weeks of the onset of liver disease is a life threatening illness associated with a rapid development of protein calorie malnutrition; even when what is calculated to be adequate amounts of calorie and nitrogen are supplied. Up to 4 times the normal rate of protein breakdown accompanied by decreased hepatic amino acid oxidation leads to the accumulation of potentially toxic levels of certain amino acids (tyrosine, phenylalanine, and methionine).

Hypoglycemia occurs commonly and serum glucose levels must be maintained with concentrated glucose infused (20–40%) to avoid the risks of exacerbating cerebral edema. Lipid emulsions may be particularly useful in this setting.

Older uncontrolled studies emphasized the importance of protein restriction in these patients. However, more recent work suggests administering at least 40–60 gm of protein to diminish the rapid depletion of protein stores in patients with Stage I and 2 encephalopathy. If necessary, the use of branched-chain amino acids may be necessary to achieve this goal in patients with more advanced stages of encephalopathy. However, the efficacy of branched-chain amino acids in this situation remains unproven. If encephalopathy should develop or worsen with protein feeding, the use of specialized formulations of branched-chain amino acids seems indicated.

5.3.2.4 Perioperative. There are a number of studies which indicate that parenteral nutrition with standard amino acid formulations are well tolerated and equally effective as branched-chain enriched formulations when used as perioperative nutritional therapy in cirrhotic patients [4,17]. However, there is only one study, which shows any clinical or financial benefits of perioperative nutrition in cirrhotic patients when compared to no nutritional therapy. In this study, perioperative nutrition decreased postoperative septic complications, weight loss, need for diuretics while improving hepatic function in patients undergoing major hepatic resection for hepatocellular carcinoma.

5.3.3. Liver transplant

Although there is no uniform approach among transplant centers regarding the management of nutrition in transplant patients, the results from a questionnaire of 16 European transplant units indicate that there is agreement that malnutrition reflects the severity of chronic liver disease and should not be considered, in general, as an exclusion for patients receiving liver transplant [18]. Most centers administer post-operative nutrition in a fashion similar to that given to other patients after gastrointestinal major surgery [6]. Therefore, the recognition that malnutrition is a significant problem has been gaining momentum.

5.3.3.1 Pre-transplant. Even though malnutrition has been shown to be a poor prognostic factor in both adults and children undergoing liver transplant, there has been only one study, which has evaluated pre-transplant nutritional therapy. In this study a formulation enriched with branched-chain amino acids was more effective than standard amino acids for improving height and body weight in pediatric patients awaiting liver transplantation.

5.3.3.2 Post-transplant. There has been only one randomized study that was performed in the post-transplant period. During the first 7 post-operative days in adult patients, isotonic glucose (500 kcal day^{-1}) was compared with standard total parenteral nutrition and a BCAA-enriched TPN solution, each containing 35 kcal kg^{-1} of non-protein calories and 1.5 g kg^{-1} day^{-1} of protein. Both the total parenteral nutrition groups had significantly better nitrogen balance with beneficial trends for a short length of stay in the intensive care unit and lower hospital costs.

A number of other benefits to nutritional therapy have been shown in uncontrolled studies as demonstrated in Table 8. As compared to conventional therapy, early enteral feeding was shown to decrease the number of viral infections and obtain better nitrogen retention post-operatively. Post-operatively, both nasogastric and jejunostomy tubes have been used successfully in these patients. The available information also indicates that both enteral and parenteral nutrition are equivalent in their ability to

Table 8. Benefits of nutritional therapy post-transplant.

Improved nitrogen balance
Less time in the ICU (Trend)
Lower hospital cost (Trend)
Fewer viral infection with early enteral feeding which is equivalent to parenteral feeding
Both nasogastric and jejunostomy tubes have been used successfully

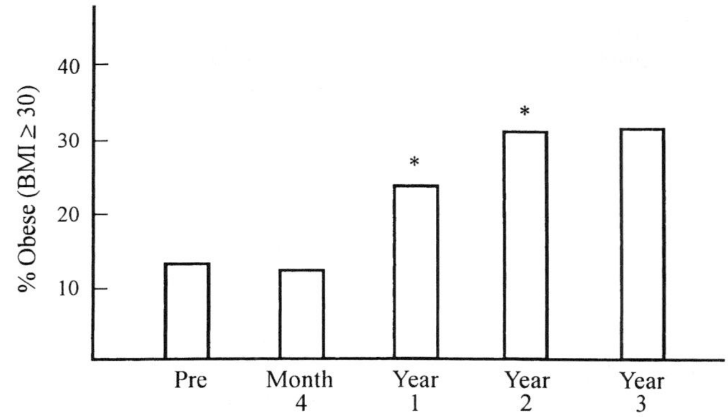

Fig. 7. These data from a four-center study show the prevalence of obesity in liver transplant recipients for the first 3 years post-transplantation.

deliver nutrients and improve nutritional status at the 10th post-operative day [19].

5.3.3.3 Long-term. In contrast to these positive results, 1 year after follow-up, protein breakdown and lipolysis in these patients have improved, but not normalized, with improvement in total body water and total body fat but no change in body cell mass. An increasingly important nutritional problem which develops in the first 1–2 years after liver transplant is obesity which has been reported to occur in 30–70% of patients. Recent data from a four-center study found that 30% of post-liver transplant patients are obese 2 years following transplant (Figure 7). Although this has been linked to the use of certain immunosuppressive agents and changes in energy expenditure post-operatively, the etiology is most likely multifactorial and has not been carefully evaluated. Therefore, it is important to follow the nutritional status of these patients post-operatively and treat obesity aggressively if it develops.

5.3.4. Principles and practical implementation

The nutritional support of patients with liver disease follows the general principles applicable to any other type of patient. However, there are a number of principles particularly relevant to liver disease patients with guidelines provided in Table 9.

5.3.4.1 Glucose requirement. Although insulin resistance and hypoglycemia are commonly observed in cirrhosis, hypoglycemia (< 50 mg/dl) occurs in up to 50% of cirrhotic patients during episodes of stress. Therefore, serum glucose must be closely monitored in patients with fulminant or decompensated chronic liver disease.

5.3.4.2 Route of nutrient administration. The least invasive route for nutritional supplements is oral which should be tried first [20]. If attempts of oral supplementation fail, enteral feedings can be administered *via* a small caliber nasogastric or nasojejunal tube. The presence of non-bleeding esophageal varices is not a contraindication to the use of enteral feeding tubes in these patients. However, feeding tubes should not be used if there is active esophageal variceal bleeding.

The placement of a gastrostomy or a jejunostomy tube in cirrhotics with ascites is not recommended due to the possible complications of peritonitis or ascitic fluid leakage. Unfortunately, this limits the potential of long-term enteral feeding in many of these patients.

Parenteral nutrition should be initiated only if nutritional requirements cannot be supplied orally or enterally in situations such as gastrointestinal bleeding, ileus, or after abdominal surgery. Because of its relatively low caloric density, peripheral parenteral nutrition cannot supply total nutritional requirements and is usually not a good choice in

Table 9. Overall guidelines for the nutritional management of patients with liver disease.

Assume protein calorie malnutrition is present in all patients Assume an inadequate dietary intake; even in hospitalized patients
Qualitative stool fat should be done intermittently; especially in patients with alcoholic or cholestatic cirrhosis. If malabsorption is present; determine the cause and treat
Treatment with either Neomycin or Lactulose for hepatic encephalopathy may exacerbate malabsorption, which should be considered in nutritional management
Treat ascites aggressively to decrease energy expenditure
Diuretic therapy is preferred over large volume paracentesis for the management of ascites in order to minimize protein loss
Balance the need for sodium restriction with nutritional considerations and diet palatability
Nutritional assessment is useful in all types of cirrhotic patients
A composite score (emphasizing anthropometry and creatinine height index) combined with overall clinical judgment should be employed.
The clinician should remember that all the methods for nutritional assessment in cirrhosis are influenced or potentially influenced by the presence of liver disease alone as well as abnormalities associated with liver disease such as renal failure, alcohol ingestion and expansion of the extracellular water compartment
Determine energy expenditure requirements with indirect calorimetry (if possible) in hospitalized patients or patients listed for liver transplantation. If energy expenditure requirements are estimated from prediction equations, calculate energy need based on ideal weight rather than actual weight if extracellular water (ascites/edema) is present
Multiple (5–6) small feedings with a carbohydrate-rich evening snack, which consists of approximately 10–15% of caloric needs, should be given. The need for breakfast feeding must also be stressed to the patient
For calories, complex rather than simple carbohydrates should be used. Lipids should supply 20–40% of caloric needs
Nutritional requirements may vary according to the specific type of patient and/or clinical situation as listed in Table 6
Severely malnourished or decompensated cirrhotics should be given oral or enteral supplements (as recommended in Table 6)
Long term nutritional supplements may be necessary to provide recommended protein and caloric supplements
Patients with severe alcoholic hepatitis should be given supplemental standard protein 1.0 gm kg^{-1} *via* an enteral or peripheral parenteral route
Peri-operative nutritional therapy should be given to those cirrhotic patients with significant malnutrition as defined by weight loss of more than 10% or for anthropometry or creatinine height index less than 5% of predicted values
Post-liver transplant, patients need higher amounts of protein and energy (see Table 6)
Pediatric patients undergoing liver transplant may benefit from branched-chain amino acids
Cirrhotics should never be treated prophylactically with protein restriction to prevent hepatic encephalopathy
Standard protein or amino acid mixtures should be supplied to meet the measured estimated nitrogen needs (as provided in Table 9)
Protein restriction should be implemented only if protein intolerance as manifested by encephalopathy occurs in the absence of precipitating factors
Protein restriction below the required amounts should not be continued for more than 3–4 days
Branched-chain amino acids should be given only if the required amount of standard feedings cannot be tolerated without precipitating hepatic encephalopathy
Monitor for hypoglycemia and treated aggressively with concentrated glucose solutions which may also decrease serum ammonia levels
Enteral feeding is the preferred route of feeding patients with insufficient oral intake. Enteral feeding tubes may be used even if non-bleeding varices are present
Do not use any nutritional product devoid of cysteine or tyrosine as the only nitrogen source for any prolonged period of time Be aware of clinically important issues related to vitamins listed in Table 7

cirrhotic patients with sodium and water retention. Peripheral parenteral nutrition may be useful in supplementing enteral or oral feeding; especially for providing amino acids in severe alcoholic hepatitis. Central parenteral nutrition is preferred in most cirrhotic patients despite the risk of central vein catheter replacement in patients with coagulopathy and thrombocytopenia.

5.3.4.3. Protein restriction. As mentioned above, there is no justification for the routine use of protein restriction as prophylaxis against precipitating hepatic encephalopathy. The data indicate that the vast majority of cirrhotic patients tolerate high quantities of protein feeding (up to 1.75 g kg^{-1} day^{-1}).

The amount of protein recommended for different types of liver disease patients in various situations is provided in Table 6. If these amounts of protein cannot be provided without precipitating hepatic encephalopathy, formulations enriched with branched-chain amino acids should be substituted for standard formulations. There are two oral or enteral feedings (Nutrihep – 50% BCAA enriched and Hepatic Aid II – 46% BCAA enriched) and two intravenous formulations (Hepatamine and Hepatasol, both 36% BCAA enriched). In addition to these formulations which have been tried in liver patients, there are also stress formulations (Freamine HBC and Aminosyn-HBC) both of which are approximately 45% BCAA enriched. However, these stress formulations have not been evaluated in patients with liver disease.

5.3.5. *Prognosis*

Table 10 lists results from a number of studies, which suggest a causal relationship between malnutrition and survival in cirrhosis. Malnutrition has prognostic value in patients undergoing liver transplantation and other surgical operations. Similar observations have been made in non-surgical liver disease patients. Malnutrition predicts impaired immunity and increased susceptibility to infection in patients hospitalized for cirrhosis and ascites. The disappearance of ascites following placement of a peritoneovenous shunt improves nutritional status and immunity. Malnutrition has also been shown to correlate with poor hepatic function and severity of disease in cirrhotic patients. These collective data suggest that the recognition and treatment of malnutrition are important considerations in the management of patients with cirrhosis, especially in those situations listed in Table 10.

5.3.5.1 PEM. Although it has been difficult to show a direct causal relationship between PEM and survival in patients with chronic liver disease many studies show the importance of PEM as a prognostic factor in the clinical outcome of patients with cirrhosis, as listed in Table 10, which includes liver transplant patients. Most, but not all studies show the importance of nutritional status on graft and/or patient morbidity and mortality. Early data showed malnutrition adversely affected survival [21]. Another recent well-performed study of patients awaiting liver transplantation also showed that PEM as well as hypermetabolism predicted decreased survival after transplantation, whereas the Child–Pugh score did not [12]. These collective data suggest that recognition and treatment of PEM should be the more important considerations in the management of patients before liver transplantation.

5.3.5.2 Obesity. There is much variability among transplant centers regarding the importance of obesity as a risk factor for patients undergoing liver transplantation. Three studies have shown that graft and patient survival are similar in patients post-transplantation. Nonetheless, many transplant physicians believe that obesity is a significant enough risk factor for liver transplantation to place certain

Table 10. Protein energy malnutrition as a poor prognostic factor in cirrhosis.

Condition or procedure	Clinical outcome measured
Cirrhotic	Survival Immunodeficiency
Cirrhosis patients undergoing abdominal surgery	Survival Post-operative complications
Hospitalized patients with ascites/cirrhosis	Survival
Alcoholic hepatitis	Survival Liver function
Liver transplantation	Patient/graft survival
Hepatectomy	Post-operative complications

Table 11. Complications in obese liver transplant patients.

	BMI < 30	BMI > 35	p
Operative blood loss (U)	9.1 ± 0.8	16.2 ± 3.5	0.004
Wound infection %	4	20	0.0001
1-year graft survival (%)	81	67	0.07
Death rate (%)			
Overall (3 yr)	20	38	0.30
Predischarge	6	15	0.10
Multiorgan failure	5	40	0.0001

Data from Sawyer *et al.* [22].

restrictions on transplantation in obese patients. These restrictions are based on the clinical impression that obese patients present significantly increased surgical difficulty and have increased perioperative morbidity compared with non-obese patients. These concerns appear most relevant in obese patients with BMIs of 35 or greater. Table 11 shows that obese patients with a BMI greater than 35 compared with patients with a BMI less than 30 required more intraoperative blood transfusions, had an increased number of wound infections, and were more likely to die of multi-organ failure, even though obese and non-obese transplant recipients had similar 3-year survivals. Therefore, it seems appropriate to study and monitor patients with severe obesity closely. However, based on the available information, obese and non-obese patients have similar long-term outcomes after liver transplantation.

6. SUMMARY

Specific recommendations for the logistics of managing PEM in patients with liver disease are provided in Tables 6 and 9. The primary directive for nutritional therapy in cirrhosis is to use standard dietary methods to assure that nutritional requirements are provided and nutritional status is well maintained. The attainment of this strategy means that long-term outpatient management is even more important to these patients than when they are hospitalized for acute illness.

REFERENCES

[1] Plauch, M., Merli, M., Kondrup, J., Weiman, A., Ferenci, P. and Müller, M.J. (1997) ESPEN guidelines for nutrition in liver disease and transplantation. *Clin. Nutr.* **16**, 43–55.

[2] McCullough, A.J., Teran, J.C. and Bugianesi, E. (1998) Guidelines for nutritional therapy in liver disease, in *The American Society of Parenteral and Enteral Nutritional Support Practice Manual*, ed. Klein, S. (Silver Spring, MD) pp. 1–12.

[3] McCullough, A.J. and Falck-Ytter, Y. (1999) Body composition and hepatic steatosis as precursors for fibrotic liver disease. *Hepatology* **29**, 1328–1330.

[4] Merli, M., Nicotini, G., Angeloni, S. and Riggio, O. (2002) Malnutrition is a risk factor in cirrhotic patients undergoing surgery. *Nutrition* **18**, 978–986.

[5] McCullough, A.J. and Bugianesi, E. (1997) Protein calorie malnutrition and the etiology of cirrhosis. *Am. J. Gastroenterol.* **92**, 734–738.

[6] McCullough, A.J. (2000) Malnutrition in liver disease. *Liver Transpl.* **6**, 585–596.

[7] Kopelman, P.G. (2000) Obesity as a medical problem. *Nature* **404**, 635–643.

[8] Campillo, B., Bories, P.P.N., Leluan, M., Pronin, B., Devanlay, M. and Fouer, P. (1995) Short-term changes in energy metabolism after 1 month of a regular oral diet in severely malnourished cirrhotic patients. *Metabolism* **44**, 765–770.

[9] Padillo, F.J., Andicoberry, B., Pera-Madrazo, C. and Sitges-Serra, A. (2002) Anorexia and malnutrition in patients with obstructive jaundice. *Nutrition* **18**, 987–990.

[10] Falck-Ytter, Y. and McCullough, A.J. (2000) Nutritional effect of alcoholism. *Curr. Gastroenterol. Rep.* **2**, 331–336.

[11] McCullough, A.J. and Raguso, C. (1999) Effect of cirrhosis on energy expenditure. *Am. J. Clin. Nutr.* **69**, 1066–1068.

[12] Selberg, O., Bottcher, J., Tusch, G., Pichlmayr, R., Henkel, E. and Müller, M.J. (1997) Identification of high and low risk patients before liver transplantation – a prospective cohort study of nutritional and metabolic parameters in 150 patients. *Hepatology* **25**, 632–637.

[13] Teran, J.C., Mullen, K.D. and McCullough, A.J. (1995) Glutamine: a conditionally essential amino acid in cirrhosis. *Am. J. Clin. Nutr.* **62**, 897–900.

[14] Patton, K.M. and Aranda-Michel, J. (2002) Nutritional aspects in liver disease and liver transplantation. *Nutr. Clin. Prac.* **17**, 332–340.

[15] Lowell, J.A. (1996) Nutritional assessment and therapy in patients requiring liver transplantation. *Liver Transpl. Surg.* **2**, 579–588.

[16] Lochs, H. and Plauth, M. (1999) Liver cirrhosis: rational and modalities for nutritional support – The European Society of Parenteral and Enteral Nutrition Consensus and Beyond. *Curr. Opin. Clin. Nutr. Metabol. Care* **2**, 345–349.

[17] Koretz, R.L., Lipman, T.O. and Klein, S. (2001) AGA technical review on parenteral nutrition. *Gastroenterology* **121**, 970–1001.

[18] Weimann, A., Kuse, E.R., Bechstein, W.O., Neuberger, J.M., Plauth, M. and Pichlmayr, R. (1998) Perioperative and enteral nutrition for patients undergoing orthotopic liver transplantation. Results of a questionnaire from 16 European transplant units. *Transpl. Int.* **11**, S289–S296.

[19] Pomposelli, J.J. and Burns, D.L. (2002) Nutrition support in the liver transplant patient. *Nutr. Clin. Prac.* **17**, 341–349.

[20] Wicks, C., Somasudaram, S., Bjarnason, I., Menzies, I.S., Routley, D., Potter, D. *et al.* (1994) Comparison of enteral feeding and total parenteral nutrition after liver transplantation. *Lancet* **344**, 837–840.

[21] Shaw, Jr., B.W., Wood, R.P., Gordon, R.D., Iwatsuki, S., Gillquist, W.W.P. and Starzl, T.E. (1985) Influence of selected patient variables and operative blood loss on six month survival following liver transplantation. *Semin. Liver Dis.* **5**, 385–393.

[22] Sawyer, R.G., Pelletier, S.J. and Pruett, T.L. (1999) Increased early morbidity and mortality with acceptable long-term function in severely obese patients undergoing liver transplantation. *Clin. Transpl.* **13**, 126–130.

Hepatology: A Practical Approach
B. Al Knawy, M.L. Shiffman, R.H. Wiesner (editors)

Chapter 2
Renal Involvement in Liver Disease

Richard K. Sterling and Todd W.B. Gehr

Divisions of Gastroenterology and Nephrology, Virginia Commonwealth University School of Medicine, Medical College of Virginia Hospitals, Richmond, VA, USA

1. Introduction 443
2. Renal Disease in Patients with Liver Disease 443
   2.1 Prerenal azotemia 444
   2.2 Acute tubular necrosis 444
   2.3 Drug-induced renal dysfunction 445
   2.4 Glomerular abnormalities 446
   2.5 Renal tubular acidosis 448
   2.6 Miscellaneous 448
3. Liver Disease in Patients with Chronic Renal Disease 449
   3.1 Hepatitis B virus 449
   3.2 Hepatitis C virus 450
References 452

1. INTRODUCTION

Renal abnormalities are common in patients with acute and chronic liver diseases. These disorders can be characterized as either those related to the underlying liver disease or those liver diseases which occur in patients with chronic renal disease. This chapter will provide a brief overview of each. The most feared renal disorder associated with severe liver disease, hepatorenal syndrome, will be discussed elsewhere.

2. RENAL DISEASE IN PATIENTS WITH LIVER DISEASE

Renal diseases are common in patients with chronic liver disease, especially in those with cirrhosis (Table 1). The best approach to the evaluation of patients who present with both should start by determining whether the patient has acute or chronic renal disease. This is an important distinction since patients with acute renal failure (ARF) often deteriorate rapidly and require complicated supportive measures such as dialysis. Causes of ARF include acute tubular necrosis (ATN), prerenal azotemia, hepatorenal syndrome, rapidly progressive glomerulonephritis (RPGN), and allergic interstitial nephritis. Causes of chronic renal disease are more diverse and include renal tubular acidosis (RTA), chronic drug-induced injury, and a variety of glomerular diseases. Often, differentiating these can be difficult and more than one process may be going on simultaneously. Evaluation requires a careful history and physical exam, serum creatinine and blood urea nitrogen (BUN), urinalysis, examination of urine sediment, and measurement of urine sodium, creatinine, and osmolarity (Table 2). In those with ARF, attention to volume status, concomitant medications, and co-morbid conditions are paramount. If correctable causes do not reverse the renal impairment, consultation with a nephrologist may be required.

Table 1. Common diseases involving the liver and kidney.

Primary liver disease	Associated kidney disease
Alcohol	IgA nephropathy, hepatic glomerulosclerosis, RTA
Hepatitis C virus	MPGN, MGN, MN, tubulointerstitial disease
Hepatitis B virus	MN, MPGN, PAN, serum sickness-like syndrome
Primary biliary cirrhosis	MN, ANCA-positive vasculitis, RTA, anti-GBM disease, tubulointerstitial disease
Primary sclerosis cholangitis	ANCA-positive vasculitis, MPGN, MN, tubulointerstitial disease
Autoimmune hepatitis	Immune complex GN, RTA
A1AT deficiency	MPGN, anti-GBM disease
Congenital hepatic fibrosis	Nephronophthisis, polycystic kidney disease (AR)
Polycystic liver disease	Polycystic kidney disease (AD)
Glycogen storage disease	Focal glomerulosclerosis
Primary hyperoxaluria	Interstitial fibrosis
Wilson's disease	Fanconi's syndrome, RTA

MPGN, mesangiocapillary or membranoproliferative glomerulonephritis; MN, membranous glomerulonephritis; MGN, mesangial proliferative glomerulonephritis; PAN, polyarteritis nodosa; RTA, renal tubular acidosis; GBM, glomerular basement membrane; ANCA, antineutrophilic cytoplasmic antibody; AR, autosomal recessive; AD, autosomal dominant; A1AT, alpha 1 antitrypsin deficiency.

2.1 Prerenal azotemia

The most common cause of prerenal azotemia in patients with chronic liver disease is overuse of diuretics in the treatment of ascites or lower extremity edema. Ascites resorption is limited to 200–900 ml/day. Thus, a diuresis in excess of this amount will eventually lead to intravascular volume depletion and a decrease in glomerular filtration rate (GFR). Prerenal azotemia can also occur in patients with excessive diarrhea induced by lactulose. Clinically, these patients present with marked elevation of BUN, increased creatinine, normal urine sediment, and a fractional excretion of sodium of less than 1% (Table 3). In patients with cirrhosis the elevation of the BUN and creatinine may go unrecognized since these patients often have baseline values which are much lower than normal owing to their low protein intake and reduced muscle mass. Prerenal azotemia is often mistaken for the hepatorenal syndrome. However, unlike the hepatorenal syndrome, it is reversible with volume repletion with normal saline with or without albumin infusion.

2.2 Acute tubular necrosis

ARF has long been known to be associated with obstructive jaundice or cirrhosis. When bile and its constituents can no longer be excreted via the liver and biliary system, it relies on the kidney for excretion. Consequently, any deterioration of renal function in patients with impaired biliary excretion

Table 2. Evaluation of the patient with renal disease who has concomitant liver disease.

Step 1. Determine if renal disease is acute or chronic (history, previous labs, symptoms)

Step 2a. If acute renal failure (ARF)
- Identify cause (volume status, medications, acute illness)
- Urinalysis including microscopic evaluation
- Urine electrolytes and osmolality, fractional excretion of sodium
- Renal ultrasound or foley catheter insertion to rule out obstruction
- Determine urine output (oliguric (<400 cm^3/day) vs. nonoliguric)

Step 2b. If chronic renal failure (CRF)
- Identify cause (HCV, HBV, cryoglobulins)
- Urinalysis including microscopic evaluation (may need to do this multiple times)
- Renal ultrasound (kidney size, rule out chronic obstruction)
- Nephrology consultation

Step 3. Correct reversible causes
- Volume expansion
- Discontinuation of medications (NSAIDS, ACE inhibitors, antibiotics)
- If oliguric may need potassium and sodium restriction
- Nephrology consultation

Table 3. Differential diagnosis of acute renal failure in patients with liver disease.

Urine sodium concentration <20 mEq/l, FENA $<1\%$
Prerenal azotemia
Benign urinary sediment
Improves with volume expansion
Improves with discontinuation of certain medications (NSAIDS, ACE inhibitors, cyclosporin A, tacrolimus)
Hepatorenal syndrome
Benign urinary sediment
No response to volume challenge (1.5 l normal saline + albumin infusion)
Rapidly progressive glomerulonephritis (RPGN)
Often oliguric with severe hypertension
Proteinuria, RBC and RBC casts in urinary sediment
HBV/HCV/cryoglobulins/ANCA may be helpful in diagnosis
Urine sodium concentration >20 mEq/l, FENA $>1\%$
Acute tubular necrosis (ATN)
Coarsely granular and tubular epithelial casts in urinary sediment
Often oliguric
Identify and discontinue toxic medications (aminoglycosides)
Allergic interstitial nephritis (AIN)
WBC/WBC casts in urinary sediment
Nonnephrotic range proteinuria (exception in NSAID induced)
Eosinophilia/eosinophiluria
Identify and discontinue toxic medications (NSAIDs, antibiotics, can be any medication)

can result in increased morbidity and mortality. The exact mechanism of ARF in obstructive jaundice or cirrhosis is unclear but may be related to endotoxemia, hyperbilirubinemia, bile salt toxicity, intravascular volume depletion, and abnormalities in renal and systemic hemodynamics. Renal failure in this setting is most commonly related to acute ATN and presents with marked reduction in GFR. Elevations of both the BUN and creatinine, a fractional excretion of sodium greater than 1%, and a urinary sediment typical for tubular damage (coarsely granular casts and tubular epithelial cells) are necessary in order to make the diagnosis (Table 3). Although ARF was reported more frequently in the past, especially in patients undergoing surgery for obstructive jaundice, it occurs less frequently today due to better medical management of volume status, treatment of underlying infections, and avoidance of nephrotoxic medications such as nonsteroidal anti-inflammatory drugs (NSAIDs) and aminoglycosides.

2.3 Drug-induced renal dysfunction

Several medications are associated with renal dysfunction in patients with advanced liver disease. NSAIDs are perhaps the most common cause of renal impairment in patients with cirrhosis. The therapeutic effect of NSAIDs is due to their ability to block the production of prostaglandin synthesis by inhibiting cyclooxygenase. In cirrhosis, there is activation of the renin–angiotensin–aldosterone system and sympathetic nervous system which results in avid sodium and fluid retention and vasoconstriction. To maintain normal renal function, renal perfusion is maintained by vasodilatory prostaglandins which act to counter the effect of vasoconstrictors such as angiotensin II. Consequently, NSAID use in this patient population is associated with decrease in GFR and renal blood flow (RBF) which results in rising creatinine. Those at highest risk are patients with ascites and/or decompensated liver disease. However, decreased GFR and RBF have also been observed in patients with compensated cirrhosis. Renal dysfunction can occur with as little as a single dose of an NSAID. Although it is usually reversible and simulates prerenal azotemia, it can progress to ATN. There is not enough data on the safety of the newer COX-2 inhibitors in patients with decompensated cirrhosis but preliminary information would suggest that the COX-2 inhibitors offer little advantage in terms of renal protection and should be used with caution if at all in this population. Occasionally, NSAIDs are also associated with allergic interstitial nephritis with concomitant nephrotic syndrome, a syndrome unique to this class of drugs. Clinically, patients present with a rising creatinine, and may have either a low fractional excretion of sodium if renal hemodynamic effects predominate or a high fractional excretion of sodium if they have ATN or interstitial nephritis (Table 3). The urinary sediment is particularly revealing with these different clinical scenarios. Due to these concerns, it is recommended that NSAIDs be avoided in patients with cirrhosis, especially those with ascites, liver decompensation, and in those with preexisting renal impairment.

Another class of drugs that have been associated with significant nephrotoxicity are aminoglycosides. Even a single dose can result in significant renal dysfunction although more typically, patients need to be exposed to these drugs for significant periods of time. These patients often are nonoliguric, may waste potassium and magnesium, have urinary sediment that suggests ATN and often improve with discontinuation of the aminoglycoside. Since the introduction of cephalosporins and quinolones in the treatment of spontaneous bacterial peritonitis and other infections, the incidence of renal failure has decreased dramatically. The poorly absorbed aminoglycoside neomycin, used in the treatment of hepatic encephalopathy, can also result in renal insufficiency. Consequently, the use of any aminoglycoside should be avoided in patients with decompensated cirrhosis.

2.4 Glomerular abnormalities

Disorders of glomerular function are common in patients with viral hepatitis and include mesangial proliferative glomerulonephritis (MGN), membranous nephropathy (MN), and mesangiocapillary or membranoproliferative glomerulonephritis (MPGN) [1–3]. Although this diverse group of glomerular diseases usually presents as a chronic kidney disease, they can occasionally present as ARF (RPGN). As a group, however, hematuria and proteinuria are common to all of these diseases (Table 3).

Hepatitis B virus (HBV) associated glomerular diseases include proteinuria and hematuria associated with a serum sickness-like syndrome, MN, MPGN and systemic necrotizing vasculitis (Table 4). MN occurs mostly in male children in areas where HBV is endemic such as Asia and presents with nephrotic range proteinuria and hematuria. Diagnosis is made with appropriate HBV serologies and variably low levels of complement (usually C3). HBV immune-complex deposits are usually seen on renal biopsy. HBV associated glomerulonephritis (GN) usually resolves spontaneously in children within months to years, often with HBV seroconversion. HBV associated MN in adults is associated with a far worse prognosis with about 30% of patients having chronic renal insufficiency and 10% progressing to end stage renal disease (ESRD). MPGN and MGN have also been reported in patients with HBV although the relationship is less clear. Treatment of HBV associated GN is not well defined. Studies using immunosuppressive agents have not been encouraging and their use may worsen the underlying liver disease. There has been mixed results on the use of interferon and little if any with the use of lamivudine. As the majority of children will spontaneously resolve renal disease over time, a conservative approach has been recommended [3]. In adults, a trial of interferon or lamivudine may be warranted.

Table 4. Differential diagnosis of glomerular disease in patients with liver disease.

Nephrotic range proteinuria (>3.5 g protein/24 h)
Membranous nephropathy (MN)
HBV, HCV serology
Slowly progressive to renal failure
Often associated with hypercoagulable state
Mesangiocapillary or membranoproliferative glomerulonephritis (MPGN)
HCV, HBV
Type 1 cryoglobulinemia common
More rapid progression to renal failure
Nonnephrotic range proteinuria (<3.5 g protein/24 h)
Mesangial proliferative glomerulonephritis (MGN)
HCV, alcoholic liver disease
IgA deposits in kidney
Gross hematuria may occur
Slowly progressive to renal failure
Polyarteritis nodosa (PAN)
HBV
pANCA
Multisystem disease with rapid progression to renal failure

The association of polyarteritis nodosa (PAN) and HBV has long been recognized. Clinically, it presents with hypertension (often malignant), eosinophilia, abdominal pain, fever, rash, livedo reticularis, polyarthritis, and can progress to involve the gastrointestinal tract, nervous system, and kidneys. Hematuria, proteinuria, and azotemia are common. Antineutrophilic cytoplasmic antibodies (ANCAs) can be seen in approximately 10% of affected individuals. The exact pathologic mechanism is unclear as immune complexes containing HBV are not always found. Pathology shows a necrotizing vasculitis of small and medium size arteries leading to aneurysms and stenosis of the vessels of the kidneys, liver, and mesentery. Prognosis is poor with mortality of 30–50% in some series, especially in those with renal involvement. Treatment is controversial as traditional therapy including immune suppression can increase HBV replication which has the possibility of worsening underlying liver disease. In uncontrolled experiences, overall prognosis appears to be improved with steroids and cyclophosphamide. Treatment with plasmapheresis and dapsone has been used successfully. Combination therapy with plasmapheresis, steroids and vidarabine antiviral therapy has been employed and appears to be promising. Use of other antiviral agents, such as interferon and lamivudine have not been well studied.

Hepatitis C virus (HCV) associated glomerular diseases include MGN, MN and MPGN with the vast majority having type I MPGN (Table 4). Perhaps the best known renal disease associated with chronic HCV is cryoglobulinemia. Cryoglobulins are immunoglobulins that precipitate in the cold and are classified into three types: type I is composed of monoclonal immunoglobulins and usually associated with malignancies of the immune system; type II is composed of polyclonal IgG and monoclonal IgM; and type III is composed of polyclonal IgG and polyclonal IgM [1]. Types II and III are referred to as mixed cryoglobulinemia (MC) and the IgM usually has rheumatoid factor activity. When no precipitating factor is identified, it is termed essential MC (EMC). Until the discovery of HCV, HBV was implicated in MC. However, since the identification of HCV, it has now emerged as the major etiology of EMC [1].

Clinically, mixed cryoglobulinemia presents as arthralgia, symmetrical arthritis, fatigue, vasculitis, palpable purpura (from a leukocytoclastic vasculitis), and neuropathy. Renal involvement occurs in up to 50% and usually presents as MPGN. Laboratory testing shows positive HCV RNA, proteinuria, microscopic hematuria, mild to moderate renal insufficiency, hypocomplementemia (especially low C4 with modest depression of CH50 and C3), and elevated C1q binding [4]. An elevated rheumatoid factor is seen in over 70% and can be used as a useful screening test. The diagnosis of MC should also include measurement of cryoglobulins. However, since many labs do not perform this test routinely, false negative results do exist and the diagnosis can still be made in the presence of other positive clinical and laboratory findings. The majority of patients with HCV associated MC have significant hepatitis or advanced fibrosis. However, there have been reports in those with normal liver enzymes and mild histology.

The prevalence of HCV in MC is estimated at 45–90%. The majority of these patients are asymptomatic. Clinically significant cryoglobulinemia occurs in only a fraction of those with chronic HCV. This discrepancy has not been fully explained and there may be both host genetic factors that predispose patients with chronic HCV to MC including HLA haplotypes B8 and DR3 as well as viral factors. HCV genotype 2a has been reported to be more prevalent in MC. Occasionally, patients with chronic HCV can develop MN in the absence of cryoglobulins or evidence of MC. In these patients, rheumatoid factor is negative and serum complement levels are normal.

The pathogenesis of GN includes glomerular deposition of immune complexes containing HCV antigens, anti-HCV IgG antibodies, and IgM rheumatoid factors (anti-IgG antibodies) [1]. This results in local complement activation and an inflammatory infiltrate. HCV RNA is concentrated over 100-fold relative to serum in the cryoprecipitate. On renal biopsy, the circulating immune complexes localize to the subendothelium and mesangium to initiate local inflammation [4]. This results in a proliferative lesion with thickening of the capillary membranes. Immunofluorescence demonstrates granular staining of the capillary walls with IgM, IgG, and C3. In addition, tubulointerstitial fibrosis and vasculitis of the small and medium arteries can be seen. In those with HCV associated MN, there is normal cellularity with basement membrane thickening, granular capillary wall deposits of IgG and C3 on immunofluorescence, and subepithelial immune deposits seen on electron microscopy.

Treatment options of HCV associated MC include corticosteroids, cytotoxic agents, plasmapheresis and direct antiviral therapy with interferon [1]. The objective is to reduce the formation and inflammation associated with cryoglobulins. Since their formation is in part related to interaction of HCV RNA and its antibodies, treatment with interferon to eradicate HCV RNA is the logical approach. Experience with interferon has been limited. Overall, there are clinical improvements in proteinuria, renal function, vasculitis, and purpura in those who achieve virologic response [1]. Unfortunately, relapse is common when therapy is discontinued. Although the sustained loss of HCV RNA is higher with interferon and ribavirin combination therapy, there are little data in patients with MC. We and others have had success in controlling MC symptoms with long-term maintenance interferon. With the development of pegylated interferon, this may now be a viable long-term option in select patients. In those that present with an acute nephritic syndrome and signs of acute vasculitis, a more aggressive approach using pulse corticosteroids, cyclophosphamide, with or without plasmapheresis has been suggested.

Cirrhosis itself has also been associated with mild glomerular disease characterized by a mild increase in glomerular matrix with no increase in cellularity and thickening of capillary walls termed hepatic glomerulosclerosis [5]. Immunofluorescence typically reveals the presence of IgA, especially in patients with alcohol-induced liver disease. Clinically significant renal disease is unusual, but patients can have proteinuria and rarely a syndrome simulating Schonlein–Henlock purpura. Resolution has been reported following liver transplantation. Cirrhosis is also associated with decreased complement levels due to impaired hepatic production and increased consumption mediated through endotoxin stimulation of the alternate complement pathways. This may enhance renal tissue injury resulting in impaired renal function. Lastly, MN can also be seen in patients with primary biliary cirrhosis and primary sclerosing cholangitis (Table 1).

2.5 Renal tubular acidosis

When the renal tubule is unable to acidify the urine in the presence of normal glomerular filtration, RTA can develop. There are two general types of RTA: type 1 or distal RTA associated with failure of the kidney to maintain an adequate pH gradient between the blood and tubular fluid in the distal tubule and type 2 or proximal RTA characterized by a lower threshold for bicarbonate resorption in the proximal tubule. RTA has been observed in patients with a variety of chronic liver diseases including autoimmune hepatitis, primary biliary cirrhosis, alcoholic liver disease, and Wilson's disease. Most patients with chronic liver disease present with an incomplete distal RTA characterized by mild hypokalemia and high urine pH after acid loading in the absence of clinically significant systemic acidosis. Spironolactone, through inhibition of the effect of aldosterone, is also associated with a mild metabolic acidosis. The clinical significance of RTA in chronic liver disease is unclear although it has been suggested to predispose patients to hepatic encephalopathy.

2.6 Miscellaneous

The adult form of polycystic kidney disease is often associated with polycystic liver disease. Hepatic cysts occur in up to 80% of patients with renal disease by age 60 while the majority of patients with polycystic liver disease have cysts in their kidneys. Often, cysts are found on routine imaging and the majority of patients are asymptomatic. Clinically, patients may complain of a protuberant abdomen with discomfort. Those with massive cysts may also have shortness of breath and post-prandial fullness. Liver chemistries are usually normal and hepatic synthetic function is preserved. Complications of hepatic cysts include intracystic hemorrhage, infection, post-traumatic rupture, cyst adenocarcinoma, or development of noncirrhotic portal hypertension. Polycystic disease is associated with renal failure and is major cause of morbidity and mortality in these patients. Consequently, all patients with this disorder should be monitored for renal dysfunction.

Calcineurin inhibitors, such as cyclosporine and tacrolimus, are associated with the development of glomerular afferent arteriolar hyalinosis, tubular atrophy, and interstitial fibrosis [5]. Consequently, patients often develop renal insufficiency following liver transplantation due to renal ischemia and extracellular matrix production. The incidence of severe renal dysfunction is approximately 20% and the development of ESRD has a negative prognostic effect in these liver transplant patients. Treatment options include minimizing exposure to these potentially nephrotoxic medications or using alternative renal sparing immunosuppressive agents such as rapamycin may be beneficial preserving renal function. As with patients with decompensated liver disease, use of NSAIDs and aminoglycosides should also be avoided in transplant recipients due to their high potential to worsen or precipitate renal dysfunction.

Many other diseases can affect both the liver and kidney and include hemochromatosis, amyloidosis, sarcoidosis, sickle cell disease, tyrosinemia, primary hyperoxaluria, acute hepatitis A, human immunodeficiency virus, leptospirosis, schistosomiasis, malaria, and cytomegalovirus. Acetaminophen toxicity associated with accidental or intentional overdose can also cause renal dysfunction due to the intrarenal effects of the toxic metabolite of acetaminophen (see section 2 chapter 20).

3. LIVER DISEASE IN PATIENTS WITH CHRONIC RENAL DISEASE

Liver disease is an important cause of morbidity and mortality in patients with ESRD on hemodialysis. Causes of abnormal liver chemistries in patients on hemodialysis include viral hepatitis, medications, alcohol, secondary iron overload for multiple transfusions, steatosis, and passive congestion from right-sided heart failure. Evaluation therefore includes careful physical exam, testing for viral hepatitis B and C, review of medications and transfusion history, and possibly liver biopsy. The risk of bleeding from percutaneous biopsy can be increased due to uremia-induced platelet dysfunction. Although no controlled trials exist, many recommend the use of DDAVP (0.3 ug/kg) prior to biopsy to help reduce post-biopsy bleeding.

3.1 Hepatitis B virus

HBV has long been recognized as a potential cause of significant liver disease and decreased survival in patients with ESRD. Prior to effective HBV screening, the prevalence of HBV was 15–20% with an annual incidence of 5–10% in patients on dialysis [6]. The overall incidence of HBV has decreased dramatically with the near elimination of HBV from the blood supply, the decreased need blood transfusions from the use of erythropoietin, and the implementation of universal precautions. Unfortunately, HBV vaccine is suboptimal in patients with ESRD with responses of 50–60% compared to over 95% in immunocompetent individuals. In addition, patients with ESRD who demonstrated a prior response to vaccination often lose antibody to HBV and may be at risk for HBV if exposed. Fortunately, HBV now plays only a minor role in patients with ESRD.

The impact of HBV on renal transplantation is associated with reduced long-term patient and graft survival. By 1993, only two-thirds of renal transplant centers performed transplants in patients with chronic HBV, mostly in patients with mild disease and normal liver function tests without evidence of HBV replication (HBV E antigen and HBV DNA negative). The spectrum of liver disease in HBV patients awaiting renal transplant is not known. Post-transplant, early reports suggested a more rapid progression of liver disease to cirrhosis associated with increased viral replication related to immune suppression. In a recent study, Mathurin and colleagues analyzed the long-term effect of HBV in renal transplant recipients and found decreased 10-year patient (55%) and graft (36%) survival compared to control patients without evidence of viral hepatitis (80 and 63%, respectively) (Figure 1) [7]. Interestingly, they found that active viral replication (HBV E antigen and HBV DNA positive) did not significantly affect long-term survival. Of note, there have also been several reports of rapid fibrosis progression in the absence of significant hepatic inflammation, the so-called fibrosing cholestatic hepatitis.

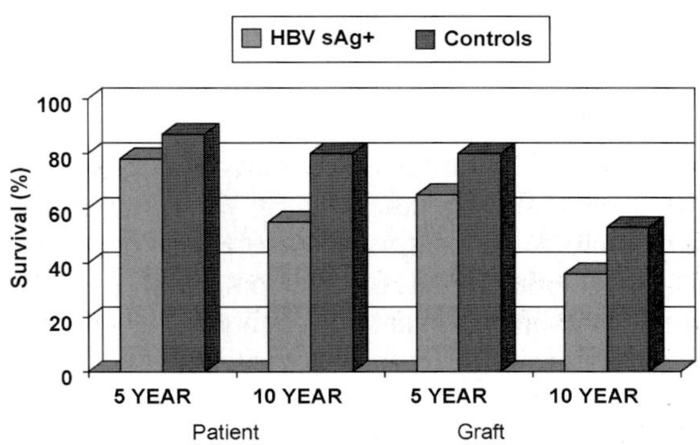

Figure 1. Five- and 10-year patient and graft survival (%) in hepatitis B virus patients following renal transplantation (adapted from Ref. [7]). *(For colored version, see Plate XLII on page 585 at the end of the book.)*

Current recommendations for patients being considered for renal transplantation include HBV testing and vaccination if negative for HBV surfaced antibody in those who have not been previously vaccinated [6]. The management of those who had responded to vaccine but lost detectable antibody is less clear. In those who are positive for HBV surface antigen, determination of replicative status with HBV E antigen and HBV DNA as well as antibodies to hepatitis D virus and HCV are needed. All patients with evidence of HBV infection require liver biopsy to determine the extent of liver damage. Those with mild disease should not be precluded from transplantation. However, they should be counseled that even mild disease has the potential to progress with immunosuppression following renal transplantation. Strategies to improve survival include minimizing immune suppression and the use of antiviral therapy. Interferon should be used with extreme caution in renal transplant recipients and may cause graft failure. Consequently, treatment options are limited in the post-transplant setting to other antiviral agents such as lamivudine. However, the long-term use of these agents and their effect on patient and graft function remain to be determined. In those with cirrhosis, the long-term effectiveness of renal transplantation is controversial and may vary from center to center. In those with advanced liver fibrosis, the risk of hepatic decompensation or eventual need for liver transplantation should be discussed. Consequently, their eventual candidacy for liver transplantation may affect their eligibility for renal transplantation.

3.2 Hepatitis C virus

Since its discovery in 1989, HCV is now recognized as an important pathogen in patients with ESRD and in patients awaiting renal transplantation. The prevalence of antibodies to HCV in patients on hemodialysis ranges from 10 to 60%. Risk factors for HCV include blood transfusion prior to 1991, previous renal transplant, intravenous and intranasal illicit drug use [8]. Hemodialysis itself has also been implicated for HCV transmission with an incidence of less than 1% per year. Modes of transmission within a dialysis unit include needle stick injuries, breakdown in standard infection control practices, the dialysis equipment itself, and possibly the physical proximity of patients [8]. Although patients with HBV are required to be dialyzed on dedicated machines, the Center for Disease Control does not recommend patients with HCV be dialyzed separately [8].

The majority of patients with HCV on hemodialysis have normal aminotransferases [9,10]. Consequently, the diagnosis of HCV requires a high index of suspicion. Given the high prevalence in the population, it seems prudent to screen all patients with ESRD on dialysis for HCV. Unfortunately, anti-HCV testing is imperfect in patients with renal failure. With first generation antibody tests, the prevalence was estimated at 10%. However, first generation tests have high false negative rates in patients with compromised immune systems. Second and now third generation antibody tests have overcome most of these limitations. Nevertheless, there have been reports of patients with detectable HCV RNA and negative anti-HCV antibodies. In addition, patients on hemodialysis can lose HCV antibodies over time. Therefore, HCV RNA testing by polymerase chain reaction is now recommended for the diagnosis of HCV in patients with ESRD. However, even this can be problematic as viral levels may fluctuate above and below the level of detectability.

The histologic spectrum of HCV in patients with ESRD can vary from mild hepatitis to cirrhosis. Several studies have focused on the clinical predictors of severe liver disease and found no significant relationship in disease severity with age, duration of hemodialysis, pattern of aminotransferase levels, number of blood units transfused, past hepatitis B infection, previous renal allograft or duration of HCV. Furthermore, because there is no relationship between HCV RNA titer, serum aminotransferase, and liver histology, liver biopsy is paramount in the evaluation of HCV in this patient population [9]. Glicklich and associates compared liver histology of HCV-positive patients awaiting transplant to those who received a transplant and found no significant differences in total histologic activity [11]. Conversely, Rao and colleagues observed progression to cirrhosis in over 60% of those with evidence of active hepatitis in patients with serial biopsies over a 4.5-year period following renal transplantation [12]. Coinfection with both HBV and HCV appears to be associated with worse

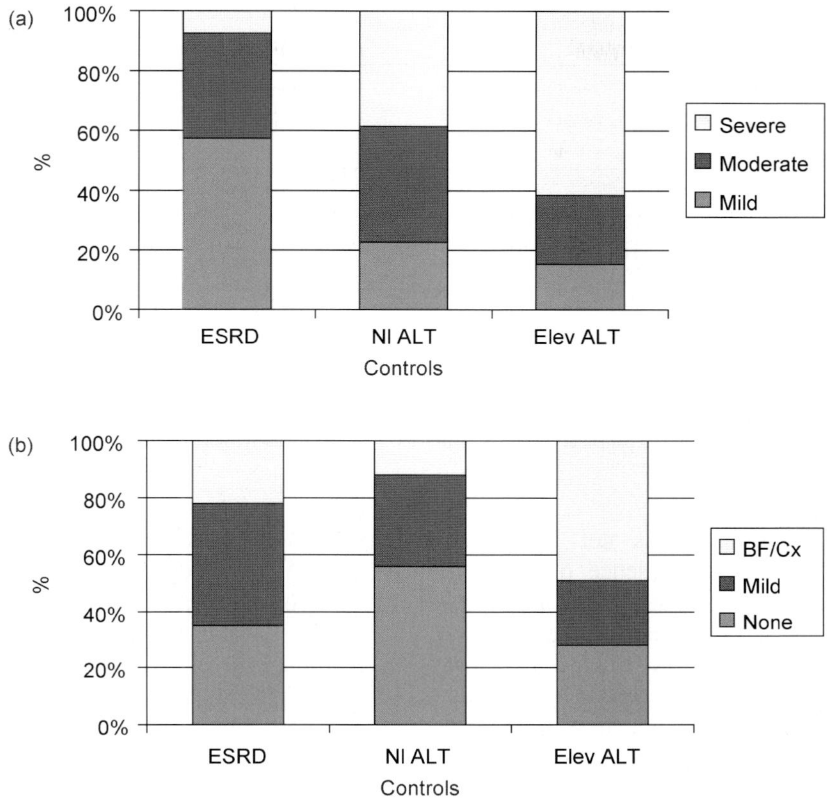

Figure 2. (a) Inflammation on liver biopsy in hepatitis C patients with end stage renal disease awaiting renal transplantation [9]. (b) Fibrosis on liver biopsy in hepatitis C patients with end stage renal disease awaiting renal transplantation [9]. ESRD, end stage renal disease; Nl ALT, normal ALT controls; Elev ALT, elevated ALT controls; BF/Cx, bridging fibrosis/cirrhosis; 0, no fibrosis; 1, portal fibrosis. *(For colored version, see Plate XLIII on page 586 at the end of the book.)*

histology. In a study that compared liver histology of patients with HCV and ESRD awaiting renal transplantation to control HCV patients, the majority of patients with ESRD had mild disease or only moderate inflammation with almost 80% with little or no fibrosis and similar to normal ALT, normal renal function controls (Figure 2a and b) [9]. However, 20–25% of these patients did have significant fibrosis (defined as bridging fibrosis or cirrhosis) despite normal aminotransferase levels underscoring the importance of liver biopsy in the evaluation of these patients.

When compared to chronic hemodialysis, patients with HCV have improved survival with renal transplantation [13,14]. Several early studies reported similar survival compared to HCV-negative patients for greater than 10 years following renal transplantation. However, recent reports have shown that HCV has a significant impact on patient and graft survival (Table 5). In fact, the impact of HCV may be even more pronounced when patients are followed for 20 years where patient and graft survivals of 64 and 35% were significantly lower compared to HCV-negative controls (88 and 64%, respectively) [15]. The increased mortality in patients with HCV appears to be related to both liver disease and infectious complications [16]. In a recent study, chronic hepatitis was observed in 36% of patients with HCV undergoing renal transplantation with cirrhosis in 5%. Interestingly, these findings were similar to pre-transplant histology observed in other studies. Because most studies of post-transplant histology have been limited by lack of pre-transplant liver biopsies, the natural history of

Table 5. Impact of HCV on survival following renal transplantation.

Author [Ref.]	Year	*N*	Group	Patient survival (%)		Graft survival (%)	
				5 years	10 years	5 years	10 years
Periera [14]	1998	23	HCV +	60	n/a	50	n/a
		80	HCV −	90	n/a	65	n/a
Legendre [16]	1998	112	HCV +	90	80	n/a	40
		387	HCV −	95	92	n/a	65
Hanafusa [15]	1998	80	HCV +	91	84	70	57
		184	HCV −	94	88	76	68
Mathurin [7]	1999	216	HCV +	85	65	71	49
		490	HCV −	87	80	78	63

HCV +/HCV − is the HCV antibody status of a patient at the time of transplant. Data are estimated from literature if specifically not stated. n/a, not available.

HCV after renal transplant has not been well characterized. However, the presence of cirrhosis pre-transplant has been associated with a marked decrease in patient survival questioning whether renal transplantation should be offered to these individuals [7]. HCV has also been a risk factor for post-transplant proteinuria which is associated with reduced graft survival [17]. Similar to HBV in the post-transplant setting, fibrosing cholestatic hepatitis has been reported with HCV.

The decision to offer renal transplant to an HCV-positive patient should depend on the liver histology. In those with mild disease, a discussion of the potential long-term reduced patient and graft survival is required. In those with cirrhosis, a discussion of the role of eventual liver transplantation should hepatic decompensation develop is required as compensated cirrhosis in itself should not preclude renal transplantation in those who are otherwise potential liver transplant candidates. In any event, patients should understand the implications of HCV on their graft and long-term outcome.

Because HCV appears to have a significant clinical impact on post-transplant patient and renal graft survival, treatment to eradicate HCV and decrease the progression to fibrosis has received increased attention. Because ribavirin is contraindicated in patients with renal insufficiency, interferon monotherapy is the only treatment option. Unfortunately, treatment after renal transplantation has limited success and has been associated with unacceptable risk of renal dysfunction and graft loss [18]. Therefore, treatment prior to transplant remains the most viable option. Several small studies have examined the effectiveness of interferon monotherapy in patients with ESRD [19,20]. Overall end of treatment and sustained response were 40–50 and 10–25%, respectively, and similar to that observed in patients with no renal dysfunction. The results of pegylated interferon in this population have not been reported and ongoing studies are anxiously awaited. Selection of patients for treatment should be based on the potential for long-term survival and should focus on those who are renal transplant candidates. Only time will tell if treatment of HCV in the pre-transplant setting will affect long-term survival.

REFERENCES

[1] Johnson, R.J., Willson, R., Yamabe, H., Couser, W., Alpers, C.E., Wener, M.H., Davis, C. and Gretch, D.R. (1994) Renal manifestations of hepatitis C virus infection. *Kidney Int.* **46**(5), 1255–1263.

[2] Gumber, S.C. and Chopra, S. (1995) Hepatitis C: a multifaceted disease. Review of extrahepatic manifestations. *Ann. Intern. Med.* **123**(8), 615–620.

[3] Willson, R.A. (1997) Extrahepatic manifestations of chronic viral hepatitis. *Am. J. Gastroenterol.* **92**(1), 3–17.

[4] Johnson, R.J., Gretch, D.R., Yamabe, H., Hart, J., Bacchi, C.E., Hartwell, P., Couser, W.G., Corey, L., Wener, M.H. and Alpers, C.E. (1993) Membranoproliferative glomerulonephritis associated with hepatitis C virus infection. *N. Engl. J. Med.* **328**(7), 465–470.

[5] Davis, C.L., Gonwa, T.A. and Wilkinson, A.H. (2002) Pathophysiology of renal disease associated with liver disorders: implications for liver transplantation. Part I. *Liver Transpl.* **8**(2), 91–109.

[6] Martin, P. and Friedman, L.S. (1995) Chronic viral hepatitis and the management of chronic renal failure. *Kidney Int.* **47**(5), 1231–1241.

[7] Mathurin, P., Mouquet, C., Poynard, T., Sylla, C., Benalia, H., Fretz, C., Thibault, V., Conrand, J.F., Bernard, B., Opolon, P., Coriat, P. and Bitker, M.O. (1999) Impact of hepatitis B and C virus on kidney transplantation outcome. *Hepatology* **29**(1), 257–263.

[8] Murthy, B.V. and Pereira, B.J. (1997) A 1990s perspective of hepatitis C, human immunodeficiency virus, and tuberculosis infections in dialysis patients. *Semin. Nephrol.* **17**(4), 346–363.

[9] Sterling, R.K., Sanyal, A.J., Luketic, V.A., Stravitz, R.T., King, A.L., Post, A.B., Mills, A.S., Contos, M.J. and Shiffman, M.L. (1999) Chronic hepatitis C infection in patients with end stage renal disease: characterization of liver histology and viral load in patients awaiting renal transplantation. *Am. J. Gastroenterol.* **94**(12), 3576–3582.

[10] Yasuda, K., Okuda, K., Endo, N., Ishiwatari, Y., Ikeda, R., Hayashi, H., Yokozeki, K., Kobayashi, S. and Irie, Y. (1995) Hypoaminotransferasemia in patients undergoing long-term hemodialysis: clinical and biochemical appraisal. *Gastroenterology* **109**(4), 1295–1300.

[11] Glicklich, D., Thung, S.N., Kapoian, T., Tellis, V. and Reinus, J.F. (1999) Comparison of clinical features and liver histology in hepatitis C-positive dialysis patients and real transplant recipients. *Am. J. Gastroenterol.* **94**(1), 159–163.

[12] Rao, K.V., Anderson, W.R., Kasiske, B.L. and Dahl, D.C. (1993) Value of liver biopsy in the evaluation and management of chronic liver disease in renal transplant recipients. *Am. J. Med.* **94**(3), 241–250.

[13] Knoll, G.A., Tankersley, M.R., Lee, J.Y., Julian, B.A. and Curtis, J.J. (1997) The impact of renal transplantation on survival in hepatitis C-positive end-stage renal disease patients. *Am. J. Kidney Dis.* **29**(4), 608–614.

[14] Pereira, B.J., Natov, S.N., Bouthot, B.A., Murthy, B.V., Ruthazer, R., Schmid, C.H. and Levey, A.S. (1998) Effects of hepatitis C infection and renal transplantation on survival in end-stage renal disease. The New England Organ Bank Hepatitis C Study Group. *Kidney Int.* **53**(5), 1374–1381.

[15] Hanafusa, T., Ichikawa, Y., Kishikawa, H., Kyo, M., Fukunishi, T., Kokado, Y., Okuyama, A., Shinji, Y. and Nagano, S. (1998) Retrospective study on the impact of hepatitis C virus infection on kidney transplant patients over 20 years. *Transplantation* **66**(4), 471–476.

[16] Legendre, C., Garrigue, V., Le Bihan, C., Mamzer-Bruneel, M.F., Chaix, M.L., Landais, P., Kreis, H. and Pol, S. (1998) Harmful long-term impact of hepatitis C virus infection in kidney transplant recipients. *Transplantation* **65**(5), 667–670.

[17] Hestin, D., Guillemin, F., Castin, N., Le Faou, A., Champigneulles, J. and Kessler, M. (1998) Pretransplant hepatitis C virus infection: a predictor of proteinuria after renal transplantation. *Transplantation* **65**(5), 741–744.

[18] Rostaing, L., Izopet, J., Baron, E., Duffaut, M., Puel, J. and Durand, D. (1995) Treatment of chronic hepatitis C with recombinant interferon alpha in kidney transplant recipients. *Transplantation* **59**(10), 1426–1431.

[19] Koenig, P., Vogel, W., Umlauft, F., Weyrer, K., Prommegger, R., Lhotta, K., Neyer, V., Stummvoll, H.K. and Gruenewald, K. (1994) Interferon treatment for chronic hepatitis C virus infection in uremic patients. *Kidney Int.* **45**(5), 1507–1509.

[20] Pol, S., Thiers, V., Carnot, F., Zins, B., Romeo, R., Berthelot, P. and Brechot, C. (1995) Efficacy and tolerance of alpha-2b interferon therapy on HCV infection of hemodialyzed patients. *Kidney Int.* **47**(5), 1412–1418.

Hepatology: A Practical Approach
B. Al Knawy, M.L. Shiffman, R.H. Wiesner (editors)

Chapter 3
Dermatologic Manifestations of Liver Disease

Julia R. Nunley

Virginia Commonwealth University School of Medicine, P.O. Box 980164, Richmond, VA 23221, USA

1. Introduction 455
2. Nonspecific Dermatologic Manifestations of Liver Disease 456
   2.1 Color changes 456
   2.2 Vascular changes 456
   2.3 Hormonal changes 457
   2.4 Signs of generalized pruritus 457
   2.5 Miscellaneous 457
3. Liver Diseases with Associated Dermatologic Manifestations 458
   3.1 Hemochromatosis 458
   3.2 Porphyria 458
   3.3 Primary biliary cirrhosis 460
   3.4 Viral hepatitis 460
   3.5 Wilson's disease 462
4. Cutaneous Diseases Which Suggest an Underlying Liver Disease 462
References 464

1. INTRODUCTION

For many years an association between the skin and the liver has been appreciated, and medical students throughout the decades have been taught to recognize the common stigmata of chronic liver disease. Cutaneous clues such as jaundice and spider angiomas, though not pathognomonic for liver disease, have long been accepted as common markers of significant liver dysfunction. Whereas jaundice can occur with both acute and chronic liver diseases, the presence of spider angiomas suggests that the liver problem is more longstanding. Although most of these cutaneous changes occur with a variety of hepatic disorders and cannot accurately predict the cause of the liver disease, some skin conditions may be better predictors than others; for example, "bronze diabetes" is a term that has been used to describe complications of hemochromatosis, which include a characteristic cutaneous discoloration. More recently, the association between porphyria cutanea tarda (PCT) and hepatitis C viral (HCV) infection has been recognized to be so significant that it is now recommended that all patients with PCT be screened for the presence of HCV [1–8].

On a daily basis, clinicians face a multitude of patients who present with innumerable subtle clues to underlying systemic diseases. Patients, frequently desperate for help, try to aid the physician by describing the tiniest of clinical details. Astute clinicians are able to sift through these details, glean those that are pertinent, correlate them with physical and laboratory findings and reach the correct diagnosis. Liver dysfunction may be suspected by either the patient's history or physical findings and confirmed through laboratory evaluation. This chapter should serve as a tool to help clinicians identify and work with patients with liver problems by recognizing the cutaneous complications of liver disease.

2. NONSPECIFIC DERMATOLOGIC MANIFESTATIONS OF LIVER DISEASE

A whole host of skin disorders (Table 1) have been deemed to be complications of liver disease. Although many of these have been described as cutaneous manifestations of cirrhosis, cirrhosis need not be present. In fact, most of the conditions listed in Table 1 are nonspecific and generally exist in the absence of liver disease. However, one cannot ignore the fact that these disorders are frequently seen in association with liver disease and patients should be evaluated when necessary.

2.1 Color changes

Jaundice is probably the most commonly recognized cutaneous marker of liver dysfunction and occurs with all types of liver disease. Color changes range from a light yellow to dark green and vary according to the bilirubin level and the patient's constitutive skin color. Mucosal surfaces are typically involved and scleral icterus is frequently the first abnormality to be noted. Conjugated bilirubin levels rise because of inadequate biliary secretion and are typically above 2.5 mg/dl when jaundice is clinically recognized [1]. Though indicative of significant liver failure, jaundice is symptom free and harmless and will resolve with resolution of the liver dysfunction.

Table 1. Nonspecific skin changes associated with liver disease.

Color changes
Jaundice
Melanosis
Vascular changes
Spider angioma
Palmar erythema
Caput Medusa
Purpura
Hormonal changes
Alopecia
Gynecomastia
Swelling of parotid gland
Testicular atrophy
Striae
Signs of generalized pruritus
Excoriations
Prurigo nodularis
Lichen simplex chronicus
Miscellaneous
Dupuytren's contractures
Terry's nails
Muehrcke's lines

Melanosis, another pigmentary change, has been described in the setting of longstanding cirrhosis and is probably more common in primary biliary cirrhosis (PBC) and hemochromatosis [9]. Patients develop a diffuse or patchy, metallic gray color change which may involve the skin and mucosa, or may be limited to the mucosa [1,9]. The pathogenesis of this pigmentary transformation is still debated though theories have suggested roles for iron overload, excessive melanin production and/or hemosiderin deposition [1].

In addition, hemochromatosis has been associated with a characteristic bronze pigmentation which reportedly occurs in approximately one-third of affected individuals. Though accentuated in sun-exposed areas, the discoloration is generally diffuse and reportedly involves mucosal surfaces in up to 20% of patients [9]. Even though the cause of this pigmentary alteration is not completely understood, phlebotomy has been reported to improve the appearance [9].

2.2 Vascular changes

Associated vascular changes occur predominately in patients with chronic liver disease and are rare in those with acute liver failure. Spider angiomas are the most widely recognized. Typical lesions consist of a central perforating vessel from which smaller vessels radiate peripherally. There is an overwhelming tendency for angiomas to develop on the face, upper trunk, and distal upper extremities. Though conjectural, this distribution suggests a possible role for either ultraviolet light or portal hypertension, since these same areas generally receive more sun exposure and are drained by the superior vena cava [9]. However, the pathogenesis of these distinctive lesions remains speculative. An alteration in estrogen metabolism, which has been implicated as causative for the characteristic palmar erythema, may also be central to the development of spider veins [1]. Palmar erythema develops as either a diffuse, exaggerated mottling over both the palms and soles, or as discrete erythematous patches on the thenar or hypothenar eminences. Muscular atrophy may be present. The true pathogenesis of these vascular changes is probably complex, due to multiple interactive factors and is yet to be elucidated.

Less common, but better understood, is the development of collateral cutaneous vessels and purpura. Collateral vessels classically demonstrate a tortuous course over the abdomen and the term "caput Medusa" has been coined to describe them [9]. If present, they are an excellent cutaneous clue that hepatic cirrhosis and significant portal hypertension exist. A deficiency in clotting factors due to impaired synthesis is another consequence of significant liver decompensation. Patients may complain of easy bruisability and the clinician may see ecchymoses and variably sized purpura as well as petechia, predominately in dependent areas due to increased hydrostatic pressure.

2.3 Hormonal changes

Several of the cutaneous and glandular anomalies (Table 1) described in patients with cirrhosis have been attributed to hormonal dysregulation. Theoretically, there is an alteration in estrogen metabolism which results in estrogen excess, although some evidence suggests that testosterone deficiency plays a role as well [1,9]. The resulting gynecomastia and testicular atrophy are associated with a loss of libido, potency and oligospermia in men [9]. A slower growth rate of facial hair may also occur in men with cirrhosis, whereas generalized hair loss may be noted in both men and women [9]. Swelling of the parotid glands has been similarly noted in both genders as has striae distensae, both with and without glucocorticoid therapy [9].

2.4 Signs of generalized pruritus

Generalized pruritus may be a manifestation of a variety of systemic conditions including atopy, end-stage renal disease, iron deficiency, pregnancy, and chronic liver disease. Frequently found in patients with HCV and PBC, pruritus is prevalent in the setting of hepatobiliary obstruction and remains one of the most debilitating and poorly understood phenomena of hepatic failure [1]. Several theories regarding pathogenesis have been conceived. Since pruritus is most common in the setting of cholestasis, retained bilirubin, bile acids and cholesterol have been implicated as pruritogenic substances. Although there is no specific proof for this theory, a reduction in bile salt levels with sequestering agents has been shown to result in partial improvement [1]. Other investigators have theorized that hepatic dysfunction results in retention of an unidentified substance with opioid-agonistic properties which is able to act centrally, stimulating the sensation of itch [1]. This theory is also supported by circumstantial evidence since opioid receptor antagonists have been shown to be effective in alleviating itch in some patients. Whatever the cause, pruritus drives patients to scratch, often to the point of drawing blood. Excoriations in all stages of healing are evident, as are hyperkeratotic papules (prurigo nodularis, Figure 1) and plaques (lichen simplex chronicus) which develop in response to chronic scratching. Lesions may be noted on all parts of the body, with the exception of the mid-back since this area is difficult for the patient to reach. Sparing of the back is a clinical clue that these lesions are self-inflicted. In addition to the therapeutic options of sequestering agents and opioid receptor antagonists, some patients may benefit from sedating antihistamines, topical anesthetics or cooling agents, phototherapy or the addition of rifampin.

2.5 Miscellaneous

Dupuytren's contractures are due to fibrosis of the palmar aponeurosis and generally appear in middle age. Though they typically begin as small nodules, they may progress and result in contracture deformities, primarily of the fingers. Their appearance has been associated with trauma and diseases such as epilepsy and alcoholic cirrhosis [9]. Partial fasciectomy may result in functional recovery, but recurrence is not uncommon.

Several nail changes have also been identified with chronic liver disease, though most are nonspecific. Initially thought to be a marker of cirrhosis, white nails or Terry's nails (Figure 2) have actually been shown to occur in up to 25% of hospitalized patients

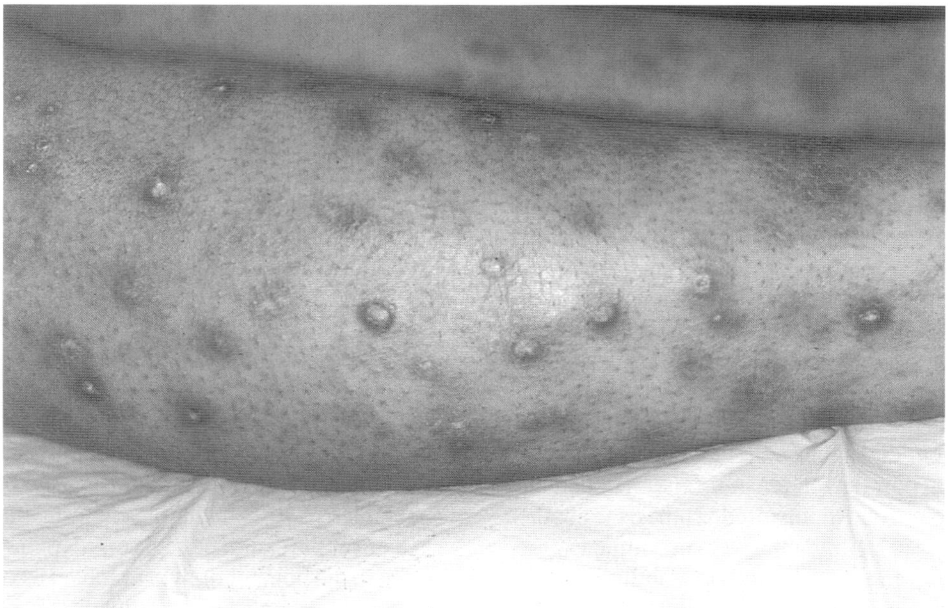

Figure 1. This patient presented with generalized pruritus which was subsequently shown to be related to HCV infection. Present here are the classic hyperkeratotic lesions of prurigo nodularis. (*For colored version, see Plate XLIV on page 587 at the end of the book.*)

with or without liver disease [1]. Clinically, one sees a diffuse whitish discoloration, with only a thin pink band at the distal most portion of the nail bed. Clubbing, though more common in pulmonary disorders, has also been described in PBC, chronic active hepatitis and cirrhosis [9]. Muehrcke's lines that appear as double transverse white bands within the nail bed have been described with hypoalbuminemia of various causes, including cirrhosis [1]. However, azure lunulae, blue discoloration of the lunula, are pathognomonic for Wilson's disease [1,9].

3. LIVER DISEASES WITH ASSOCIATED DERMATOLOGIC MANIFESTATIONS

Table 2 lists several liver diseases which frequently have cutaneous markers. Though most of these skin changes are nonspecific (see Table 1), some are relatively unique and should raise the clinician's suspicion that a hepatic process may be present. In addition, those who work with patients with liver diseases, must recognize and understand these cutaneous complications.

3.1 Hemochromatosis

Hemochromatosis is a heritable disorder of iron uptake. Multiple organ systems may be affected and two discrete genetic defects have been identified [2,8]. Whereas most patients with hemochromatosis are homozygous, approximately 20% of those who are heterozygous may also manifest iron overload [8]. The diagnosis of hemochromatosis should be suspected when the classic clinical triad of hyperpigmentation, cirrhosis and diabetes mellitus are present in a Caucasian. Interestingly, a significant association between the presence of one of the genetic mutations for hemochromatosis and the acquired form of PCT has recently been recognized [2,8]. Screening for these genetic mutations should be considered in Caucasian patients with PCT.

3.2 Porphyria

The porphyrias are a group of systemic disorders caused by specific enzyme defects in the pathway of heme biosynthesis [9,10]. Accumulation of certain porphyrins and their precursors results in distinctly different clinical scenarios. Currently, the diagnosis

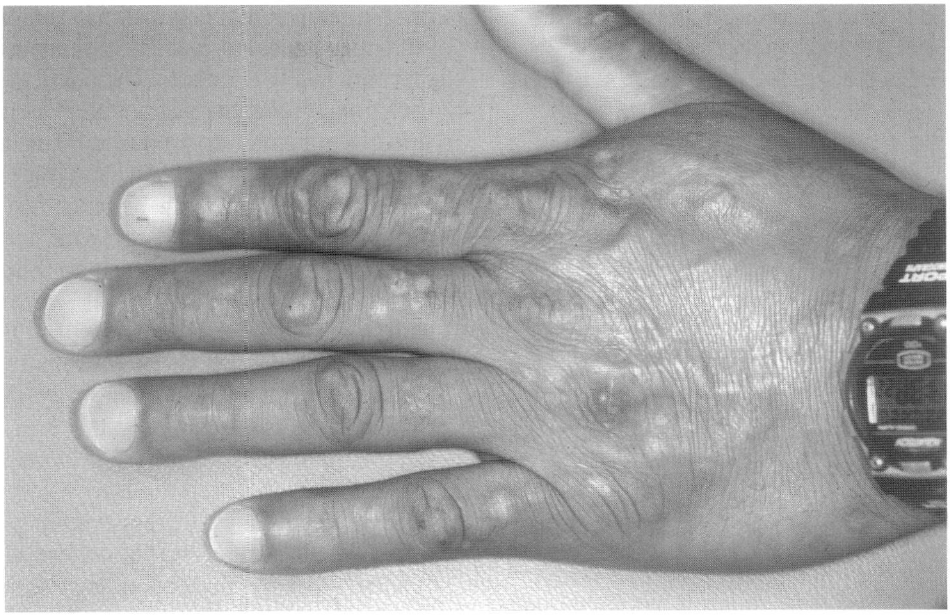

Figure 2. This hand demonstrates two cutaneous changes associated with liver disease. The nails have the classic white, or Terry's nails. The erosions are evidence of the underlying porphyria cutanea tarda. (*For colored version, see Plate XLV on page 587 at the end of the book.*)

of the specific type of porphyria requires quantification and profiling of porphyrins secreted or excreted in the urine and/or stool. All of the porphyrias, with the exception of acute intermittent porphyria, may demonstrate cutaneous changes.

PCT, the most common of the porphyrias, is due to a defect in the enzyme uroporphyrinogen decarboxylase and may be inherited or acquired [10].

Table 2. Liver diseases which have characteristic skin findings.

- Hemochromatosis
- Porphyria
  - Porphyria cutanea tarda
  - Variegate porphyria
  - Hereditary coproporphyria
  - Hepatoerythropoietic porphyria
  - Erythropoietic protoporphyria
  - Congenital erythropoietic porphyria
- Primary biliary cirrhosis
- Viral hepatitis
  - Hepatitis A virus
  - Hepatitis B virus
  - Hepatitis C virus
- Wilson's disease

The enzyme defect is present in both the liver and red corpuscles in the heritable forms, but only in the liver in the more common acquired or sporadic form. As a consequence, excessive amounts of uroporphyrin and its precursors are in the circulation and may trigger a photosensitivity reaction upon exposure to ultraviolet A light (UVA). Interestingly, a combination of comorbid factors (Table 3) appears to be necessary before the clinical picture may become manifest [2]. Patients present with blisters and erosions in sun-exposed areas, predominately on the dorsal hands (Figure 2), forearms and face. Frequently, the blisters go unnoticed by the patient who complains only of skin fragility. Lesions heal with scarring which over time may result in scleroderma-like skin changes, milia formation and pigmentary loss. Facial hypertrichosis is a peculiar cutaneous finding that typically develops between the lateral eyebrows and the hairline. Treatment for PCT includes phlebotomy, and sun protection [2]. Ultraviolet A light is a major component of natural sunlight, so patients must be instructed to avoid sun exposure whenever possible, and to use a sunscreen on a daily basis which contains a sunscreen specifically for UVA and has a high sun protective

Table 3. Comorbid factors associated with the development of PCT.

Alcohol consumption
Dialysis
Hepatitis C virus
Hepatitis B virus
Human immunodeficiency virus
Hemochromatosis genetic mutation
Iron overload
Medications/toxins
Aromatic hydrocarbons
Estrogens
Phenytoin

factor (SPF). Since UVA may pass through glass, patients sitting in cars and in rooms with windows are also at risk.

Cutaneous changes seen in variegate porphyria and hereditary coproporphyria are identical to those found in PCT. Although these conditions are rare, they must be properly identified through laboratory studies since phlebotomy is not indicated for treatment of either of these types of porphyria [10].

Phlebotomy is also not indicated for hepatoerythropoietic porphyria, erythropoietic protoporphyria or congenital erythropoietic porphyria. Each of these metabolic disorders is very rare and present in childhood, compared to those above which generally present in adults. Photosensitivity remains a predominate component in these disorders and patients frequently develop erythema, blisters, and significant scarring with minimal exposure to the sun. Ultraviolet A light is the major trigger, so these patients must be educated in the same manner as are those with PCT [10].

3.3 Primary biliary cirrhosis

PBC is a chronic, progressive cholestatic liver disease for which a pathognomonic cutaneous tetrad has been recognized: pruritus, hyperpigmentation, jaundice, and xanthomas. If all four are present, the diagnosis is generally readily confirmed. The associated pruritus has been attributed to retained bile acids and may be the presenting symptom. Patients frequently manifest a generalized brown discoloration with accentuation in sun-exposed areas, but unlike patients with hemochromatosis, there is no mucosal involvement. As with other liver diseases, the etiology of hyperpigmentation is poorly understood. Xanthomas are produced by the accumulation of lipid-laden histiocytes within the skin [9–12]. Several patterns of xanthoma exist and though each pattern frequently correlates with a specific lipid abnormality, many of these patterns also occur in the setting of normal plasma lipids. Examples of each pattern have been reported with PBC, although xanthelasmas, which develop around the eyes, are the most common [9–11]. Curiously, though cholesterol may be mild to moderately elevated in PBC, there is no correlation between the development of xanthomas in PBC and the level of cholesterol [11]. In fact, lesions may regress despite progression of disease. Unfortunately, each of these skin changes is generally nonspecific and rarely are all four clues simultaneously present.

Yet, there are other cutaneous changes which have also been reported with PBC. Believed to be autoimmune in etiology, PBC may coexist with a number of other autoimmune disorders, most commonly Sjogren's syndrome (SS) [11]. Patients frequently complain of dry eyes or mouth. Damage of the lacrimal and salivary glands has been attributed to an alteration in the immune system similar to that seen in chronic graft versus host disease (cGVH) [9,11]. Though less common than SS, patients may also develop skin changes indistinguishable from lichen planus (LP) and systemic sclerosis, which are also identical to those found in cGVH [9,11]. The most common form of systemic sclerosis to be associated with PBC is CREST (calcinosis cutis, Raynaud's phenomenon, esophageal dysmotility, sclerodactyly and telangiectasias), though full blown scleroderma has also been reported [11].

3.4 Viral hepatitis

Hepatitis A virus (HAV) generally causes a self-limited disease, rarely associated with skin findings. However, there are reports of HAV precipitating a serum sickness-like illness with arthralgias, arthritis and a rash, which is usually urticarial. There are also a few cases of HAV-induced cryoglobulinemia and vasculitis [1,9].

In comparison, acute hepatitis B virus (HBV) triggers a serum sickness-like illness in up to 20–30% of affected individuals and approximately 10% of those infected progress to a chronic carrier state [1,9]. The systemic and cutaneous complications of chronic HBV have been attributed an immunologic response to the infection [1]. Cases of vasculitis, most commonly systemic polyarteritis nodosa (sPAN), have been attributed to chronic or subacute HBV [13]. Up to 30% of patients with sPAN are shown to have active HBV. Generally, these individuals are systemically ill with fever, abdominal pain, hypertension and/or acute renal failure. Persistent HBV has also been implicated in two other types of vasculitis: mixed cryoglobulinemia (types II and III) and cutaneous polyarteritis nodosa (cPAN) [1,9]. Whereas mixed cryoglobulinemia (MC) frequently has systemic manifestations such as arthralgias, glomerulonephritis, neuropathy and Raynaud's, cPAN is limited to the skin. Cutaneous lesions in all three diseases reflect the size of the vessel involved. The most common cutaneous lesions seen with MC are palpable purpura, due to immune complex deposition and subsequent inflammation of the small arterioles and venules. Cutaneous ulceration, generally on the lower extremities, may result if the vascular damage is extensive. Livedo reticularis, a lacy blue mottling of skin color, may also develop in association with circulating cryoglobulins. Though livedo reticularis occurs most frequently on the lower extremities as well, it may also be generalized. Although patients with either sPAN or cPAN may develop identical purpura and punctate ulcers, cutaneous nodules and larger ulcers can also occur, since the caliber of affected vessels include larger sized arteries as well as smaller ones. Both sPAN and cPAN have also been associated with HCV infection in the absence of HBV.

Miscellaneous cutaneous conditions such as erythema multiforme, pyoderma gangrenosum and erythema nodosum have been anecdotally attributed to HBV and HCV. However, considerable evidence exists connecting the childhood illness Gianotti–Crosti with HBV infection [9,14]. Gianotti–Crosti, otherwise called papular acrodermatosis of childhood, is an asymptomatic eruption which occurs primarily in children under the age of 6 years [14]. It consists of monomorphic, variably sized, flesh-colored papules predominately on the face, extremities, palms and soles. Many patients have constitutional symptoms with malaise, low grade fever and adenopathy; some have hepatomegaly and/or splenomegaly. Though this condition was initially reported to occur with HBV infection, HBV is now only one of its infectious associations [14].

A myriad of cutaneous conditions (Table 4) have similarly been attributed to hepatitis C (HCV) since it was first identified in 1989 [3–7,15,16]. However, cause and effect have been proven in only one, mixed cryoglobulinemia (types II and III) as HCV RNA has been repeatedly documented in the cryoprecipitate (Figure 3) [7]. Most of the other cutaneous associations are presumed to be a manifestation of either immune alteration and/or liver disease triggered by HCV. Of these, acquired PCT is probably the most commonly encountered. Between 17 and 91% of cases of PCT have been associated with HCV infection, depending on geographic locality and prevalence HCV within the particular region [3,7]. Though HCV is one of the more common trigger factors, most patients with PCT and HCV generally have other comorbid factors (Table 3) present as well [2,7]. The cutaneous changes associated with these conditions are discussed above. Phlebotomy is effective in this setting, however, lesions of HCV-induced PCT, may also respond favorably to therapy for HCV without phlebotomy.

Pruritus is probably one of the other more widely accepted conditions associated with HCV. It is reported in about 15% of affected individuals [5,11,15], and patients with generalized pruritus

Table 4. Cutaneous conditions associated with HCV.

Mixed cryoglobulinemia
Pruritus
Porphyria cutanea tarda
Lichen planus
Sialadenitis
Polyarteritis nodosa
Necrolytic acral erythema

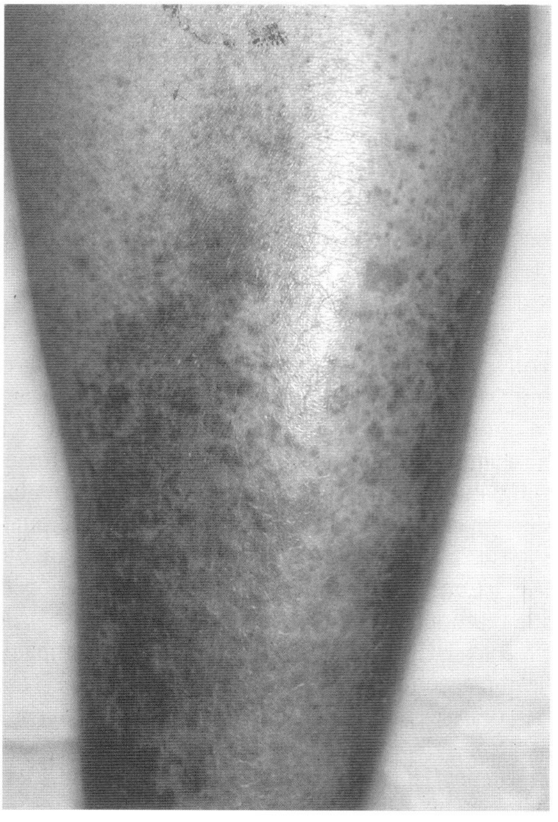

Figure 3. The leg of this patient demonstrates the classic palpable purpura of small vessel vasculitis from HCV-induced mixed cryoglobulinemia. (*For colored version, see Plate XLVI on page 588 at the end of the book.*)

should be evaluated for HCV infection as well as other metabolic abnormalities.

Though the link between LP and HCV remains somewhat controversial, up to 35% of patients with LP have some sort of chronic liver disease [6,7]. Originally attributed to chronic active hepatitis of unknown etiology, data now suggest that the most common cause of liver disease in patients with LP is HCV [7]. Depending upon geographic location, the prevalence of HCV in LP ranges from 4 to 38% [7]. Lichen planus is a chronic cutaneous disorder consisting of pruritic, polygonal, purple papules, that are generally found on the volar aspect of the wrists, though lesions may be generalized and mucosal involvement is common. The cutaneous and histologic findings are similar to those seen with cGVH disease. A lymphocytic sialadenitis similar to SS and cGVH has also been attributed to HCV infection. Though the pathogenesis of LP is unknown, it is believed to be an immunologically mediated. How HCV may trigger LP is yet unknown. Treatment options for LP include immunologic manipulation with topical corticosteroids and phototherapy.

Another rare and unique cutaneous finding that should raise the suspicion of HCV infection is the presence of necrolytic acral erythema [16]. Dusky erythematous plaques, often with blisters, develop in an acral distribution. These lesions are similar to other forms of necrolytic erythemas, such as necrolytic migratory erythema associated with glucagonomas. Anecdotal data suggest that these changes may resolve with effective treatment for HCV [16].

3.5 Wilson's disease

Wilson's disease, also known as hepatolenticular degeneration, is a genetic disorder of copper metabolism which results in excessive copper accumulation, predominately within the liver, cornea, kidneys and brain. Though not always present, two visible signs of the disease exist: azure lunula (described above) and Kayser–Fleischer rings [9]. Kayser–Fleischer rings, which may also been seen in argyria, are greenish-gold to brown rings of Descemet's membrane of the cornea.

4. CUTANEOUS DISEASES WHICH SUGGEST AN UNDERLYING LIVER DISEASE

Table 5 lists the distinct cutaneous disorders which may be found in a variety of liver diseases. Most of these conditions have been discussed above and will not be repeated. The exception is the group of diseases classified as neutrophilic dermatoses.

Neutrophilic dermatoses have been linked with disorders of the gastrointestinal tract for many years.

Table 5. Skin diseases which may suggest an underlying liver disease.

Gianotti–Crosti
Lichen planus
Mixed cryoglobulinemia
Neutrophilic dermatoses
Sweet's syndrome
Pyoderma gangrenosum
Vesiculopustular eruption of hepatobiliary disease
Polyarteritis nodosa
Porphyria cutanea tarda
Scleroderma
Xanthomas

Though they occur more commonly with inflammatory bowel disease and rheumatologic conditions, these conditions have also been reported in chronic liver disease [17–20]. The etiology of these disorders is unknown, but they may have infectious or immunologic triggers. In fact, antibiotics and immunosuppressive agents are frequently utilized to treat these conditions.

Sweet's syndrome, also called acute febrile neutrophilic dermatosis, consists of painful red to purple nodules which range in size from about 1 cm to several centimeters in diameter. The surface of the lesions is generally studded with vesiculopustules. Histologic examination reveals a sea of neutrophils, and patients frequently have a leukocytosis. The syndrome typically presents with an abrupt fever which may be accompanied by arthralgias. Though frequently idiopathic, Sweet's syndrome has been associated with both benign and malignant underlying diseases. Recent data suggest that Sweet's syndrome may also be associated with autoimmune and viral hepatitis [19–20].

Pyoderma gangrenosum (PG) has a histologic picture similar to Sweet's syndrome though the clinical lesions are discernibly different. The typical lesion of PG begins as an ordinary pustule. Rather quickly, however, it can enlarge into a large excruciatingly painful ulcer which has a classic shaggy, violaceous and overhanging border. Associated most commonly with inflammatory bowel disease and rheumatoid arthritis, cases have been attributed to chronic persistent hepatitis [18].

A distinctive vesiculopustular eruption has recently been reported in association with hepatobiliary disease [17]. Histologically, these lesions resemble PG, though clinically they are more similar to Sweet's syndrome (Figure 4). Uniformly, all reported cases occur in the setting of hepatobiliary disease of various etiologies. The pathologic mechanism, though yet undetermined, is thought to be an abnormal immunologic reaction to an infection, an autoimmune process or an unknown toxin [17]. Patients who present with one of the neutrophilic dermatoses should be evaluated for an underlying hepatic disorder.

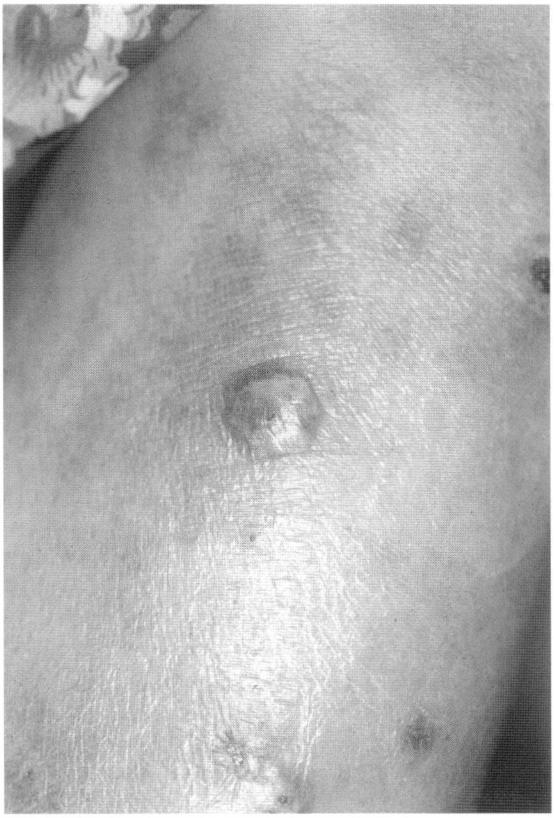

Figure 4. This patient presented with episodes of hepatic decompensation associated with skin lesions. Seen here are Sweet's syndrome-like lesions of the vesiculopustular eruption of hepatobiliary disease. (*For colored version, see Plate XLVII on page 588 at the end of the book.*)

REFERENCES

[1] Ward, S.K., Roenigk, H.H. and Gordon, K.B. (1998) Dermatologic manifestations of gastrointestinal disorders. *Gastroenterol. Clin. N. Am.* **27**, 615–636.

[2] Bonkovsky, H.L., Poh-Fitzpatrick, M., Pimstone, N., Obando, J., Di Bisceglie, A., Tattrie, C., Tortorelli, K., LeClair, P., Mercurio, M.G. and Lambrecht, R.W. (1998) Porphyria cutanea tarda, hepatitis C and HFE gene mutations in North America. *Hepatology* **27**, 1661–1669.

[3] Chuang, T.Y., Brashear, R. and Lewis, C. (1999) Porphyria cutanea tarda and hepatitis C virus: a case-control study and meta-analysis of the literature. *J. Am. Acad. Dermatol.* **41**, 31–36.

[4] Carpintero, P., DeCastro, M., Garcia-Monzon, C., Garcia-Buey, L., Borque, M.J., Garcia-Diez, A. and Moreno-Otero, R. (1997) Hepatitis C virus infection detected by RNA analysis in porphyria cutanea tarda. *J. Infect.* **34**, 61–64.

[5] Cordel, N., Chosidow, O. and Frances, C. (2000) Cutaneous disorders associated with hepatitis C virus infection. *Ann. Med. Interne (Paris)* **151**, 46–52.

[6] Hadziyannis, S.J. (1998) Skin diseases associated with hepatitis C virus infection. *J. Eur. Acad. Dermatol. Venereol.* **10**, 12–21.

[7] Pawlotsky, J.M., Dhumeaux, D. and Bagot, M. (1995) Hepatitis C virus in dermatology. *Arch. Dermatol.* **131**, 1185–1193.

[8] Bulaj, Z.J., Phillips, J.D., Ajioka, R.S., Franklin, M.R., Griffen, L.M., Guinee, D.J., Edwards, C.Q. and Kushner, J.P. (2000) Hemochromatosis genes and other factors contributing to the pathogenesis of porphyria cutanea tarda. *Blood* **95**, 1565–1571.

[9] Graham-Brown, R.A.C. and Sarkany, I. (1999) The hepatobiliary system and the skin, in *Dermatology in General Medicine*, eds. Freedberg, I.M., Eisen, A.Z., Austen, K.F., Goldsmith, L.A., Katz, S.I. and Fitzpatrick, T.B., 5th edition (McGraw-Hill, Health Professions Division, New York) pp. 1918–1929.

[10] Black, M.M., Gawkrodger, D.J., Seymour, C.A. and Weisman, K. (1998) Metabolic and nutritional disorders, in *Textbook of Dermatology*, eds. Champion, R.H., Burton, J.L., Burns, D.A. and Breathnach, S.M., 6th edition (Blackwell Science, Oxford) pp. 2577–2677.

[11] Heathcote, J. (1997) The clinical expression of primary biliary cirrhosis. *Semin. Liver Dis.* **17**, 23–33.

[12] Peters, M.G., Hoffnagle, J.H., McGarvey, C., Fox, I., Gregg, R.E. and Jones, E.A. (1989) Primary biliary cirrhosis: management of an unusual case with severe xanthomata by hepatic transplantation. *J. Clin. Gastroenterol.* **11**, 694–697.

[13] Gocke, D.J., Morgan, C., Lockshin, M., Hsu, K., Bmbardieri, S. and Christian, C.L. (1970) Association between polyarteritis and Australian antigen. *Lancet* **2**, 1149–1153.

[14] Hurwitz, S. (1993) Papulosquamous and related disorders, in *Clinical Pediatric Dermatology: A Textbook of Skin Disorders of Childhood and Adolescence*, ed. Hurwitz, S., 2nd edition (W.B. Saunders, Philadelphia, PA) pp. 105–135.

[15] Lebovics, E., Seif, F., Kim, D., Elhosseiny, A., Dworkin, B.M., Casellas, A., Clark, S. and Rosenthal, W.S. (1997) Pruritus in chronic hepatitis C: association with high serum bile acids, advanced pathology and bile duct abnormalities. *Dig. Dis. Sci.* **42**, 1094–1099.

[16] Khanna, V.J., Shieh, S., Benjamin, J., Somach, S., Zaim, M.T., Doener, Jr., W., Still, M. and Wood, G.S. (2000) Necrolytic acral erythema associated with hepatitis C: effective treatment with interferon alfa and zinc. *Arch. Dermatol.* **136**, 755–757.

[17] Magro, C.M. and Crowson, A.N. (1997) A distinctive vesiculopustular eruption associated with hepatobiliary disease. *Int. J. Dermatol.* **36**, 837–844.

[18] Koskinas, J., Raptis, I., Manika, Z. and Hadziyannis, S. (1999) Overlapping syndrome of autoimmune hepatitis and primary sclerosing cholangitis associated with pyoderma gangrenosum and ulcerative colitis. *Eur. J. Gastroenterol. Hepatol.* **11**, 1421–1424.

[19] Tan, E., Yospovitch, G., Giam, Y.C. and Tan, S.H. (2000) Bullous Sweet's syndrome associated with acute hepatitis B infection: a new association. *Br. J. Dermatol.* **143**, 914–916.

[20] Kumar, A., Helwig, K. and Komar, M.J. (1999) Sweet's syndrome in association with probably autoimmune hepatitis. *J. Clin. Gastroenterol.* **29**, 349–350.

Hepatology: A Practical Approach
B. Al Knawy, M.L. Shiffman, R.H. Wiesner (editors)

Chapter 4
Immune-Mediated Manifestations of Chronic Liver Diseases

Stephanie Straley and Norah Terrault

University of California, San Francisco, San Francisco, CA, USA

1. Multisystem Conditions 467
 1.1 Polyarteritis nodosa 467
  1.1.1 General aspects of the disease 467
  1.1.2 Pathophysiology 468
  1.1.3 Clinical features 468
  1.1.4 Diagnosis 469
  1.1.5 Management 469
  1.1.6 Prognosis 469
 1.2 Mixed cryoglobulinemia 469
  1.2.1 General aspects of the disease 469
  1.2.2 Pathophysiology 470
  1.2.3 Clinical features 470
  1.2.4 Diagnosis 470
  1.2.5 Management 470
  1.2.6 Prognosis 471
2. Musculoskeletal Diseases 471
 2.1 Pseudogout (calcium pyrophosphate crystal-induced inflammatory arthritis, CPPD) 471
  2.1.1 General aspects of the disease 471
  2.1.2 Pathophysiology 472
  2.1.3 Clinical features 472
  2.1.4 Diagnosis 472
  2.1.5 Management 473
  2.1.6 Prognosis 473
 2.2 Rheumatoid-type arthritis 473
  2.2.1 General features of the disease 473
  2.2.2 Pathophysiology 473
  2.2.3 Clinical features 474
  2.2.4 Diagnosis 474
  2.2.5 Management 474
  2.2.6 Prognosis 474
 2.3 Viral hepatitis-associated arthropathy 474
  2.3.1 General aspects 474
  2.3.2 Pathophysiology 474
  2.3.3 Clinical features 475
  2.3.4 Diagnosis 475
  2.3.5 Management 475
  2.3.6 Prognosis 476
3. Renal Diseases 476
 3.1 Glomerulonephritis 476

3.1.1 General aspects of the disease 476
3.1.2 Pathophysiology 476
3.1.3 Clinical features 477
3.1.4 Diagnosis 478
3.1.5 Management 478
3.1.5.1 Treatment of HCV-associated GN 479
3.1.5.2 Treatment of HBV-associated GN 480
3.1.6 Prognosis 480
3.2 IgA nephropathy 481
3.2.1 General aspects of the disease 481
3.2.2 Pathophysiology 481
3.2.3 Clinical features 482
3.2.4 Diagnosis 482
3.2.5 Management 482
3.2.6 Prognosis 482
4. Skin 483
4.1 Scleroderma 483
4.1.1 General aspects of the disease 483
4.1.2 Pathophysiology 483
4.1.3 Clinical features 483
4.1.4 Diagnosis 483
4.1.5 Treatment 483
4.1.6 Prognosis 483
5. Endocrine and Exocrine Glands 483
5.1 Hypothyroidism 483
5.1.1 General aspects of the disease 483
5.1.2 Pathophysiology 484
5.1.3 Clinical features 484
5.1.4 Diagnosis 484
5.1.5 Management 484
5.1.6 Prognosis 485
5.2 Sjogren's syndrome 485
5.2.1 General aspects of the disease 485
5.2.2 Pathophysiology 485
5.2.3 Clinical features 485
5.2.4 Diagnosis 486
5.2.5 Management 486
5.2.6 Prognosis 487
6. Gastrointestinal Diseases 487
6.1 Inflammatory bowel disease 487
6.1.1 General aspects of the disease 487
6.1.2 Pathophysiology 487
6.1.3 Clinical features 487
6.1.4 Diagnosis 487
6.1.5 Management 487
6.1.6 Prognosis 488
6.2 Celiac disease 488
6.2.1 General aspects of the disease 488

6.2.2 Pathophysiology 488
6.2.3 Clinical features 488
6.2.4 Diagnosis 489
6.2.5 Management 489
6.2.6 Prognosis 489
References 489

The immune-mediated manifestations of chronic liver disease are diverse in terms of the sites of involvement, clinical presentation and response to specific treatments. Recognition of these immune-mediated extrahepatic conditions is important for at least two reasons. First, extrahepatic manifestations often provide the first clue as to the presence of undiagnosed and untreated chronic liver disease. Secondly, the extrahepatic conditions, in some cases, can be more severe and associated with greater morbidity than the chronic liver disease, so prompt diagnosis and treatment are important. Table 1 lists the extrahepatic manifestations of chronic liver diseases with a well-established immune association. These are reviewed in detail by body system (see below). Conditions with a more questionable immune basis are listed in Table 2.

1. MULTISYSTEM CONDITIONS

1.1 Polyarteritis nodosa

1.1.1 General aspects of the disease

Polyarteritis nodosa is a systemic necrotizing vasculitis involving the small and medium-sized arteries. Involvement of the kidney, peripheral nervous system, skin, muscle and gastrointestinal tract predominate. Hepatitis B virus (HBV) is a well-recognized cause of PAN [1]. The prevalence of chronic HBV infection in patients with PAN varies considerably across series from 0 to 70%. Studies from the 1970s in the US estimated that 20–30% of patients with PAN had detectable HBsAg. However, this proportion has decreased to <10% and likely reflects the declining incidence of HBV in the

Table 1. Well-recognized immune-mediated manifestations of chronic liver disease.

Chronic liver disease	Specific immune-mediated condition
Alcoholic liver disease	IgA nephropathy
Autoimmune hepatitis	Autoimmune hemolytic anemia
	Hashimoto's thyroiditis
Hemochromatosis	Inflammatory arthritis (pseudogout)
HBV	Glomerulonephritis (membranous and membranoproliferative)
	Polyarteritis nodosa
	Viral-associated arthritis
HCV	Essential mixed cryoglobulinemia
	Glomerulonephritis (membranous and membranoproliferative)
	Viral-associated arthritis
PBC	Sjogren's syndrome
	Rheumatoid arthritis
	Hashimoto's thyroiditis
	Scleroderma
	Celiac disease
PSC	Inflammatory bowel disease
Wilson's disease	Inflammatory arthritis (pseudogout)

Table 2. More controversial extrahepatic manifestations of chronic liver disease with possible immune-mediated basis.

Chronic liver disease	Specific immune-mediated condition	Strength of association
HCV	Diabetes mellitus	++
	Idiopathic pulmonary fibrosis	±
	Immune-mediated thrombocytopenia	++
	Lichen planus	++
	Lymphoma (NHL)	++
	Polyarteritis nodosa	±
	Sjogren's syndrome	+++
	Thyroid dysfunction	+
HBV	Mixed essential cryoglobulinemia	+
Alcoholic liver disease	Minimal change nephropathy	±
PBC	Pulmonary fibrosis	+
Autoimmune hepatitis	Sjogren's syndrome	++
	Systemic sclerosis	+
	Celiac disease	±

population as a consequence of vaccination and modification of risk behaviors [2]. In addition to a reduced incidence of HBV-associated PAN during the past two decades, there have been significant strides made in the management of this disease with improved diagnostics and broader experience with antiviral and cytotoxic therapies.

1.1.2 Pathophysiology

Immune complexes (ICs) containing HBsAg, IgM and complement are found in the blood vessel walls of patients with PAN. This supports the etiological relationship of HBV to PAN. However, in experimental studies of serum sickness and IC-associated glomerulonephritis, only ICs of 1 million kDa or less induce such lesions, raising the issue of whether HBsAg is the critical element in disease pathogenesis. HBsAg is more than 300 million kDa without immunoglobulin. HBeAg, in contrast, circulates in free form as a 19 kDa protein and complexed with immunoglobulin is 300 kDA. Thus, HBeAg seems more likely to be the trigger PAN than HBsAg. Most but not all cases of HBV-associated PAN occur in patients with wild-type HBV infection and circulating HBeAg, which would support the importance of HBeAg [2]. There may be other circulating HBV-related antigens distinct from HBeAg that are involved. Thus, the exact antigenic triggers for HBV-associated PAN have not been clearly defined.

1.1.3 Clinical features

This is primarily a disease of adults. HBV-associated PAN has been described following acute hepatitis, typically developing weeks to several months after the clinical symptoms of acute hepatitis. The majority of patients with HBV-associated PAN, however, are unaware of their HBV status at the time of the diagnosis of PAN. The multisystem nature of PAN is a clue to its diagnosis. Initial symptoms can resemble a serum-sickness-type syndrome with fever, urticaria, purpura, polyarthritis and polyarthralgias. This prodrome evolves into a full-blown vasculitis within weeks with involvement of multiple organs. The kidney is the organ most commonly affected, typically presenting with hypertension or renal insufficiency. Involvement of the musculoskeletal and peripheral nervous systems occurs in 50–60%, gastrointestinal tract and skin in 40–45% and heart, genitourinary and central nervous systems in 20–35% of patients.

Differentiating PAN from other vasculitis syndromes is important, as optimal treatment requires the correct diagnosis. Microscopic polyangiitis, Wegner's granulomatosis, temporal arteritis and Takayasu's arteritis can be distinguished from PAN by the organ(s) involved predominantly with the disease, specific arteriography abnormalities and characteristic findings on tissue biopsy.

1.1.4 Diagnosis

There are no diagnostic laboratory tests for PAN. An elevated white cell count and ESR are frequent findings. ANCA is positive in less than 20% of patients with PAN; a positive ANCA is more suggestive of microscopic polyangiitis (p-ANCA type) or Wegner's granulomatosis (c-ANCA type). A definite diagnosis of PAN requires a biopsy of the involved tissue. If tissue cannot be easily accessed for biopsy, angiographic findings can be highly suggestive of the diagnosis. Microaneurysms, arterial stenoses and vessel occlusions involving small and medium-sized renal and abdominal arteries are consistent with the diagnosis. The diagnosis of HBV infection is established by testing for HBsAg and anti-HBc. Additionally, measurement of HBV DNA titers and HBeAg status is useful in guiding treatment decisions.

1.1.5 Management

No controlled trial has addressed the optimal treatment strategy for patients with HBV-associated PAN. However, antiviral therapies have emerged as an essential component of therapy. In several cases, spontaneous or treatment-related eradication of HBV infection led to resolution of PAN complications. Suppression of HBV replication (without loss of HBsAg) using interferon or lamivudine results in clinical improvement and stabilization [2]. There are no reports of using adefovir in patients with HBV-associated PAN but similar efficacy to lamivudine can be anticipated with lower rates of virological breakthrough with long-term therapy.

Since PAN is a relatively rare condition, no controlled trials have been conducted to compare antiviral therapy with immunosuppressive therapy. However, the accumulated experience with immunosuppressive and antiviral therapies suggests antiviral therapy alone may be sufficient in patients with mild clinical disease but combination cytotoxic therapy or plasmapheresis plus antivirals are needed for patients with more severe symptoms. Once PAN symptoms have improved, plasma exchange, corticosteroids or cytotoxic agents can be stopped and antiviral therapy alone continued until HBeAg or HBsAg seroconversion occurs (the former more frequent than the latter) [2]. The concurrent administration of antiviral therapy (lamivudine or adefovir) and immunosuppressive agents will prevent the increase in HBV viremia and associated flare of hepatitis associated with withdrawal of immunosuppression.

1.1.6 Prognosis

The natural history and prognosis of this HBV-associated disease is closely linked with suppression of viral replication. Spontaneous or drug-induced clearance of HBeAg or HBsAg and reductions in HBV viral levels are associated with improved clinical parameters. Severe untreated PAN carries a significant risk of mortality. Up to 50% may die as a consequence of their disease. Renal failure, catastrophic gastrointestinal complications (infarcts, hemorrhage and perforation) and cardiovascular failure are the major causes of morbidity and mortality. Additionally, liver-related complications were not infrequent in the era when corticosteroids and cytotoxic therapy were used primarily [1,2]. However, with the use of antiviral agents, the outcome of HBV-associated PAN appears to be much improved [2].

1.2 Mixed cryoglobulinemia

1.2.1 General aspects of the disease

Mixed cryoglobulinemia (MC) is one of the most common extrahepatic manifestations of chronic HCV infection. The relationship between HBV and MC is less well-established and will not be discussed further. The prevalence of mixed cryoglobulins in patients with chronic HCV varies from 35 to 90% in different geographical areas [3]. HCV infection is regarded as the most common condition associated with MC, and HCV testing is mandatory in any patient diagnosed with cryoglobulinemia. There is a female predominance. Patients with HCV-associated MC are older and more likely to be cirrhotic compared to patients with HCV without MC suggesting long-standing disease is a risk factor [3]. MC is considered a lymphoproliferative disorder and in 5–8% of cases may evolve to a frank B-cell malignancy.

1.2.2 Pathophysiology

There are two types of MC: mixtures of monoclonal and polyclonal Igs (type II); and polyclonal Igs only (type III). In MC, a polyclonal IgG is bound to another immunoglobulin that acts as an anti-IgG rheumatoid factor. Circulating ICs activate the complement system and ICs are deposited in small vessels. The main evidence favoring a causal relationship between HCV and MC is that the cryoprecipitates contain anti-HCV antibodies, HCV proteins and HCV RNA (the latter in 85% of cases) [3]. Additionally, the concentration of HCV RNA in the cryoprecipitates is higher than in the supernatant, so passive precipitation is unlikely. Furthermore, the response to interferon therapy provides indirect evidence of the link between HCV and MC.

The production of MCs in HCV infection is believed to be related to the immune response to HCV (antibody production), liver alterations related to chronic HCV disease, and a genetic predisposition. The virus presumably acts as the trigger for production of immunoglobulins and during the course of chronic infection, ICs form. These ICs reach lymph nodes and act as antigen-presenting cells to amplify the production of immunoglobulins, especially IgM-WA (initials of person who first identified the protein). The latter is the most common idiotype of IgM-RF found in HCV patients with MC. The production of IgM-RFs is key in the production of cryoglobulins. The production of these temperature-sensitive proteins leads to a myriad of clinical symptoms related to small-vessel vasculitis. Glomerulonephritis, peripheral neuropathy, arthritis, cerebral vasculitis and purpura can occur.

1.2.3 Clinical features

The frequency of clinical symptoms in patients with MC and chronic HCV infection is reported to be 3–15% with severe symptoms found in <5% [3]. Cutaneous manifestations are most common (~25%). Articular involvement is the second most common manifestation, present in ~20%. Joint pains are usually symmetrical and not migratory with the proximal interphalangeal (PIPs) joints, metacarpophalangeal (MCPs) joints and knees most frequently involved. Renal involvement occurs in 8–58%, depending upon the series, and the most common lesion is membranoproliferative glomerulonephritis (MPGN) (see Section 4.3). Peripheral neuropathy is reported in 8% of patients with HCV-associated MC. The classic lesion is a moderate axonal sensory polyneuropathy. These neuropathies present with pain and can evolve over years to affect motor function. Central nervous system, pulmonary and gastrointestinal involvements are rare, occurring in 2% or less of patients.

1.2.4 Diagnosis

The triad of laboratory findings in patients with MC includes detectable cryoglobulins, positive rheumatoid factor and low complement levels (C4 and CH50 notably). Methods of measuring cryoglobulins are not standardized and improper handling of the specimen may lead to false negative results. A negative test for cryoprecipitates in the right clinical setting should prompt retesting, especially if rheumatoid factor is positive. Despite the frequent finding of HCV in patients with MC, a positive test for cryoglobulins is also found in a variety of other diseases, including other chronic liver diseases. Cryoglobulins are present in 45% of patients with alcohol hepatitis and 50% of patients with autoimmune hepatitis. Exclusion of other causes of MC is important, particularly chronic infections and malignancies.

The clinical manifestations of MC are the result of a leukocytoclastic vasculitis. To make this diagnosis, a tissue biopsy is needed. The skin is frequently involved and easiest to biopsy. Pathological specimens demonstrate a mixed inflammatory infiltrate with a predominance of mononuclear cells in the walls of the affected vessels, with some patients also having fibrinoid necrosis of the arteriolar walls with vascular thrombi.

1.2.5 Management

In asymptomatic patients with HCV and MC, the management should be the same as HCV-infected patients without MC. In patients with symptomatic MC disease, antiviral therapy is indicated [3,4]. Studies have shown a close relationship between suppression of viral replication and resolution of MC symptoms, so the primary goal of therapy is viral eradication. To this end, the most effective antiviral therapy should be used. Although there are no published data on the use of pegylated interferon and ribavirin, this would be the treatment of choice in most patients. The available data using standard interferon and ribavirin indicate that combination therapy is superior to interferon monotherapy. However, relapse is common when treatment is discontinued and longer courses of treatment (at least 24 months) may be needed for management of symptoms. Maintenance therapy has been used successfully in some patients, especially those with cutaneous complications of MC. Additionally, studies have shown that clinical improvement can be seen even when there is only a partial virological and biochemical response to antiviral therapy. For patients who are intolerant or unable to take interferon-based therapy, ribavirin monotherapy may be considered.

1.2.6 Prognosis

Eradication of HCV viremia results in resolution of cryoglobulinemia and many of the associated clinical manifestations; clinical improvement and stabilization can be achieved with partial virological responses. The reversibility of the clinical manifestations may be related to the severity of the disease at the time of treatment initiation and the specific organ involved. HCV-infected patients with MC-associated peripheral neuropathy appear to be relatively resistant to the effects of antiviral therapy but this may be related to an insufficient duration of antiviral therapy [3]. The risk of end-stage renal disease in patients with MC-associated GN is 14% in the first year after diagnosis [5]. Since MC is associated with long-standing HCV disease, liver-related complications may be more frequent in these patients and serve as a competing cause of mortality. Studies comparing the natural history and outcome of patients with HCV and clinically apparent MC disease versus patients with HCV without MC disease are needed.

2. MUSCULOSKELETAL DISEASES

Pseudogout, rheumatoid arthritis (RA) (erosive polyarthritis), non-erosive polyarthritis and cryoglobulinemia-associated mono- or pauciarticular arthritis are seen in patients with chronic liver disease. Pseudogout is found in patients with hemochromatosis (HHC) and Wilson's disease; RA in patients with primary biliary cirrhosis (PBC), autoimmune cholangitis and autoimmune hepatitis; and non-erosive polyarthritis and monoarthritis in patients with chronic HBV and HCV infection. The pathogenesis of these inflammatory arthropathies varies considerably from one disease to another. The arthropathies associated with HHC, PBC and viral hepatitis will be reviewed in detail.

2.1 Pseudogout (calcium pyrophosphate crystal-induced inflammatory arthritis, CPPD)

2.1.1 General aspects of the disease

Arthritis is the most common extrahepatic clinical manifestation of HHC and can precede symptoms of liver disease. In studies of patients with clinically apparent HHC, the prevalence of arthritis is approximately 50% [6]. In a recent study of persons newly identified as homozygous for the C282Y mutation in population screening studies, 82% complained of chronic joint pain and 47% had a prior diagnosis of arthritis and these complaints tended to be more common than age- and gender-matched controls (62% and 38% with joint pain and an arthritis diagnosis, respectively) [7].

Given the frequency of this extrahepatic complication in patients with HHC, screening for HHC should be considered in any person presenting with crystal-induced arthritis. One study found that in 11% of persons with HHC, arthritis was the primary clinical condition leading to the diagnosis of iron overload. In patients screened in a rheumatology clinic, the prevalence of HHC was 1.5%, a prevalence much higher than the general population. Among 128 patients recruited from an orthopedic clinic, 1.6% were homozygous for the C282Y mutation and 3.1% were compound heterozygotes for the C282Y/H63D mutations, indicating a 3.4 higher relative risk than European population controls [8].

2.1.2 Pathophysiology

The trigger for this inflammatory arthritis is the accumulation of calcium pyrophosphate crystals within the cartilage and synovium. Iron deposition in synovial lining cells is believed to inhibit pyrophosphatase leading to calcium pyrophosphate crystal accumulation. The release of these crystals into the joint space is followed by phagocytosis by neutrophils, which initiates the inflammatory response. The normal aging of cartilage also favors calcium pyrophosphate deposition and can compound the symptoms in patients with HHC.

2.1.3 Clinical features

In HHC-associated arthritis, the second and third MCPs and proximal PIPs are most commonly affected. Involvement may be confined to the hands and wrist, but may also progress to larger joints such as the knees and hips. The arthritis is typically polyarticular and symmetrical but unilateral presentations can occur. Early in the disease course, the symptoms are mainly pain and stiffness with objective evidence of joint inflammation seen later. Joint space loss (particularly at the MCP joints), subchondral cysts and squaring of the metacarpal heads are seen on plain X-rays. While joint swelling, deformity, restricted range of motion and nodule formation are seen, synovial thickening is atypical (in contrast to RA). Acute episodes can be superimposed on chronic joint changes and acute episodes may be confused with gout.

2.1.4 Diagnosis

Patients may present with acute, subacute, chronic or acute superimposed on chronic arthritis (Figure 1). In patients with HHC, pseudogout should be the first consideration but other causes of arthritis common in the population must be considered (osteoarthritis, gout, infectious arthritis). Involvement of the MCPs and PIPs would be typical, although larger joints can be involved. Radiological clues include the presence of punctate or linear calcifications in the fibrocartilaginous joint menisci or articular hyaline cartilage, and in the absence of joint fluid analysis can be used to make a presumptive diagnosis of pseudogout [6]. Other radiological findings include loss of joint space and presence of osteophytes. Definitive diagnosis is based on synovial fluid analysis and the identification of short, rhomboid-shaped and positively birefringent crystals. For the patient with an acute monoarthritis,

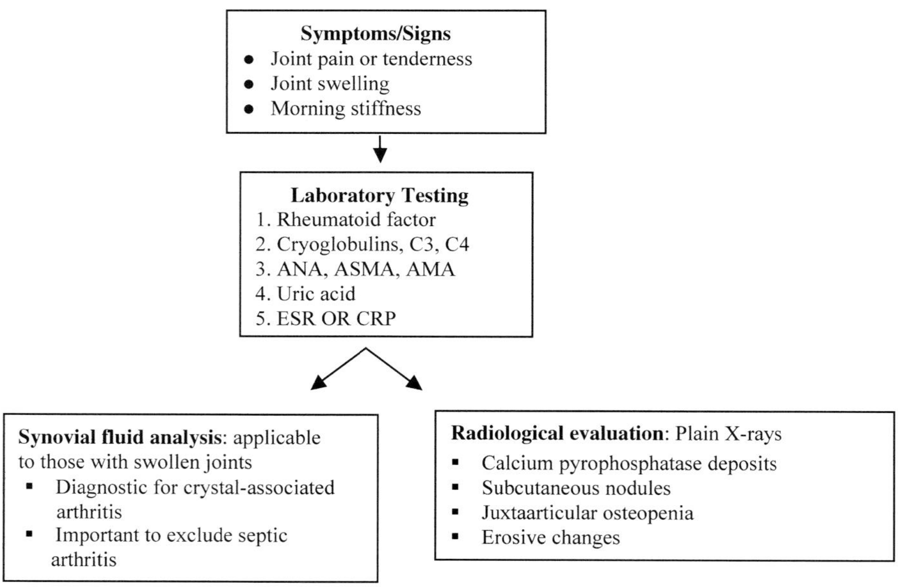

Figure 1. Patient with chronic liver disease and suspected arthropathy diagnostic algorithm.

aspiration of the joint is always indicated, as infection must be excluded.

In patients with newly diagnosed CPPD arthritis, testing for underlying metabolic conditions is important. This is especially true for patients with early onset, atypical arthralgias, a family history of HHC, or other HHC-associated conditions (atypical cardiac disease, diabetes mellitus, elevated liver enzymes and/or hepatomegaly). Patients should be screened with fasting iron studies. Those who have a transferrin saturation >45% should undergo further evaluation with ferritin, genetic testing and possibly a liver biopsy with quantitation of iron content. On a final note, Wilson's disease is another chronic liver disease that is associated with pseudogout, and testing for this condition should be performed in any patient under the age of 40 years.

2.1.5 Management

Therapies for patients with HHC-associated crystal-induced arthritis are the same as for patients without HHC with pseudogout. Joint immobilization and non-steroid anti-inflammatory drugs are the mainstay of treatment. Intraarticular corticosteroids and colchicine are also commonly used. For patients with severe polyarticular symptoms, a short course of systemic corticosteroids may be necessary.

The mainstay of treatment for HHC is phlebotomy. The goals of therapy are a normal ferritin level and a transferrin saturation below 50%. Patients should avoid vitamin C, which can increase iron absorption. Genetic testing of all first-degree relatives is recommended.

2.1.6 Prognosis

Aggressive iron reduction, while the mainstay of therapy, does not always result in resolution of joint symptoms. Earlier studies found that symptoms gradually worsened in 75%, improved in 12.5% and remained unchanged in 12.5% [6]. Studies did not distinguish between acute pseudogout versus chronic or acute on chronic presentations. The latter may be less responsive to iron reduction therapy as structural abnormalities and osteoarthritis are present. The additional difficulty in defining the natural history of HHC-associated pseudogout relates to the increasing prevalence of non-HHC-associated pseudogout in an aging population. Thus, a lack of resolution of joint symptoms with phlebotomy may be related to concomitant age-related joint disease. Nonetheless, phlebotomy is an important component of treatment, both to potentially reduce joint symptoms and future joint injury as well as to prevent damage to other organs.

2.2 Rheumatoid-type arthritis

2.2.1 General features of the disease

Approximately 25% of patients with PBC will have a positive rheumatoid factor but only a small proportion have symptoms compatible with RA. However, a higher than expected frequency of RA is found in patients with PBC compared to the general population (4–42 versus 0.2–2.1%, respectively) [9]. PBC shares with RA a predilection for females and clinical disease onset in the fourth and fifth decades of life.

Among patients with RA, liver test abnormalities are present in 18–50% of patients, which is higher than in the general population [10]. However, the interpretation of abnormal alkaline phosphatase levels in this population may be problematic as the source may be bone or liver. Liver biopsy studies report heterogeneous histological findings including non-specific hepatitis, steatosis, nodular regenerative hyperplasia as well as normal histology.

2.2.2 Pathophysiology

The pathogenesis of RA involves a combination of innate immune activation, a genetic predisposition and an adaptive immune response directed against autologous antigens. Similar factors are of importance in the pathogenesis of PBC, but with the bile ductules being the target rather than the synovium. A specific pathogenetic link between PBC and RA has not been elucidated.

2.2.3 Clinical features

The clinical features of RA in the setting of PBC do not appear to differ from those in RA patients without PBC. The arthritis is usually symmetrical and involves multiple joints with greater involvement of small and large joints of the extremities than the axial skeleton. Morning stiffness, the presence of rheumatoid nodules and constitutional symptoms further support the diagnosis.

2.2.4 Diagnosis

The diagnosis of RA is based upon a combination of clinical, radiological and laboratory findings (Figure 1). Rheumatoid factor lacks specificity and is elevated in 5% of healthy persons and in a greater proportion of patients with certain chronic liver diseases (i.e., PBC, autoimmune hepatitis, HBV, HCV). In the right clinical setting, however, a high titer of rheumatoid factor is highly suggestive. ESR and CRP are usually elevated. Synovial fluid analysis is consistent with an inflammatory arthritis but is non-specific. Characteristic radiological signs include juxtaarticular osteopenia, loss of articular cartilage and bone erosions.

2.2.5 Management

The management of patients with RA and chronic liver disease is similar to that of patients with RA alone with a few caveats. Drug hepatotoxicity induced by non-steroid anti-inflammatory agents and methotrexate is well recognized. Persons with pre-existing liver disease, especially those with advanced stages of fibrosis, may be at a higher risk of drug-induced hepatotoxicity. Thus, patients with RA and chronic liver disease may have fewer treatment options than patients without chronic liver disease, and greater vigilance in following liver tests during treatment is required.

Though data are limited, there is no evidence that treatment directed at the underlying liver disease influences the course of RA. In patients with PBC and joint symptoms, the use of ursodeoxycholic acid has no measurable effect on the rates of resolution of joint symptoms over a 2-year treatment period [11].

2.2.6 Prognosis

Whether the natural history of RA in patients with and without PBC differs is unknown. A fluctuating course over decades is typical of RA. Predictors of joint deformities and disability include a markedly elevated ESR, radiographic evidence of bone erosions, the presence of rheumatoid nodules, high titer of rheumatoid factor, persistent inflammation and advanced age at time of onset.

2.3 Viral hepatitis-associated arthropathy

2.3.1 General aspects

Arthalgias are a frequently cited extrahepatic manifestation of chronic viral hepatitis, but arthritis is uncommon. Arthalgias and arthritis are more frequently linked with chronic HCV than chronic HBV infection. An estimated 2–20% of patients with HCV have complaints of arthritis versus 5% of patients with HBV infection. While these prevalence rates are higher than the general population, controlled studies are lacking.

At least two types of arthritis are reported in association with chronic HCV infection: an RA-like polyarthritis and a less common mono-oligoarthritis involving medium-sized and large joints. The latter form is associated with the presence of serum cryoglobulins and has a more intermittent course. Chronic HBV has been associated with arthritis, most frequently an RA-like polyarthritis. HBV-associated PAN can present with arthritis but other organ involvement is present. Whether HBV is a cause of RA remains unknown. Case reports of acute followed by chronic erosive polyarthritis in patients with acute HBV infection are suggestive of an association but case control studies are lacking.

2.3.2 Pathophysiology

The proposed immune mechanisms underlying arthritis in patients with cryoglobulinemia and PAN have been described (see Section 4.1). The pathophysiology of arthritis in patients with viral hepatitis who lack cryoglobulins is poorly understood. In HCV, HCV RNA has been detected in synovial fluid of patients with arthritis suggesting the possibility of direct invasion of synovial cells, with the virus eliciting a local inflammatory response and cytokine-associated or IC-type disease, particularly in genetically susceptible individuals [12]. An increased prevalence of autoantibodies in patients with chronic viral hepatitis (especially HCV) is also evident [13]. The positive correlation between viral eradication with interferon therapy and resolution of arthritis in some patients with chronic viral hepatitis (HBV and HCV) supports the contention that the virus plays a pathogenic role, either directly or indirectly in this form of arthritis.

2.3.3 Clinical features

If multisystem disease is present, cryoglobulinemia (HCV-associated) and PAN (HBV-associated) need to be considered in the differential diagnosis. The majority of patients with viral-associated arthropathy have evidence of a symmetric polyarthritis, but up to one-third of patients may have a mono- or oligoarticular arthritis. In cryoglobulinemia-associated arthritis, the presenting picture is more likely to be a mono- or oligoarthritis involving the medium and large joints [12]. The level of cryoglobulins is correlated with the presence or absence of symptoms. In one study of 114 patients with HCV and cryoglobulinemia, the cryocrit was more than 0.5% in 72% of arthritis cases (mean concentration 2.6%) versus 50% of patients without rheumatologic symptoms ($p = 0.02$) [14]. In patients without cryoglobulins, the arthritis is usually RA-like involving small joints [15]. Morning stiffness is common, but rheumatoid nodules and radiographic evidence of erosions are lacking and the presence of these latter findings should prompt consideration of coexisting RA.

2.3.4 Diagnosis

In patients with known chronic viral hepatitis, screening for serum cryoglobulins should be performed for those with arthalgias or arthritis (Figure 1). In patients who present with RA-type symptoms, HCV and HBV should be in the differential diagnosis, especially when the arthritis is non-erosive. RA is often misdiagnosed in patients with viral hepatitis, as rheumatoid factor positivity is prevalent in patients with some chronic liver diseases. Careful evaluation of these patients to determine whether other criteria for RA are present will help to clarify whether a patient has two distinct diseases, RA and viral hepatitis or an RA-like polyarthritis. Testing for the presence of antikeratin antibodies may be useful also. In one study, antikeratin antibodies were detected in 20/33 patients with RA (60.6%) versus 2/25 patients (8%) with HCV-associated RA-like arthritis ($p < 0.0001$).

2.3.5 Management

For patients with viral-associated arthropathy, the management strategy focuses on both symptom control as well as consideration of antiviral therapy. Control of symptoms may require non-steroidal anti-inflammatory drugs, hydroxychloroquine, sulfasalazine and low doses of corticosteroids, even in those who respond to antiviral therapy. Corticosteroids should be used with caution as an increase in viremia occurs in association with their use and this may exacerbate the underlying liver disease or impact on the subsequent response to antiviral therapy. Disease-modifying antirheumatic drugs are not necessary as the arthritis is non-erosive [12]. Antiviral therapy is most applicable to patients with viral-associated arthropathy and the presence of cryoglobulins. In HBV-infected patients with cryoglobulinemia, lamivudine and adefovir would be first-line antiviral agents; interferon should be avoided due to its potential to exacerbate autoimmune conditions. In HCV patients who have positive serum cryoglobulins, treatment with interferon and ribavirin leads to a reduction in symptoms associated with suppression of virus and circulating cryoglobulins. Longer-term suppressive therapy may be required for those patients who fail to achieve viral eradication with a defined course of therapy.

In the absence of cryoglobulins, the applicability of antiviral therapy is less clear. In patients with chronic HCV infection who require antiviral therapy for management of their liver disease, such therapy is reasonable to consider. Antiviral therapy may be considered in selected cases of isolated arthritis that are unresponsive to other drugs. In the largest published series of HCV-infected patients with arthritis treated with antiviral therapy, out of 25 anti-HCV positive, HCV RNA positive patients (12 with cryoglobulinemia, 13 without detectable cryoglobulins), 11 (44%) experienced a significant improvement in arthritis-related symptoms within 6–12 weeks of initiating treatment with interferon (alfa-2a or 2b; 3 MU three times weekly) [15]. All patients had been previously treated with non--steroidal anti-inflammatory drugs ($N = 22$), corticosteroids ($N = 12$), gold salts ($N = 3$), methotrexate ($N = 4$), azathioprine ($N = 1$) hydroxychloroquine ($N = 3$), sulfasalazine ($N = 2$), and colchicine ($N = 2$) alone or in combination, and in only three patients (12%) was a satisfactory response obtained. Sustained remission of arthritic symptoms appeared to more likely in those obtaining a sustained virological response. In this series, patients with cryoglobulinemia tended to respond better than patients without cryoglobulinemia (58% versus 31%) but the difference was not statistically significant [15]. Despite these encouraging results, the potential of interferon to exacerbate arthritis and other autoimmune conditions is well known, and careful consideration of the risks and benefits of interferon therapy should be discussed with the patient prior to initiating therapy [12]. The role of antiviral therapy in patients with HBV infection and arthritis without cryoglobulinemia is similarly unclear. However, since non-interferon therapies (i.e., lamivudine, adefovir) are available for suppression of HBV viremia, undertaking a trial of antiviral therapy is less risky in HBV than HCV patients.

2.3.6 Prognosis

Viral-associated arthritis usually runs a relatively benign course that, in contrast to RA, is typically non-deforming and not associated with articular bony erosions. Nonetheless, symptoms can be debilitating for some patients. Prognosis for HCV and HBV patients with cryoglobulinemia-associated arthritis, who achieve a sustained virological response to antiviral therapy, is good since symptoms generally resolve with eradication of virus.

3. RENAL DISEASES

The most common immune-mediated renal diseases identified in patients with chronic liver disease are membranous glomerulonephritis (MGN), MPGN, mesangial proliferative glomerulonephritis, IgA nephrophathy, and the vasculitic syndromes, including PAN and mixed essential cryoglobulinemia. PAN and cryoglobulinemia have been previously reviewed (see Section 4.1 above). MGN and MPGN are most frequently associated with HBV and HCV infections. IgA nephropathy is most consistently linked with alcoholic liver disease. Table 3 summarizes the different renal lesions that have been linked with chronic liver diseases, including those with and without a postulated immune-mediated mechanism of injury.

3.1 Glomerulonephritis

3.1.1 General aspects of the disease

MGN and MPGN are the most common forms of glomerulopathy associated with HBV infection. The prevalence of these glomerulopathies mirrors generally the prevalence of HBV infection in the world. HBV-associated MPGN is seen in both adults and children but a more severe clinical form is seen in adults [1,16]. The past prevalence of HBsAg among children presenting with MGN was 20% in the US, 42–60% in Western Europe, and >80% in Eastern Europe, African and South Asia. However, there has been a decline in HBV-associated GN over the past 1–2 decades, likely reflecting the declining incidence of HBV infection in endemic and other regions of the world in relationship to vaccination.

Cryoglobulinemic GN is the most common type of renal disease associated with HCV infection, although non-cryoglobulinemic MPGN is recognized. Renal involvement in patients with MC is reported in 2–50%. In the US, 10–20% of MPGN is HCV-associated; in Japan and other countries in Southeast Asia as many as 60% of adults with MPGN have HCV-associated disease [3,16]. The higher prevalence in Japan and other Southeast Asian countries likely reflects the higher prevalence of HCV in those countries. In one study from Southern Europe, ~80% of patients with cryoglobulinemia-associated MPGN were HCV RNA positive versus 25% of patients with non-cryoglobulinemia MPGN.

3.1.2 Pathophysiology

ICs are a central feature of the viral-associated glomerulopathies. In the classic model, circulating

Table 3. Renal diseases in patients with underlying chronic liver disease.

Chronic liver disease	Specific renal lesions associated with each liver disease	
	Strong evidence for association	Questionable association
Immune-mediated mechanism		
HCV	Membranoproliferative GN (with/without cryoglobulinemia)	Polyarteritis nodosa
	Membranoproliferative GN	IgA nephropathy
		Focal glomerulosclerosis
HBV	Polyarteritis nodosa	IgA nephropathy
	Mesangial proliferative GN	Focal glomerulosclerosis
	Membranoproliferative GN (with/without cryoglobulinemia)	Minimal change nephropathy
	Membranoproliferative GN	
Alcoholic liver disease	IgA nephropathy	
Non-immune mechanisms		
PBC	Renal tubular acidosis	IgA nephropathy
Autoimmune cholangitis	Interstitial nephritis	
Wilson's disease	Renal tubular acidosis	
Polycystic liver disease	Polycystic kidney disease	

ICs involving viral antigens and host antiviral antibodies form in the circulation and are captured in the glomeruli thereby setting off a cascade of events leading to inflammation and injury. In patients with HCV-associated glomerulopathies, IC-containing HCV antigens, HCV antibodies and complement (mainly C3) have been identified in the mesangium and subendothelium. However, viral antigen and antibodies are not always identified. Similar pathophysiological processes underlie HBV-associated GN.

An alternative model has the ICs forming *in situ* when viral antigens become bound to glomerular structures and trigger the inflammatory cascade. Viral proteins may also cause inflammatory renal disease through the synthesis of various mediators that may cause sclerosis and worsen the glomerulopathy. A direct cytopathic effect of viral proteins has also been proposed but the mechanism of glomerular injury has not been defined. Finally, another proposed mechanism is the induction of autoantibodies by the virus that cross-reacts with specific glomerular antigens. Portosystemic shunting related to advanced liver disease may enhance the systemic circulation of IC and the deposition in the glomeruli. However, the latter is unlikely to be a major factor in the pathogenesis of GN, as the severity of renal disease is not correlated with that of liver disease.

3.1.3 Clinical features

MGN usually presents as nephrotic syndrome or with non-nephrotic range proteinuria. Microscopic hematuria is frequently present; macroscopic hematuria is rare. Hypertension is present in less than 25% at presentation [16]. MGN associated with HBV infection affects children more frequently than adults and among children there is a predilection for the condition to affect males. HCV-associated MGN appears to be more common in adults. Liver tests are more likely to be elevated in viral-associated than idiopathic MGN patients. There is no correlation between severity of renal disease and liver disease.

MPGN may or may not be associated with cryoglobulinemia. Cryoglobulinemia-associated MPGN (predominantly due to HCV) presents most commonly with microscopic hematuria and non-nephrotic range proteinuria. Approximately 50% will have some degree of renal insufficiency at presentation and 20–25% will present acutely with hypertension and nephritic syndrome [16]. While epidemiological studies indicate cryoglobulinemia is more common in patients with longer duration of HCV disease, the severity of the renal disease is frequently disproportionate to that of the liver disease.

Extra-renal symptoms related to cryoglobulinemia involving the skin, peripheral nerves and joints are present in less than half of the patients.

3.1.4 Diagnosis

In any patient presenting with proteinuria and/or microscopic hematuria, the diagnosis of viral-associated GN must be considered. Initial steps are focused on confirming the glomerular origin of the urine abnormalities and characterizing the degree of renal dysfunction (Figure 2). Viral serology is an essential component of the work-up and should be obtained in all patients with suspected glomerular disease regardless of whether risk factors for viral hepatitis are present or absent. In immunocompetent persons, anti-HCV testing is sufficient to exclude HCV infection. However, measurement of HCV RNA is recommended to exclude infection in immunocompromised patients and assess for viremia in HCV antibody positive patients. HBsAg and anti-HBc are the screening tests used to assess for HBV infection and the vast majority of patients with HBV-associated GN have serological markers of chronic HBV infection and, in earlier reported series, 60–80% of patients had HBeAg. In patients with MPGN, other common laboratory abnormalities include positive rheumatoid factor, reduced C3 and C4 levels and elevated levels of c1q binding assay. Cryoglobulins may be present. In contrast, patients with MGN typically have normal complement levels and lack cryoglobulins and rheumatoid factor.

Since more than one type of GN is associated with HBV and HCV, a renal biopsy is frequently required to make a specific diagnosis. Moreover, since patients with viral hepatitis can develop renal diseases unrelated to their viral status, a renal biopsy is frequently needed to confirm the diagnosis. Additionally, the renal biopsy provides prognostic information that may be important in determining the urgency and aggressiveness of treatment.

3.1.5 Management

There is a paucity of controlled trials of sufficient sample size to inform physicians regarding the optimal treatment strategy for viral-associated GN. Additionally, interpretation of available studies is hampered by heterogeneity of renal lesions within treatment groups. Antiviral therapy, however, is increasingly viewed as the primary therapy,

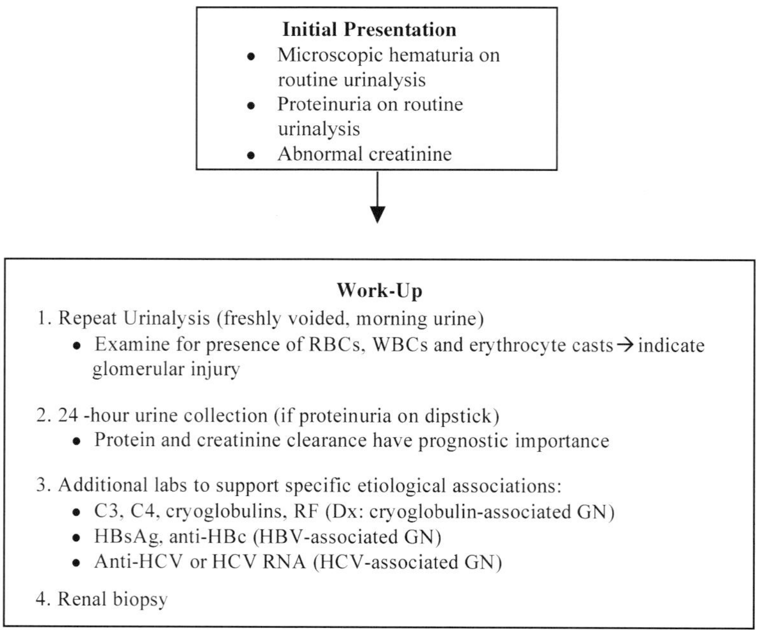

Figure 2. Diagnostic approach to a patient with chronic liver disease and suspected renal disease.

especially in patients with cryoglobulinemia GN and HBV-associated GN [2,3]. The use of antiviral therapy in these specific diseases is supported by the demonstration of clinical improvement in renal status in association with virological response, i.e., decline in levels of HCV RNA or HBV DNA. The use of antiviral therapy in the management of non-cryoglobulinemic GN (typically associated with HCV) is more controversial as the outcomes of treatment have not been consistently positive.

3.1.5.1 Treatment of HCV-associated GN. Combination treatment using interferon (standard or pegylated) and ribavirin is approved for the treatment of patients with chronic HCV infection (Figure 3). In the treatment of patients with HCV-associated cryoglobulinemic GN, standard interferon has been effective in some but not all patients [3]. Genotype and pretreatment viral load likely influence response to treatment, similar to patients with chronic HCV without GN. Studies to data have been of limited sample size and thus, preclude evaluation of predictors of response. Clinical remission of proteinuria and hematuria and stabilization of renal function correlates with the decline in HCV RNA levels and subsequent clearance of virus in most studies. Unfortunately, relapse following discontinuation of antiviral therapy may be more common in this patient population than in chronic HCV-infected patients without GN. Use of ribavirin in combination with interferon increases efficacy and is recommended in patients with preserved renal function. There are no published studies using pegylated interferons but since they are more efficacious than standard interferons in patients without GN, the use of pegylated interferons in patients with renal disease may enhance response rates. As with other severe or rapidly progressive end-organ complications related to cryoglobulinemia (see Section 4.1), combination therapy with cytotoxic drugs and sometimes cryoapheresis followed by antiviral therapy may be required. Regarding the impact of interferon in preventing progression of renal damage, results are inconsistent. Response to treatment in terms of proteinuria and stabilization of renal function may depend upon the stage of renal disease at the time of initiation of antiviral therapy. For patients unable to tolerate interferon, ribavirin monotherapy may be considered.

The efficacy of interferon-based therapy in HCV-infected patients with non-cryoglobulinemic GN (membranous, membranoproliferative and mesangial proliferative) is less consistent. Several case

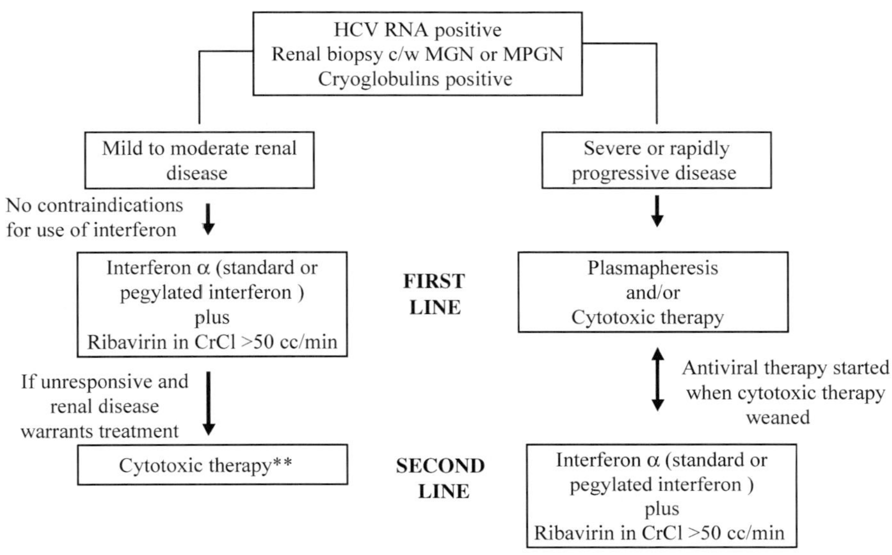

** Cyclophosphamide superior to corticosteroids in controlled trials

Figure 3. Treatment of HCV-associated glomerulonephritis.

series report an improvement in proteinuria that correlates with virological response, supporting the use of antiviral therapy. However, this response is not uniform. Consequently there may be a greater role for combination antiviral and cytotoxic therapy in these patients. If a combination approach is undertaken, experts recommend introducing antiviral therapy as the immunosuppressive therapy is being weaned in order to prevent steroid-induced flares of viremia.

3.1.5.2 Treatment of HBV-associated GN. Resolution of renal disease seems closely related to elimination of viral replication (Figure 4). While mixed results were reported with the use of interferon, more recent case reports using lamivudine are encouraging. In patients with mild disease, antiviral therapy alone may be successful. However, use of antiviral therapy does not prohibit the use of cytotoxic therapy. In fact, cytotoxic drugs and sometimes plasmapheresis followed by antiviral therapy may be needed for those with severe or rapidly progressive disease. Whenever cytotoxic drugs are used (especially prednisone), concurrent use of antiviral agents is recommended to prevent a flare in viremia, and possible worsening of liver disease that can occur when cytotoxic drugs are weaned or withdrawn [2].

In patients with chronic HBV disease, lamivudine and adefovir have been shown to reduce serum HBV DNA levels by 3–4 $\log_{10}$ within the first 3–6 months of treatment. Interferon may achieve viral load reductions more rapidly but the drug is associated with more frequent side effects, and viral responses are less uniform. Thus, oral nucleoside analogues may be the drugs of choice in the management of viral-associated GN. Both lamivudine and adefovir doses need to be adjusted for renal insufficiency.

3.1.6 Prognosis

In children with HBV-associated MGN, a high rate of spontaneous remission is seen; 85% of children are in remission 2 years after diagnosis and 95% after 7 years. Clinical remission typically occurs in conjunction with reduced levels of viral replication

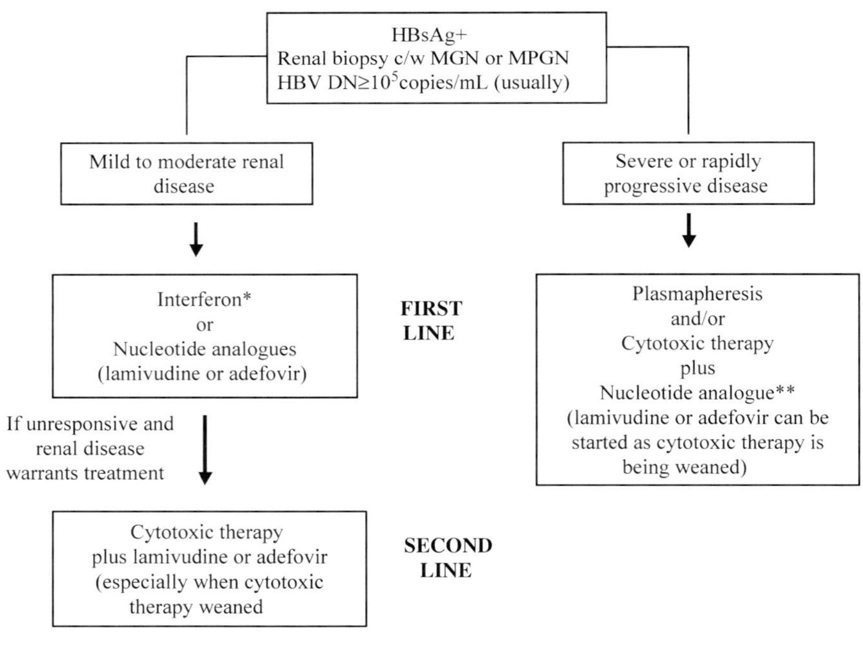

* If no contraindications; ** doses must be adjusted if renal dysfunction

Figure 4. Treatment of HBV-associated glomerulonephritis.

related to HBeAg seroconversion. The spontaneous remission rate appears to be lower for adults. While antiviral therapy is recommended for both HBV-associated MGN and MPGN, response to antiviral therapy appears to be better for those with MGN versus MPGN.

In patients with HCV-associated MPGN, approximately 10% will ultimately progress to chronic renal failure. Another 30% will have a more indolent course with minimal evidence of progression in renal disease over several decades despite persistent urinary abnormalities (hematuria or proteinuria). Spontaneous partial or complete remissions occur, possibly in up to 30% of patients whereas the final 20–30% of patients will have intermittent exacerbations and remissions. Among treated patients, the severity of disease and rate of progression is closely linked with the success of viral suppression or eradication.

3.2 IgA nephropathy

3.2.1 General aspects of the disease

IgA nephropathy is an IC-mediated glomerulonephritis defined immunohistochemically by the presence of glomerular IgA deposits in the mesangial region of the glomeruli. Primary IgA nephropathy is now recognized to be the most common form of glomerulonephritis in the world [17]. Purported secondary causes of IgA nephropathy are numerous (Table 4). Of the several different chronic liver diseases linked with IgA nephropathy, alcoholic liver disease is the most frequently cited. Experimental models support a role for alcohol and possibly nutritional deficiencies in disease pathogenesis. In an autopsy series from the 1980s, 64% of those consuming alcohol regularly had evidence of IgA nephropathy; cirrhosis was not a prerequisite and was present in only 9% of cases [16]. Whether the incidence of the alcohol-associated IgA nephropathy has changed in recent decades is unknown.

Table 4. Secondary causes of IgA nephropathy.

Liver diseases: alcoholic, PBC, cryptogenic, HBV
Luminal GI diseases: Crohn's disease, ulcerative colitis, celiac disease
Respiratory diseases: sarcoidosis, idiopathic pulmonary hemosiderosis, cystic fibrosis, bronchiolitis obliterans
Neoplasia: carcinoma of lung, larynx, pancreas; mycosis fungoides
Infectious: chronic schistosomiasis, HIV, leprosy
Diseases of skin: dermatitis herpetiformis, psoriasis

Source: Ref. [4].

3.2.2 Pathophysiology

The pathogenic mechanisms underlying the relationship between IgA nephropathy and chronic liver disease are not completely known [16,17]. The glomerular deposits in IgA nephropathy are of IgA1 subtype exclusively. IgA1 is produced by plasma cells, the gastrointestinal and respiratory tracts. A defect of the mucosal immune system with a possible compensatory increase in the production of IgA1 by the bone marrow may contribute to increased circulating IgA1 levels. In patients with IgA nephropathy, a defect in galactosylation of IgA1 is seen and mesangial cells may possess a receptor for IgA1 with a high specificity for the undergalactosylated type. Hepatic clearance of IgA1 is decreased and whether the asialoglycoprotein receptor in the liver recognizes and effectively clears undergalactosylated IgA1 has not been fully defined. Once deposited in the kidney, IgA1 ICs are associated with glomerular inflammation. The activation of complement, cytokines and growth factors likely plays a central role in disease pathogenesis and renal damage.

IgA production and catabolism is altered in patients with alcoholic liver disease. Alcohol is proposed to increase the permeability of the intestinal mucosa leading to increased circulating levels of IgA. Patients with liver disease have impaired immune responses leading to increased production of IgA in the lamina propria with increased secretion and absorption into the circulation, and reduced clearance of IgA and IgA IC from the circulation via inhibition of the hepatic asialoglycoprotein receptor, which is the main catabolic pathway for IgA. Additionally, the deposition of IgA in the space of Disse leads to further impairment in blood flow, which is important for IgA degradation.

3.2.3 Clinical features

In the early stages of the disease, the majority of patients are asymptomatic. Indeed, unless urinalysis is performed, this diagnosis may be missed. Microscopic hematuria with and without proteinuria is the most common presentation. Urine abnormalities can be present persistently or intermittently for years before the onset of additional clinical symptoms. Macroscopic hematuria is less common and, when present, is often associated with an intercurrent infection. In published series, ~5% had nephrotic syndrome at presentation and the remainder had lesser degrees of proteinuria.

3.2.4 Diagnosis

The presence of microscopic hematuria with or without proteinuria should raise suspicions regarding this diagnosis (Figure 2). Confirmation of a glomerular source for red blood cells is best performed on freshly voided morning urine. Once confirmed, additional laboratory tests are used to exclude non-IgA nephropathy etiologies. Some but not all patients have elevated IgA levels; this finding does not have sufficient specificity or sensitivity for IgA nephropathy to be useful diagnostically. Complement levels may be reduced, but are usually normal. A renal biopsy is the only definitive way to make diagnosis. Other secondary causes of IgA nephropathy should be considered once the diagnosis is made (Table 4).

Light microscopy reveals focal or diffuse mesangial expansion. However, since these deposits are not specific for IgA nephropathy, additional immunofluorescence or immunoperoxidase studies are needed to identify the presence of IgA. Deposits of C3, IgG and less commonly IgM may be seen. Other features including BM thickening, increased mesangial matrix and subendothelial deposits are less common.

3.2.5 Management

No treatment is indicated if renal disease is mild (normal renal function and proteinuria <1 g/d) but annual follow-up is needed [17]. While the specific effects of continued alcohol use versus abstinence on renal disease progression and proteinuria in patients with alcohol-associated IgA nephropathy have not been determined, abstinence is recommended. In patients with heavy proteinuria and reasonably well-preserved renal function, corticosteroids have been shown to protect against progression and reduce proteinuria. Other immunosuppressive agents such as cyclosporine, mycophenolate mofetil, azathioprine and cyclophosphamide have not been evaluated in controlled trials of sufficient size to assess superiority of one therapy over another. Anticoagulant and antithrombotic agents were hypothesized to be potentially beneficial in decreasing intraglomerular deposition of fibrinogen and platelet antigens. Most clinical trials with these agents have been uncontrolled and the therapeutic regimens have included corticosteroids or other drugs, confounding the interpretation of the findings. There was much enthusiasm for fish oils as a dietary therapy. Possible effects include alterations in cytokine and eicosanoid production and decreased platelet aggregation. A meta-analysis of five controlled trials found no benefit.

General measures such as mild restriction of protein and strict control of blood pressure are recommended to slow renal progression [16]. Angiotensin converting enzyme inhibitors (ACEI) and angiotensin-II receptor antagonists (ATRA) appear to be the agents of choice. A recent study provided evidence that the combination of ACEI and ATRA in normotensive patients with IgA nephropathy reduces proteinuria more than either drug alone. For patients with cirrhosis, low doses of ACEI and ATRA have been used safely without complications but use of these agents in patients with decompensated cirrhosis is not recommended as there is significant risk of precipitating renal failure and hepatorenal syndrome.

3.2.6 Prognosis

Prognosis is highly variable, but disease progression is typically slow. Actuarial renal survival after 10 years is approximately 80% in most European and Asian studies. The strongest predictors of an unfavorable outcome in patients with primary IgA nephropathy are impairment of renal function, severe proteinuria and arterial hypertension. The histological features on renal biopsy predictive of progressive disease are glomerulosclerosis and interstitial fibrosis. In some patients, the severity of the liver disease has a strong influence on long-term survival [17]. Combined liver and kidney transplantation in patients with end-stage liver disease and renal failure due to IgA nephropathy is controversial because the recurrence rate for IgA nephropathy is high post-transplantation [16].

4. SKIN

4.1 Scleroderma

4.1.1 General aspects of the disease

PBC has been linked with several autoimmune conditions including systemic sclerosis (SSc) [9,18]. SSc, a disease characterized by tissue fibrosis and small vessel abnormalities, has a reported frequency in PBC patients of 3–50% depending upon the series [18]. PBC-associated SSc is generally mild and of more limited involvement [6]. CREST syndrome (Calcinosis, Raynaud's phenomenon, Esophageal dysfunction, Sclerodactyly, Telangiectasia) is rarely seen in its complete form. Both PBC and SSc are much more common in women and usually diagnosed in middle age.

4.1.2 Pathophysiology

The antigenic targets in PBC are epitopes on proteins of the pyruvate dehydrogenase and other 2-oxo-acid dehydrogenase complexes within mitochondria. Some of these proteins appear to be aberrantly expressed at the surface of cholangiocytes in PBC. The basis for breakdown in tolerance remains uncertain. The cause of SSc is equally inexplicable. A common autoimmune mechanism may underlie PBC and SSc but the specific factors associated with these apparently diverse presentations are unknown.

4.1.3 Clinical features

In PBC patients with associated SSc, the first signs and symptoms include Raynaud's phenomenon, finger and hand edema and tightening and thickening of the skin. Gastrointestinal involvement including submucosal fibrosis, lower esophageal sphincter weakness and hypomotility of the lower esophagus can present as chronic reflux esophagitis, dysphagia and upper GI bleeding.

4.1.4 Diagnosis

The diagnosis of SSc is largely based on clinical symptoms and signs. Antinuclear antibodies (ANA) are positive in more than 90% of patients and rheumatoid factor (RF) is positive in approximately one-third [19]. Anticentromere antibodies may also be present and, in one Italian study, was found to be the best predictor of connective tissue disease in PBC patients. Among patients with SSc, anticentromere antibodies are more frequent in patients with PBC than those without liver disease (15.8 versus 0%).

4.1.5 Treatment

SSc treatment is also largely symptomatic, as no disease-modifying agents have been identified. Raynaud's phenomenon may respond to calcium channel blockers such as nifedipine. Esophagitis is helped by proton pump inhibitors and periodic dilatation may be required if esophageal strictures develop. There has been no proven benefit to corticosteroids or other immunosuppressive agents. Finally, the limited data available indicate there is no improvement in the SSc symptoms with use of ursodeoxycholic acid [11].

4.1.6 Prognosis

PBC-associated SSc is generally mild and in patients with both diseases (PBC and SSc), the cause of mortality is more frequently related to liver disease than complications of SSc.

5. ENDOCRINE AND EXOCRINE GLANDS

5.1 Hypothyroidism

5.1.1 General aspects of the disease

PBC, autoimmune hepatitis and chronic hepatitis C have been associated with autoimmune hypothyroidism and an increased prevalence of thyroid autoantibodies. In the general population, the incidence of hypothyroidism is 0.8–1%. In PBC patients, the incidence may be as high as 25% [9,18]. One study of 95 patients found that 26% of PBC patients had circulating thyroid antibodies, approximately 50% of whom had biochemical evidence of hypothyroidism. Another study of 58 PBC patients found that 12% had a prior diagnosis of hypothyroidism and 22% had biochemical evidence of hypothyroidism (elevated TSH, elevated thyroid hormone binding capacity and/or decreased free T4) [20]. The diagnosis of hypothyroidism can precede the diagnosis of PBC by many years. Thus, PBC should be high on the differential in a hypothyroid patient manifesting signs and symptoms of cholestatic liver disease. In patients with autoimmune hepatitis, the frequency of Hashimoto's thyroiditis is reported to be 2–12%. In two prospective studies of HCV patients the prevalence of antithyroid antibodies was found to be 7–31% [13,21]. There was a female predominance in patients with chronic HCV and detectable autoantibodies. There is also an increased risk of thyroid dysfunction associated with HCV treatment with interferon alfa. This risk is highest in patients with detectable thyroid autoantibodies prior to treatment, indicating immune stimulation can unmask this disorder.

5.1.2 Pathophysiology

Hashimoto's thyroiditis is characterized by the immune-destruction of thyroid follicules ultimately resulting in thyroid follicle atrophy and fibrosis. This is predominantly T-cell-mediated. Autoantibodies (especially antithyroid peroxidase and antithyroglobulin) may augment the immune response by binding exposed autoantigens, fixing complement and triggering the complement cascade or inhibition of thyroid cell function. As with other autoimmune diseases, genetic susceptibility and the presence of specific environmental triggers are required for disease expression. The precise mechanisms linking HCV and hypothyroidism are unknown. Both direct (via molecular mimicry) and indirect (activation of auto-reactive T- and B-cells) mechanisms have been proposed [3].

5.1.3 Clinical features

There is potential overlap in the symptoms of hypothyroidism and chronic liver disease, especially in patients with cirrhosis. Symptoms of hypothyroidism include fatigue, increased sleep requirement, bradycardia, constipation, delayed tendon reflexes, weight gain, cold intolerance and dry skin. Patients in the early stages of Hashimoto's thyroiditis may have symptoms of hyperthyroidism including weight loss, tachycardia, heat intolerance and insomnia. On physical examination, the thyroid may be normal or enlarged.

5.1.4 Diagnosis

The frequent association of hypothyroidism with PBC has led some experts to recommend that all PBC patients should be screened for thyroid dysfunction [20]. Such a recommendation has not been made for patients with chronic HCV infection. Elevated TSH and reduced FT4 are indicative of primary hypothyroidism, and Hashimoto's thyroiditis is the most common cause of primary hypothyroidism. The presence of antithyroglobulin antibodies and antimicrosomal antibodies confirm the diagnosis of Hashimoto's thyroiditis. Low or normal TSH in combination with low free T4 is consistent with secondary hypothyroidism; an elevated TSH and FT4 are indicative of thyroid hormone resistance. The latter two scenarios, uncommon in hypothyroidism associated with chronic liver disease, should prompt referral to an endocrinologist for further diagnostic testing and treatment.

5.1.5 Management

The management of hypothyroidism associated with PBC or HCV is the same as that for patients without liver disease. Thyroid replacement with oral levothyroxine is typically started at doses of 50–100 mcg per day. Patients with comorbidities, especially heart disease, should be started at lower doses. TSH, FT4 and T3 levels should be checked in 2–3 weeks and the dose titrated as indicated. The goal would be normal TSH, FT4 and T3 levels. TSH improvement may lag behind FT4 and T3 improvement by 2–4 weeks. Once a euthyroid state is achieved, TSH, FT4 and T3 should be checked every 6–12 months or more frequently if clinical symptoms dictate. Thyroid replacement is typically required life-long.

5.1.6 Prognosis

There are no studies to indicate that the presence of hypothyroidism has any impact on the natural history of PBC, autoimmune hepatitis or HCV. Patients who developed thyroid abnormalities on interferon therapy may return to the euthyroid state once interferon is discontinued. The presence of antithyroglobulin and antithyroperoxidase antibodies at the end of interferon therapy correlates with persistence of thyroid dysfunction.

5.2 Sjogren's syndrome

5.2.1 General aspects of the disease

Sjogren's syndrome usually presents with symptoms of dryness of the eyes and mouth, due to impaired secretion of the lacrimal and salivary glands, respectively, and swelling of salivary glands. Salivary gland enlargement is uncommon in secondary Sjogren's syndrome; keratoconjunctivitis and xerostomia (sicca syndrome) are the primary manifestations. Sicca syndrome has been linked with several chronic liver diseases including PBC, autoimmune hepatitis and, most recently, chronic HCV infection. The association between Sjogren's syndrome and PBC is well established. About 10% of patients with Sjogren's syndrome and 42% of those with Sjogren's syndrome and RA have a positive antimitochondrial antibody (AMA) and either clinical or biochemical evidence of liver disease. Among patients with PBC, Sjogren's syndrome is the most common extrahepatic manifestation, present in up to two-thirds of patients [9].

Whether sicca syndrome is an extrahepatic manifestation of chronic HCV remains controversial [3]. The prevalence of HCV infection among patients with sicca syndrome is higher than the general population in most studies from Europe [22]. In these European studies, anti-HCV is present (confirmed by RIBA-2) in 5–19% of patients whereas the prevalence of HCV in the population is only 1%. In contrast, US studies have found anti-HCV in only ~1% of patients with sicca syndrome, a prevalence which is similar to the 1.8% prevalence of anti-HCV in the population. Epidemiological studies with appropriate controls are needed to firmly establish the causal relationship between HCV and sicca syndrome. Nonetheless, there are accumulating experimental data that HCV may be a sialotropic virus. Among European HCV-infected patients presenting for liver biopsy, sicca syndrome was present in 62%; all had oral dryness and half had both oral and ocular dryness.

5.2.2 Pathophysiology

Sjogren's syndrome is an autoimmune disease affecting the exocrine glands. Glandular dysfunction is thought to arise from destruction associated with lymphocytic infiltration but the degree of glandular destruction does not correlate with the severity of sicca symptoms, suggesting that other mechanisms are involved. Abnormalities in parasympathetic neurotransmission (autoantibodies against the muscarinic acetylcholine receptor have been implicated), alterations related to the cytokine milieu and dysregulation of apoptosis have been identified. A genetic predisposition is suggested by familial clustering.

Viruses have been suspected to play a role in triggering autoimmune and lymphoproliferative disorders. The pathogenic role of HCV in sicca syndrome is the subject of much debate but there are experimental data to support a relationship between HCV and autoimmune sialadenitis. Transgenic mice carrying the HCV envelope genes have been shown to develop an exocrinopathy involving salivary and lacrimal glands, which strongly resembles Sjogren's syndrome. Additionally, parotid B-cell non-Hodgkin's lymphoma may arise in patients with sialadenitis and is typically seen in patients with type II cryoglobulinemia with which HCV is frequently associated.

5.2.3 Clinical features

The clinical presentation of Sjogren's syndrome in patients with chronic liver disease reflects the reduced lacrimal and salivary gland function. Dryness of the mouth, increased dental caries and problems wearing dentures are common features of xerostomia. Dry eyes are typically manifest as a sandy or gritty sensation, redness or itchiness of the eyes and increased photosensitivity. While no unique features of sicca syndrome have been identified in patients with PBC, patients with sicca syndrome and HCV may have a lower prevalence of clinical symptoms of dryness, an absence of classical systemic manifestation observed in primary SS and an absence of anti-SSA or anti-SSB antibodies (Table 5). Predictably, liver involvement as indicated by liver enzyme tests or histology is more common in SS patients with PBC or HCV than those with primary Sjogren's syndrome. While one study found that biopsies of salivary glands in HCV-associated SS showed localization of lymphocytes to pericapillary regions rather than periductal regions and less prominent lymphocytic infiltrates compared to those with primary SS [21], the weight of the data suggests the morphological differences are minor and related more to the stage of disease than to primary versus secondary SS.

5.2.4 Diagnosis

A definitive diagnosis of sicca syndrome requires specialized testing (Table 5). In those with symptoms of dry eyes, measurement of tear flow (Schirmer's test) and slit-lamp examination of the cornea and conjunctiva after rose Bengal staining to assess for the presence of punctuate corneal ulceration and attached filaments of corneal epithelium are used. Diagnostic tests for xerostomia include sialometry, sialography and scintigraphy and salivary gland biopsy of the labial minor gland. The latter will show focal lymphocytic infiltrates.

5.2.5 Management

Patients with Sjogren's syndrome and chronic liver disease are managed the same as patients with Sjogren's syndrome without liver disease. Ophthalmic and oral solutions to replace deficient tears and saliva are available; frequent application is necessary. Drug therapies, which stimulate lacrimal flow, include pilocarpine and cevimeline, and judicious short-term use of steroid-containing drugs may be necessary. For patients with xerostomia, regular dental visits are essential. High-dose oral interferon alpha shows promise. In one study, 150 IU three times daily for 6 months resulted in improvement of saliva flow and symptomatic relief in 50% of patients versus 3% of controls. Other agents under study include zidovudine, androgen replacement and herbs such as primrose oil.

In patients with PBC and sicca syndrome, the use of ursodeoxycholic acid had no measurable effect on the rates of resolution of symptoms over a 2-year treatment period [11]. The precise role of anti-HCV therapy in patients with HCV and sicca syndrome needs to be defined. *De novo* sicca syndrome has been reported in an HCV-infected patient treated with interferon but there are no data on the effect of

Table 5. Clinical and diagnostic features of primary Sjogren's syndrome (SS) versus liver-associated SS.

	Primary SS	PBC and SS	HCV and SS
Age	Predominant in middle-aged women	Predominant in middle-aged women	Females > males
Severity of symptoms	++ to +++	+ to ++	+ to ++
Sjogren-specific autoantibodies	Ro/SS-A ++	±	–
	La/SS-B ++	+	–
Associated serological markers	AMA <5%	AMA positive >90%	Anti-HCV + (HCV RNA +)
	RF ++	RF +++	RF ++
	Cryoglobulins +	Cryoglobulins +	Cryoglobulins ++
Pulmonary or renal diseases	+	±	–
Liver involvement[a]	<10%	>90%	>90%

[a]Based on liver enzymes abnormalities or histology.

anti-HCV therapy on sicca symptoms in patients with pre-existing disease.

5.2.6 Prognosis

Sjogren's syndrome is not regarded as a curable disease and no therapy has been identified that modifies disease progression. Based upon currently available data, it appears that the natural history of Sjogren's syndrome is independent of the clinical course of the chronic liver disease. Salivary gland lymphoma is a rare but recognized complication of long-standing Sjogren's syndrome.

6. GASTROINTESTINAL DISEASES

6.1 Inflammatory bowel disease

6.1.1 General aspects of the disease

Inflammatory bowel disease (IBD) is the most common extrahepatic manifestation of primary sclerosing cholangitis (PSC); IBD is present in 50–70% of patients with PSC. Ulcerative colitis (UC) is more common than Crohn's disease (CD) in most series [23]. One study found that patients with PSC and CD have milder liver disease than patients with PSC and UC, perhaps because large-duct PSC is less common in patients with CD. Among patients with IBD, 2.5–7.5% have PSC, with the strongest association in those with pancolitis. Among patients with UC, the presence of PSC is a marker of increased risk of colorectal dysplasia and cancer [24].

6.1.2 Pathophysiology

The pathogenic mechanisms that underlie the association between IBD and PSC are unknown. The majority of patients with PSC and UC have the HLA-DR3 B8 haplotype, and low titer autoantibodies to smooth muscle, parietal cells and nuclear antigens are seen. Cross-reacting epitopes between colonic and biliary epithelia are proposed. Portal bacteremia is believed to be important, acting as a potential antigen source in genetically susceptible individuals. Endotoxins from intestinal bacteria may be absorbed abnormally through diseased bowel wall and promote production of TNFα which in turn promotes inflammatory responses in the liver. Additionally, studies show reduced T-cell responsiveness of liver-derived lymphocytes to TNFα; this altered immune response may further contribute to liver injury.

6.1.3 Clinical features

Common symptoms related to UC or Crohn's colitis include diarrhea, cramping and hematochezia. Additionally, CD symptoms can include abdominal pain (especially right lower quadrant), nausea, vomiting. The clinical features of IBD in patients with PSC are similar to that of patients without PSC. Some but not all studies have found that PSC-associated colitis is typically a pancolitis rather than limited (in UC) or segmental (in CD) colitis [23].

6.1.4 Diagnosis

Since colitis in patients with PSC is frequently mild and can even be asymptomatic, screening on the basis of symptoms will lead to under-diagnosis. Given the high prevalence of IBD in patients with PSC, screening sigmoidoscopy or colonoscopy is recommended. The diagnosis of IBD in patients with PSC is undertaken in the same way as in patients without PSC. A combination of endoscopic and radiological tests will confirm the diagnosis. Sigmoidoscopy with biopsy is usually sufficient to make the diagnosis of UC, but colonoscopy is used to determine the extent of disease and to differentiate CD from UC when the former diagnosis is a consideration. Laboratory tests are not pathognomic. Common abnormalities with active pancolitis include elevated acute phase reactants (e.g., CRP) and ESR, hypoalbuminemia (can also be related to liver disease) and anemia.

6.1.5 Management

IBD management is largely independent of PSC treatment. Whether patients with PSC and UC derive chemopreventive benefits from treatment with ursodeoxycholic acid is controversial. In a study of 52 patients followed for a total of 335 person-years, those treated with ursodeoxycholic acid showed a 74% reduction in risk of colorectal neoplasia compared to patients not treated with ursodeoxycholic acid [24]. However, not all studies have confirmed this finding. Colectomy for UC does not alter the natural history of PSC.

6.1.6 Prognosis

PSC has been found to be an independent risk factor for colorectal dysplasia and neoplasia. An estimated 5-fold higher risk of cancer and dysplasia is seen in UC patients with PSC compared to those with UC alone [24,25]. Whether the presence of IBD influences the natural history of PSC is more controversial. Factors predictive of survival in PSC include older age, serum bilirubin levels, albumin level, hemoglobin level. splenomegaly, variceal bleeding and histological stage of liver disease. Early survival models found IBD also to be an independent predictor of survival, but more recent survival models have not. Finally, a recent large European multicenter study of 394 PSC patients found that a diagnosis of IBD was more common and the duration of IBD was longer in patients with cholangiocarcinoma than those without, and concluded that IBD was a risk factor for cholangiocarcinoma [26]. Additional cohort studies are needed to confirm or refute this association.

6.2 Celiac disease

6.2.1 General aspects of the disease

Studies suggest the frequency of celiac disease in patients with PBC is greater than expected by chance. In a 12-year study of a stable 250,000 Northern European population, the prevalence of PBC was 3% in 143 patients with celiac disease, and the prevalence of celiac disease was 6% in 67 patients with PBC. Similar prevalence rates are reported in other European and North American populations [27]. The evidence linking celiac disease and autoimmune hepatitis is less convincing but large-scale epidemiological studies are lacking.

Among patients with newly diagnosed celiac disease, liver test abnormalities are not uncommon. In a study of 132 Northern European patients, 47% had at least one liver test abnormal; in 10.6% an isolated elevation of alkaline phosphatase was seen. However, liver biopsies most commonly show nonspecific changes, and chronic cholestatic liver diseases were very infrequent. In another study, sera from 108 adult celiac disease patients from Italy were tested for AMA and positivity was found in four patients (3.7%); all had normal liver biochemistry tests [28].

6.2.2 Pathophysiology

The pathogenic mechanisms that underlie the association between PBC and celiac disease are poorly understood. Both a genetic predisposition and an environmentally triggered immune response are likely important in disease pathogenesis. Both PBC and celiac disease have specific HLA associations but a shared haplotype that might confer susceptibility to both diseases has not been identified to date.

6.2.3 Clinical features

Celiac disease is an inflammatory disease of the small intestine associated with variable malabsorption of nutrients. The clinical hallmark of the disease is improvement in symptoms and small bowel histology with removal of dietary gluten from the diet. Typical symptoms include chronic diarrhea, weight loss, flatulence and abdominal distention. Extraintestinal manifestations include such diverse presentations as osteopenia, peripheral neuropathy, amenorrhea, edema and dermatitis herpetiformis. Laboratory abnormalities may include anemia (secondary to iron, folate and occasionally vitamin B12 deficiency), hypocalcemia and hyperprothrombinemia.

Osteopenia/osteoporesis, fatigue, amenorrhea, steatorrhea and skin changes are clinical symptoms common to both PBC and celiac disease. Bone disease, in particular, can be a significant complication, especially in post-menopausal women; bone pain and pathological fractures can be seen. While dermatitis herpetiformis is not a skin condition associated with PBC, pruritus is common in patients with cholestatic liver disease. Steatorrhea related to PBC is a manifestation of advanced disease and most commonly reflects impaired bile acid delivery to the small intestine.

6.2.4 Diagnosis

Experts recommend screening for celiac disease with antiendomysium antibodies in patients with PBC. For patients with positive results, duodenal biopsy is recommended to confirm the diagnosis and determine the severity of disease.

6.2.5 Management

The management of patients with PBC and celiac disease is the same as patients with celiac disease alone. A gluten-free diet is the cornerstone of treatment. Supplemental therapies to correct nutritional deficiencies are frequently required early in the treatment period. Fat-soluble vitamin deficiencies related to celiac disease may be compounded by deficiencies related to PBC. In patients with PBC, vitamin A deficiency is most common followed by vitamin D deficiency.

6.2.6 Prognosis

Liver biochemistry does not improve when PBC patients with celiac disease are treated with a gluten-free diet [27]. However, the complications of untreated celiac disease alone warrant the early identification and treatment of the condition. There are no data to address the question of whether survival among PBC patients is impacted by coexistent celiac disease.

REFERENCES

[1] Lai, K.N. and Lai, F.M. (1991) Clinical features and the natural course of hepatitis B virus-related glomerulopathy in adults. *Kidney Int. Suppl.* **35**, S40–S45.

[2] Trepo, C. and Guillevin, L. (2001) Polyarteritis nodosa and extrahepatic manifestations of HBV infection: the case against autoimmune intervention in pathogenesis. *J. Autoimmun.* **16**, 269–274.

[3] Loustaud, V. and Lunel, F. (2002) Extrahepatic manifestations of HCV infection, in HCV Viral Infection, vol. 1, eds. A. Di Bisceglie and A. Zignego (UTET, Milano) pp. 28–54.

[4] Zuckerman, E., Keren, D. *et al.* (2000) Treatment of refractory, symptomatic, hepatitis C virus related mixed cryoglobulinemia with ribavirin and interferon-alpha. *J. Rheumatol.* **27**, 2172–2178.

[5] Tarantino, A., Campise, M. *et al.* (1995) Long-term predictors of survival in essential mixed cryoglobulinemic glomerulonephritis. *Kidney Int.* **47**, 618–623.

[6] Walker, N.J., Zurier, R.B. *et al.* (2002) Liver abnormalities in rheumatic diseases. *Clin. Liver Dis.* **6**, 933–946.

[7] Waalen, J., Felitt, V. *et al.* (2002) Prevalence of hemochromatosis-related symptoms among individuals with mutations in the HFE gene. *Mayo Clin. Proc.* **77**, 522–530.

[8] Timms, A.E., Sathananthan, R. *et al.* (2002) Genetic testing for haemochromatosis in patients with chondrocalcinosis. *Ann. Rheum. Dis.* **61**, 745–747.

[9] Culp, K., Fleming, C. *et al.* (1982) Autoimmune associations in primary biliary cirrhosis. *Mayo Clin. Proc.* **59**, 365–370.

[10] Youssef, W.I. and Tavill, A.S. (2002) Connective tissue diseases and the liver. *J. Clin. Gastroenterol.* **35**, 345–349.

[11] Zukowski, T., Jorgensen, R. *et al.* (1998) Autoimmune conditions associated with primary biliary cirrhosis: response to ursodeoxycholic acid therapy. *Am. J. Gastroenterol.* **6**, 958–961.

[12] Olivieri, I., Palazzi, C. *et al.* (2003) Hepatitis C virus and arthritis. *Rheum. Dis. Clin. North Am.* **29**(1), 111–122.

[13] Pawlotsky, J., Yahia, M. *et al.* (1994) Immunological disorders in C virus chronic active hepatitis: a prospective case-control study. *Hepatology* **19**, 841–848.

[14] Leone, N., Pellicano, R. *et al.* (2002) Mixed cryoglobulinaemia and chronic hepatitis C virus infection: the rheumatic manifestations. *J. Med. Virol.* **66**, 200–203.

[15] Zuckerman, E., Yeshurun, D. *et al.* (2001) Management of hepatitis C virus-related arthritis. *BioDrugs* **15**, 573–584.

[16] Wong, F. (2002) Liver and kidney diseases. *Clin. Liver Dis.* **6**, 981–1011.

[17] Donadio, J.V. and Grande, J.P. (2002) IgA nephropathy. *N. Engl. J. Med.* **347**(10), 738–748.

[18] Clark, A., Galbraith, R. *et al.* (1978) Rheumatic disorders in primary biliary cirrhosis. *Mayo Clin. Proc.* **37**, 42–47.

[19] Marasini, B., Gagetta, M. *et al.* (2001) Rheumatic disorders and primary biliary cirrhosis: an appraisal of 170 Italian patients. *Ann. Rheum. Dis.* **60**, 1046–1049.

[20] Elta, G., Sepersky, R. *et al.* (1983) Increased incidence of hypothyroidism in primary biliary cirrhosis. *Dig. Dis. Sci.* **28**(11), 971–975.

[21] Tran, A., Quaranta, J.F. *et al.* (1993) High prevalence of thyroid autoantibodies in a prospective series of patients with chronic hepatitis C before interferon therapy. *Hepatology* **18**, 253–257.

[22] Ramos-Casals, M., Garcia-Carrasco, M. *et al.* (1999) Sjogren's syndrome and hepatitis C virus. *Clin. Rheumatol.* **18**, 93–100.

[23] Rasmussen, H., Fallingborg, J. *et al.* (1997) Hepatobiliary dysfunction and primary sclerosing cholangitis in patients with Crohn's disease. *Scand. J. Gastroenterol.* **32**, 604–610.

[24] Pardi, D., Loftus, E.J. *et al.* (2003) Ursodeoxycholic acid as a chemopreventive agent in patients with ulcerative colitis and primary sclerosing cholangitis. *Gastroenterology* **124**, 889–893.

[25] Soetikno, R., Lin, O. *et al.* (2002) Increased risk of colorectal neoplasia in patients with primary sclerosing cholangitis and ulcerative colitis: a meta-analysis. *Gastrointest. Endosc.* **56**, 45–48.

[26] Boberg, K., Rodrigo, L. *et al.* (2002) Cholangiocarcinoma in primary sclerosing cholangitis: risk factors and clinical presentation. *Scand. J. Gastroenterol.* **37**, 120.

[27] Volta, U., Betterle, C. *et al.* (2002) Celiac disease in autoimmune cholestatic liver disorders. *Am. J. Gastroenterol.* **97**, 2609–2613.

[28] Floreani, A., Betterle, C. *et al.* (2002) Prevalence of coeliac disease in primary biliary cirrhosis and of antimitochondrial antibodies in adult coeliac disease patients in Italy. *Dig. Liver Dis.* **34**, 258–261.

Hepatology: A Practical Approach
B. Al Knawy, M.L. Shiffman, R.H. Wiesner (editors)

Chapter 5
The Liver in Systemic Diseases

L. Balart

Center for Digestive Diseases, 2820 Napolean Avenue Suite 700, New Orleans, LA 70115, USA

1. Cardiovascular Disorders 492
   1.1 Budd–Chiari syndrome 492
   1.2 Congestive heart failure 492
      1.2.1 Introduction 492
      1.2.2 Pathophysiology 492
      1.2.3 Clinical features 492
      1.2.4 Diagnosis 492
      1.2.5 Management 493
      1.2.6 Prognosis 493
   1.3 Ischemic hepatitis 493
      1.3.1 Clinical features 493
      1.3.2 Laboratory features 494
      1.3.3 Histologic features 494
      1.3.4 Treatment 494
   1.4 Constrictive pericarditis 494
2. Granulomatous Disease 494
   2.1 Sarcoidosis 494
      2.1.1 Introduction 494
      2.1.2 Pathophysiology 494
      2.1.3 Clinical features 495
      2.1.4 Diagnosis 495
      2.1.5 Management 495
      2.1.6 Prognosis 495
   2.2 Amyloidosis 495
      2.2.1 Pathophysiology 495
      2.2.2 Clinical features 496
      2.2.3 Diagnosis 496
      2.2.4 Treatment 496
   2.3 Collagen vascular diseases 496
      2.3.1 Introduction 496
      2.3.2 Pathophysiology 496
      2.3.3 Clinical features 497
      2.3.4 Diagnosis 497
      2.3.5 Management 497
      2.3.6 Prognosis 497
   2.4 Liver disease in diabetes mellitus 497
   2.5 Glycogen deposition 497
   2.6 Cholelithiasis and cholecystitis 498
   2.7 Liver disease due to treatment of diabetes 498

2.8 Diabetes occurring as a complication of chronic liver disease 498
2.9 Cirrhosis and glucose homeostasis 499
References 499

The liver can frequently become involved in systemic diseases and this can lead to manifestations which can be easily detected. Liver abnormalities can then lead to the correct diagnosis in many instances. These disorders can be divided into cardiovascular causes, infectious causes, connective tissue causes and granulomatous causes. These in turn can be subdivided into different components (Table 5.1).

1. CARDIOVASCULAR DISORDERS

1.1 Budd–Chiari syndrome

(Please see elsewhere.)

1.2 Congestive heart failure

1.2.1 Introduction

There are two main hepatic manifestations: congestion and ischemia. While the changes due to congestion are chronic and evolve slowly, the changes due to ischemia are usually acute and are due to decreased cardiac output. These changes are usually asymptomatic unless they occur in a patient with chronic congestion in which case severe liver failure may ensue.

1.2.2 Pathophysiology

Pathophysiologically, the changes in congestive failure resemble those in Budd–Chiari syndrome: zone 3 congestion and necrosis, "nutmeg" appearance of the liver, injured hepatic veins, fibrosis and bridging fibrosis. This bridging fibrosis is not the usual portal–portal bridging fibrosis; rather, it extends from central vein to central vein creating what has been called cardiac cirrhosis. There is research to suggest that hepatic vein and portal vein intimal fibrosis with intraluminal thrombosis causes cirrhosis in this setting [1].

In the setting of ischemia, the insult is hypoperfusion due to a decrease in cardiac output, sepsis or trauma. Histologically, there is zone 3 necrosis as in congestive failure. However, normal architecture is maintained with ischemia. Rearrangement of the architecture is one of the steps in the development of cirrhosis.

1.2.3 Clinical features

Hepatic congestion is usually asymptomatic, found on routine evaluation. Mild jaundice is common. Hepatomegaly, hepatojugular reflux (absent in venous outflow obstruction) and ascites are also found. Ascites is usually due to the congestive heart failure rather than liver disease.

Hepatic ischemia is usually asymptomatic as well and detected only because a hypotensive episode preceded it, thus provoking a physician to look for its effects on liver biochemistry. Asymptomatic elevation of transaminases is the rule. However, in a patient with cirrhosis or congestion due to heart failure, the ischemic episode may present with jaundice, nausea, vomiting, anorexia and right upper quadrant pain. Depending on the degree of hepatic reserve, the patient may recover uneventfully or progress to fulminant failure.

1.2.4 Diagnosis

Blood test. Hepatic congestion usually presents with a very mild biochemical profile. Serum bilirubin may be elevated but is rarely above 3 mg/dl. Transaminases may be elevated by about 2–3 times the upper limit of normal. Serum alkaline phosphatase may be normal or may show minimal elevation. Serum albumin is usually decreased but not below 2.5 g/dl. Coagulation abnormalities are common.

Table 5.1. Components of cardiovascular disorders.

Cardiovascular disorders	Infections	Collagen diseases	Others
Budd–Chiari	Tuberculosis	Systemic lupus	Sarcoidosis
Congestive failure	Leptospirosis	Rheumatoid arthritis	Amyloidosis
Ischemic hepatitis	Q fever	Polyarteritis	
Constrictive pericarditis	AIDS	Cryoglobulinemia	
	Sepsis		

The prothrombin time is prolonged in 80–90% of patients and it does not get corrected with vitamin K supplementation.

On the other hand, the biochemical pattern of liver ischemia is quite different. The most striking difference is the elevation of the transaminases, which could be as high as 100–200 times upper limit of normal. Transaminases usually peak rapidly (about 2–4 days) and then return to normal in 7–10 days. Serum bilirubin increases as the transaminases are on their way down. Serum bilirubin usually does not go above four times the upper limit of normal. There is also a very rapid rise in LDH prior to the transaminase elevation. This biochemical profile could also represent acute viral hepatitis. A useful way to differentiate between the two, other than viral hepatitis serology, is an ALT to LDH ratio <1.5, which tends to support ischemia as opposed to viral hepatitis [2].

Imaging studies. Non-specific finding accompanies congestion. Ultrasound or CT examinations would detect hepatomegaly with a homogeneous pattern. No focal lesions should be seen. Imaging studies may show an area of infarction in the setting of ischemia if the insult has been severe enough.

Pathological studies. Paracentesis usually shows a high gradient fluid (serum albumin–ascites albumin gradient >1.1) with total protein >2.5 g/dl.

1.2.5 Management

Medical therapeutics. The management of hepatic congestion consists mostly of treating the heart failure. This is achieved by maintaining cardiac output and avoiding excessive diuresis. The management of ischemia is non-specific. Many strategies have been employed like dopamine, dobutamine and ACE inhibitors but no clear benefit has been seen as of now.

1.2.6 Prognosis

Hepatic congestion depends mostly on the underlying cardiac problem. Even when cirrhosis is established, improvement of pump failure may help improve hepatic function. Hepatic ischemia is usually asymptomatic and self-limited unless it happens in the setting of chronic liver disease where it could be lethal.

1.3 Ischemic hepatitis

1.3.1 Clinical features

This term refers to acute hepatocellular injury occurring in the setting of biventricular failure, usually occurring in the setting of severe valvular disease or cardiomyopathy. The clinical picture is that of an abrupt fall in cardiac output which has been reversed but which causes increases in aminotransferases. In many cases, these increases are sufficiently high enough (over 1000 IU/ml) to cause concern about acute viral hepatitis. There is usually evidence of an arrhythmia or myocardial infarction complicating the cardiac picture and leading to the ischemic event. The majority of patients do not develop congestive failure and aminotransferase levels return to near normal within several days, thus helping in the differential with acute viral hepatitis. The development of hepatic failure is rare [15].

1.3.2 Laboratory features

Aminotransferases are elevated 10–12 × the limits of normal; total bilirubin and alkaline phosphatase levels increase slightly. Acute hepatitis A and B markers are negative. When appropriate HCV-RNA can be done to exclude acute hepatitis C.

1.3.3 Histologic features

There is hepatocellular necrosis most prominently in zone 3 and there is no portal or hepatocellular necrosis.

1.3.4 Treatment

The outcome of ischemic hepatitis is largely predetermined as the cardiac failure leading to it has usually been treated, therefore the hepatic course is usually benign. The course of the cardiac condition will determine the final outcome. Only in the instances of severe underlying liver disease will ischemic hepatitis lead to a more severe liver picture such as fulminant failure [16].

1.4 Constrictive pericarditis

Constructive pericarditis, Budd–Chiari and right-side heart failure share similar hemodynamic characteristics that produce similar hepatic pathology. Zone 3 congestion and necrosis are seen histologically. This leads to bridging fibrosis and cirrhosis similar to that seen in chronic hepatic congestion. However, in constrictive pericarditis the rate of development of cirrhosis seems to be accelerated in comparison to heart failure.

Ascites, peripheral edema and hepatomegaly are common. Pulsus paradoxus and distended neck veins that do not collapse with inspiration are helpful clinical signs. However, a high index of suspicion is needed to make the diagnosis since there may only be subtle indicators of heart disease. Calcified deposits in pericardium, EKG changes and 2D echocardiography can help establish a strong suspicion of pericarditis. Cardiac catheterization continues to provide the best basis for the diagnosis but care should be taken to assure that the right information is obtained.

Pericardiectomy is the only definitive treatment for cure. However, if cardiac cirrhosis has developed this will not be reversible.

2. GRANULOMATOUS DISEASE

2.1 Sarcoidosis

2.1.1 Introduction

Sarcoidosis is a systemic granulomatous disease characterized by fever, skin rash, uveitis and lung involvement. Part of the systemic effects includes liver involvement in the majority of patients. The incidence of granulomas in the liver of patients with sarcoidosis has been reported to be between 21 and 79%. Granulomatous involvement of the liver, however, is usually asymptomatic with only serum alkaline phosphatase elevation as an indication of liver involvement. There is no one test that is diagnostic for sarcoidosis, so a combination of blood work, radiographs, biopsy and high index of suspicion is necessary to make the diagnosis.

It is important to mention that sarcoidosis, tuberculosis and primary biliary cirrhosis account for the majority of granulomatous diseases of the liver in immunocompetent patients. Granulomatous disease of the liver cannot always be attributed to sarcoidosis; a meticulous diagnostic work-up must be undertaken to rule out tuberculosis every time granulomas are found on liver biopsy. Certain medications can also present with granulomatous infiltration. Tuberculosis and medications will be discussed elsewhere in this book.

2.1.2 Pathophysiology

Sarcoidosis is characterized by non-caseating granulomas affecting portal areas. These usually consist of giant, multinucleated cells surrounding a non-necrotic center. These granulomas usually cause damage to interlobular bile ducts but may also compress central veins or cause an obliterative terminal venulitis causing Budd–Chiari syndrome.

2.1.3 Clinical features

The spectrum of disease in sarcoidosis goes from asymptomatic for the majority of patients to cirrhosis and end-stage liver disease for a minority of patients [3]. Patients with sarcoidosis, as part of the systemic disease, present with fever, uveitis, skin rash, anorexia and hepatomegaly. Jaundice may be present as well. However, there are instances in which sarcoidosis will present with clinical symptoms such as Budd–Chiari. There is a primary biliary cirrhosis-like syndrome consisting of hepatomegaly, pruritus, increased serum cholesterol and jaundice but no fever, uveitis or skin rash. Most of these patients test negative for the presence of anti-mitochondrial antibodies, which will differentiate it from classic primary biliary cirrhosis. A part of this syndrome is damage to the interlobular bile ducts, which could be so severe as to cause the vanishing bile duct syndrome (VBDS). Patients may also present with portal hypertension, nodular regenerative hyperplasia and, as stated before, Budd–Chiari syndrome.

2.1.4 Diagnosis

Blood test. There is no pathognomonic test to diagnose sarcoidosis. The diagnosis is made by finding granulomas in liver biopsy along with a suggestive clinical picture. As mentioned before, tuberculosis must be ruled out.

Usually serum alkaline phosphatase is the most frequent biochemical abnormality. Serum bilirubin may be elevated with severe disease, as in VBDS. ACE levels are increased in up to 85% of patients. However, this is not a specific finding for sarcoidosis and cannot be used as a diagnostic test.

Imaging studies. Sarcoidosis would show as multiple, low attenuation lesions involving the liver and on contrast-enhanced CT. The spleen may be involved as well. The granulomas would show as hypointense lesions on T2-weighted images on MRI.

Pathological studies. Non-caseating granulomas with Kupffer cell proliferation is common.

2.1.5 Management

Medical therapeutics. Since liver involvement is mostly asymptomatic, treatment is only rarely indicated. Steroids, ursodeoxycholic acid and liver transplantation have been used for progressive disease.

2.1.6 Prognosis

In the asymptomatic patient, prognosis is excellent. However, in the progressive form of the disease, prognosis is guarded and usually depends on the systemic nature of the disease.

2.2 Amyloidosis

Hepatic amyloidosis can result from overproduction of at least six different proteins which can assume a fibrillar form and are deposited in association with glycoprotein subunits. Amyloidosis can be divided into primary and secondary and by the types of proteins produced (Table 5.2).

2.2.1 Pathophysiology

Amyloid fibrils are deposited along pre-existing fibers which may be collagen or reticulin. This then

Table 5.2. Classification of amyloidosis.

Type	Pathologic involvement	Protein	Hepatic involvement
Primary	Pericollagen	AL	Rarely
Multiple myeloma	Pericollagen	AL	Rarely
Secondary	Perireticulin	AA	Usual
FamMedFever	Perireticulin	AA	Usual

gives rise to a pattern of either pericollagen or perireticular amyloidosis. Pericollagen amyloidosis is mostly a disease of blood vessels, connective tissue around vessels, the stroma of various organs, neurilemna and sarcolemna. Perireticulin amyloidosis involves primarily small blood vessels, capillaries and sinusoids.

2.2.2 Clinical features

Most patients with hepatic involvement developed hepatomegaly but aminotransferase levels are usually normal. Alkaline phosphatase is usually elevated as it is in other infiltrative diseases; jaundice develops only in a minority. Occasionally severe intrahepatic cholestasis can develop in kappa and lambda AL amyloidosis and this may augur a poorer prognosis. Presumably the cholestasis is due to intense amyloid deposition in the canaliculi and small bile ducts. Other organs are involved leading to splenomegaly, renal insufficiency and proteinuria [4].

2.2.3 Diagnosis

Liver biopsy is the best way to diagnose hepatic amyloidosis. Findings include a homogeneous, amorphous, eosinophilic material, which is an amyloid infiltrating between the liver cords and the space of Disse. The liver cells themselves are not infiltrated. Occasionally amyloid is only found infiltrating the walls of the arterioles in the portal tracts and at the interlobular level. This deposit stains positive with Congo red. Polarization reveals the amyloid as birefringent green fibrils.

2.2.4 Treatment

AA amyloid can be treated by primary control of the underlying disease causing it, for instance, tuberculosis or rheumatoid arthritis. AL amyloidosis can be treated with melphalan and prednisone. Amyloidosis secondary to familial Mediterranean fever is treated with colchicines. Liver transplantation may be an option for some patients but multiorgan involvement (heart, renal) usually precludes successful transplantation.

2.3 Collagen vascular diseases

2.3.1 Introduction

Collagen vascular diseases (CVD) involve a group of diseases such as systemic lupus erythematosus, rheumatoid arthritis, polymyositis/dermatomyositis and mixed connective tissue disease. Patients with these diseases have elevated liver enzymes about 49% of the time. Most of the biochemical abnormalities is explained by drug-induced damage (NSAID), and hemolysis.

Actual liver damage related to CVD occurs in a minority of patients. A study by Arnett *et al.* found a prevalence of 3% in patients with SLE after excluding all other known factors for elevated liver enzymes [5].

2.3.2 Pathophysiology

CVD affect many organ systems. Liver involvement is characterized by a myriad of disease processes. In a recent study by Kobayaki *et al.*, 16.9% of patients were diagnosed with hepatic arteritis [6]. Histologically, the lesions resemble polyarteritis nodosa. SLE was the most common of the CVD, causing hepatic arteritis with an incidence of 15.1% followed by MCTD, systemic sclerosis, RA and PM/DM. SLE had been associated with hepatic infarction, hepatic rupture and Budd–Chiari syndrome [7]. In the same study by Kobayaki *et al.*, other liver diseases, such as primary biliary cirrhosis, nodular regenerative hyperplasia and autoimmune hepatitis were associated with CVD. Primary biliary cirrhosis was found in 5.6% of patients, 78% of which were anti-mitochondrial antibody positive. Nodular regenerative hyperplasia was found in 4.4% of patients. Autoimmune hepatitis was found in 1.9% of patients. SLE and autoimmune hepatitis share a number of autoimmune phenomena including anti-nuclear antibodies. The term “lupoid hepatitis” referred to liver involvement with autoimmune phenomena. Histologically, periportal hepatitis with lymphocyte and plasma cell infiltration suggest autoimmune hepatitis [8]. Today “lupoid hepatitis” represents autoimmune hepatitis.

Other findings associated with CVD include hepatic congestion, fatty liver, non-specific reactive hepatitis (lupus hepatitis), viral hepatitis and drug-induced hepatitis. NSAID, cyclophosphamide and azathioprine are common offenders. CVD are also associated with hypercoagulable syndromes due to the anti-phospholipid antibody syndrome and anti-cardiolipin antibodies. Budd–Chiari is a serious complication in SLE patients. We mentioned earlier the report of a patient with Budd–Chiari syndrome due to SLE. Portal hypertension has also been associated with CVD [9]. Veno-occlusive disease is also associated with SLE as well as with bone marrow transplantation, chemotherapy and irradiation of the liver.

2.3.3 Clinical features

Signs and symptoms of liver involvement depend on the underlying process; hepatomegaly, ascites, abdominal pain would be present with Budd–Chiari syndrome. Jaundice and pruritus would be present with primary biliary cirrhosis; fever, arthralgias, photosensitivity, alopecia, malar rash, cerebritis would be present with SLE.

In general, jaundice could be due to cholestasis but most often it will be due to hemolysis in which case the biochemical abnormality would be unconjugated hyperbilirubinemia.

2.3.4 Diagnosis

Blood test. Due to the wide range of liver involvement, there is no diagnostic pattern of elevated liver enzymes in CVD. Transaminases are usually elevated with active disease. Anti-mitochondrial antibodies are positive in the vast majority of patients with primary biliary cirrhosis. Anti-nuclear antibodies, anti-smooth muscle antibodies are usually present in patients with autoimmune hepatitis.

2.3.5 Management

Medical therapeutics. Since drug-induced hepatitis is a common problem, a thorough drug history with discontinuation of NSAID, cyclophosphamide or azathioprine, if possible, should be the first step. In the case of Budd–Chiari syndrome, thrombolysis has been used in the past with success. Otherwise, management is mostly supportive.

2.3.6 Prognosis

Prognosis depends on the underlying problem. For fatty infiltration, prognosis is excellent but for Budd–Chiari syndrome, surgical intervention may be a necessity. Since most of the damage comes from drug-induced hepatitis, as long as the offending agent can be removed prognosis would depend on the underlying CVD.

2.4 Liver disease in diabetes mellitus

The liver plays a central role in the regulation of carbohydrate homeostasis, which helps understand the many biochemical and physical alterations that occur in the liver of diabetics. It also helps understand how liver disease may affect glucose metabolism.

In type 2 diabetes, excessive hepatic output of glucose contributes to the fasting hyperglycemia. Majority of this excess glucose comes from gluconeogenesis rather than from glycogenolysis. Hypoglycemia, sometimes intractable, is due to the reduction of hepatic glucose release and is most commonly seen in patients with acute liver failure from any cause [10].

2.5 Glycogen deposition

Eighty percent of diabetics have excess accumulation of glycogen in the liver but there is no correlation between hepatic glycogen content and fasting blood glucose levels. Glycogen can be deposited in the nuclei of hepatocytes where it is synthesized. It has been found in approximately 75% of diabetics and is probably of no clinical significance. Usually this finding is discovered at the time of liver biopsy and may be of help identifying patients with diabetes and accompanying fatty liver. Glycogen infiltrates the nuclei of liver cells, which shows on a hematoxylin and eosin stain as vacuolated nuclei. Clinically these patients may exhibit hepatomegaly and abnormalities of liver enzymes.

2.6 Cholelithiasis and cholecystitis

There appears to be an increased incidence of cholelithiasis in diabetics, however, there is a significant confounding influence from the presence of obesity and hyperlipidemia in these patients. The literature supports a two to three-fold increased incidence of gallstones but some studies have failed to demonstrate a significant association. The presumed pathogenesis is the secretion of lithogenic bile by the liver of type II diabetics, thus predisposing these patients to form gallstones. The role of obesity in this model is probably of importance and again it is difficult to ignore this as a cofactor. In acute cholecystitis, neither the relative risk of mortality nor the risk of serious complications is thought to be greater in diabetic patients than in non-diabetics. Because of this, prophylactic cholecystectomy is no longer advised for diabetic patients with asymptomatic gallstones. It is most likely that any increase in morbidity and mortality is due to the presence of vascular and renal diseases [11].

2.7 Liver disease due to treatment of diabetes

Oral hypoglycemic agents are used extensively in the Western world, and the metabolism and potential toxicities need to be kept in mind when treating diabetics.

Biguanides, such as metformin (Glucophage), and the sulfonylurea, diabenese, do not undergo hepatic metabolism and are excreted in the urine unchanged. Other sulfonylureas such as glyburide (Glynase, Diabeta, Micronase) are excreted in bile. Another sulfonylurea, glipizide (Glucotrol) is metabolized mostly by the liver and, at least in theory, may be a problem in patients with underlying chronic liver disease.

From a practical point of view the association between oral hypoglycemic agents and liver injury remains rare. Sulfonylureas can cause chronic hepatitis and necroinflammatory changes as well as granulomatous changes but the mechanism of injury is unknown. Of the drugs mentioned above, chlorpropamide is most commonly hepatotoxic with a reported incidence of cholestatic hepatitis in 0.5% of those taking the drug. Typically, jaundice develops within 2–5 weeks of initiation of therapy and resolves in the vast majority of patients when stopped. The rate of liver toxicity with others in this class (Orinase, Tolinase) appears to be rare. Glyburide can rarely cause acute hepatocellular necrosis and deaths have been reported with this agent. Till very recently there have not been any reports of significant liver injury with biguanides use. However, lactic acidosis is one of the known complications of this group and this may occur more frequently in patients with underlying chronic liver disease due to a decreased ability of the liver to clear lactate. Of the newer agents, the thiazolidinediones, which act primarily by decreasing insulin resistance, have mixed data on the potential for liver toxicity. Troglitazone (Rezulin) has been withdrawn from the market following reports of severe liver injury resulting in death or the need for liver transplantation. These reactions were thought to be idiosyncratic and thus unpredictable. The other drugs in this class, pioglitazone and rosiglitazone appear not to have the same risk of severe liver injury as they have continued to be used extensively with no serious reports of liver toxicity. Rare cases of hepatocellular injury in older men have been reported with pioglitazone. In all cases liver enzymes improved rapidly after discontinuation of the drug. Therefore it is still recommended that liver enzymes be checked every 2 months while patients are on either of these medications.

2.8 Diabetes occurring as a complication of chronic liver disease

There appears to be an increased prevalence of viral hepatitis in diabetics and this may be explained by the exposure to needles for injection and frequent blood testing. There was a reported outbreak of hepatitis B in a nursing home where transmission was thought to have been due to the use of a spring-loaded device for fingerstick glucose testing.

There have been a number of reports outlining the association between hepatitis C infection and diabetes. However, in most of these studies the control population was not matched for body mass index, race, severity of liver disease and known risk factors for the development of type II diabetes. Data from the Third National Health and Nutrition Examination Survey in the US showed that persons 40 years or older with hepatitis C infection were more than three times more likely, than those without hepatitis C, to have type II diabetes. In this study no increase in the prevalence of type II diabetes was found in patients with hepatitis B virus infection [12]. In a prospective analysis (case cohort study), the overall prevalence of hepatitis C in patients who acquired type II diabetes was 0.8%; however, if patients were at high risk for diabetes the prevalence was 11 times higher in those with hepatitis C than in those without it. This means that pre-existing hepatitis C may increase the risk of type II diabetes in patients with recognized risk factors [13]. Finally, in one of the most recent studies, the prevalence of type II diabetes was higher in patients with hepatitis C cirrhosis compared to a matched control group of patients with cirrhosis from other causes [14]. This was found to be secondary to a higher prevalence of diabetes in blacks with hepatitis C infection. Proposed mechanisms for this relationship include insulin resistance by direct pancreatic beta cell damage or an autoimmune process mediated by molecular mimicry.

The role of hepatitis C in the pathogenesis of type II diabetes remains at this time purely speculative and we must await larger and more conclusive studies that address the biologic basis for this relationship.

2.9 Cirrhosis and glucose homeostasis

Patients with cirrhosis can have elevated insulin levels, which may in turn be indicative of insulin resistance or a decrease in the degradation of insulin because of compromised hepatic function. This will likely be associated with glucose intolerance and hyperglycemia. The pathogenesis of insulin resistance is unknown but a receptor or postreceptor abnormality is likely. Another proposed mechanism is impaired insulin secretion by the pancreatic beta cells. Patients with cirrhosis may conversely develop fasting hypoglycemia through an autoimmune mechanism associated with high levels of insulin antibodies. Patients with cirrhosis and fulminant hepatic failure may have lower levels of blood glucose than matched controls but more profound hypoglycemia may not occur due to the decreased utilization of glucose and an increased utilization of non-glucose fuels such as fats. The development of hypoglycemia in fulminant hepatic failure implies a poor prognosis and increased mortality. These patients need close monitoring and continuous supplementation of glucose intravenously. In patients with hepatocellular carcinoma, hypoglycemia can occur through the production of insulin-like growth factor-II by the carcinoma cells. Therefore, diabetic patients that develop hepatocellular carcinoma may need less insulin.

REFERENCES

[1] Wanless, I., Liu, J.J. and Butany, J. (1995) Role of thrombosis in the pathogenesis of congestive hepatic fibrosis (cardiac cirrhosis). *Hepatology* **21**, 1232–1237.

[2] Cassidy, W.M. and Reynolds, T.B. (1994) Serum lactic dehydrogenase in the differential diagnosis of acute hepatocellular injury. *J. Clin. Gastroenterol.* **19**, 118–121.

[3] Devaney, K., Goodman, Z.D., Epstein, M.S., Zimmerman, H.J. and Ishak, K.G. (1993) Hepatic sarcoidosis. Clinicopathologic features in 100 patients. *Am. J. Surg. Pathol.* **17**, 1272–1280.

[4] Kyle, R.A. and Greipp, P.R. (1983) Amyloidosis (AL): clinical and laboratory features in 229 cases. *Mayo Clin. Proc.* **58**, 665.

[5] Arnett, F. and Reichlin, M. (1995) Lupus hepatitis; an under-recognized disease feature associated with auto antibodies to ribosomal p. *Am. J. Med.* **99**, 465–472.

[6] Matsumoto, T., Kobayashi, S., Shimizu, H., Nakajima, M., Watanabe, S., Kitami, N., Sato, N., Abe, H., Aoki, Y., Hoshi, T. and Hashimoto, H. (2000) The liver in collagen diseases: pathologic study of 160 cases with particular reference to hepatic arteritis, primary biliary cirrhosis, autoimmune hepatitis and nodular regenerative hyperplasia of the liver. *Liver* **20**, 366–373.

[7] Cosnes, J., Robert, A., Levy, V.G. and Darnis, F. (1980) Budd–Chiari syndrome in a patient with mixed connective tissue disease. *Dig. Dis. Sci.* **25**, 467–469.

[8] van Hoek, B. (1996) The spectrum of liver disease in systemic lupus erythematosus. *Neth. J. Med.* **48**, 244–253.

[9] Hirasahi, S. (1997) Mixed connective tissue disease associated with idiopathic portal hypertension and chronic thyroiditis. *J. Gastrol.* **32**, 808.

[10] Sherlock, S. (1997) *Diseases of the Liver and Biliary System*, 10th edition (Blackwell Sciences, Oxford) pp. 485–495.

[11] Stone, B.E. and Van Thiel, D.H. (1985) Diabetes mellitus and the liver. *Semin. Liver Dis.* **5**, 8–28.

[12] Thuluvath, P.J. and John, P.R. (2003) Association between hepatitis C, diabetes mellitus, and race: a case-control study. *Am. J. Gastroenterol.* **98**(2), 438–441.

[13] Mehta, S.H. and Brancati, F.L. (2000) Prevalence of type II diabetes mellitus among persons with hepatitis C virus infection in the United States. *Ann. Intern. Med.* **133**, 592–599.

[14] Mehta, S.H. and Brancati, F.L. (2003) Hepatitis C virus infection and incident type II diabetes. *Hepatology* **38**, 50–55.

[15] Gibson, P.R. and Dudley, F.J. (1984) Ischemic hepatitis: clinical features, diagnosis and prognosis. *Aust. N. Z. J. Med.* **14**, 822–825.

[16] Nouel, O., Henrion, J., Bernuau, J., Degott, C., Rueff, B. and Benhamou, J.P. (1980) Fulminant hepatic failure due to transient circulatory failure in patients with chronic heart disease. *Dig. Dis. Sci.* **25**, 49–52.

Hepatology: A Practical Approach
B. Al Knawy, M.L. Shiffman, R.H. Wiesner (editors)

Chapter 6
Use and Misuse of Medications in Patients with Liver Disease

R. Todd Stravitz

Section of Hepatology, Virginia Commonwealth University, Richmond, VA 23298-0341, USA

1. Introduction 501
2. Analgesics 502
   2.1 Acetaminophen 502
   2.2 Other non-steroidal anti-inflammatory drugs 502
   2.3 Opioids 504
3. Sedatives and Hypnotics 505
4. Diuretics 505
5. Antihypertensives 506
6. Lactulose 508
7. Antibiotics 508
   7.1 Aminoglycosides 508
   7.2 Other antibiotics 508
8. Hypolipidemic Agents 509
9. Hypoglycemic Agents 511
10. Antidepressants 512
References 512

1. INTRODUCTION

This chapter will review the practical use, and emphasize examples of misuse, of the most commonly prescribed drugs in patients with chronic liver disease. Measures to avoid iatrogenic drug toxicity in patients with cirrhosis will be discussed, since the inappropriate administration of drugs constitutes a major source of morbidity in such patients. Algorithms for treating complications of chronic liver disease will not be offered as these topics are covered in previous chapters; similarly, the reader is referred to preceding chapters for systematic discussion of drug-induced liver injury.

As with all patients, the overriding question in prescribing a drug to patients with chronic liver disease must be whether the benefit of a drug outweighs the potential risk of toxicity. With a few noteworthy exceptions, drugs prescribed in standard doses to patients with chronic liver disease are well tolerated and do not pose an increased risk of toxicity until the stage of decompensated cirrhosis. Severe chronic liver disease in some instances increases the susceptibility of a patient to drug-induced liver toxicity, but extrahepatic toxicity often dominates the clinical presentation because other organ systems are functionally impaired by liver failure, and therefore are vulnerable. In cirrhotic patients, the kidneys and central nervous system usually endure the greatest injury from drugs, while the gastrointestinal and hemostatic systems are also at increased risk of toxicity.

Although all phases of hepatic drug metabolism may be affected by severe chronic liver disease, normal drug elimination persists until very late in the disease process. In general, hepatic degradation of drugs by glucuronidation and/or sulfation remains relatively unaffected even in the most advanced stages of cirrhosis, while oxidative biotransformation through cytochrome P-450 enzymes decreases earlier. Porto-systemic shunting of blood around the liver, a result of portal hypertension, decreases hepatic blood flow, impairing the clearance of drugs with high first-pass metabolism, thereby increasing their oral bioavailability. Diminished hepatic synthesis of plasma proteins, particularly albumin, may increase the risk of extrahepatic drug toxicity because of lower protein binding, and thus, higher free levels. Finally, excretion or inactivation of drugs and their metabolites may be delayed because of a higher volume of distribution in patients with ascites and edema.

The risk of drug hepatotoxicity in a patient with chronic liver disease also depends on the mechanism by which the drug causes liver damage. Intrinsic hepatotoxins, which injure the liver by predictable, dose-dependent effects, may accumulate in the setting of severe chronic liver disease, thereby increasing the *incidence* of liver injury. Conversely, drugs that cause idiosyncratic hepatotoxicity do so independently of dose or drug levels, as a result of biotransformation of the drug into toxic or immunogenic molecules. Chronic liver disease may, therefore, increase the *severity* of liver injury from an idiosyncratic drug reaction, but should not influence the incidence of liver injury. However, the functional reserve of a diseased liver to recover from any drug injury may be compromised.

2. ANALGESICS

2.1 Acetaminophen

The analgesic/antipyretic, acetaminophen (APAP), is an intrinsic hepatotoxin and overdose can cause severe liver injury in healthy patients without pre-existing liver disease. Several features of patients with chronic liver disease may increase their susceptibility to APAP hepatotoxicity. Patients with active alcoholic liver disease are particularly prone to APAP toxicity even in therapeutic ($\leq$4 g/d) doses [1], as a result of the induction of cytochrome P-450 2E1 activity by chronic ethanol ingestion, which increases the production of the toxic metabolite, *N*-acetyl-*p*-benzoquinone imine (NAPQI; Figure 1). Malnutrition, which often accompanies alcoholism and cirrhosis, depletes stores of reduced glutathione, the endogenous antidote, and thus increases the risk of APAP hepatotoxicity; inactive alcoholic cirrhosis, however, may not increase this risk [2]. Patients with inherited disorders of UDP-glucuronyltransferase (e.g., Gilbert's syndrome) metabolize more APAP into NAPQI, also increasing the risk of hepatotoxicity (Figure 1). Conversely, patients with severe chronic liver disease may be less susceptible to APAP hepatotoxicity because of the preservation of glucuronidation relative to oxidation (Figure 1).

Currently, there is no convincing data to suggest that patients with stable chronic liver disease are at increased risk of APAP hepatotoxicity. The metabolism of APAP into glucuronides, sulfates, and mercapturic acid conjugates does not significantly differ between patients with severe chronic liver diseases and patients without liver disease. One study exploring the potential toxicity of APAP in chronic liver disease included patients with alcoholic, viral and cholestatic diseases, some of whom had cirrhosis [2]. Patients received 4 g/d of APAP for 2 weeks. Maximal plasma concentrations of APAP never exceeded recognized toxic levels; furthermore, no patient experienced an elevation of serum transaminases or creatinine. Therefore, APAP appears to be safe when used in therapeutic doses ($\leq$4 g/d) in patients with stable chronic liver disease who do not regularly consume ethanol. Malnourished patients or active alcoholics with or without chronic liver disease should receive APAP in reduced doses (perhaps $\leq$2 g/d). APAP should probably be avoided in patients with chronic liver disease who require other drugs which induce the activity of cytochrome P-450 2E1, such as isoniazid, rifampin, phenytoin and phenobarbital.

2.2 Other non-steroidal anti-inflammatory drugs

Non-steroidal anti-inflammatory drugs (NSAIDs) may also be used safely by most patients with chronic liver disease, with specific exceptions. Although NSAIDs cause idiosyncratic drug hepatitis frequently relative to other drugs, the presence of chronic liver disease should not increase the incidence of hepatotoxicity, which remains low [3]. Certain NSAIDs more often induce idiosyncratic

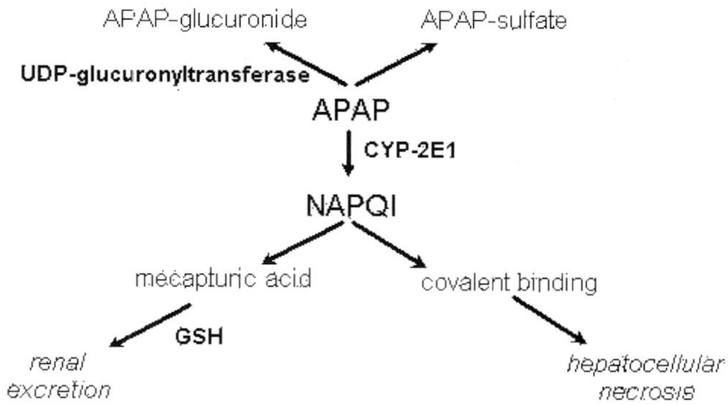

Figure 1. Risk factors for liver injury in patients using acetaminophen. Acetaminophen (APAP) may be metabolized to harmless glucuronides or sulfates or to the reactive electrophile, *N*-acetyl-*p*-benzoquinone imine (NAPQI). NAPQI may be detoxified by reduced glutathione (GSH) and excreted as a mercapturic acid or may covalently bind to hepatocellular components and induce necrosis. Patients who chronically consume ethanol, whether or not they have overt alcoholic liver disease, and patients receiving certain drugs (isoniazid, rifampin, phenytoin, phenobarbital) are at increased risk of toxicity because these agents induce the activity of cytochrome P-450 2E1 (CYP-2E1). Patients who abuse alcohol, or are acutely or chronically malnourished, are at increased risk of toxicity because of decreased GSH stores. Patients with decreased UDP-glucuronyltransferase activity (malnutrition, Gilberts syndrome) are at increased risk of toxicity because of deficient glucuronidation of APAP, channeling more into the oxidative pathway to NAPQI.

drug hepatitis than others, and may be less desirable for use in patients with chronic liver disease. Ibuprofen and naproxen very rarely cause idiosyncratic hepatitis, while sulindac and diclofenac precipitate liver injury more frequently as a result of metabolism into hepatotoxic or immunogenic molecules (Table 1). Only few cases of suspected hepatotoxicity (presumably idiosyncratic) due to selective cyclo-oxygenase-2 (COX-2) inhibitors have been reported, but collective experience with these drugs is small. The mechanism of liver toxicity due to aspirin (ASA) differs from other NSAIDs, as high doses are intrinsically (dose-dependently) hepatotoxic. The risk of salicylate hepatotoxicity correlates best with serum levels, as 90% of cases occur when concentrations exceed 15 mg/dl [3]. Consequently, high doses (>4–8 g/d) of ASA should probably be avoided in patients with chronic liver disease.

The administration of all NSAIDs to patients with cirrhosis presents the greatest risk to extrahepatic tissues. Impairment of renal perfusion is one of the primary pathogenetic mechanisms of ascites formation in cirrhosis; hence, the presence of ascites implies renal arterial constriction. Prostaglandins of the E type, endogenously produced by the kidneys, counteract the action of circulating renal vasoconstrictors and are critical to preserving renal perfusion in cirrhosis. In such patients, the inhibition of renal prostaglandin synthesis by NSAIDs leaves renal artery vasoconstriction unopposed, leading to decreased renal blood flow, creatinine clearance, urine volume and sodium excretion. NSAIDs are among the most common precipitating agents of ascites and renal failure in cirrhotic patients. Similarly, cirrhotic patients with ascites, refractory to diuretics, should always be queried about NSAID use before increasing the dose of diuretics, since NSAIDs blunt the natriuresis of both furosemide and spironolactone [4]. COX-2 inhibitors (celecoxib and rofecoxib) may induce renal dysfunction and edema formation in patients without chronic liver or kidney disease, and therefore must also be avoided in cirrhotic patients with ascites. NSAIDs should also be avoided in patients with cirrhosis who have thrombocytopenia, coagulopathy or a prior history of bleeding from gastroduodenal ulceration, portal hypertensive gastropathy or esophageal varices.

In summary, a history of ascites is an absolute contraindication to the use of all NSAIDs in patients with chronic liver disease, including selective COX-2 inhibitors. In well-compensated cirrhotic patients without risk factors for upper GI bleeding, COX-2 inhibitors may be analgesics of choice because of their lower propensity to cause gastroduodenal ulceration.

Table 1. Use of non-steroidal anti-inflammatory drugs in patients with chronic liver disease.

Drug	Mechanism of liver injury	Incidence of liver injury	Recommendation for use in patients with cirrhosis
Acetaminophen	Intrinsic	Dose-dependent	$\leq$4 g/d; high risk, $\leq$2 g/d[a]
ASA	Intrinsic	Dose-dependent	Avoid in cirrhotic patients with:
Sulindac	Idiosyncratic	Low	1. Renal insufficiency
Diclofenac	Idiosyncratic	Low	2. A history of ascites (past or present)
Piroxicam	Idiosyncratic	Very low	3. A history of upper GI bleeding
Indomethacin	Idiosyncratic	Very low	4. Known esophageal varices or portal hypertensive gastropathy
Naproxen	Idiosyncratic	Very low	5. Thrombocytopenia
Ibuprofen	Idiosyncratic	Very low	6. Coagulopathy
Celecoxib	?Idiosyncratic	Five case reports	Avoid if $\uparrow S_{Cr}$ or history of ascites

[a]See text and Figure 1 for patients at higher risk of acetaminophen hepatotoxicity.

2.3 Opioids

The liver catabolizes all opioids, and severe chronic liver disease can result in accumulation of drug as well as active metabolites, resulting in excessive sedation and respiratory depression (Table 2). In healthy patients, morphine is metabolized predominantly by glucuronidation with high first-pass extraction; consequently, its oral bioavailability is low. Although patients with cirrhosis exhibit only a modest (~25%) decrease in hepatic metabolism of morphine because of the relative sparing of glucuronidation, plasma clearance rates can be greatly reduced in patients with porto-systemic shunting, which also greatly increases its oral bioavailability. Patients with cirrhosis complicated by portal hypertension should therefore receive morphine in lower doses or longer dosing intervals. Morphine may otherwise be the drug of choice for severe pain in cirrhotic patients because of its short half-life, safety and relatively preserved hepatic biotransformation.

Most other opioids, including meperidine, tramadol and codeine, undergo oxidative catabolism, and may therefore accumulate earlier in cirrhosis than morphine (Table 2; [5]). Repetitive doses of meperidine should not be used in patients with concomitant liver and renal disease, which results in the accumulation of normeperidine and can precipitate seizures. In contrast, codeine must undergo bioactivation to morphine, and liver failure may thereby compromise its analgesic effect. Tramadol (Ultram®), a centrally acting synthetic ligand of the μ-opioid receptor, provides effective analgesia with less respiratory depression than morphine. Oxidative metabolism of tramadol decreases with advanced cirrhosis, and doses must be reduced [5]. It should be emphasized, however, that patients with chronic liver disease and a history of hepatic encephalopathy are predisposed to

Table 2. Use of commonly prescribed opioids in patients with chronic liver disease.

Drug	Primary hepatic metabolism	Relative contraindications	Potential toxicity[a]
Morphine	Conjugation	None	None
Meperidine	Oxidation	Renal failure. Chronic administration not recommended	Seizures
Codeine	Oxidation	Severe liver failure (decreased activation to morphine)	None
Propoxyphene	Oxidation	Severe liver failure	Hepatotoxicity
Tramadol	Oxidation	Severe liver failure	Seizures

[a]Dose reduction and increased dosing intervals are recommended in all patients with severe chronic liver disease (cirrhosis) because of increased CNS sensitivity to the sedating effects of opioids and the risk of respiratory depression.

excessive sedation by all opioids regardless of the effect of liver disease on clearance of the drug.

3. SEDATIVES AND HYPNOTICS

The presence of cirrhosis increases the risk of over-sedation from benzodiazepines. The metabolism of many benzodiazepines, especially those eliminated by oxidation (diazepam and chlordiazepoxide), may be impaired in cirrhosis, as may elimination of their active metabolites (Table 3). In addition, all benzodiazepines are extensively protein-bound, and hypoalbuminemia increases free levels and, thus, brain uptake of the drugs. Most importantly, cirrhotic patients with hepatic encephalopathy accumulate endogenous benzodiazepines derived from gut bacteria, increasing inhibitory neurotransmission through the gamma aminobutyric acid (GABA) receptor complex [6]. Therefore, even benzodiazepines that undergo glucuronidation (lorazepam, midazolam and oxazepam) and have near-normal elimination kinetics in cirrhosis, may result in prolonged and excessively deep sedation. All members of this class of drug should be used with caution in severe chronic liver disease, and avoided in patients with a history of recurrent hepatic encephalopathy. The benzodiazepine antagonist, flumazenil, has been shown to ameliorate the neuropsychiatric syndrome of hepatic encephalopathy [7], presumably by blocking the binding of endogenously produced benzodiazepines to the GABA receptor. Since the improvements in encephalopathy after flumazenil administration are incomplete and transient, the drug cannot be advocated as a first-line agent. However, flumazenil may be useful in patients with chronic liver disease and over-sedation from the injudicious use of benzodiazepines.

Patients with chronic liver disease commonly complain of insomnia, which may represent early hepatic encephalopathy. As discussed above, benzodiazepines should be avoided, and lactulose rarely improves insomnia (day–night reversal) in such patients. Other drugs with little tendency to induce dependence or exacerbate encephalopathy include antihistamines or antidepressants with sedating side effects (Table 3). Even in patients with decompensated cirrhosis, diphenhydramine 25–50 mg or trazodone 25–100 mg at bedtime, will often improve insomnia without prolonged sedation. The short-acting hypnotic, zolpidem (Ambien®), may also be considered; however, studies have documented increased levels of unbound drug in hypoalbuminemic patients with cirrhosis, which may lead to higher brain levels and prolonged sedation. In addition, zolpidem is believed to act on the benzodiazepine receptor and should therefore be avoided in patients with a history of hepatic encephalopathy.

4. DIURETICS

Patients with chronic liver disease frequently require diuretics to control ascites and edema. Typically, a

Table 3. Use of sedatives and hypnotics in patients with chronic liver disease.

Drug(s)	Primary hepatic metabolism	Indications for use in chronic liver disease	Recommendations for use in chronic liver disease
Diazepam, chlordiazepoxide	Oxidation	None	Not recommended
Lorazepam, oxazepam, midazolam	Conjugation	Sedation	Avoid in patients with a history of HE
Flumazenil		Reversal of over-sedation from BDZ	May precipitate seizures. Not indicated for treating HE
Diphenhydramine		Hypnotic	Drug of choice in severe liver disease
Trazodone		Hypnotic	Dose reduction in severe liver disease
Zolpidem		Hypnotic	Avoid in patients with a history of HE

BDZ, benzodiazepines; HE, hepatic encephalopathy.

Table 4. Complications of diuretic therapy in patients with chronic liver disease.

Complication	Diuretic(s) responsible	Proposed correction
Azotemia	F/S	
$S_{Cr} > 2$ or 2-fold increase		Decrease dose of diuretics by one step[a]
$S_{Cr} > 2.5$		Hold diuretics
Hyponatremia	F/S	Decrease free water intake
< 130 mEq/l		Decrease dose of diuretics by one step[a]
< 125 mEq/l		Hold diuretics
Hypokalemia	F	Replete; increase dose of S
Hyperkalemia	S	Decrease dose of S
Hypomagnesemia, hypocalcemia	F	Replete
Encephalopathy	F > S	
w/hypokalemia		Replete K to 5–5.5 mEq/l
w/azotemia		Hold diuretics
Gynecomastia	S	Substitute amiloride

F, furosemide; S, spironolactone.
[a]One step refers to spironolactone 100 mg and furosemide 40 mg p.o. (see text).

combination of a loop diuretic and spironolactone provides the most effective diuresis by sequentially inhibiting sodium reabsorption from the lumen of the loop of Henle and distal convoluted tubule of the nephron, respectively. A useful ratio of oral furosemide/spironolactone, which usually preserves normokalemia, is 40 mg/100 mg (step 1), increasing the dose successively by 40 mg/100 mg to a maximum of 160 mg/400 mg (step 4). Doses beyond step 4 should usually not be administered as they rarely improve diuresis and imply inadequate renal perfusion due to renal arterial constriction. Spironolactone and its active metabolites have extremely long half-lives in patients with cirrhosis, and therefore, the drug can be given in a single daily dose; dose adjustments should be made slowly (2–3 week intervals) to avoid over-diuresis due to the accumulation of active metabolites [8]. Male patients with cirrhotic ascites and edema do not often tolerate spironolactone because of painful gynecomastia. Other potassium-sparing diuretics, which inhibit sodium reabsorption from the distal tubule, such as amiloride or triamterene, may be substituted. In one randomized trial, however, amiloride (up to 60 mg/d) was decidedly less effective than an active metabolite of spironolactone.

Patients with decompensated cirrhosis are particularly vulnerable to the complications of diuretic treatment, including electrolyte depletion, dehydration, hepatic encephalopathy and azotemia (Table 4). Hypomagnesemia is particularly underrecognized, and may precipitate seizures. Hyponatremia results from the hypersecretion of antidiuretic hormone from the posterior pituitary and may be greatly exacerbated by the use of diuretics. Diuretic doses should be decreased when serum sodium falls below ~130 mEq/l, and held below ~125 mEq/l. Cirrhotic patients become hypokalemic due to secondary hyperaldosteronemia, malnutrition and through gastrointestinal losses (use of cathartics, vomiting, diarrhea). Further potassium depletion from loop diuretics frequently precipitates hepatic encephalopathy by decreasing renal excretion of ammonium, thereby increasing arterial ammonia concentrations. Based upon these observations, some authors have suggested that patients with cirrhosis, ascites and recurrent hepatic encephalopathy receive potassium supplementation to serum levels of highest normokalemia (5.4–5.5 mEq/l). Doses of diuretics should not be increased to treat unresponsive ascites or edema in the setting of progressive azotemia (rise of serum creatinine of 100% or increase >2.0 mg/dl).

5. ANTIHYPERTENSIVES

Patients with chronic liver disease occasionally require antihypertensives, although they usually become normotensive with progression of their liver disease to cirrhosis. Most commonly prescribed antihypertensive agents are well tolerated and do not require dose adjustment in chronic liver disease until the stage of cirrhosis, when they may be required to treat portal hypertension rather than systemic hypertension (Table 5). As the severity of chronic liver disease advances, patients become increasingly sensitive to antihypertensive agents and increasingly intolerant of side effects, especially postural hypotension and fatigue. All antihypertensive agents occasionally cause liver injury, with the incidence highest for L-methyldopa, which increases liver transaminases in up to 30% of patients, and may lead to cirrhosis [9].

Non-selective β-blockers have gained wide acceptance in primary and secondary prophylaxes against esophageal variceal hemorrhage in cirrhotic patients, in whom they decrease portal pressure modestly (~15%). The hepatic clearance of propranolol, the most commonly used β-blocker for these indications, is 44% reduced in patients with cirrhosis due to decreased hepatocellular oxidative enzyme activity and decreased hepatic blood flow. Consequently, propranolol may be taken only twice daily in cirrhotic patients as prophylaxis against variceal bleeding. As a result of decreased cardiac output and decreased mesenteric blood flow, non-selective β-blockers may slow the clearance of other hepatically metabolized drugs by decreasing hepatic blood flow, especially drugs with high first-pass metabolism such as morphine. Although non-selective β-blockers decrease cardiac output, renal function has not been shown to be adversely affected, even in advanced cirrhosis.

Most patients with portal hypertension do not achieve adequate reduction in portal pressures after β-blocker administration to prevent variceal bleeding. Accordingly, long-acting nitrates such as isosorbide-5-mononitrate, which decrease portal pressure by vasodilating porto-systemic collaterals and intrahepatic vessels, have been added to β-blockers. Most studies support an additive effect of combined nitrate/β-blocker therapy over β-blocker monotherapy; however, the combination often induces symptomatic hypotension and may worsen renal and systemic hemodynamics [10]. In addition, nitrates should not be used as monotherapy for prophylaxis against variceal hemorrhage, since one randomized, long-term study clearly indicated that overall survival in patients over 50 years of age was reduced as compared to patients on β-blocker monotherapy [11].

Drugs which inhibit the renin–angiotensin–aldosterone axis have become first-line agents in the treatment of systemic hypertension, and have been tested in patients with cirrhosis to counteract the adverse effects of hypersecretion of angiotensin II (ATII). Although angiotensin-converting enzyme (ACE) inhibitors such as enalapril may improve natriuresis

Table 5. Use of antihypertensives in chronic liver disease.

Drug	Indications in chronic liver disease	Potential toxicity in patients with chronic liver disease
Methyldopa	None	Avoid due to high incidence of chronic hepatitis (up to 30%)
Beta blockers (non-selective)	Prophylaxis against variceal bleeding	Fatigue; may slow metabolism of other drugs
ISMN	Prophylaxis against variceal bleeding with β-blockers	Not indicated as monotherapy (increased mortality)
ACE inhibitors	Antihypertensives	Avoid in cirrhotic patients with ascites (adverse hemodynamic effects)
ATII receptor antagonists	Antihypertensives	Avoid in cirrhotic patients with portal hypertension (adverse hemodynamic effects)
Calcium channel blockers	Antihypertensives	Generally safe

in cirrhotic patients by decreasing aldosterone synthesis and partially relieving ATII-mediated renal vasoconstriction, they may also precipitate marked hypotension and are generally poorly tolerated. Recently, the ATII receptor antagonist, losartan (25 mg PO), was tested in a pilot study of cirrhotic patients with portal hypertension and reported to dramatically decrease the hepatic venous pressure gradient without adversely affecting systemic or renal hemodynamics. Unfortunately, in two subsequent randomized studies, ATII receptor antagonists decreased hepatic venous pressure gradient minimally and frequently led to hypotension and decreased creatinine clearances [12]. Thus, all inhibitors of the renin–angiotensin system should be used cautiously in cirrhotic patients and cannot be recommended as prophylactic agents to treat portal hypertension.

6. LACTULOSE

For 35 years, the non-absorbable, non-hydrolyzable disaccharide, lactulose, has remained the treatment of choice for hepatic encephalopathy. In patients with hepatic encephalopathy, lactulose should not be administered without a careful search for precipitating causes, such as gastrointestinal bleeding, infection and electrolyte abnormalities. Lactulose may then be titrated to oral doses producing 2–4 loose stools per day. Overdose, while uncommon, can have detrimental effects in patients with severe chronic liver disease. Although lactulose itself is not absorbed from the gut lumen, preparations contain other carbohydrate contaminants that may adversely affect glucose homeostasis. Large doses can exacerbate hepatic encephalopathy by causing diarrhea, hypokalemia, acidosis and hypernatremic dehydration [13]. Some patients can neither tolerate the excessively sweet taste of lactulose nor the flatulence and bloating. These unpleasant side effects must not be ignored, for they may contribute to anorexia and further malnutrition in a cirrhotic patient.

7. ANTIBIOTICS

7.1 Aminoglycosides

Once prescribed as the most effective class of antibiotics against gram-negative bacilli, aminoglycosides have become second-line therapy as a result of their narrow therapeutic window, the need for blood level monitoring and the hazards of nephro- and ototoxicity. Perhaps no patient is at greater risk of aminoglycoside toxicity than the patient with cirrhosis, where the risk of acute renal failure has been shown to increase 32-fold over cephalosporin-treated patients without liver disease and 6-fold over patients with chronic liver disease treated with cephalosporins [14]. Surprisingly, even 10–15 years after these reports, cirrhotic patients continue to receive aminoglycosides and develop renal failure [15]. Aminoglycoside nephrotoxicity appears to be particularly frequent in cirrhotic patients with ascites, the presence of which reflects decreased renal blood flow and glomerular filtration rate. These characteristics predispose the kidney to acute tubular necrosis from aminoglycosides, and also to the hepatorenal syndrome. For these reasons and since effective alternatives now exist for serious gram-negative infections (e.g., fluoroquinolones), aminoglycosides should be considered contraindicated in patients with serious chronic liver disease, especially if accompanied by ascites (Table 6).

The "non-absorbable" aminoglycoside, neomycin, was the first oral agent introduced to treat hepatic encephalopathy, and functions to suppress gut bacterial production of ammonia. Although effective, neomycin levels can accumulate in blood and precipitate sensorineural deafness and acute renal failure [16]. The total oral dose of neomycin responsible for deafness ranges between 500 and 2500 g used over months (1–5 g/d). Chronic use of oral neomycin can also injure small bowel mucosa and induce a malabsorptive syndrome, exacerbating malnutrition in some cirrhotic patients. These adverse effects mandate close follow-up of creatinine clearance and hearing tests in patients receiving the drug chronically. Neomycin may be used acutely to treat hepatic encephalopathy in doses of up to 6 g/d, but chronic dosing should be decreased to 2–4 g/d; neomycin should be avoided in cirrhotic patients with renal insufficiency (Table 6).

7.2 Other antibiotics

Oral metronidazole may be considered as a second-line drug to treat hepatic encephalopathy in cirrhotic patients who have either incompletely responded to, or cannot tolerate the side effects of, lactulose.

Table 6. Use of antibiotics in patients with chronic liver disease.

Drug	Indication in chronic liver disease	Potential toxicity in chronic liver disease	Recommendation in chronic liver disease
Aminoglycosides (i.v.)	Gram-negative infection	Nephrotoxicity, ototoxicity	Avoid in cirrhosis
Neomycin (p.o.)	Hepatic encephalopathy	Nephrotoxicity, ototoxicity, malabsorption	Lowest effective dose; monitor renal function and hearing tests
Metronidazole (p.o.)	Hepatic encephalopathy	GI symptoms, peripheral neuropathy	Lowest effective dose (≤750 mg/d)
Cephalosporins	Infection	Coagulopathy (second-generation)	Reduce dose in renal failure; monitor PT
Rifampin	Pruritis in cholestasis	Drug hepatitis, coagulopathy (rare)	Monitor ALT and PT
Nitrofurantoin	None	Chronic hepatitis	Not recommended
Fluoroquinolones	Infection	Well tolerated	Drugs of choice to replace aminoglycosides

Similar to neomycin, metronidazole suppresses ammonia production by gut bacteria. Few clinical data support the use of metronidazole in hepatic encephalopathy; however, one study suggests that an oral dose of 800 mg/d may be as effective as 4 g/d of neomycin, and that the two drugs may have an additive effect [17]. Although the use of metronidazole in hepatic encephalopathy appears to have fewer serious side effects than neomycin, unpleasant gastrointestinal symptoms such as anorexia, nausea and a metallic taste may contribute to malnutrition (Table 6). These side effects occur more often in cirrhotic patients, in whom hepatic oxidation of the parent compound and renal elimination of metabolites are both impaired [18]. Consequently, the dose of metronidazole should not exceed 250 mg p.o. thrice daily when used chronically.

Most penicillins and cephalosporins are renally excreted and therefore do not require dose reduction in cirrhotic patients unless significant renal insufficiency co-exists. Some β-lactam antibiotics, in particular, second-generation cephalosporins containing an *N*-methylthiotetrazole side chain (moxalactam, cefamandol and cefoperazone) undergo impaired hepatobiliary elimination in cirrhosis, and have been incriminated in exacerbating the coagulopathy of chronic liver disease, especially in malnourished patients. Multiple mechanisms may account for this effect, including decreased gut bacterial synthesis of vitamin K_2 and a warfarin-like inhibition of hepatic vitamin K metabolism. Prothrombin times should be monitored accordingly and vitamin K supplemented orally or subcutaneously.

The antibiotic rifampin has been used increasingly in the treatment of pruritis associated with chronic cholestatic liver diseases such as primary biliary cirrhosis (PBC). Presumably, rifampin functions by inducing cytochrome P-450 metabolism of unidentified pruritogens. Chronic administration of rifampin (300 mg/d) has been reported to cause reversible coagulopathy in patients with PBC and may have a direct warfarin-like effect. In addition, rifampin induced a drug hepatitis in 12.5% of PBC patients treated for pruritis, requiring follow-up of both prothrombin time and liver enzymes during rifampin therapy [19].

Nitrofurantoin is a bacteriostatic antibiotic commonly prescribed to prevent recurrent urinary tract infection. Nitrofurantoin can cause a severe chronic drug hepatitis with immunologic features, including high titers of antinuclear antibodies. Its use on a long-term basis in patients with chronic liver disease is thus probably unwise.

8. HYPOLIPIDEMIC AGENTS

Patients with severe, non-cholestatic, chronic liver diseases uncommonly require hypolipidemic agents, as most have low hepatic biosynthesis of lipids. Patients with non-alcoholic steatohepatitis (NASH), however, frequently have hypertriglyceridemia with or without hypercholesterolemia, reflecting the fundamental metabolic abnormality of insulin resistance in this disorder. All hypolipidemic agents, except for bile acid binding resins that are not absorbed from the gut, can cause hepatotoxicity (Table 7). However, patients with hyperlipidemia and chronic liver disease should receive treatment for their lipid disorders; indeed, the increased risk of cardiovascular events from not treating such patients clearly outweighs the small risk of hepatotoxicity. Patients with predominant hypercholesterolemia may receive HMG-CoA reductase inhibitors ("statins") as initial therapy, with or without a bile acid sequestrant (cholestyramine or colestipol). Although all statins cause mild dose-dependent drug hepatitis, pravachol may have advantages over other reductase inhibitors in patients with chronic liver disease: reduced effects on cytochrome P-450 activities, greater fractional renal excretion (60%) and no requirement for hepatic activation because it is not a prodrug [20]. Monitoring transaminases during statin therapy is recommended at baseline, 3 months and 6 months thereafter, but may not prevent the rare cases of severe hepatotoxicity.

Most NASH patients have a mixed lipid disorder, and persistent hypertriglyceridemia on a statin may be treated by the addition of a fibric acid derivative, such as gemfibrozil or fenofibrate. Gemfibrozil has a long track record of use and only very rarely induces significant liver injury, usually reversible mild cholestatic hepatitis. Less information exists for fenofibrate, but this agent has been reported to cause progressive liver fibrosis with autoimmune features [9]. Therefore, gemfibrozil may be the preferred agent to treat hypertriglyceridemia in patients with underlying liver disease; fish oils high in Ω-3 fatty acids also improve serum triglyceride levels with no risk of toxicity. Patients on combination statin/fibric acid therapy should be counseled about myalgias, as this symptom may herald severe rhabdomyolysis. Since liver transaminases are typically mildly elevated (~2–3-fold) in patients with NASH before the administration of hypolipidemic agents, ALT as well as CPK activities should be routinely monitored, and drugs should be stopped if significant increases of transaminases occur or biochemical signs of myopathy appear.

Nicotinic acid causes dose-dependent hepatic dysfunction in approximately 30% of patients without pre-existing liver disease. Sustained-release forms of niacin are far more likely to cause severe liver injury than the short-acting forms and should be avoided in patients with chronic liver disease.

Patients with chronic cholestatic liver diseases such as PBC commonly become hypercholesterolemic, especially in the later stages of their disease. The hyperlipidemia of PBC has been ascribed to the presence of lipoprotein-X, an abnormal LDL that refluxes into the blood from an obstructed biliary tree. The hyperlipidemia observed in PBC, however, does not confer the same cardiovascular risk as observed in hyperlipidemic patients without liver disease. Although scant long-term data exist, the risk of cardiovascular death in hyperlipidemic patients with PBC is similar to that of the general population. Therefore, the hyperlipidemia of PBC does not require treatment unless a patient has risk factors for, or a personal history of, atherosclerosis. Such patients may be safely treated with statins, and bile acid sequestrants (cholestyramine, colestipol) may be

Table 7. Use of hypolipidemic agents in patients with chronic liver disease.

Drug class	Indication	Potential toxicities	Use in chronic liver disease
Bile acid sequestrants	Hypercholesterolemia	None; may bind other oral medications	Safe; dose other medications 1–2 h after
HMG-CoAR inhibitors	Hypercholesterolemia	Hepatitis (usu. mild); myopathy	Pravachol preferred?
Fibrates	Hypertriglyceridemia	Hepatitis; myopathy	Gemfibrozil preferred?
Fish oils (Ω-3 fatty acids)	Hypertriglyceridemia	None	Safe
Niacin, Niacin-SR	Mixed lipid disorders	Drug hepatitis, acute liver failure	SR-niacin not recommended

HMG-CoAR, hydroxy-methyl-glutaryl coenzyme A reductase inhibitor (statin); Niacin-SR, sustained release formulation.

added, but should be given at least 1–2 h after their daily dose of ursodiol.

9. HYPOGLYCEMIC AGENTS

Insulin resistance commonly complicates cirrhosis and underlies the pathophysiology of NASH. Moreover, several epidemiological studies have documented an increased incidence of diabetes in patients with chronic hepatitis C, although the mechanism of the association has not been determined. Consequently, oral hypoglycemic agents are required in many patients with chronic liver disease. Most oral hypoglycemic agents have been rarely reported to cause idiosyncratic hepatotoxicity, including sulfonylureas, thiazolidinediones and metformin. Apart from the risk of toxicity of the drugs themselves, all oral antidiabetic drugs risk serious hypoglycemia in patients with advanced cirrhosis because of deficient caloric intake, decreased glycogen stores in the liver and impaired gluconeogenesis. All such drugs should therefore be used with caution in patients with serious chronic liver disease (Table 8).

First-generation sulfonylureas such as chlorpropamide cause cholestatic hepatitis rarely, but more frequently than second-generation agents. The pharmacokinetics of glipizide and glyburide, two second-generation sulfonylureas, remains largely unchanged in patients with chronic liver diseases. Both very rarely induce intrahepatic cholestasis or cholestatic hepatitis, and may be the preferred hypoglycemic agents in cirrhotic patients because of their long track records and relative safety [9]. Glimepiride (Amaryl®), a newer sulfonylurea, is eliminated entirely by oxidative biotransformation. Although no data exist on its pharmacokinetics in cirrhotic patients, doses of glimepiride in patients with severe chronic liver disease should also be reduced. Similar to sulfonylureas, repaglinide (Prandin®) improves serum glucose control by stimulating insulin secretion by pancreatic β-cells and undergoes oxidative biotransformation and conjugation to glucuronide in the hepatocyte. Accordingly, clearance of repaglinide and its metabolites decreases with the severity of chronic liver disease, and dosage and dose intervals should be appropriately modified.

All the thiazolidinedione class of insulin-sensitizing agents have been reported to cause severe idiosyncratic liver injury, and the first of this class of drug, troglitazone (Rezulin®), was withdrawn from the US market for this reason. Troglitazone caused at least 90 cases of acute liver failure, and in clinical trials, was associated with a 3-fold higher incidence of significant ALT elevation than placebo. In contrast, rosiglitazone (Avandia®) and pioglitazone (Actos®) have both been incriminated in very few cases of severe liver injury, and in controlled trials, the incidence of significant elevations of ALT in patients receiving these agents was similar to placebo. Thus, rosiglitazone and pioglitazone appear to be less likely to cause liver injury than troglitazone at this time and are probably safe for use in type II diabetics with stable chronic liver disease. However, as it has not been clearly established whether liver toxicity is a

Table 8. Use of oral hypoglycemic agents in patients with chronic liver disease.

Drug class	Potential toxicity	Use in chronic liver disease[a]
First-generation sulfonylureas	Cholestatic hepatitis	Second generation preferred
Second-generation sulfonylureas: glipizide, glyburide, glimepiride	Mild ALT elevation	?Drugs of choice in chronic liver disease
Thiazolidinediones: rosiglitazone, pioglitazone	Rare drug hepatitis	Reduce dose. Follow LFTs
Metformin	Drug hepatitis, metabolic acidosis	Follow LFTs, HCO_3, and Cr. Avoid in renal insufficiency

[a]The use of all oral hypoglycemic agents in patients with severe chronic liver disease (cirrhosis) risks hypoglycemia. Doses of all agents should be decreased, and doing intervals increased, with close follow-up of serum glucose.

class effect of all thiazolidinediones, patients treated with these agents should receive regular screening for hepatotoxicity.

Both thiazolidinediones and metformin (Glucophage®) have been explored in preliminary studies as possible treatments for NASH as both improve insulin resistance. Metformin rarely causes drug hepatitis, but more frequently induces severe lactic acidosis (50% mortality), usually in patients with renal insufficiency. Since the presence of NASH may increase the risk of lactic acidosis because of hepatocellular mitochondrial dysfunction, patients receiving metformin should be closely monitored for biochemical evidence of acidosis as well as liver injury and renal insufficiency. Moreover, clearance of the drug decreases with progressive renal insufficiency; therefore, patients with cirrhosis and elevated serum creatinine should not receive metformin.

10. ANTIDEPRESSANTS

Patients with chronic liver disease should receive treatment for depression, particularly dysphoric patients undergoing interferon therapy for chronic viral hepatitis in whom antidepressants may increase the odds of successful completion of the antiviral regimen. Selective serotonin reuptake inhibitors (SSRIs) now comprise most of the American demand for antidepressants, and are drugs of choice for dysphoric patients on interferon. Although all SSRIs very rarely cause overt hepatocellular injury, the incidence of asymptomatic liver chemistry elevation may be as high as 0.5% for fluoxetine (Prozac®; [9]). The incidence of subclinical hepatitis in patients treated with citalopram (Celexa®) or paroxetine (Paxil®), however, approximates placebo. The doses of all SSRIs must be reduced in patients with liver dysfunction, since oxidative metabolism decreases by roughly 50%, yielding higher blood levels and increasing the risk of adverse reactions. Trazodone may be used at bedtime for depression with insomnia in patients with chronic liver disease, but has been reported to cause acute liver injury as well as chronic active hepatitis, mandating follow-up liver chemistries [9]. Nefazodone (Serzone®) has been reported to cause several cases of acute liver failure and should probably be avoided in patients with chronic liver disease.

REFERENCES

[1] Zimmerman, H.J. and Maddrey, W.C. (1995) Acetaminophen (paracetamol) hepatotoxicity with regular intake of alcohol: analysis of instances of therapeutic misadventure. *Hepatology* **22**, 767–773.

[2] Benson, G.D. (1983) Acetaminophen in chronic liver disease. *Clin. Pharmacol. Ther.* **33**, 95–101.

[3] Fry, S.W. and Seeff, L.B. (1995) Hepatotoxicity of analgesics and anti-inflammatory agents. *Gastroenterol. Clin. North Am.* **24**, 875–905.

[4] Mirouze, D., Zipser, R.D. and Reynolds, T.B. (1983) Effect of inhibitors of prostaglandin synthesis on induced diuresis in cirrhosis. *Hepatology* **3**, 50–55.

[5] Tegeder, I., Lotsch, J. and Geisslinger, G. (1999) Pharmacokinetics of opioids in liver disease. *Clin. Pharmacokinet.* **37**, 17–40.

[6] Jones, E.A. (1989) NIH Conference: the γ-aminobutyric acid A receptor complex and hepatic encephalopathy. *Ann. Intern. Med.* **110**, 532–546.

[7] Barbaro, G., DiLorenzo, G., Soldini, M., Giancaspro, G., Bellomo, G., Belloni, G., Grisorio, B., Annese, M., Bacca, D., Francavilla, R. and Barbarini, G. (1998) Flumazenil for hepatic encephalopathy grade III and IVa in patients with cirrhosis: an Italian multicenter double-blind, placebo-controlled, cross-over study. *Hepatology* **28**, 374–378.

[8] Sungaila, I., Bartle, W.R., Walker, S.E., DeAngelis, D., Uetrecht, J., Pappas, C. and Vidins, E. (1992) Spironolactone pharmacokinetics and pharmacodynamics in patients with cirrhotic ascites. *Gastroenterology* **102**, 1680–1685.

[9] Chitturi, S. and George, J. (2002) Hepatotoxicity of commonly used drugs: non-steroidal anti-inflammatory drugs, antihypertensives, antidiabetic agents, anticonvulsants, lipid-lowering agents, psychotropic drugs. *Semin. Liver Dis.* **22**, 169–183.

[10] Salmerón, J.M., Del Arbol, L.R., Ginès, A., Arroyo, V. and Rodés, J. (1993) Renal effects of acute isosorbide-5-mononitrate administration in cirrhosis. *Hepatology* **17**, 800–806.

[11] Angelico, M., Carli, L., Piat, C., Gentile, S. and Capocaccia, L. (1997) Effects of isosorbide-5-mononitrate compared with propranolol on first bleeding and long-term survival in cirrhosis. *Gastroenterology* **113**, 1632–1639.

[12] González-Abraldes, J., Abillos, A., Banares, R., Del Arbol, L.R., Moitinho, E., Rodríguez, C., González, M., Escorsell, A., García-Pagán, J.C. and Bosch, J. (2001) Randomized comparison of long-term losartan versus propranolol in lowering portal pressure in cirrhosis. *Gastroenterology* **121**, 382–388.

[13] Kaupke, C., Sprague, T. and Gitnick, G.L. (1977) Hypernatremia after the administration of lactulose. *Ann. Intern. Med.* **86**, 745–746.

[14] Moore, R.D., Smith, C.R. and Lietman, P.S. (1986) Increased risk of renal dysfunction due to interaction of liver disease and aminoglycosides. *Am. J. Med.* **80**, 1093–1097.

[15] Hampel, H., Bynum, G.D., Zamora, E. and El-Serag, H.B. (2001) Risk factors for the development of renal dysfunction in hospitalized patients with cirrhosis. *Am. J. Gastroenterol.* **96**, 2206–2210.

[16] Greenberg, L.H. and Momary, H. (1965) Audiotoxicity and nephrotoxicity due to orally administered neomycin. *JAMA* **194**, 237–238.

[17] Morgan, M.H., Read, A.E. and Speller, D.C. (1982) Treatment of hepatic encephalopathy with metronidazole. *Gut* **23**, 1–7.

[18] Loft, S., Sonne, J., Dossing, M. and Buch Andreasen, P. (1987) Metronidazole pharmacokinetics in patients with hepatic encephalopathy. *Scand. J. Gastroenterol.* **22**, 117–123.

[19] Bachs, L., Pares, A., Elena, M., Piera, C. and Rodes, J. (1992) Effects of long-term rifampicin administration in primary biliary cirrhosis. *Gastroenterology* **102**, 2077–2080.

[20] Blum, C.B. (1994) Comparison of properties of four inhibitors of 3-hydroxy-3-methylglutaryl-coenzyme A reductase. *Am. J. Cardiol.* **73**, 3–11D.

Section V
Liver Transplantation

Section Editor – R. Wiesner

Hepatology: A Practical Approach
B. Al Knawy, M.L. Shiffman, R.H. Wiesner (editors)

Chapter 1

Assessment and Timing of Liver Transplantation

Abdulmajeed Alabdulkareem

Department of Hepatobiliary Sciences and Liver Transplantation, Liver Center, King Abdulaziz Medical City, National Guard, P.O. Box 22490, Riyadh 11246, Saudi Arabia

1. Introduction 517
2. Indications and Contraindications 518
3. Hepatitis C 519
4. Hepatitis B 520
5. Alcohol-Related Cirrhosis 520
6. Primary Biliary Cirrhosis 520
7. Primary Sclerosing Cholangitis 521
8. Fulminant Hepatic Failure 521
9. Hepatic Malignancy 521
10. Metabolic Diseases 522
11. Assessment of the Liver Transplant Potential Candidate 523
12. Selection, Listing and Prioritization for Liver Transplantation 527
13. Timing of Liver Transplantation 528
References 529

1. INTRODUCTION

The landmark paradigm shift in the practice of liver transplantation occurred in 1983 when the National Institute of Health consensus development conference issued a statement indicating that liver transplantation is not an experimental procedure but an effective therapy that deserves broader application [1]. This was followed by an accelerated increase in the number of centers and cases of orthotopic liver transplantation (OLT) in North America and worldwide. The introduction of cyclosporine and other immunosuppressant drugs, the University of Wisconsin allograft preservation solution (UW) and refinement of surgical technique resulted in a significant improvement of liver transplantation outcome. One-year survival rates of 85% or higher are reported by many centers [2]. This success and expansion has brought with it the new dilemma of a widening gap between the number of available cadaveric organs and the expanding waiting list of candidates with an increasing number of deaths among patients waiting to be transplanted (Figure 1). Under these circumstances, cadaveric organs become a scarce and valuable resource.

The goals of liver transplantation are to prolong life and improve its quality in patients with end-stage liver disease and to do this in the most cost-effective and efficient manner, with a focus on proper utilization of available scarce resources. The achievement of these goals is challenging but attainable, to varying extents, in many centers as indicated by recent survival data [2], quality of life analysis [3] and cost reduction if transplantation is done before patients deteriorate [4], or by exploring cost-saving therapeutic alternatives [5]. To achieve these goals, however, the difficult process of tedious assessment, careful selection of appropriate patients and proper timing of transplantation is required. In the absence of uniformly agreed upon national or international standards and with the present crises of the widening gap between supply and demand for organs (Figure 1), this process becomes even more difficult and inexact. It requires a judicious blend of medical science (and art), judgment and experience

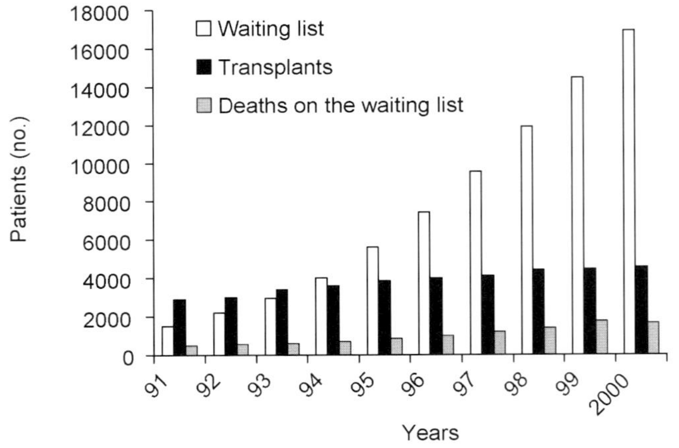

Figure 1. The widening gap between the number of transplants (supply) and the number of patients on the waiting list (demand) and the number of deaths on the waiting list annually for the last decade (1991–2000). (Based on United Network of Organ Sharing (UNOS) data accessed at www.unos.org on May 24, 2001.)

in a team approach. Many aspects of liver transplantation remain unexplored in "uncharted territories". This chapter will provide an overview of indications and contraindications for liver transplantation and the process of patients' evaluation, selection for and timing of the operation.

2. INDICATIONS AND CONTRAINDICATIONS

In principal, liver transplantation is indicated whenever it is proven to significantly prolong survival and improve the quality of life in a cost-effective manner over the natural history of liver disease or other non-transplant medical/surgical management. As more experience has been gained with liver transplantation, the list of indications has been refined and changed. The majority of diseases for which liver transplantation is considered appropriate can be categorized into seven groups (Table 1). However, some of these entities are controversial (e.g., hepatic malignancies, hemochromatosis, alcoholic liver disease (ALD) and hepatitis B cirrhosis). Since there is no standardized list of indications that is uniformly followed by all centers and given the absence of randomized trials that prove the efficacy of liver transplantation for various conditions, medical communities have to rely on the available registries and large single-center or multi-center experience to draw upon for some form of guidelines. One example is The American Association for the Study of Liver Disease (AASLD) clinical practice guidelines [6]. These non-peer-reviewed guidelines were based on a formal review of the medical literature over the past decade and suggest the preferred approach to different major categories of liver disease in a flexible manner. The recommendation of liver transplantation for each major category of liver disease is given with a rating of the strength of that recommendation and the available evidence to support it.

Contraindications for OLT are usually classified into absolute and relative (Tables 2 and 3). As more experience has been gained with OLT, the list of contraindications to transplantation has been refined and even shortened but not agreed upon universally by all centers. As an example, advanced age is considered by some to be a contraindication for OLT, but the cut-off limit is difficult to define. Many studies have shown that survival in patients older than 60 with low-risk factors is the same as for those younger than 60. There are also many reports of successful OLT in octogenarians. The acceptable approach is to rely on the physiologic rather than the chronologic age as a guide. There is even a consensus among some recognized authorities in OLT that there should be no absolute contraindications to the placement of patients on the waiting list but only relative contraindications [7].

Table 1. End-stage liver diseases for which OLT may be indicated.

Hepatocellular
Viral hepatitis: A, B, C
Alcoholic liver disease
Autoimmune hepatitis
Cryptogenic cirrhosis
Chronic drug-induced
Cholestatic
Primary and secondary biliary cirrhosis
Primary and secondary sclerosing cholangitis
Biliary atresia
Alagille's syndrome
Byler's syndrome
Familial cholestasis
Metabolic disorders
Alpha-1-antitrypsin deficiency
Glycogen storage disease type I, IV
Hemochromatosis
Crigler-Najjar syndrome
Wilson's disease
Familial hypercholesterolemia
Primary hyperoxaluria
Urea cycle deficiency
Fulminant hepatic failure
Acute intoxication
Viral hepatitis
Metabolic liver disease
Acute fatty liver of pregnancy
Hepatic tumors
Slow-growing endocrine tumors
Hepatocellular carcinoma
Hepatoblastoma
Epithelioid hemangioendothelioma
Hepatic adenomatosis
Lymphangiomatosis
Nodular regenerative hyperplasia
Vascular
Budd–Chiari syndrome
Veno-occlusive disease
Giant hemangiomas
Anatomic
Polycystic liver disease
Caroli's disease
Trauma

Currently 80% of liver transplants in the USA are done for eight entities [2]. These are classified into non-cholestatic cirrhosis, cholestatic cirrhosis and acute hepatic necrosis (Table 4). Some indications are worth examining in some detail as certain aspects of these diseases have relevance to the outcome of OLT and thus should be considered during the clinical evaluation phase for liver transplantation, which will be discussed later in this chapter.

Table 2. Absolute contraindications for liver transplantation.

Multisystem organ failure
Extrahepatic malignancy
Active uncontrolled extrahepatic sepsis
Advanced cardiopulmonary disease
Active substance abuse

3. HEPATITIS C

Hepatitis C virus (HCV) liver cirrhosis is becoming the leading indication for OLT worldwide. In addition to the direct effect of HCV, there is evidence to suggest that HCV infection in the presence of other forms of liver disease like alcoholic hepatitis or hepatitis B may exacerbate liver injury caused by the latter. HCV infection can also lead to extrahepatic manifestations of cryoglobulinemia in the form of renal (glomerulonephritis), dermatologic (porphyria cutanea tarda), hematologic and autoimmune diseases [8]. These aspects are to be kept in mind during the pretransplant workup.

Recurrence of HCV infection post-OLT is almost universal with graft hepatitis developing in as many as 80% of patients, and 20% of these patients develop allograft cirrhosis at 5 years [9]. Although earlier small studies showed that graft and patient survival for the first decade after OLT appeared to be unaffected by this universal recurrence, a recent analysis of a large cohort of patients in the UNOS database showed significant reduction of survival at 5 years post-primary OLT in HCV-positive patients [10]. Retransplantation remains the only viable option for recurrent allograft decompensated cirrhosis. The results of retransplantation, however, are poor, especially when done at a later stage of decompensation [9]. The challenges ahead are to identify pre-OLT risk factors for recurrence so that better selection of patients can be done before transplantation and an effective treatment given before and/or after OLT.

Table 3. Relative contraindications for liver transplantation.

Primary hepatobiliary malignancy
Renal failure
HIV infection
Hemochromatosis
Anatomical, e.g., portal vein thrombosis, previous extensive upper abdominal surgery
Unwillingness and inability to accept OLT and comply with follow-up care
Advanced age

Table 4. The most common entities for which 80% of liver transplants are currently done in the USA.

Non-cholestatic cirrhosis
Hepatitis C
Alcoholic
Cryptogenic
Autoimmune
Hepatitis B
Cholestatic
Primary biliary cirrhosis
Primary sclerosing cholangitis
Acute hepatic necrosis

Based on the United Network of Organ Sharing (UNOS) data – 2001 annual report accessed at www.unos.org on May 24, 2002.

4. HEPATITIS B

Earlier experience with liver transplantation for patients with hepatitis B (HBV) cirrhosis was associated with poor outcome due to the common reinfection and development of allograft cirrhosis in 1–3 years, especially in patients who are HBeAg positive and have HBV DNA in their serum. This dismal result led to a significant decline in the number of OLTs done for HBV cirrhosis in the USA through the early 1990s [9]. After recognizing the prognostic significance of active HBV replication pre-OLT and the protective effect of high-dose hepatitis B immunoglobulin (HBIG), new strategies evolved to prevent graft reinfection. Recent strategies include using nucleoside analogues, e.g., Lamivudine, either alone or in combination with HBIG. The concern, however, is the high cost of high-dose HBIG that may have to be continued for months or years post-OLT since there is no solid recommendation on when it can be safely stopped. These changes over the last decade made it possible to offer OLT for candidates with HBV infection with a low likelihood of serious reinfection [9].

5. ALCOHOL-RELATED CIRRHOSIS

ALD is the leading cause of cirrhosis in the USA and the second most common indication for OLT, but the number of patients receiving OLT each year represents only 5% of the estimated deaths from ALD. Moreover, rates of graft and patient survival after OLT are excellent and similar to those for other chronic liver diseases [11]. These results alleviated the early concerns that extrahepatic diseases of ALD such as cardiomyopathy, malnutrition and neurologic impairment may have a detrimental effect on the results of OLT. However, these should be investigated during the workup of ALD patients.

Recidivism after OLT remains a chief concern in ALD patients, and attempts to accurately predict it in individual patients have had limited success. However, some studies have shown that the duration of abstinence prior to transplantation correlates inversely with the risk of subsequent recidivism [12]. Based on these studies a period of abstinence of 6 months is one of the listing criteria in as many as 85% of the OLT centers in the USA [11]. Other psychosocial factors that help predict recidivism are also considered with the 6-months rule [13].

6. PRIMARY BILIARY CIRRHOSIS

Primary biliary cirrhosis (PBS) was among the first diseases accepted as a prototype indication for liver transplantation. OLT is the best alternative for PBS patients with end-stage disease, achieving a 5-year survival higher than 80% in most centers. To achieve this result, however, early referral is important before life-threatening complications develop. Quality of life indications for OLT are prominent in this disease and are manifested as pruritus, fatigue and jaundice [14]. Osteopenic bone disease with predisposition to spontaneous fractures is a common complication and should be investigated and documented with bone densitometry study during the workup for OLT as a guide to active management and a base line for post-OLT follow-up. To predict survival with and without OLT as well as to determine the best time for the transplant, several prognostic models have been reported; the Mayo model is the most widely used [15]. Post-OLT recurrence of this disease is a controversial issue but most recent studies support the existence of recurrence although it is not yet confirmed to have a significant detrimental effect on survival [16].

7. PRIMARY SCLEROSING CHOLANGITIS

Primary sclerosing cholangitis (PSC) has a disease course that is often punctuated intermittently by bouts of cholangitis or jaundice. The most important aspect of this disease is the predisposition to the development of cholangiocarcinoma with an annual incidence of about 1% and a prevalence of up to 42% [14]. Ulcerative colitis is associated with PSC in up to 75% of patients and is not a contraindication of OLT; in fact it may improve with posttransplant immunosuppressive therapy. With this association there may be an increased risk of colon cancer pre- and post-OLT. These malignant potential aspects should be considered during the workup process by careful screening. Although the natural history of PSC is not as well defined as that of PBS, several prognostic models have also been developed to predict survival, define optimum time for and predict outcome of OLT [15]. Recurrence of PSC after OLT has been reported but is difficult to diagnose because of the lack of diagnostic gold standard, and patient and graft survival does not appear to be affected in the intermediate term [16].

8. FULMINANT HEPATIC FAILURE

The majority of acute hepatic failure cases are caused by viral hepatitis, drug-induced hepatitis or toxin ingestion. Brain edema, coagulopathy, sepsis and renal failure are the main complications that lead to death. Despite advances in supportive care the mortality for most patients is around 80% without transplantation. Since 15–20% of patients will recover without OLT, it is essential to identify this subset of patients who will recover only with supportive care. Various prognostic features have been suggested such as the widely cited King's College Liver Unit criteria [17]. The key to maximum possible success, however, is early referral to a tertiary center where OLT is available. Despite maximum efforts the 1-year survival after OLT is around 60% [18].

9. HEPATIC MALIGNANCY

The number and percentage of OLT for malignant neoplasms has declined in the USA over the last decade from 130 cases (4.4% of all liver transplants) in 1991 to 108 cases (2.4% of liver transplants) in 2000 despite the increase in the total number of OLTs done each year [2]. Hepatocellular (HCC) carcinoma complicates liver cirrhosis of any etiology, but it most commonly occurs in cirrhotic patients with HCV, HBV, hemochromatosis or tyrosinemia. These patients generally cannot tolerate surgical resection due to the underlying cirrhosis. Results of surgical resection when possible or other non-surgical therapy have been disappointing. During the early era of OLT and because of the dismal life expectancy of these patients, liver transplantation was endorsed as a form of life-saving procedure [1]. However, it was soon discovered that the outcome with OLT was poor and may not be justified in the face of severe organ shortage. Later analysis of results in the subset of patients who were transplanted with incidental small HCC detected by modern imaging or in the explanted liver showed a similar survival to other non-malignant cirrhosis. It was obvious that better patient selection is a key in obtaining good results to justify OLT in this disease. The criteria accepted now are solitary tumor ≤5 cm or up to three tumor foci each ≤3 cm and no vascular invasion or extrahepatic metastasis. The exception to the size criteria is the fibrolamellar-type hepatomas, which have a better result when surgical resection is not possible and the disease is not advanced.

Other hepatic malignant neoplasms like cholangiocarcinoma or liver metastatic tumors are not usually considered for OLT due to the poor outcome. Exceptions, however, are given to epithelioid hemangioendothelioma, hepatoblastoma and hepatic metastasis from slow-growing neuroendocrine tumors when the extrahepatic disease is controlled [19]. Finally it should be emphasized that OLT should not be done with just palliative intent in hepatic malignant neoplasms.

10. METABOLIC DISEASES

Inborn errors of metabolism are recognized as a cause of acute or chronic liver disease presenting either as fulminant hepatic failure (Wilson's disease), cirrhosis (hemochromatosis and alpha-1 antitrypsin deficiency), hepatocellular carcinoma (tyrosinemia) or a second organ failure without structural liver disease (primary hyperoxaluria) [20].

Wilson's disease is an autosomal recessive disorder of copper excretion characterized by the accumulation of toxic levels of copper in various tissues and organs including the liver. Fulminant hepatic failure may be the first presenting clinical picture in some patients. Copper toxicity in the brain is manifested by motor disturbances but rarely sensory or cognitive deficits. OLT is indicated when progressive hepatic dysfunction occurs despite intense medical therapy or in fulminant hepatic failure. The 1-year survival is 70–90% with reversal of most of the associated metabolic abnormalities [20].

Hereditary hemochromatosis is a disorder of iron metabolism. The iron deposition in different tissues, and particularly in the liver, leads in time to cellular toxicity and functional failure. Hepatocellular carcinoma is a common complication of established hemochromatosis. In addition to liver cirrhosis, iron-induced damage to the heart and the pancreas may lead to cardiac complications and diabetes mellitus, each accounting for 10% of deaths [20]. Other endocrine glands may also be affected. These aspects of the disease should be considered during the assessment of potential candidates for OLT. The initial results of OLT in hereditary hemochromatosis were disappointing. Sepsis was identified as the main cause of death after transplantation. The recent strategy of pretransplant aggressive iron-depleting therapy improved the 1-year posttransplant survival to 75–83% [20].

Alpha-1 antitrypsin (alpha-1AT) deficiency is an autosomal recessive disorder characterized by abnormally low levels of this protease inhibitor. While the lung disease in alpha-1AT deficiency is caused by decreased serum levels of this enzyme, the liver disease appears to be due to accumulation of an abnormal variant of the enzyme in the hepatocytes. The disease is usually evident in early childhood. Individuals who escape severe liver disease during childhood are free of clinical liver disease until the 4th or 5th decade of life. Adults presenting with cryptogenic cirrhosis should be evaluated for alpha-1AT. OLT is the only proven therapy when end-stage liver disease develops. One-year survival of 70% has been reported with the main cause of mortality in the posttransplant period being sepsis. The associated lung disease is usually mild and the effects of OLT on pulmonary function have not yet been fully studied [20].

Primary hyperoxaluria is a rare autosomal recessive disorder that represents a unique indication for combined liver–kidney transplantation. Although the liver is structurally normal it has an abnormal alanine glyoxylate aminotransferase activity that leads to the production of large amounts of oxalate. Calcium oxalate crystals are then deposited in various tissues, particularly the kidneys and heart, leading to progressive renal failure and cardiomyopathy. Kidney transplantation invariably leads to recurrent kidney allograft failure. Liver–kidney transplantation simultaneously or sequentially is considered the treatment of choice. Liver transplantation before kidney failure is a possible management strategy but the difficulty lies in the timing of OLT because the time for renal failure to develop is variable and may take years. The key, however, is early referral to a tertiary center for assessment [20].

Urea cycle deficiency (ornithine transcarbamylase deficiency), familial hypercholesterolemia and hypercoagulable enzyme deficiency states (protein C, protein S and antithrombin III deficiency) are other life-threatening metabolic diseases that can be cured with liver transplantation. The appropriate timing of the transplant before significant irreversible end-organ damage or serious complications occur is of prime importance for OLT to succeed [20].

11. ASSESSMENT OF THE LIVER TRANSPLANT POTENTIAL CANDIDATE

The evaluation of potential candidates for liver transplantation is a tedious process that requires a systematic approach in a standardized flexible fashion. At the King Abdulaziz Medical City Liver Center in Riyadh, Saudi Arabia, the following general principles are emphasized in our protocol, which we have been following for the last 150 transplants. (1) All aspects of evaluation are to be done in the same center where the transplant is going to be performed whenever possible. (2) The evaluation is done in a sequential step-wise fashion from simple screening tests and assessments to more extensive or invasive (expensive) ones. This sequence leads to more appropriate utilization of resources and saves some patients who are found to be unfit for transplantation by the simpler tests from undergoing unnecessary invasive or expensive tests. (3) There is always a recognized team leader who is either the hepatologist or the surgeon. (4) It is emphasized that during the evaluation process the health care providers who are going to manage the selected patients pre-, peri- and postoperatively have an active role in the assessment. (5) A multidisciplinary team approach is followed. (6) There is a clear understanding by the evaluating team members and the patients and their family that this is a dynamic process that blends evaluation with management when necessary and that the current results can change over time. (7) Speed without haste is necessary in finalizing the evaluation since undue delay can cause a significant level of anxiety and uncertainty among patients and their family.

The goals of the evaluation process are to establish the need for OLT, determine its feasibility and estimate the likelihood of success in the individual patient. This process should address several important issues. First, establish or confirm the diagnosis of end-stage liver disease. Second, evaluate the degree of hepatic dysfunction. Third, obtain anatomic information that has relevance to surgery and outcome. Fourth, evaluate the overall physical, psychosocial and emotional fitness of the recipient and identify any coexistent disorder. Finally, identify any contraindications to OLT and if none, clarify conditions that may have to be addressed before the transplantation.

As shown in Figure 2, the process begins after the initial referral to the center with the first visit. During this "phase one evaluation" visit, a complete history and physical examination is done in addition to a review of the referring physician's report. The patient and his/her family meet the hepatologist or the surgeon, the transplant nurse coordinator, the social worker and the financial advisor. Routine phase one tests are requested (Figure 2). This first encounter is also utilized to educate the patient and the family about the upcoming process and to gain an initial impression about the need for any special consultation or investigation. Moreover, obvious contraindications may be detected thus leading to termination of the evaluation for OLT. Relative contraindications may also be identified and investigated for further management and possible reversal. These early deferred patients continue to receive further evaluation and management tailored to their clinical status, and if at any time the original contraindication is resolved, they proceed to the second phase (Figure 3).

The second phase of the evaluation process focuses on more invasive tests and specialized consultations, which are tailored to individual systems and guided by the results of phase one evaluation. Some of the important aspects of possible co-morbid conditions are:

Cardiovascular system: End-stage liver cirrhosis is associated with a unique hyperdynamic cardiovascular syndrome characterized by low systemic vascular resistance and high cardiac output. After transplantation, the systemic vascular resistance increases, leading to increased after-load. Sudden cardiac failure and/or myocardial ischemia can occur, especially with underlying cardiac disease [21]. Cardiac evaluation is recommended for patients 45 years of age or older or those who have a history of cardiovascular abnormality. Smokers, diabetics and patients with other liver diseases that are associated with cardiomyopathy (e.g., alcoholic liver disease, hemochromatosis) are candidates for in-depth evaluation. A stress test or

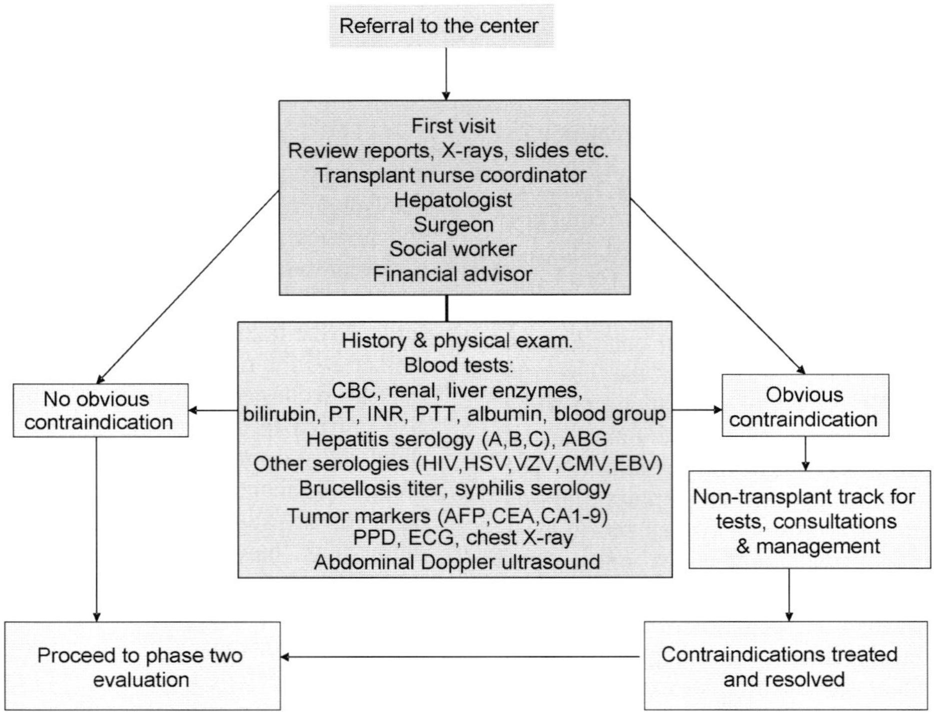

Figure 2. Phase one evaluation of OLT potential candidate. These are obtained for all patients.

cardiac catheterization and angiography may be necessary. There are, however, no precise guidelines for workup or limits below which OLT should not be done. Consultation and discussion with the cardiologist and the anesthesiologist is mandatory.

Pulmonary system. Patients with symptoms or signs of pulmonary disease, smokers and patients with abnormal arterial blood gases should undergo more extensive pulmonary evaluation. Cirrhosis of the liver is associated with circulatory abnormalities in the pulmonary vasculature. In some patients hypoxemia and pulmonary vasodilatation and intrapulmonary shunting characterize these changes. This condition is known as hepatopulmonary syndrome. The diagnostic criterion on arterial blood gases is a PaO2 $<$ 70 mmHg or arterial–alveolar gradient $>$15–20 mmHg. Contrast-enhanced echocardiography is the most sensitive modality to detect this syndrome. Liver transplantation can reverse this abnormality albeit slowly. However, there is a limit to this statement in that patients who fail to increase their PaO2 to $>$ 80 mmHg on 100% FIO2 have a very high risk for transplantation.

The other associated abnormality is portopulmonary hypertension in which there is an elevated mean pulmonary artery pressure, normal capillary wedge pressure and elevated pulmonary vascular resistance. OLT may reverse this condition when it is mild but it is associated with high mortality when the mean pulmonary artery pressure is higher than 50 mmHg. Infusion of prostacycline has been shown to improve the hemodynamics in these patients and has been used pre-OLT and continued post-OLT with good outcome [22].

Renal disorders: Renal dysfunction of varying degrees and types is not uncommon in patients with end-stage liver disease. It is important to distinguish among the different types as each has a different prognosis with OLT. Hepatorenal syndrome is a functional disorder of the kidney without intrinsic structural abnormality. The renal function returns to normal in the majority of cases after OLT. On the

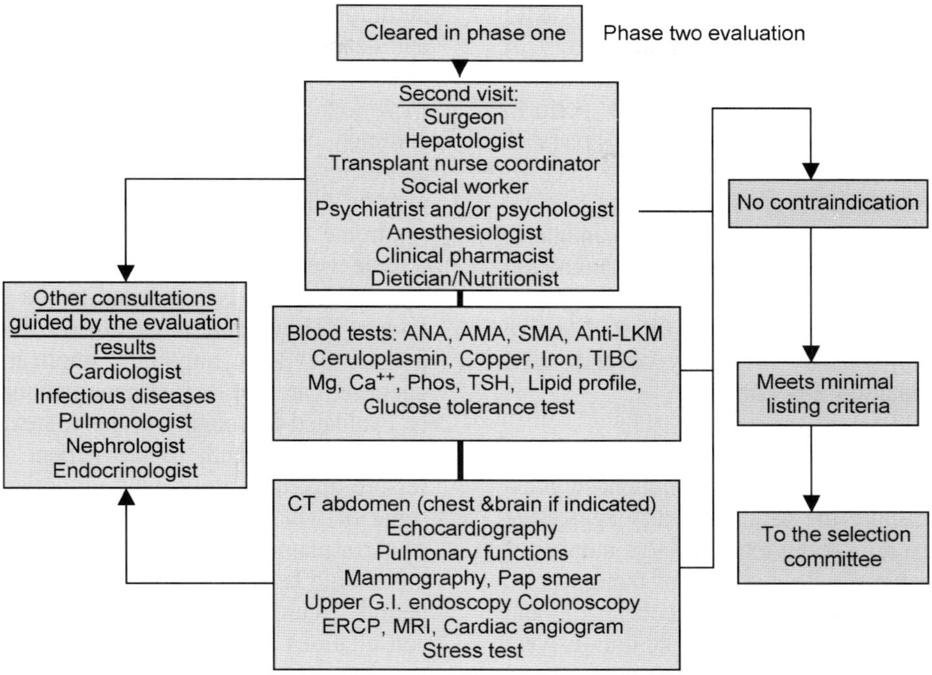

Figure 3. Phase two evaluation of potential OLT candidate.

other hand, acute or chronic renal insufficiency due to intrinsic structural changes is associated with significant increase in mortality, and kidney transplantation may be required. In general, potential candidates for OLT who have renal impairment should undergo a similar evaluation to patients without liver disease. Renal biopsy may be recommended when the diagnosis is obscure. Consultation with the nephrologist is essential [23].

Infectious diseases: All potential candidates are screened for the presence of active sepsis and immunologic evidence of prior exposure to certain infections. Some positive results may have to be clarified by further tests like HBsAg, which will need the clarification of HBeAg and HBV DNA status. The presence of antibodies to certain viruses may predict the risk of primary infection with these viruses after OLT and defines possible prophylactic measures. Patients with positive PPD should be treated with isoniazid. Other tests for rare disease, e.g., brucellosis and schistosmiasis, should be tailored to the regional prevalence of these diseases. The immunization history for these patients should be obtained and updated for influenza, measles–mumps–rubella, pneumococcus, tetanus–diphtheria, hepatitis A and hepatitis B. Dental assessment for dental or periodontal disease is carried out on all patients to treat any existing source of infection. Ear, nose and throat examination is done to rule out any ongoing infection with emphasis on the paranasal sinuses. Patients with ascites should be investigated for spontaneous bacterial peritonitis. Urinalysis and cultures are done to rule out urinary tract infection.

Endocrine diseases: Patients with long-standing diabetes mellitus should be evaluated for end-organ disease like renal, cardiac, vascular and retinal diseases. Thyroid dysfunction is common in PBC, autoimmune hepatitis and hemochromatosis and should be treated before transplantation. Osteoporosis affects many patients with chronic liver disease and is particularly seen in female patients with cholestatic cirrhosis. Vitamin D measurement and bone densitometry should be done as a baseline and a guide to therapy.

Gastrointestinal diseases. Upper gastrointestinal endoscopy is performed on all patients to investigate the existence and degree of esophageal varices as well as gastroduodenal ulcers. Colonoscopy should be performed on all patients with PSC, history of colonic polyps, guaiac-positive stool and family history of colon cancer. Some centers perform routine sigmoidoscopy on all patients 40 years or older.

Gynecologic examination: All female candidates should have a mammogram, pelvic examination and pap smear. Some centers limit mammography to patients 40 years of age and older. Elective gynecologic surgery may preferably be performed before transplantation if possible.

Previous malignancies: Past history of malignancy is of concern since major surgery and immunosuppression may predispose the patient to early aggressive recurrence. In a registry review of a large number of transplanted patients with a history of malignancies before transplantation, some general conclusions and recommendations were given [24]. The tumors were classified into three categories: low, intermediate and high recurrence rates. It was concluded that a minimum 2-year waiting period between the "curative" treatment of cancer and transplantation is appropriate for most cancers. The longer period of 5 years is needed for malignant melanoma, breast cancer and colon carcinoma. In this context these patients should have a rigorous review of previous malignancy with review of the histopathology report, slides if possible, details of treatment given and outcome. Current focused history, physical examination, blood test, endoscopy and imaging examinations are also done.

Hematologic disorders: Thrombocytopenia, anemia and, leukopenia are usual findings in patients with cirrhosis. A complete blood count with indices is screened to identify the type of anemia, and a reticulocyte count is done when necessary as iron deficiency or megaloblastic anemia may exist. Blood coagulation abnormalities are manifested by prolongation of prothrombin time, international normalized ratio and activated partial thromboplastin. These changes are due to malabsorption of vitamin K and decreased production of several coagulation factors by the diseased liver. Patients with Budd–Chiari syndrome or a history of thrombosis should undergo a full work-up for antithrombin III, protein C and protein S deficiency and hematology consultation.

Neurological disorders: Hepatic encephalopathy is a common complication of decompensated cirrhosis and is reversible with OLT. Subtle encephalopathy may be difficult to differentiate from organic brain syndrome or other organic brain disorders. Ataxia, muscle weakness and other neurological disorders may or may not be attributed to the patient's liver disease. These and other irreversible intellectual deficits have an important implication on postoperative care and long-term compliance, and should be evaluated thoroughly in the context of the available support system to the patient. Patients with seizure disorders are usually on antiepileptic drugs, some of which have a significant interaction with posttransplant immunosuppression medication and this should be kept in mind during the postoperative period. Neurological and psychiatric/psychological consultations are required.

Nutritional assessment: The liver plays a central role in all nutrients' metabolism and thus liver disease causes alterations in protein, calorie, carbohydrate, fat, fluid and vitamin and mineral requirements. The assessment of the nutritional status of liver disease patients using objective anthropometric measurements and blood tests is difficult due to the overall systemic derangements and fluid shifts. The subjective global assessment method should be considered. It is based on a thorough history, physical examination and existing conditions [25]. Using this global assessment, more than 70% of patients with end-stage liver disease are found to have some degree of malnutrition. The dietician/nutritionist has a pivotal role in the assessment and advice of appropriate nutritional support pre- and posttransplantation.

Anatomical evaluation: Doppler ultrasound and triphasic CT scan or MRI are used to evaluate the liver for HCC or any other space-occupying lesions. Assessment of the portal, mesenteric and hepatic veins and IVC is done looking for thrombosis and, if found, to define its extent as this has a significant technical impact on the operative feasibility. Patients with transjugular intrahepatic portosystemic shunt (TIPS) should have the shunt evaluated with emphasis on its location and whether there is any migration into the suprahepatic cava or distally into the portal vein. Any surgical portosystemic shunt should be evaluated for patency as this may have to be ligated at the time of transplantation. Liver biopsy to establish the specific etiology of liver disease is not always critical and its risk must be weighed against the benefit of histologic examination. Using a transjugular approach can minimize the potential risk of biopsy. Biopsy of HCC is often discouraged because of the possibility of tumor spread and is not always required as the diagnosis is invariably made with ultrasound, CT or MRI.

12. SELECTION, LISTING AND PRIORITIZATION FOR LIVER TRANSPLANTATION

Once the pretransplantation evaluation is complete the patient is usually presented to the institution's liver transplantation selection committee for categorization and listing. This committee consists of the entire transplant team of transplant surgeons, hepatologists, anesthesiologists, psychiatrist and/or psychologist, transplant nurse coordinator, social worker, dietician, clinical pharmacist and others.

Selection and categorization: After presentation and review and deliberation by the committee, patients are usually assigned to one of the four categories: (1) suitable and ready for transplantation; (2) suitable but too well and early and thus deferred to inactive status and continue follow-up; (3) deferred due to certain reversible contraindication that needs further management or some issues in the patient condition that warrant further investigation and clarification. The patient is to be represented once these issues are dealt with; (4) existence of absolute contraindication that leads to denial of transplantation.

Listing and prioritization. The question of when to place the patient with end-stage liver disease on the transplantation waiting list is a contentious one. The existing severe shortage of organs has fueled a controversy about the regional marked differences in the number of waiting days on the list before receiving a liver. The concern is about the possibility that some patients are placed on the list at different points in the natural history of their liver disease resulting in getting a priority based only on how long they were on the list. The present reality of long waiting times on the list, which can reach up to 1–2 years for about 60% of patients [2], may lead to a pressure to list patients early before they actually need a transplant. This practice has been referred to as "waiting list inflation" [7]. To address these issues, UNOS invited the leaders in liver transplantation to develop criteria for entry into the national waiting list. On February 21, 1997, The American Society of Transplant Physicians and the American Association for the Study of Liver Diseases organized a national conference and issued the "minimal listing criteria for placement of adults on the liver transplant waiting list" [7]. After extensive review of the literature the consensus was to use a two-criteria set: non-disease specific and disease specific. For the non-disease-specific criterion, the Child–Turcotte–Pugh (CTP) scoring system for prediction of survival of chronic liver disease patients is used (Table 5). This scoring system defines the non-disease-specific criterion of ≤90% chance of survival for 1 year, which is equivalent to a CTP score of ≥7 and is the minimum score required for a patient to be placed on the list. Other complications that influence predicted survival were also incorporated in the criteria (Table 6).

For conditions in which survival and outcome may be inadequately scored by the CTP system, disease-specific criteria were delineated (Table 6). These criteria cover PBC, PSC, fulminant hepatic failure, alcoholic liver disease and hepatic malignancies. For PBC and PSC, the Mayo mathematical models

Table 5. Child–Turcotte–Pugh classification.

	1 point	2 points	3 points
Bilirubin (mg/dl)	<2	2–3	>3
For PBC and PSC patients	<4	4–10	>10
Albumin (g/dl)	>3.5	2.8–3.5	<2.8
PT (prolonged in seconds)	1–3	4–6	>6
Or INR	<1.7	1.8–2.3	>2.3
Ascites	None	Slight	Moderate
Encephalopathy	None	1–2	3–4

PBC, primary biliary cirrhosis; PSC, primary sclerosing cholangitis; PT, prothrombin time; INR, international normalized ratio. Child–Turcotte–Pugh class: A, 5–6 points; B, 7–9 points; C, 10–15 points.

Table 6. Minimal listing criteria.

Non-disease-specific
Child–Turcotte–Pugh (CTP) score >7 or
History of gastrointestinal variceal bleed regardless of CTP score or
History of spontaneous bacterial peritonitis regardless of CTP score
Disease-specific
Mayo Risk Score which predicts >10% 1-year mortality for PBC and PSC or CTP score >7 using PBC and PSC bilirubin scoring points.
Hepatic malignancy confined to the liver
Fulminant hepatic failure
CTP >7 and minimum of 6 months abstinence and evaluation substance abuse professional for alcoholic liver disease

Adapted from Lucey, M.R., Brown, K.A., Everson, G.T. *et al.* (1997) Minimal criteria for placement of adults on the liver transplant waiting list: a report of a national conference organized by the American Society of Transplant Physicians and the American Association for the Study of Liver disease. *Liver Transpl. Surg.* **3**, 628–637.

were suggested [15]. However, due to the complexity of the calculation, modified bilirubin levels in CTP scores for PBC and PSC were recommended (Table 6). Any patient with other diseases that are not amenable to this scoring system, e.g., Budd–Chiari syndrome or primary hyperoxaluria, or exceptional cases, should be brought to the regional review committee.

When an organ becomes available a system of prioritization and allocation should be in place to select a recipient. In an effort to allocate organs in the order of medical urgency and minimize the role of waiting time, the UNOS allocation policy came under scrutiny and review. Identifying the shortcomings and limitations of the CTP score for prioritization and the UNOS allocation algorithm, which was in use until recently, a new model was developed and published in 2001 [26]. In February 2002 this model was adopted by UNOS to prioritize patients waiting for liver transplantation. This model for end-stage liver disease (MELD) uses serum creatinine, total serum bilirubin and international normalized ratio (INR) as its parameters. It has been validated and found to be reproducible, objective and applicable to a heterogeneous group of patients with end-stage liver disease to predict the risk of dying at any certain point in time. The MELD model development was based on data from adult patients and is not applicable for pediatric patients, and thus a pediatric end-stage liver disease (PELD) model was developed [27].

13. TIMING OF LIVER TRANSPLANTATION

Optimal timing for liver transplantation was conceptually addressed by the NIH consensus development conference on liver transplantation in 1983 in the following statement: "The procedure should be performed in a late enough phase of the disease to offer the patient all opportunity for spontaneous stabilization and recovery but in an early enough phase to give the surgical procedure a fair chance of success" [1].

In clinical practice, however, defining the optimal time for liver transplantation is an arduous task that is influenced by multidimensional factors. The first of these is the fact that the conditions for which liver transplantation is indicated is a heterogeneous group of diseases, each of which has a different natural history and different response and outcome to treatment with or without transplantation. The second is that the medical non-transplant treatments and transplantation are continuously changing and improving in outcome, making it difficult to study each disease entity over an extended period of time and come up with an everlasting applicable model. Last but not least is the multiplicity of variables that have to be considered with and without transplantation. These factors are survival, morbidity, quality of life and resource utilization (funds and organs) [28]. The ultimate objective then is to have a "net gain outcome" of these variables with liver transplantation.

Figure 4 illustrates oversimplified hypothetical curves of survival (and possible morbidity and quality of life), cost and severity of disease. Curve A depicts the natural course of the disease indicating the progressive deterioration of survival probability as the disease severity increases as depicted by curve C. In parallel, curve B depicts the survival curve with liver transplantation at different times of disease severity. If the transplant is done "too early", the mortality at that stage may exceed that of the natural course of the disease leading to a "net loss outcome"

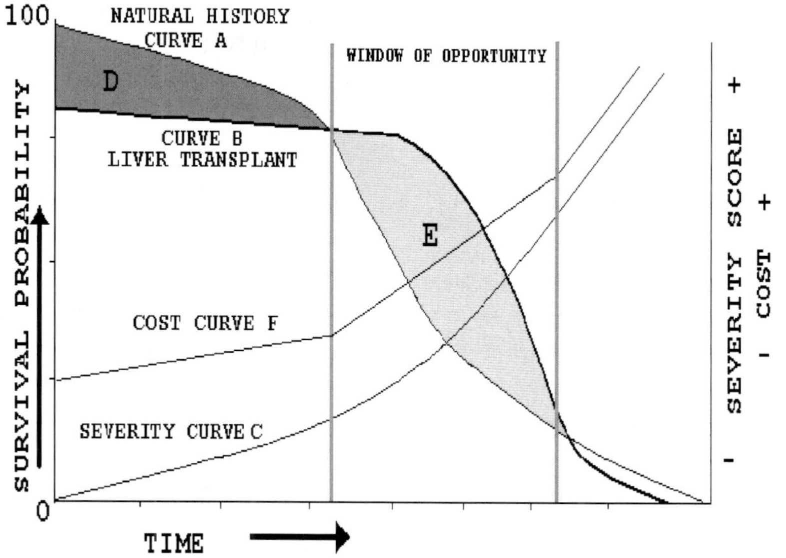

Figure 4. Hypothetical curves of survival for end-stage liver disease patients with and without liver transplantation over time. Curves and differences are accentuated to illustrate the concept of ideal time for liver transplantation as discussed in the text. Adapted with modification from Kim, W.R. and Dickson, E.R. (2000) Timing of liver transplantation. *Semin. Liver Dis.* **20**, 451–464.

illustrated by area D. Following the curves, a point in time will come when curves A and B approach each other and cross leading to a "net gain outcome" depicted by area E. Further down the two curves and as disease severity increases (curve C), the outcome of transplantation deteriorates and becomes a futile exercise with high cost (curve F). The optimal time of liver transplantation falls somewhere between these two points where there is a net gain in outcome, and this is the "window of opportunity" for that specific disease during which liver transplantation should be performed.

In summary, the process of assessment, selection and timing is a challenging exercise that has to incorporate multiple variables that are changing with time. The development of different prognostic models (e.g., minimal listing criteria [7], Mayo models for cholestatic liver diseases [15], MELD model [27]) for the common diseases where OLT is indicated is a valuable contribution to this field. These "computerized" models, however, cannot replace the "human touch" of the clinician who should make a decision by using them with knowledge, experience and proper clinical judgment for the individual patient. The art of our science should prevail.

REFERENCES

[1] National Institute of Health Consensus Development Conference Statement: liver transplantation, June 20–23, 1983. *Hepatology* **4**, S107–S110, 1984.

[2] Annual report of the US Scientific Registry of Transplant Recipients and the Organ Procurement and Transplantation Network: Transplant Data, 1991–2000 (2001, August 1) (HHS/HRSA/OSP/DOT and UNOS, Rockville, MD and Richmond, VA). Accessed May 23, 2002 from the World Wide Web: http://www.unos.org.

[3] Bravata, D.M., Oklin, I. and Keefe, E.B. (2001) Quality of life and employment after liver transplantation. *Liver Transpl.* **7**, S119–S123.

[4] Muto, P., Freeman, R.B., Haug, C.E., Lu, A. and Rohrer, R.J. (1994) Liver transplant candidates stratification systems: implication for third-party payers and organ allocation. *Transplantation* **57**, 306–307.

[5] Lake, J.R., Gorman, K.J., Esquivel, C.O., Wiesner, R.H., Klintmalm, G.B., Miller, C.M., Shaw, B.W. and Gordon, J.A. (1995) The impact of immunosuppressive regimens on the cost of liver transplantation – results from the US. FK-506 multicenter trial. *Transplantation* **60**, 1089–1095.

[6] Carithers, Jr., R.L. (2000) Liver transplantation. *Liver Transpl.* **6**, 122–135.

[7] Lucey, M.R., Brown, K.A., Everson, G.T., Fung, J.J., Gish, R., Keeffe, E.B., Kneteman, N.M., Lake, J.R., Martin, P., McDiarmid, S.V., Rakela, J., Shiffman, M.L., So, S.K. and Wiesner, R.H. (1997) Minimal criteria for placement of adults on the liver transplant waiting list: a report of a national conference organized by the American Society of Transplant Physicians and the American Association for the Study of Liver disease. *Liver Transpl. Surg.* **3**, 628–637.

[8] Dickson, R.C. (1997) Clinical manifestations of hepatitis C. *Clin. Liver Dis.* **1**(3), 569–585.

[9] Rosen, H.R. (2001) Hepatitis B and C in the liver transplant recipient: current understanding and treatment. *Liver Transpl.* **7**, S87–S98.

[10] Forman, L.M. and Lucey, M.R. (2001) Orthotopic liver transplantation for hepatitis C: analysis of allograft survival using the UNOS database [abstract 82]. *Am. J. Transpl.* **1**, S156A.

[11] Hoofnagle, J.H., Kresina, T., Fuller, R.K., Lake, J.R., Lucey, M.R., Sorrell, M.F. and Beresford, T.P. (1997) Liver transplantation for alcoholic liver disease: executive statement and recommendations. Summary of a National Institute of Health Workshop held December 6–7, 1996, Bethesda, Maryland. *Liver Transpl. Surg.* **3**, 347–350.

[12] Bravata, D.M., Olkin, I., Barnato, A.E., Keefe, E.B. and Owens, D.K. (2001) Employment and alcohol use after liver transplantation for alcoholic and nonalcoholic liver disease: a systematic review. *Liver Transpl.* **7**, 191–203.

[13] Maldonado, J.R. and Keefe, E.M. (1997) Liver transplantation for alcoholic liver disease: selection and outcome. *Clin. Liver Dis.* **1**, 305–321.

[14] Angulo, B. and Lindor, K.D. (1999) Primary biliary cirrhosis and primary sclerosing cholangitis. *Clin. Liver Dis.* **3**, 529–570.

[15] Kim, W.R. and Dickson, E.R. (1997) The role of prognostic models in the timing of liver transplantation: application in cholestatic liver diseases. *Clin. Liver Dis.* **1**, 263–279.

[16] Faust, T.W. (2001) Recurrent primary biliary cirrhosis, primary sclerosing cholangitis, and autoimmune hepatitis after liver transplantation. *Liver Transpl.* **7**, S99–S108.

[17] Dickson, E.R., Murtaugh, P.A., Wiesner, R.H., Grambsch, P.M., Fleming, T.R., Ludwig, J., LaRusso, N.F., Malinchoc, M., Chapman, R.W. and Kaplan, M.M. (1992) Primary sclerosing cholangitis: refinement and validation of survival models. *Gastroenterology* **103**, 1893–1901.

[18] O'Grady, J.G., Alexander, G.J., Hayllar, K.M. and Wiliams, R. (1989) Early indicators of prognosis in fulminant hepatic failure. *Gastroenterology* **97**, 439–445.

[19] Bismuth, H., Samuel, D., Castaing, D., Adam, R., Saliba, F., Johann, M., Azoulay, D., Ducot, B. and Chiche, L. (1995) Orthotopic liver transplantation in fulminant and subfulminant hepatitis. The Paul Brousse experience. *Ann. Surg.* **222**, 109–119.

[20] Suarez, Y., Franca, A.C.V., Llovet, J.M., Fuster, J. and Bruix, J. (2000) The current status of liver transplantation for primary hepatic malignancy. *Clin. Liver Dis.* **4**, 591–605.

[21] Goss, J.A., Stribling, R. and Martin, P. (1998) Adult liver transplantation for metabolic liver disease. *Clin. Liver Dis.* **2**, 187–210.

[22] Rubin, D.A., Schulman, D.S., Edwards, T.D., Starzl, T.E. and Curtiss, E.I. (1994) Myocardial ischemia after orthotopic liver transplantation. *Am. J. Cardiol.* **74**, 53–56.

[23] Narayanan Menon, K.V. and Kamath, P.S. (2001) Regional and systemic hemodynamic disturbances in cirrhosis. *Clin. Liver Dis.* **5**, 617–627.

[24] Pham, P.-T.T., Pham, P.-C.T. and Wilkinson, A.H. (2000) The kidney in liver transplantation. *Clin. Liver Dis.* **4**, 567–590.

[25] Penn, I. (1993) The effect of immunosuppression on pre-existing cancers. *Transplantation* **55**, 742–747.

[26] Hasse, J., Strong, S., Gorman, M.A. and Liepa, G. (1993) Subjective global assessment – an alternative nutritional assessment technique for liver transplant candidates. *Nutrition* **9**, 339–343.

[27] Wiesner, R.H., McDiarmid, S.V., Kamath, P.S., Edwards, E.B., Malinchoc, M., Kremers, W.K., Krom, R.A. and Kim, W.R. (2001) MELD and PELD: application of survival models to liver allocation. *Liver Transpl.* **7**, 567–580.

[28] Kim, W.R. and Dickson, E.R. (2000) Timing of liver transplantation. *Semin. Liver Dis.* **20**, 451–464.

Hepatology: A Practical Approach
B. Al Knawy, M.L. Shiffman, R.H. Wiesner (editors)

Chapter 2
Surgical Issues in Cadaveric and Living Donor Liver Transplantation Recipients

James F. Trotter

Division of Gastroenterology/Hepatology, University of Colorado Health Sciences Center, 4200 E. 9th Avenue, B-154, Denver, CO 80262, USA

1. Introduction 532
  1.1 Definition 532
  1.2 General demographics 532
2. Operative Issues 533
  2.1 Cadaveric transplantation 533
  2.2 LDLT 533
3. Post-operative Complications 534
  3.1 Primary non-function 534
    3.1.1 Clinical features 534
    3.1.2 Blood tests 534
    3.1.3 Imaging studies 534
    3.1.4 Pathologic studies 535
    3.1.5 Management 535
    3.1.6 Prognosis 536
  3.2 Acute cellular rejection 536
    3.2.1 Clinical features 536
    3.2.2 Blood tests 536
    3.2.3 Imaging studies 536
    3.2.4 Pathologic studies 536
    3.2.5 Management 537
    3.2.6 Prognosis 537
  3.3 Hepatic artery thrombosis 537
    3.3.1 Clinical features 537
    3.3.2 Blood tests 537
    3.3.3 Imaging studies 537
    3.3.4 Pathologic studies 538
    3.3.5 Management 538
    3.3.6 Prognosis 538
  3.4 Post-operative bleeding 538
    3.4.1 Clinical features 538
    3.4.2 Blood tests 538
    3.4.3 Imaging and pathologic studies 538
    3.4.4 Management 538
    3.4.5 Prognosis 539
  3.5 Biliary tract complications 539
    3.5.1 Blood tests 539
    3.5.2 Imaging studies 539
    3.5.3 Pathologic studies 539

3.5.4 Management 539
3.5.5 Prognosis 540
3.6 Cytomegalovirus infections 540
3.6.1 Blood tests 540
3.6.2 Imaging studies 540
3.6.3 Pathologic studies 540
3.6.4 Management 540
3.6.5 Prognosis 540
3.7 Immunosuppression 541
4. Perioperative Issues and Complications Specific to LDLT 541
4.1 Hepatic regeneration 541
4.2 Immunosuppressive levels 541
4.3 Hypophosphatemia in LDLT donors 542
References 542

1. INTRODUCTION

1.1 Definition

The surgical period is defined as the time from the operation to 3 months after surgery [1]. This perioperative period is characterized by a wide variation in outcomes and complications for each recipient. Some patients are discharged after a very short hospitalization while other patients require prolonged intensive care hospitalization or recurrent readmissions to the hospital. This chapter will focus on the common clinical problems which occur in cadaveric and living donor liver transplant (LDLT) recipients in the perioperative period.

1.2 General demographics

The number of liver transplants performed each year is shown in Figure 1 [2]. Over the past 10 years the number of liver transplants has increased over two-fold. However, the number of patients listed has increased nearly 10-fold over the same period. As a result, the shortage of donor organs has intensified in recent years. In response to the organ shortage, adult–adult right hepatic lobe living donor liver transplantation was introduced in 1997 in the United States. The number of LDLTs performed in the US has increased nearly 10-fold in the past 5 years, as shown in Figure 2. In 2001, 10% of all liver transplants in the United States (over 500 cases) were performed using a live donor.

Compared to cadaveric recipients, LDLT patients are currently selected for favorable outcome which is reflected in the patient demographics shown in Table 1 [2]. LDLT patients are thinner, younger and less sick in contrast to the cadaveric recipients. In addition, the proportion of ICU-bound patients and patients with prior transplantation is much higher in

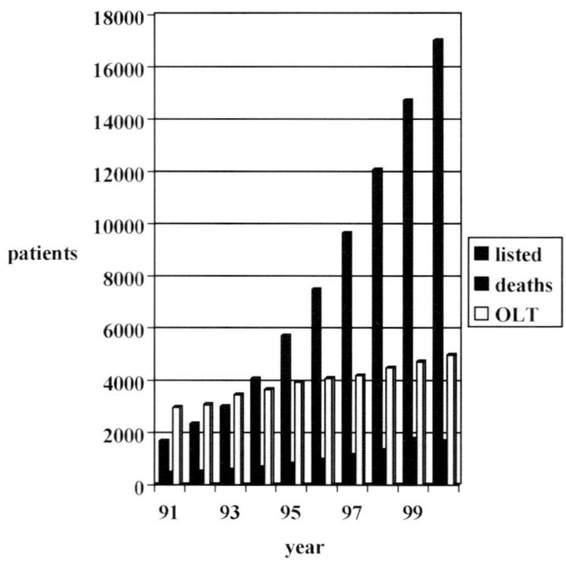

Figure 1. US liver transplant list.

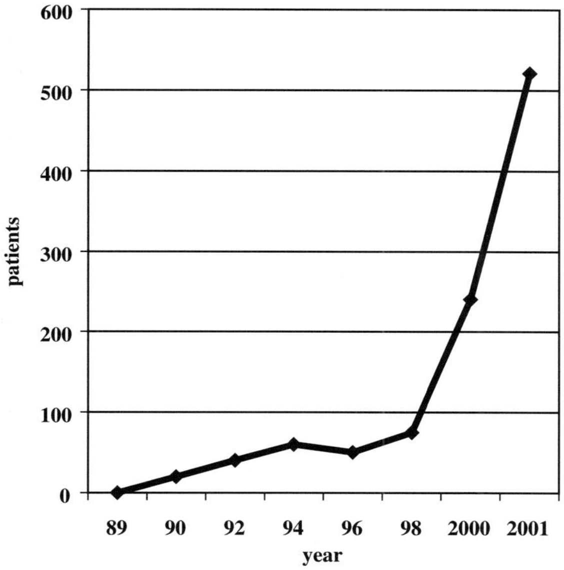

Figure 2. US living donor liver transplants.

cadaveric recipients. All of these features adversely impact survival and post-transplant outcome in cadaveric patients. As a result, cadaveric survival and outcomes' data may not be directly comparable to LDLT.

Table 1. Demographics of cadaveric and LDLT recipients.

	LDLT	Cadaveric
Race		
White	88	86
Black	5	9
Asian	3	3
Other	3	2
Age		
<18	23	11
18–34	9	6
35–49	29	32
50–64	34	43
>64	6	7
Gender		
Male	56	63
Female	44	37
Prior transplant		
Yes	3	10
No	97	90
Body mass index		
≤ 25	41.3	36.4
26–30	21	23
≥ 31	9	18
Unknown	30	23
Condition at time of transplant		
Not hospitalized	62	54
Hospitalized	14	11
ICU	6	26
Unknown	18	10

2. OPERATIVE ISSUES

2.1 Cadaveric transplantation

The most important determinant in the outcome following liver transplantation is the skill of the surgical team. A recent study by the United Network for Organ Sharing (UNOS) showed that the mortality rates were 28% higher for patients transplanted at centers performing fewer than 20 liver transplants per year [3]. Another important predictor in the outcome of the transplant recipient is the severity of illness of the recipient at the time of surgery. Patients who are ICU-bound with chronic liver disease have a 1-year mortality of 25% compared to a 10% mortality rate for patients not in the ICU. Therefore, recipient outcome is improved if transplantation occurs before the patient becomes so ill that transplantation is unlikely to provide a clinical benefit. Finally, the recipient age is an important predictor for outcome after transplantation. The 5-year mortality rate for liver transplant recipients over the age of 65 is 38% compared to 22% for patients between the ages of 18 and 49 [2]. With the increasing organ shortage, the consideration of elderly patients for liver transplantation is becoming increasingly difficult.

2.2 LDLT

LDLT is an even more complex surgery, compared to cadaveric transplantation [4]. Recommendations by the American Society for Transplant Surgeons dictate that LDLT should only be performed at centers with a vast experience in hepatobiliary and liver transplant surgery [5]. The donor and recipient surgeries are performed simultaneously in adjacent operating rooms. The recipient undergoes complete hepatectomy and removal of the entire diseased liver while the right hepatic lobe (including the gall bladder) is simultaneously removed from the donor (see Figure 3A and B). The right hepatic lobe is then implanted in the recipient. The following vascular anastomoses are performed: donor right portal vein to recipient portal vein; donor right hepatic artery to recipient hepatic artery remnant. In most LDLT recipients, the donor right hepatic duct(s) is(are) connected through a Roux-en Y anastomosis. Alternatively, the donor right hepatic duct may be anastomosed to the recipient common bile duct.

LDLT offers several advantages over cadaveric transplantation, the most important of which is a significant reduction in the waiting time prior to transplantation [6]. Once a suitable donor has been identified, the LDLT may proceed within days to weeks. At our center the waiting time for LDLT recipients is approximately 1/2 of cadaveric recipients. The reduction in waiting time allows patients to be transplanted before complications develop which could compromise outcome or result in death prior to surgery. Another advantage of LDLT over cadaveric transplantation is the elective nature of the surgery. The date of LDLT surgery is often anticipated for days or weeks. As a result, intensive therapy may be administered to the recipient to maximize their medical condition prior to the surgery. For example, patients with poorly controlled ascites and/or renal insufficiency benefit from recurrent paracentesis and albumin infusion in the pre-operative period, which may mitigate post-operative complications. The unanticipated nature of conventional transplantation precludes coordinated treatment for the cadaveric recipients.

The most appropriate candidates for LDLT are patients with an urgent need for transplantation, i.e., decompensated liver disease with ≥ 10 Child-Turcotte-Pugh points. However, not all patients who are medically in need of LDLT are suitable for the procedure. Patients with multiple comorbid conditions which could jeopardize the success of the LDLT are generally considered unsuitable for the procedure.

3. POST-OPERATIVE COMPLICATIONS

The chronology of the common complications after liver transplantation are shown in Figure 4.

3.1 Primary non-function

3.1.1 Clinical features

Primary non-function (PNF) of the transplanted liver is the most common cause of graft failure in the immediate post-operative period. The clinical presentation is dramatic and represents an emergency for the patient and the transplant team. The patient develops rapidly progressive acute liver failure usually occurring within the first 48 h after transplantation characterized by encephalopathy, coagulopathy and multiorgan system failure. Without emergency, retransplantation or death occurs within days. Risk factors for PNF include donor hypernatremia (serum sodium >170 mEq/l), advanced age in the donor and steatosis $>30\%$.

3.1.2 Blood tests

The most common laboratory abnormalities in PNF are marked elevations in liver function tests. PNF is defined by serum aspartate aminotransferase (AST) >2500 IU/l, coagulopathy (prothrombin time INR >2.0), elevated serum bilirubin and often elevated serum creatinine, characteristic of renal failure. In addition, the blood ammonia levels are elevated.

3.1.3 Imaging studies

Imaging studies are critical in the diagnosis of PNF. While PNF is defined by clinical findings and laboratory tests, imaging studies are important to rule out hepatic artery thrombosis (HAT) and portal vein thrombosis, which has a similar clinical picture as PNF. Hepatic artery and portal vein thromboses must be excluded by Doppler ultrasonography.

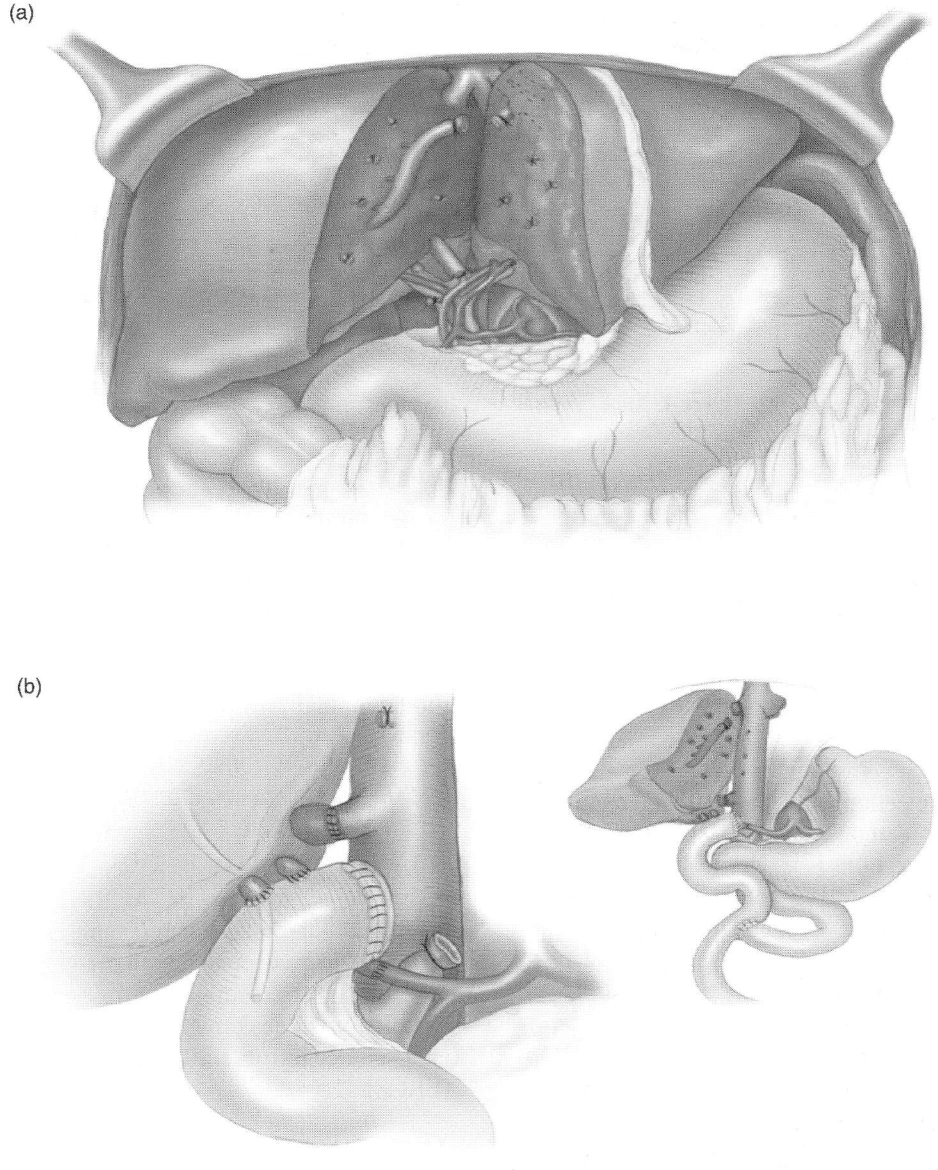

Figure 3. (a) Donor hepatectomy. (b) Implantation of donor right hepatic lobe. (*For colored version, see Plate XLVIII on page 589 at the end of the book.*)

3.1.4 Pathologic studies

Liver biopsy with histologic examination is rarely indicated for the diagnosis of PNF and may be prohibitively risky because of the associated coagulopathy. However, in the cases where biopsy is performed the histologic findings are of massive hepatic necrosis.

3.1.5 Management

The only effective therapy for PNF is retransplantation without which virtually all patients die within days. Once the patient is re-listed for transplantation continuous intensive medical support is required with mechanical ventilation and hemodialysis for most patients.

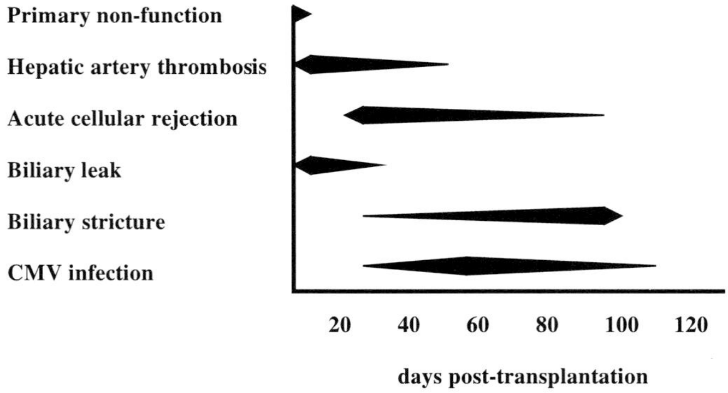

Figure 4. Time course of liver transplant complications.

3.1.6 Prognosis

Without timely retransplantation essentially all patients with PNF die within days of progressive acute liver failure.

3.2 Acute cellular rejection

3.2.1 Clinical features

Acute cellular rejection (ACR) is a clinical condition characterized by damage to the transplanted liver by host immune reaction [7]. Up to 60% of liver transplant recipients develop ACR, which may occur at any time after transplantation, but typically occurs between 10 and 90 days after surgery. In most cases, there are no clinical symptoms and the diagnosis is suspected based on elevated liver function tests. On occasion, patients may develop low-grade fever, lassitude and, if left untreated, jaundice. Other complications may mimic ACR. HAT, portal vein thrombosis, biliary obstruction, biliary leak, cytomegalovirus infection (CMV), hepatitis C and drug reaction may cause elevated liver function tests and must be excluded prior to the institution of therapy for ACR.

3.2.2 Blood tests

The diagnosis of ACR is suspected based on elevated liver function tests. For this reason liver transplant recipients must have liver function tests drawn at regular intervals after transplantation. In the immediate post-operative period (first week), labs are drawn daily and then twice a week for the first month. Thereafter, liver function tests are performed at least every month. The most common patterns of LFT abnormality in ACR are elevated alanine aminotransferase (ALT) and AST. Alkaline phosphatase and total bilirubin may also be elevated. Following treatment (see below) the LFTs rapidly improve and should normalize if the rejection has been adequately controlled.

3.2.3 Imaging studies

There are no imaging tests which are necessary to make the diagnosis of ACR. However, other conditions that have a similar presentation as ACR may need to be excluded with imaging studies. HAT is excluded by Doppler ultrasonography, biliary obstruction or leak by hepatic ultrasonography or endoscopic retrograde cholangiopancreatography (ERCP).

3.2.4 Pathologic studies

The diagnosis of ACR is confirmed by the histologic findings on liver biopsy. The three histologic features which are characteristic of ACR are: endothelialitis (inflammatory disruption of the endothelium of the portal and hepatic venules), lymphocytic biliary duct damage and portal tract pancellular inflammatory cellular infiltrate. In addition, other conditions, which mimic ACR (CMV, HAT, drug reaction or cholangitis), may be excluded by the histologic findings on liver biopsy. In some cases where a liver biopsy is prohibitively risky due to coagulopathy and the likelihood of ACR is high, empiric treatment is given without confirmation by liver biopsy.

3.2.5 Management

The treatment for ACR is typically high dose of intravenous corticosteroids. The regimen used varies from transplant center to center, but one of the most common protocols is daily intravenous methylprednisolone 1 g followed by 0.5 g on two successive days. This therapy may be given in the outpatient setting unless other medical issues are present which require hospitalization. In approximately 90% of cases, high-dose corticosteroids are adequate treatment for ACR. In the remaining 10% of cases additional treatment using more aggressive therapies may be required including anti-lymphocyte globulin (ALG) or anti-thymocyte globulin (ATG or OKT3). The differentiation between hepatitis C and ACR is extremely problematic, because the histologic features of ACR and HCV are very similar [8]. In addition, the treatment strategies for ACR and recurrent HCV are different. With recurrent HCV, the immunosuppression is decreased to prevent further progression of the viral infection, whereas the treatment for ACR is increased immunosuppression through massive dose of corticosteroid.

3.2.6 Prognosis

In almost all cases, ACR is readily reversible with treatment and there are no long-term sequelae. In fact, there is evidence demonstrating that one episode of ACR may improve patient and graft survival. In general, ACR is rarely a significant clinical problem after liver transplantation and can usually be easily controlled by a course of intravenous corticosteroids.

3.3 Hepatic artery thrombosis

3.3.1 Clinical features

HAT occurs in fewer than 10% of liver transplant recipients and is the second most common cause of graft failure in the immediate post-operative period [9]. There are three typical clinical presentations of HAT: rapidly progressive liver failure, recurrent bacteremia and biliary complications [10]. In most cases, HAT results in complete loss of all arterial blood flow to the transplanted liver, which rapidly leads to acute liver failure. HAT in the immediate post-operative period causes rapidly progressive acute liver failure that requires immediate retransplantation or surgical revascularization of the graft. The blood supply to the biliary tree is exclusively by the hepatic artery. When the arterial blood supply is interrupted, significant biliary injury occurs which can result in biliary leaks, bilomas and biliary strictures. As a result, some patients with HAT present with biliary complications. Finally, hepatic ischemia and biliary complications may lead to the formation of hepatic abscess, which may clinically present as recurrent bacteremia. Therefore, liver transplant recipients who develop unexplained sepsis should be evaluated from HAT with imaging studies (see below). The patients at greatest risk are children (because of diminutive arteries which are more likely to thrombose), patients with clotting disorders or patients requiring hepatic arterial grafts. HAT typically occurs within the first few weeks after transplantation and very rarely occurs more than 2 months post-operatively.

3.3.2 Blood tests

Liver function tests typically become markedly elevated in HAT. Patients with normal or near-normal liver function test who suddenly develop marked elevations in AST and ALT should be evaluated for HAT. In this setting the AST and ALT may rapidly rise to >2000 in 24 h. Patients who develop biliary complications have a cholestatic profile with elevated alkaline phosphatase and bilirubin. The white blood cell count is elevated when sepsis, hepatic abscess or biliary infection is present.

3.3.3 Imaging studies

The diagnosis of HAT is made by either Doppler ultrasonography demonstrating the absence of blood flow in the hepatic artery or thrombosis in the artery. In cases where the diagnosis cannot be made with ultrasonography or where confirmation is required after ultrasonography, hepatic artery angiography is performed. In some cases, HAT may be identified on a computed tomography scan of the abdomen. HAT may be more common in LDLT recipients because of the smaller size of the arterial anastomosis. At our center, we routinely interrogate the hepatic artery in LDLT recipients in the immediate post-operative period to exclude HAT.

3.3.4 Pathologic studies

HAT does not require liver biopsy for confirmation of the diagnosis. When liver biopsy is performed the histologic findings are central lobular ischemia and bile duct damage. In addition, large bilomas with extensive inflammation and bacterial or fungal elements are often present.

3.3.5 Management

For most patients with HAT the treatment of choice is retransplantation; very few patients may be managed with alternative modalities. Some grafts may be salvaged by immediate surgical revascularization of the clotted hepatic artery or with percutaneous balloon angioplasty. Prior to retransplantation many patients require the placement of percutaneous biliary drains and intravenous antibiotic therapy to manage biliary and hepatic infections. Once hepatic bilomas or abscess have developed, retransplantation is almost always indicated. Infections in the ischemic liver are refractory to treatment because of the inability of antibiotics to reach the infection and the absence of blood flow to the liver which prevents clearance of established hepatic infections.

3.3.6 Prognosis

Most patients develop progressive liver failure or refractory biliary sepsis and die without retransplantation. Retransplantation is almost always indicated when HAT occurs in the immediate post-operative period or in patients with established hepatic abscess or biloma. Some patients may develop HAT and experience no significant clinical problems. These patients typically develop HAT more than 8 weeks after transplantation and may have developed significant collateral arterial blood flow.

3.4 Post-operative bleeding

3.4.1 Clinical features

The most common surgical complication after liver transplantation is post-operative bleeding. The source of bleeding is located either in or around the transplanted liver or in the peritoneum. Approximately 10–15% of patients require re-exploration for bleeding. In about half of the cases a point source of bleeding is identified and in the other half no source is found. In these cases, bleeding is often due to coagulopathy. The diagnosis of post-operative bleeding is usually clinically apparent from increased bloody output from peritoneal drains in the immediate post-operative period and a significant drop in hematocrit (see below). If the bleeding is profound, the patient may become hypotensive.

3.4.2 Blood tests

The hematocrit or hemoglobin is the blood test which is of greatest value in the diagnosis of post-operative bleeding. In cases where the hematocrit drops more than 10 points in 24 h (with no other apparent source of bleeding), intra-abdominal post-operative bleeding should be suspected. In addition, the hematocrit from the peritoneal drains is elevated (greater than 10%) when bleeding is in the peritoneal space.

3.4.3 Imaging and pathologic studies

Radiologic and pathologic studies are not necessary to diagnose post-operative bleeding. In cases where abdominal imaging is performed, hematoma may be seen in the peritoneum or within the transplanted liver, usually as a subcapsular hematoma.

3.4.4 Management

The management of most cases is re-exploration of the abdomen. During re-exploration a point source of bleeding may be identified and surgically repaired. In addition, intraperitoneal hematoma may be evacuated. Peritoneal hematoma may serve as a nidus of infection if not evacuated. Liquified intraperitoneal hematomas may be drained in some patients with a percutaneous drain. However, subcapsular hepatic hematoma is typically managed conservatively (blood transfusion, monitoring hematocrit) without surgical intervention. Percutaneous drains of subcapsular hepatic hematoma are rarely effective, unless the hematoma is liquefied or infected.

3.4.5 Prognosis

In our experience, the prognosis of patients with postoperative bleeding is generally good if there are no other intercurrent problems identified (HAT, ruptured visceral artery aneurysm).

3.5 Biliary tract complications

Biliary problems occur in 10–20% of cadaveric transplant recipients [11,12]. There are two types of biliary problems: leaks and strictures. In cadaveric transplantation, the most common site of a biliary leak or stricture is the anastomosis. Leaks are usually evident within the first few days after transplantation and present with bile drainage from peritoneal drains, jaundice and abdominal pain. Undrained bile collections may become infected which can cause systemic infection. Strictures may occur later with 90% developing between 3 weeks and 6 months after transplantation. Typical clinical findings in patients with biliary complications include: elevated liver function test, infection, jaundice and/or abdominal pain.

Biliary complications may be more common in LDLT recipients [13]. During the donor right hepatectomy, thousands of biliary radicles are transected. Despite meticulous surgical technique a fraction of recipients may develop bile leaks from the cut surface of the liver. In addition, LDLT recipients often require more than one biliary anastomosis to the donor right hepatic lobe. This increases the likelihood of anastomotic leak or stricture.

3.5.1 Blood tests

The diagnosis of biliary complications is suspected when a cholestatic pattern of liver function tests is present. Leukocytosis is present when infection occurs.

3.5.2 Imaging studies

Several imaging modalities are useful in the diagnosis and treatment of post-transplant biliary problems. Hepatic ultrasound may identify bile fluid collections around the liver (consistent with a biliary leak) or intrahepatic biliary dilation (present in cases of biliary obstruction). In addition, the hepatic artery may be simultaneously interrogated to rule out HAT as the cause of bile leak. Computed tomographic scan of the abdomen can identify biliary dilation and bilomas. ERCP is useful as a diagnostic and therapeutic modality (stent placement) for biliary strictures and leaks. In some cases, a HIDA scan may help to identify biliary leak into the peritoneal space.

3.5.3 Pathologic studies

Histology is not required and often not clinically useful in the diagnosis of biliary complications. There are no characteristic histologic features of biliary leak. However, the biliary stricture may be suspected when bile duct reduplication and microscopic evidence of cholangitis are evident on liver biopsy.

3.5.4 Management

A comprehensive discussion of the management of biliary complications is beyond the scope of this chapter. However, in general, biliary strictures are treated with stent placement and dilation of the stricture by either an endoscopic or percutaneous approach. In some patients, stenting and balloon dilatation of the stricture may result in significant improvement or resolution of the stricture. For patients with recurrent strictures that are refractory to conservative treatment and continue to cause significant clinical problems (recurrent cholangitis), surgical repair with a Roux-en Y anastomosis may be required. Biliary leak may be treated with percutaneous drains. Isolated biliary leaks may benefit from placement of an endoscopic stent, which allows improved biliary drainage. Small biliary leaks may resolve spontaneously after percutaneous drainage. Biliary leaks that occur immediately after surgery and those that do not resolve with percutaneous drainage may require surgical repair.

3.5.5 Prognosis

The prognosis for patients depends on the severity and type of biliary problem. In most cases, biliary problems may be successfully treated by conservative or surgical therapy.

3.6 Cytomegalovirus infections

CMV is the most common infection after liver transplantation [14]. There are three possible mechanisms of acquiring CMV after transplantation: acquisition from the transplanted liver, newly acquired infection from a non-hepatic source (blood transfusion) or reactivation of previous infection. Up to 90% of adults have had previous exposure to CMV, which is determined by the presence of the CMV IgG antibody. The patients at the greatest risk of CMV after liver transplantation are those who have never been exposed to CMV and receive a liver from a donor who had a prior CMV infection. Recipients who have previously been exposed to CMV may reactivate the virus immediately after transplantation when immunosuppression is the greatest. CMV infection typically occurs 4–12 weeks after transplantation. The clinical findings in patients with CMV infection include: low-grade fevers, malaise, thrombocytopenia, leukopenia and anemia. Another common manifestation of CMV is gastrointestinal involvement, most commonly in the esophagus, colon and stomach. In severe cases, pneumonitis may occur. Patients who are highly immunosuppressed, e.g., after receiving OKT3 therapy or high-dose corticosteroid therapy for ACR, are at higher risk for CMV.

3.6.1 Blood tests

The diagnosis of CMV infection is based on the level of CMV viremia in the blood and associated clinical findings. CMV may be detected in the blood using PCR. While low viral titers (<3000 Eq/l) may be present in many patients after transplantation without CMV infection, titers greater than 3000 Eq/ml are strongly suggestive of CMV infection. Clinical findings present in CMV infection include leukopenia, anemia and thrombocytopenia. The CMV antibody test plays no role in the diagnosis of active CMV infection. If CMV is present in the liver, the liver function tests may be elevated.

3.6.2 Imaging studies

Imaging studies are rarely useful in the diagnosis of CMV. In patients with lung involvement, pulmonary infiltrates may be seen on a standard chest radiograph. Endoscopic findings consistent with CMV infection include ulcerations of the GI tract.

3.6.3 Pathologic studies

Histologic evaluation of tissue may be helpful in the diagnosis of CMV. Tissue (most commonly from the liver or GI tract) may be tested for CMV using immunohistochemical techniques. Histologic findings suggestive of CMV infection on liver biopsy include granuloma formation of microabscesses which should prompt the pathologist to perform immunohistochemical stains for CMV.

3.6.4 Management

The treatment for CMV infection is ganciclovir. In most cases, CMV infection warrants intravenous therapy for at least 2 weeks followed by 4–6 weeks of oral ganciclovir. Recently, valganciclovir has become available as an oral therapy, which may be as effective as intravenous ganciclovir. To prevent CMV infection in high-risk patients (no prior exposure to CMV, receiving a liver from a donor who has been exposed to CMV), prophylactic oral ganciclovir is administered for 4–8 weeks after transplantation. This practice is followed by most centers in the United States. In addition, prophylactic treatment with intravenous ganciclovir is typically administered for 2 weeks for patients receiving lympholytic immunosuppressive therapy (OKT3).

3.6.5 Prognosis

Most patients with CMV infection respond rapidly to intravenous ganciclovir. Therefore, the overall prognosis of the patient is generally excellent unless there are other concomitant conditions present.

3.7 Immunosuppression

All liver transplant recipients require immunosuppression to prevent rejection of the transplanted liver [15]. A comprehensive discussion of immunosuppression in the liver transplant recipient is beyond the scope of this chapter. However, there are several basic principles regarding the administration of immunosuppressants. First, almost all current immunosuppressive regimens for liver transplant recipients in the United States include either cyclosporine A (with azathioprine and prednisone) or tacrolimus (with prednisone). The specific immunosuppressive regimen varies greatly from center to center and has become much more complex with the addition of new highly effective immunosuppressive agents such as sirolimus, daclizumab, basiliximab and mycophenolate mofetil (Table 2). Second, the level of immunosuppression required to prevent acute and chronic rejection is greatest immediately after transplantation and decreases with time. Within 6 months after transplantation, the level of immunosuppression (and therefore the dose of specific immunosuppressive agents) is reduced by approximately two-thirds from the initial perioperative period. Third, the oral doses of the two most commonly prescribed immunosuppressive agents, cyclosporine A and tacrolimus, are adjusted to achieve target blood levels. Therefore, patients require recurrent and frequent blood draws and dose adjustments to achieve the proper blood level of immunosuppression. Cyclosporine A and tacrolimus (as well as sirolimus) are metabolized through the hepatic cytochrome P450 pathway. As a result, concurrently administered medications, which alter cytochrome P450 metabolism, may alter the blood level of these immunosuppressants and the level of immunosuppression in the patient. Commonly used medications which alter the blood levels of tacrolimus and cyclosporine A are listed in Table 2. Third, corticosteroids are used less frequently and weaned more quickly than in previous years. Most centers completely wean liver transplant recipients off prednisone (or to 5 mg per day) within 6 months after transplantation. At our center we have entirely discontinued the use of prednisone from our immunosuppressive regimen.

Table 2. Common immunosuppressives used in liver transplantation.

Agent	Class
Tacrolimus	Calcineurin inhibitor
Cyclosporine A	Calcineurin inhibitor
Prednisone	Corticosteroid
Mycophenolate mofetil	Anti-metabolite
Azathioprine	Anti-metabolite
Sirolimus	mTOR inhibition
Daclizumab	Interleukin-2 receptor antagonist
Basiliximab	Interleukin-2 receptor antagonist
OKT3	Monoclonal anti-CD 3 antibody
Anti-thymocyte globulin	Polyclonal anti-thymocyte antibody
Anti-lymphocyte globulin	Polyclonal anti-lymphocyte antibody

4. PERIOPERATIVE ISSUES AND COMPLICATIONS SPECIFIC TO LDLT

4.1 Hepatic regeneration

The transplanted right hepatic lobe is approximately 60% the volume of a cadaveric organ. However, LDLT graft undergoes intense regeneration, growing to normal size in a few weeks. Marcos *et al.* reported the increase in mean liver mass in LDLT recipients 7, 14, 30 and 60 days post-operatively [16]. Recipients demonstrated an increase in liver graft size of 87% at 7 days post-operatively, from 862 cc at the time of donation to 1614 cc at day 7. Remarkably, the graft had reached 94% of its final regenerated volume by the seventh post-operative day.

4.2 Immunosuppressive levels

While hepatic regeneration occurs rapidly and appears to be complete within weeks of the surgery, there is initial data which suggests that the transplanted right hepatic lobe may not function as well as a full cadaveric organ. The metabolism of immunosuppressants (which occurs through hepatic metabolism) may be impaired compared to cadaveric recipients. Data from our center showed that LDLT patients achieved higher blood levels of immunosuppressant, given the same oral dose. In LDLT recipients, the mean level/dose ratio was 26% higher in the LDLT recipients compared to cadaveric patients [17]. This difference was observed for up to 6 months after transplantation when hepatic regeneration is supposed to be completed. The explanation for the higher immunosuppressive levels in LDLT patients is that either the donor graft does not regenerate fully or the regenerated graft does not metabolize immunosuppressants normally. These findings may have important implications for LDLT recipients. The immunosuppressive requirements may be less than that of cadaveric patients. In addition, without adjustments in the oral dosage of immunosuppressant, the level of immunosuppression achieved in LDLT recipients may be significantly higher in the perioperative period compared to cadaveric patients.

4.3 Hypophosphatemia in LDLT donors

A recent publication identified hypophosphatemia as a common and often severe post-operative complication in donors following right hepatectomy for LDLT [18]. All the reported donors received post-operative total parenteral nutrition (TPN). Of an initial group of 10 donors, 70% developed "life-threatening" hypophosphatemia (serum phosphorous <1.0 mg/dl) and the remaining 30% experienced "severe" hypophosphatemia (serum phosphorous 1.0–1.5 mg/dl). A subsequent group of 10 donors received supplemental phosphorous in the TPN and only 8% developed life-threatening hypophosphatemia and 30% developed severe hypophosphatemia. There were no complications, which could be directly related to hypophosphatemia in any of the donors. The recipients of the donor right hepatic lobe grafts did not develop hypophosphatemia. The mechanism of post-operative hypophosphatemia in these donors includes administration of TPN and increased phosphorous flux into the regenerating liver. Whether hypophosphatemia is found in donors at our center and the clinical significance of this interesting observation awaits further studies.

REFERENCES

[1] Everson, G.T. (2001) Immediate postoperative care, in *Transplantation of the Liver*, eds. Maddrey, W.C., Schiff, E.R. and Sorrell, M.F. (Williams and Wilkins, Baltimore, MD) pp. 131–162.

[2] United Network for Organ Sharing, data, 2002.

[3] Edwards, E.B., Roberts, J.P., McBride, M.A., Schulak, J.A. and Hunsicker, L.G. (1999) The effect of the volume of procedures at transplantation centers on mortality after liver transplantation. *N. Engl. J. Med.* **341**, 2049–2053.

[4] Trotter, J., Wachs, M., Everson, G. and Kam, I. (2002) Adult-to-adult transplantation of the right hepatic lobe from a living donor. *N. Engl. J. Med.* **346**, 1074–1082.

[5] Anonymous (2001) American Society of Transplant Surgeons' position paper on adult-to-adult living donor liver transplantation. *Liver Transpl.* **6**, 815–817.

[6] Trotter, J. (2000) Selection of donors and recipients for living donor liver transplantation. *Liver Transpl.* **6**, S52–S58.

[7] Batts, K.P. (1999) Acute and chronic hepatic allograft rejection: pathology and classification. *Liver Transpl.* **5**, S21–S29.

[8] Scheiner, P.A. (2000) Hepatitis C after liver transplantation. *Semin. Liver Dis.* **20**, 201–209.

[9] Langnas, A.N., Marujo, W., Stratta, R.J., Wood, R.P. and Shaw, B.W. (1991) Vascular complications after orthotopic liver transplantation. *Am. J. Surg.* **161**, 76–83.

[10] Tzakis, A.G., Gordon, R.D., Shaw, B.W., Iwatsuki, S. and Starzl, T.E. (1985) Clinical presentation of hepatic artery thrombosis after liver transplantation in the cyclosporine era. *Transplantation* **40**, 667–671.

[11] Moser, M.A. and Wall, W.J. (2001) Management of biliary problems after liver transplantation. *Liver Transpl.* **7**, S46–S52.

[12] Ostroff, J.W. (2001) Post-transplant biliary problems. *Gastrointest. Endosc. Clin. N. Am.* **11**, 163–183.

[13] Testa, G., Malago, M., Valentin-Gamazo, C., Lindell, G. and Broelsch, C.E. (2000) Biliary anastomosis in living-related liver transplantation using the right hepatic lobe: techniques and complications. *Liver Transpl.* **6**, 710–714.

[14] Kusne, S., Shapiro, R. and Fung, J. (1999) Prevention and treatment of cytomegalovirus infection I organ transplant recipients. *Transpl. Infect. Dis.* **1**, 187–203.

[15] Cattral, M.S., Lilly, L.B. and Levy, G.A. (2000) Immunosuppression in liver transplantation. *Semin. Liver Dis.* **20**, 523–531.

[16] Marcos, A., Fisher, R.A., Ham, J.M., Shiffman, M.L., Sanyal, A.J., Luketic, V.A., Sterling, R.K., Fulcher, A.S. and Posner, M.P. (2000) Liver regeneration and function in donor and recipient after right lobe adult to adult living donor liver transplantation. *Transplantation* **69**, 1375–1379.

[17] Trotter, J.F., Stolpman, N., Wachs, M., Bak, T., Kugelmas, M., Kam, I. and Everson, G.T. (2002) Living donor liver transplant recipients achieve relatively higher immunosuppressant blood levels than cadaveric recipients. *Liver Transpl.* **8**, 212–218.

[18] Pomposelli, J.J., Pomfret, E.A., Burns, D.L., Lally, A., Sorcini, A., Gordon, F.D., Lewis, W.D. and Jenkins, R.L. (2001) Life-threatening hypophosphatemia after right hepatic lobectomy for live donor adult liver transplantation. *Liver Transpl.* **7**, 637–642.

Hepatology: A Practical Approach
B. Al Knawy, M.L. Shiffman, R.H. Wiesner (editors)

Chapter 3
Long-Term Management of the Liver Transplant Recipient

Jayant A. Talwalkar and Michael R. Charlton

Division of Gastroenterology/Hepatology, Mayo Medical School, Mayo Clinic and Foundation, Rochester, MN, USA

1. Introduction 545
2. Immunosuppression Related 546
3. Specific Immunosuppression Issues 547
4. Renal Dysfunction 547
5. Arterial Hypertension 548
6. Diabetes Mellitus 549
7. Hyperlipidemia 550
8. Metabolic Bone Disease 550
9. Obesity 551
10. Late Hepatic Allograft Dysfunction 552
    10.1 Allograft rejection 552
    10.2 Vascular complications 552
    10.3 Biliary stricture formation 553
    10.4 Recurrent hepatic disease 553
        10.4.1 Hepatitis C 553
        10.4.2 Hepatitis B 555
        10.4.3 Autoimmune liver diseases 556
        10.4.4 Infectious hepatitis/PTLD 556
11. Contraception and Pregnancy 556
12. Health Maintenance Strategies 557
    12.1 Immunizations 557
    12.2 Cancer screening 558
    12.3 Depression 558
    12.4 Substance abuse 558
References 558

1 INTRODUCTION

Since Thomas Starzl performed liver transplantation in a human for the first time in 1963, the procedure has become a standard of care in the management of not only decompensated acute and chronic liver disease but also for some tumors and metabolic disorders. The increasing acceptance of liver transplantation as a therapy reflects the dramatic improvement in outcomes following this procedure. One-year patient survival has improved from ~30 to 88% in the last 20 years. Five-year patient survival is currently 74%. Graft survival rates are generally ~10% less than patient survival (the United Network of Organ Sharing, UNOS). The basis for improved patient and graft survival rates is complex but undoubtedly includes advances in

(1) patient selection (most of the early recipients had metastatic liver disease);
(2) immunosuppression (less than 2% of livers are currently lost to chronic rejection);
(3) surgical technique;
(4) expertise in related fields (e.g. intensive care, anesthesia, infectious diseases, etc.).

In 1999 there were 4954 cadaveric liver transplant recipients (cf. 2676 in 1990), of which 6.8% were children. The total number of transplants has increased relatively rapidly since 1999, primarily due to the dramatic increase in living donor transplants in adults. Recipients between the ages of 35 and 64 accounted for 52% of all living donor liver transplants in 1999, up from 19% in 1998. The increase in adult living donor liver transplantation reflects the acuity of the liver transplant cadaveric organ shortage. There are currently over 15,000 patients listed for liver transplantation with a median waiting time of over 600 days for adults. The waiting list and the median waiting time both increased more than 10-fold in the 1990s. This chapter will review the diagnosis and management of long-term complications among liver transplant recipients.

2 IMMUNOSUPPRESSION RELATED

A summary of the most commonly used immunosuppressive agents, their mechanisms of action, and their adverse effects [1] are listed below:

Corticosteroids: The mechanism of action for systemic corticosteroids involves inhibition of lymphocyte activation through binding with intracellular receptors. Differentiation of T and B lymphocytes is also suppressed. Intravenous bolus therapy remains the standard of care in the treatment of acute cellular rejection. Adverse effects from systemic corticosteroids are dose dependent and influenced by duration of therapy. Specific complications include the development of hirsutism and Cushingoid features, arterial hypertension, diabetes mellitus, hyperlipidemia, osteoporosis, avascular necrosis, and gastroesophageal reflux disease.

Azathioprine: Azathioprine is an imidazole derivative of 6-mercaptopurine which inhibits the differentiation and propagation of T and B lymphocytes through interference with DNA synthesis. Long-term use of azathioprine is usually restricted to recipients who fail to tolerate steroid tapering (e.g. patients with multiple episodes of rejection, pre-transplant history of autoimmune hepatitis or ulcerative colitis). Adverse effects are generally dose dependent including bone marrow suppression leading to leucopenia and aplastic anemia. Drug-induced hepatotoxicity, including veno-occlusive disease and pancreatitis may occur idiosyncratically.

Mycophenolate mofetil: Mycophenolate mofetil (MMF) is an inhibitor of the *de novo* pathway of guanine nucleotide synthesis for DNA synthesis through non-competitive inosine monophoshate dehydrogenase inhibition. Based on the exclusive reliance on this synthetic pathway by lymphocytes, MMF is observed to deliver targeted suppression of lymphocyte proliferation. Adverse effects include bone marrow suppression (anemia and thrombocytopenia) and gastrointestinal complaints including nausea and diarrhea. At the recommended doses, there does not appear to be an increased risk of opportunistic infections, including CMV, or lymphoproliferative disorders.

Cyclosporine: Cyclosporine is a hydrophobic endacapeptide derived from the fungus *Tolypocladium inflatum*. Its mechanism of action involves binding to the intracellular protein immunophylin which in turn selectively inhibits the phosphatase activity of calcineurin. Subsequent inhibition of calcineurin inhibits the release of cytokines such as interleukin-2 (IL-2) which activate T lymphocytes. Variability in drug bioavailability with bile production led to the development of a microemulsion formulation. Both formulations have equal prevalences of adverse effects. These include hypertension, diabetes mellitus, renal insufficiency, dyslipidemia, tremor, headache, gingival hyperplasia, and hirsutism.

Tacrolimus: Tacrolimus (Prograf) is a macrolide analog originally isolated from the fungus *Streptomyces tsukubaensis*. It is also a calcineurin-based inhibitor of T cell activation acting through intracellular FK-binding protein 12. Adverse effects also include hypertension, diabetes mellitus, renal insufficiency, dyslipidemia, tremor, headache and, in contrast to cyclosporine, alopecia. Tacrolimus is not associated with gingival hyperplasia or hirsutism. When compared to cyclosporine, tacrolimus use is associated with a greater frequency nephro- and neurotoxicity [2].

Sirolimus: Sirolimus (Rapamycin) is a macrolide compound isolated from the fungus *Streptomyces hygroscopis*, with affinity to FK-binding protein

12 and subsequent inhibition of the intracellular protein mammalian target of rapamycin (mTOR) resulting in T cell inactivation. The anti-proliferative properties associated with rapamycin can manifest clinically as impaired wound healing. Current immunosuppressive strategies after liver transplantation include its use in steroid-free protocols or as a calcineurin-sparing agent for individuals with renal insufficiency. Dose-dependent side effects including dyslipidemia and bone marrow toxicity (especially thrombocytopenia) are observed. Sirolimus has been associated with increased frequency of hepatic artery thrombosis and late infections.

3 SPECIFIC IMMUNOSUPPRESSION ISSUES

Tumorigenesis: Only three types of tumors are definitively more prevalent in liver transplant recipients: skin cancer (squamous and basal cell), carcinoma of the cervix and lymphoma. Over 40% of liver transplant recipients eventually develop a skin cancer and ~10% will develop post-transplant lymphoproliferative disease/lymphoma. Annual dermatological evaluation is mandatory among liver transplant recipients. Post-transplant lymphoproliferative disease is associated with Epstein–Barr infection and administration of OKT3.

Steroid withdrawal: Early discontinuation of oral corticosteroids has been reported to reduce the incidence of hypertension, diabetes mellitus, metabolic bone disease, and dyslipidemia. Patients who discontinue steroid therapy in a tapering format (e.g. decrease dose by 1 mg/day per month until off) may experience arthralgia-type symptoms especially in the setting of long standing use, particularly at doses less than 3 mg/day. Although usually self-limiting, reinstitution of previous dosing may be necessary.

Drug interactions: Cytochrome P450 3Y4 enzyme comprises nearly 50% of total hepatic activity. This enzyme is directly involved with the metabolism of immunosuppressive agents such as cyclosporine, tacrolimus, and sirolimus. Agents which interfere with the metabolism of these drugs can result in elevated serum levels (resulting in adverse events including renal dysfunction) or sub-therapeutic levels resulting in cellular rejection (Table 1). Other important interactions include reduced azathioprine metabolism by allopurinol resulting in bone marrow depression. The frequency of rhabdomyolysis from HMG-CoA reductase inhibitors after liver transplantation appears rare. Chronic use of non-steroidal anti-inflammatory agents and COX-2 inhibitors further reduces effective renal arterial blood flow which may aggravate or lead to renal dysfunction. Transplant recipients should be encouraged to seek advice regarding the initiation of any drug to determine if effective immunosuppression will be altered.

4 RENAL DYSFUNCTION

Renal insufficiency increases in prevalence with duration of post-LT follow-up. While renal dysfunction is often reversible in the early post-operative period, a majority of recipients develop some degree of chronic renal dysfunction [3].

Pathophysiology: A number of factors contribute to renal dysfunction after liver transplantation. Hepatorenal syndrome (HRS) affects approximately 10% of liver transplant candidates. HRS usually reverses soon after liver transplantation with a minority of patients experiencing delayed, persistent recovery requiring intermittent hemodialysis. Comorbid illness such as diabetes mellitus and hypertension is likely to contribute to prolonged post-LT renal dysfunction. Patients with pre-transplant tubuloglomerular diseases such as IgA nephropathy and

Table 1. Agents which alter therapeutic serum levels of cyclosporine and tacrolimus.

Increase serum levels	Decrease serum levels
Clarithromycin	Carbamazepine
Clotrimazole	Rifampin
Erythromycin	Phenytoin
Fluconazole	Phenobarbital
Itraconazole	Rifabutin
Ketoconazole	
Grapefruit juice	
Verapamil	
Diltiazem	
Ranitidine	

membranous glomerulonephritis are more likely to require prolonged renal support after transplantation.

In the long-term recipient, a deterioration in renal function is most commonly caused by calcineurin inhibitor nephrotoxicity. Cyclosporine and tacrolimus increase resistance in the afferent glomerular arteriole and reduce renal blood flow. Other medications causing early post-transplant renal insufficiency include aminoglycosides, vancomycin, amphotericin B, and acyclovir. Non-steroidal anti-inflammatory drugs may also be associated with acute and chronic renal dysfunction. Renal dysfunction may be associated with recurrent hepatic disease. Patients transplanted for hepatitis C (HCV) have an increased risk of proteinuria based on membranoproliferative glomerulonephritis. Allograft cirrhosis may also progress to end-stage liver disease, recreating the setting for HRS and renal dysfunction.

Clinical features: Immediate post-transplant renal insufficiency occurs in up to 73% of liver recipients. The GFR declines to approximately 60% of pre-transplant levels within 6 weeks of surgery and then remains relatively stable for at least 4 years. Serum creatinine is typically elevated between 1.5 and 2.0 mg/dl after liver transplantation. No report of symptom development from chronic renal insufficiency has been reported among liver transplant recipients to date.

Diagnosis: Despite renal insufficiency, malnourished transplant recipients often have a low serum creatinine. Even well-nourished patients with cirrhosis maintain a normal creatinine until GFR decreases by more than 50%. Glomerular filtration rate and creatinine clearance can be easily estimated using various formulas, but the formulas tend to overestimate the true GFR because of the increase in tubular creatinine secretion as GFR decreases. Standard renal clearance tests measuring surrogate markers including iothalamate provide the most accurate results.

Management: There are several strategies for managing immunosuppression-based nephrotoxicity. Dose reduction is essential although renal dysfunction may not always respond. Persistent renal dysfunction should lead to appropriate dosing adjustments (e.g. decreasing calcineurin inhibitor) and consideration of non-nephrotoxic alternatives (e.g. MMF) and aggressive management of hypertension. Lower doses of calcineurin inhibitors are usually well tolerated among recipients with renal insufficiency.

Renal tubular acidosis from calcineurin inhibitors does not usually require therapy but may be associated with long-term hypomagnesemia and hyperkalemia. Hypomagnesemia must be corrected aggressively because it acts synergistically with calcineurin inhibitors to reduce seizure threshold. Correction of hyperkalemia involves diet control and the occasional use of sodium polystyrene sulfonate (Kayexalate). Angiotensin converting enzyme (ACE) inhibitors and potassium-sparing diuretics should be avoided after liver transplantation because they aggravate hyperkalemia.

Prognosis: Although renal dysfunction is common after liver transplantation, the majority of patients do not develop end-stage renal failure. Among 834 liver transplant recipients followed for a mean duration of 8 years, the incidence of chronic renal failure and end-stage renal disease was 4.9 and 6%, respectively. Individuals experiencing a significant increase in serum creatinine at 1 year following liver transplantation despite immunosuppression reduction appear at greatest risk for advanced renal disease.

5 ARTERIAL HYPERTENSION

Introduction: Arterial hypertension affects 25–85% of OLT recipients. Hypertension is caused or exacerbated by immunosuppression therapy but can be controlled with pharmacotherapy [4].

Pathophysiology: Cyclosporine, tacrolimus, and corticosteroids are most commonly associated with the development of hypertension. Hypertension occurs less frequently and with delayed onset using tacrolimus compared with cyclosporine. Both agents cause renal vasoconstriction resulting in increased sodium chloride retention, fluid overload, and arterial hypertension. Endothelial dysfunction is the dominant mechanism of immunosuppression-induced hypertension. Cyclosporine inhibits endothelial nitrous oxide synthesis and increases thromboxane A_2 production, which further leads to widespread vasoconstriction. Immunosuppression-induced hypomagnesemia also aggravates hypertension.

Management: Managing hypertension after liver transplantation usually requires the initial strategy of reducing dietary sodium intake. Oral diuretic therapy with furosemide is used to manage fluid overload when present. Calcium channel blockers, based on their ability to inhibit endothelin and cause smooth muscle vasodilatation, are considered optimal drugs for treatment. The dihydroperidine class of agents including nifedipine and amlodipine are most commonly used because verapamil and diltiazem increase calcineurin-based drug levels. Edema and headache are side effects associated with these agents. Beta blocker agents have also been effective in treating hypertension but are also limited by side effects including fatigue and sexual dysfunction. Central acting agents including clonidine may be useful but are associated with drowsiness. ACE inhibitors are ineffective and frequently worsen cyclosporine-induced hyperkalemia.

Conversion to a tacrolimus-based regimen may help improve treatment-resistant hypertension among select patients taking cyclosporine. Early withdrawal of corticosteroid therapy with calcineurin inhibitor tapering has been associated with the declining incidence of post-transplant hypertension.

Prognosis: Hypertension frequently develops within a few weeks of transplantation. Long-term pharmacological therapy is often required but effective in preventing end-organ target damage. Reduction of immunosuppression doses is not necessarily curative but assist in reducing hypertension severity. The impact of post-transplant hypertension on developing cardiac disease or stroke in long-term survivors after liver transplantation appears small when controlled.

6 DIABETES MELLITUS

Introduction: Diabetes mellitus is found in 10–15% of patients with advanced cirrhosis and primarily related to insulin resistance. Putative mechanisms include impaired insulin-stimulated glucose transport with skeletal muscle glycogen synthesis and defective pancreatic beta cell insulin secretion. Following liver transplantation, the prevalence of diabetes mellitus ranges between 4 and 14% [5].

Pathophysiology: The pathogenesis of diabetes mellitus after liver transplantation is multifactorial. Patients may have a genetic susceptibility to diabetes mellitus. Corticosteroids, cyclosporine, tacrolimus, azathioprine, and mycophenolic acid all have hyperglycemic effects. Reductions in insulin synthesis are also observed with calcineurin inhibitor use. There seems to be no difference in the prevalence of glucose intolerance between OLT recipients maintained on cyclosporine or tacrolimus. Obesity also contributes to the development of impaired glucose tolerance.

Clinical features: In the post-operative period, hyperglycemia is related to stress, calcineurin inhibitors, corticosteroids, and infection. Long-term diabetes mellitus is related to pre-existing hyperglycemia and multiple episodes of acute cellular rejection requiring corticosteroids. The majority of affected individuals are known to have pre-existing diabetes mellitus. In addition, *de novo* diabetes mellitus develops in about one-third of recipients although this declines to less than 5% at 3 years follow-up. In contrast to the pre-OLT situation, more than 90% of post-OLT diabetics are insulin dependent. Formal glucose tolerance testing may identify as many as 50% of individuals.

Management: The management of diabetes mellitus after liver transplantation includes strategies found in the non-transplant setting. Dietary and lifestyle modifications, exercise, and control of obesity are initial treatment measures. Oral hypoglycemic agents are being increasingly used but potential interactions with immunosuppressive agents and inherent hepatotoxicity warrant caution with their use. Short and long-acting insulin preparations remain useful for patients with difficult to control hyperglycemia. Maintenance immunosuppression regimens using lower doses of prednisone or steroid-free regimens are associated with a lower frequency of diabetes mellitus. MMF and/or sirolimus with calcineurin inhibitor tapering can also be used to provide further control. Preventive health measures including education are recommended.

Prognosis: The impact of diabetes mellitus on outcomes after liver transplantation remains controversial. While previous studies are inconclusive, a recent analysis of UNOS data strongly suggests the presence of a reduced patient and graft survival with pre-existing diabetes mellitus. Complications related to microvascular disease appear responsible given the strict exclusion of patients with significant macrovascular complications from liver transplantation. The natural history of diabetic nephropathy, retinopathy, and neuropathy is unknown but some reports suggest an increased frequency of nephropathy in type 1 insulin-dependent diabetic recipients.

7 HYPERLIPIDEMIA

Introduction: While more common in heart and kidney transplant recipients, the development of hyperlipidemia after liver transplantation is well recognized. Prevalence rates for hypercholesterolemia range between 16 and 40% with hypertriglyceridemia occurring in 40% of individuals [6].

Pathophysiology: The cause of post-transplant hyperlipidemia is multifactorial. Abnormal lipid profiles before liver transplantation are associated with post-transplant hyperlipidemia. Increased caloric intake, diabetes mellitus, and increased low density lipoprotein (LDL) production are associated with corticosteroids. Calcineurin inhibitors reduce cholesterol transport into bile (raising serum levels) and increase LDL production. Tacrolimus may be less hyperlipidemic as conversion from cyclosporine may improve lipid profiles in select individuals.

Clinical features: The majority of patients are asymptomatic with serial blood testing documenting abnormal cholesterol and triglyceride levels. The risk of developing complications from atherosclerosis related to untreated hyperlipidemia is felt to be unaltered in the post-transplant setting.

Management: Dietary and lifestyle modifications including exercise are first-line therapies for improving lipid profiles. Improved glucose control in patients with diabetes mellitus is mandatory to improve hypertriglyceridemia. Pharmacological therapy may still be required despite adherence to initial measures. Bile acid binding resins are not optimal as they may interfere with absorption of immunosuppressive agents resulting in reduced serum levels and increased risk of rejection. Nicotinic acid is considered as a second-line agent given its potential for hepatotoxicity. HMG-CoA reductase inhibitors or "statins" are safe and effective in reducing LDL. Drug-induced hepatotoxicity, myositis, and rhabdomyolysis are potential adverse events. Gemfibrozil and other fibric acid derivatives are effective in treating hypertriglyceridemia but may cause myositis when given with HMG-CoA reductase inhibitors. In terms of immunosuppressive management, sirolimus is associated with hyperlipidemia and thus requires serial monitoring. Reduction of calcineurin inhibition and steroid withdrawal may also improve lipid profiles.

Prognosis: An increased frequency of clinical atherosclerotic disease related to hyperlipidemia after liver transplantation remains to be demonstrated. In one study, the survival of liver OLT recipients up to 7 years was not decreased because of atherosclerotic events, even though the estimated coronary risk index increased over time. Based on the known association of hyperlipidemia with atherosclerotic disease, however, it is reasonable to evaluate hyperlipidemic OLT recipients and consider therapy when indicated.

8 METABOLIC BONE DISEASE

Introduction: Metabolic bone disease is common among patients with end-stage liver disease awaiting liver transplantation. Patients with chronic cholestatic liver disease (primary biliary cirrhosis, PBC; primary sclerosing cholangitis, PSC) are at highest risk for reduced bone mineral density (BMD). Osteopenia and/or osteoporosis is observed in 10–60% of cases. While a significant decrease in BMD occurs in the immediate post-operative period, bone demineralization usually continues throughout the post-transplant period [7].

Pathophysiology: The mechanisms related to bone disease after liver transplantation are multiple in nature. They include pre-existing bone disease, micronutrient deficiency, immobility, immunosuppressive medications including corticosteroids and calcineurin inhibitors, and secondary hyperparathyroidism from chronic renal insufficiency.

Clinical features: In the first 3–6 months following liver transplantation, the fracture rate is between 25 and 65%. Over the next 6 months, a gradual rise in BMD is observed but often remains below the fracture threshold in one-third of patients with a fracture rate of 7.5%. Fractures usually occur in areas of trabecular bone such as vertebrae and ribs. In contrast to osteoporosis, select individuals may develop avascular osteonecrosis related primarily to corticosteroid use. Pain originating from the proximal femur and hip is most commonly observed. Diagnosis is made by magnetic resonance imaging (MRI). Osteotomy and/or hip replacement is indicated in severe cases.

Management: Measurement of serum calcium and phosphate levels, thyroid function tests, parathyroid hormone level, 25-hydroxyvitamin D level, and testosterone (men) or estradiol/luteinizing hormone should be performed to exclude correctable etiologies of metabolic bone disease. In addition to weight-bearing exercise, the use of calcium and vitamin D supplementation decreases the incidence of atraumatic fractures. Steroid withdrawal has also been associated with improvements in BMD. Hormone replacement therapy appears safe in the post-menopausal setting despite the absence of controlled data supporting its use. Corticosteroid-dependent individuals may benefit from oral bisphosphonate therapy. A recent study failed to recognize calcitonin as an effective treatment for bone disease after liver transplantation. Surveillance BMD measurement is indicated to assess the effectiveness of therapeutic interventions.

Prognosis: Bone density after the second post-transplant year is anticipated to remain stable but may remain below the fracture threshold. Prognosis is based primarily on fracture-related outcomes which can be mild or severe in nature.

9 OBESITY

Introduction: Few individuals prior to liver transplantation are affected by obesity based on the protein-calorie malnutrition state associated with end-stage liver disease. Following transplantation, however, an estimated two-thirds of patients are identified with elevated body mass indices consistent with obesity [8].

Pathophysiology: The pathogenesis of post-transplant weight gain is multifactorial. Similar factors associated with diabetes mellitus and hyperlipidemia also predispose to obesity including dietary indiscretions and physical inactivity. Corticosteroids are associated with increased hunger and food cravings. A reduced likelihood of post-transplant weight gain may be related to tacrolimus when compared to cyclosporine yet this remains unproven.

Clinical features: In the first post-operative year, weight gain is rapid and then reaches a plateau. Continued weight gain is associated with pre-transplant obesity. The risk for obesity after 2 years from transplantation is estimated at 20%. Independent post-transplant risk factors include the absence of acute cellular rejection, cyclosporine-based immunosuppression, and higher cumulative prednisone dose during the second year. Of concern is the growing recognition of hepatic allograft steatohepatitis related to obesity.

Management: In addition to the management of obesity-related comorbidities including hypertension, diabetes mellitus, and hyperlipidemia, the institution of a controlled diet and exercise program with the goal of gradual but consistent weight loss is mandatory. Behavioral management techniques utilized among non-transplant recipients would also appear effective in this setting. Corticosteroid reduction or withdrawal has been associated with significant weight loss. Conversion from cyclosporine to tacrolimus, which may further assist in weight reduction, is likely related to subsequent corticosteroid tapering or discontinuation. Pharmacological agents (sibutramine, orlistat) for the treatment of obesity are difficult to use based on potential reductions in calcineurin inhibitor drug absorption. The safety and effectiveness of bariatric surgery following liver transplantation remains unknown.

Prognosis: The morbidity from obesity after liver transplantation is primarily based on the severity of body mass index. Long-term survival among patients developing obesity appears similar to unaffected patients. In contrast, patients with pre-transplant obesity have a greater risk for peri-operative complications and death.

10 LATE HEPATIC ALLOGRAFT DYSFUNCTION

The occurrence of hepatic allograft dysfunction can be classified based on its temporal existence to liver transplantation. Evidence to suggest abnormal liver function 2 months and beyond has been defined as late hepatic allograft dysfunction. The persistence of elevations in serum hepatic biochemical parameters warrants subsequent evaluations to reveal an underlying cause. Testing often includes the use of allograft ultrasonography with Doppler flow studies, cholangiography, and/or liver biopsy. Common reasons of late allograft hepatic dysfunction include acute cellular or chronic ductopenic rejection, hepatic artery thrombosis, biliary tract complications, malignancy, and recurrent hepatic disease (Table 2).

Table 2. Causes of late hepatic allograft dysfunction.

Category	Etiology
Immunologic rejection	Acute (cellular) and chronic (ductopenic)
Vascular compromise	Hepatic artery, portal vein, hepatic vein
Biliary complications	Strictures (anastamotic, non-anastamotic) Stones Ischemic cholangiopathy
Recurrent disease	Hepatitis B and C Autoimmune disease (PBC, PSC, AIH) Non-alcoholic steatohepatitis Alcoholic liver disease
Infections	Bacterial cholangitis Fungal Cytomegalovirus Epstein–Barr virus *De novo* hepatitis (B and C)
Malignancy	PTLD Recurrent hepatocellular carcinoma (HCC)
Drug induced	Similar to non-transplant experience

10.1 Allograft rejection

Acute cellular rejection occurs in 30–60% of patients within the initial 30 days following liver transplantation. Late-onset acute cellular rejection, however, has also been observed in up to 20% of recipients beyond the first post-operative month. Causes include a reduction or withdrawal of immunosuppression, poor absorption of medications, or non-compliance. Risk factors for late-onset acute cellular rejection include age <30 years and prior autoimmune hepatitis or fulminant hepatic failure as the cause of transplantation. Tacrolimus-based regimens are associated with lower rates of late rejection compared to cyclosporine. Based on less rigorous follow-up, the diagnosis of late rejection is often delayed and more often resistant to corticosteroid therapy [9].

Chronic ductopenic rejection occurs in 3% of recipients. Declining rates are based on improved use of immunosuppression. One or more episodes of corticosteroid-resistant acute cellular rejection usually predate the onset of ductopenic rejection. Liver biopsy findings include cholestasis and the disappearance of interlobular and septal bile ducts in greater than 50% of portal tracts examined. Among patients on cyclosporine, the switch to tacrolimus in early stages of chronic ductopenic rejection may lead to biochemical and histological improvement [10].

10.2 Vascular complications

Hepatic artery thrombosis is the most common vascular complication after liver transplantation occurring in 10% of adults and up to 40% of pediatric recipients. Both early and late thrombosis (after post-operative month 1) have been observed. Risk factors include donor–recipient artery size mismatch, arterial anastamotic reconstruction, hypercoaguable state, and prolonged ischemic time. In late thrombosis, the development of biliary symptoms including cholangitis and hepatic abscesses results from ischemic cholangiopathy and biliary strictures. The diagnosis is made by Doppler ultrasonography and hepatic angiography. Ultimately, the development of progressive graft failure warrants consideration for hepatic retransplantation. Hepatic artery stenosis (5% of cases) is managed by percutaneous angioplasty and/or segmental resection in refractory cases.

Portal vein thrombosis or stenosis may be asymptomatic or result in clinical manifestations including ascites, variceal bleeding, and hepatic encephalopathy. Risk factors include native portal vein thrombosis, the use of interposition vein grafting, and previous portocaval shunt surgery. The diagnosis is made by Doppler ultrasonography and subsequent hepatic venography. Percutaneous angioplasty and/or stenting has provided benefit for portal vein stenosis with operative therapy reserved for refractory cases.

Hepatic vein or inferior vena cava thrombosis/stenosis may present with refractory ascites after liver transplantation. The diagnosis is again made by Doppler ultrasonography and subsequent hepatic venography. Percutaneous angioplasty, stent placement, and operative repair are therapeutic options.

10.3 Biliary stricture formation

The most common site for biliary stricturing is at the surgical anastomosis. These strictures occur sporadically and on a technical basis. Over 80% occur during the first post-operative month and only rarely after the first year. Although both duct-to-duct and Roux-en-Y anastomoses can develop strictures, they are most common among duct-to-duct anastomoses. Clinical manifestations include asymptomatic elevations of liver biochemistries, jaundice, or a clinical syndrome of bacterial cholangitis. Intrahepatic biliary tract dilatation may be missed on ultrasonography. Endoscopic retrograde cholangiopancreatography (ERCP) provides both diagnostic and therapeutic measures including balloon dilatation and/or stent placement. Refractory cases require operative anastamotic reconstruction. Two-thirds of anastamotic strictures will respond to endoscopic therapy and one-third will ultimately require surgical revision of the anastomosis/conversion to a Roux-en-Y [11].

Non-anastamotic strictures are more likely with longer cold and warm ischemia times, following ABO incompatible liver transplantation, following hepatic artery thrombosis and in patients whose original liver disease was PSC. The median time for development of non-anastomotic strictures is 11 weeks post-transplantation vs. 2 weeks for anastomotic stricturing. Stenting and external biliary drainage are performed as needed. Approximately half of patients with non-anastomotic biliary strictures will either die or undergo retransplantation due to stricture associated complications event.

Biliary leaks previously occurred with T-tube removal yet recent use of donor cystic duct for tube placement has reduced the frequency of this event.

Anastamotic strictures may occur early or late. Non-anastamotic strictures may occur in the presence or absence of hepatic artery thrombosis within 3 months of transplantation. Additional risk factors include ABO incompatibility, prolonged ischemic time >12 h, CMV infection, chronic rejection, and recurrent PSC. ERCP with balloon dilatation and/or stenting is the preferred method of treatment. In 20% of cases where diffuse intrahepatic stricturing is present, hepatic retransplantation is the only option. Empiric therapy with antibiotics and/or ursodeoxycholic acid may prevent recurrent cholangitis.

10.4 Recurrent hepatic disease

10.4.1 Hepatitis C

The most common cause of late allograft dysfunction is recurrent hepatic disease. As the most common indication for liver transplantation, chronic hepatitis C (HCV) is also the most important recurrent disease. Post-transplant HCV recurrence is essentially universal in patients who have viremia prior to undergoing liver transplantation. The two most common causes of death among HCV recipients are non-HCV infections and allograft failure secondary to HCV recurrence. Serum levels of HCV RNA increase rapidly from week 2 post-transplantation, peaking at 1–3 months, and eventually achieving 1 year post-transplant levels that are 16- to 17-fold higher than pre-transplant levels. Following reinfection, between over 80% of patients will develop histological evidence of chronic hepatitis C infection within 1–4 years of undergoing transplantation. Up to 30% of patients will develop cirrhosis within 5 years post-transplantation. A small proportion of recipients with post-transplant HCV infection (4–7%) experience an accelerated course of liver injury ("fibrosing" cholestatic hepatitis C) leading to rapidly progressive allograft failure.

The majority of patients with post-transplant HCV infection, however, experience mild medium-term allograft injury. Several risk factors have been identified that are associated with an increased risk of more severe HCV recurrence.

Risk factors associated with severity of HCV recurrence and/or diminished graft survival can be grouped in the following four classifications: (1) viral factors, (2) recipient factors, (3) donor factors, and (4) clinical variables [12].

High pre-transplant viral load in both the serum and explant tissue has been associated with both fibrosis progression and relatively poor 5-year patient and graft survival. Higher post-transplant serum and tissue HCV RNA levels have been associated with early acute recurrence of HCV and more rapid histological progression. Patients who develop fibrosing cholestatic HCV almost always have very high levels of HCV RNA, often with minimal necroinflammatory activity on liver biopsy.

Although HCV genotypes 1 and 4 are associated with pre-transplant failure of interferon therapy, the impact of genotype on post-transplant recurrence of HCV is less clear. Some investigators have reported genotype 1a or 1b is associated with more severe disease recurrence while others have found that HCV genotype does not influence post-transplant outcomes. Pre-transplant HCV quasispecies, reflecting amino acid diversification in the HVR1 epitope of HCV, have also been reported to be predictive of a poor outcomes following liver transplantation. Mutations in the HVR1 area have been associated with a low likelihood of viral clearance, the development of acute HCV, lack of response to antiviral therapy and a higher likelihood of developing hepatocellular cancer. At least one study has suggested that pre-transplant failure to respond to interferon therapy may be a associated with more severe recurrence of HCV.

Host factors that can be associated with poor outcomes in HCV-infected liver transplant recipients include greater recipient age and non-Caucasian recipient race. Donor factors associated with adverse outcomes in HCV liver recipients include: (1) donor age, (2) donor fat content, (3) greater warm ischemia time, and (4) utilizing live donors. Older donors and organs with higher fat content should be used with caution in recipients with HCV infection. The preliminary data concerning adverse outcomes in living donor recipients needs confirmation.

Post-transplant clinical factors associated with more severe recurrence of HCV and/or poorer overall patient and graft survival include: (1) average daily steroid dose, (2) treatment for rejection, (3) use of antilymphocyte preparations, (4) the early recurrence of acute hepatitis C, and (5) cytomegalovirus infection. A strong correlation between rejection episodes, treated with bolus corticosteroids, and increased severity of histological recurrence of HCV has been well documented. The relationship between treated rejection and attenuated patient survival among HCV recipients is in contrast to the non-HCV infected recipient in whom treatment of single episodes of acute cellular rejection is associated with a diminished mortality (relative risk 0.58, $p < 0.007$).

No difference in the severity of HCV recurrence or in patient or graft survival has been found between tacrolimus and cyclosporine-based immunosuppressive regimens. The impact of mycophenolic acid mofetil on the severity of HCV recurrence is a matter of some debate. The only large multicenter, controlled trials, in which recipients were randomized to receive MMF or non-MMF based protocols, including the registration study for MMF, found no significant difference in clinical parameters of HCV recurrence. Corticosteroids are known to increase levels of HCV viremia and to be associated with more severe histological injury in the non-transplant setting. This finding also holds true for liver transplant recipients with HCV infection. Bolus IV methylprednisolone therapy for the treatment of acute rejection is associated with a 4–100-fold increase in HCV RNA levels. These high HCV RNA levels are associated with increased necroinflammatory activity at 1 year post-transplantation. Conversely, early withdrawal of corticosteroids has been associated with and increased frequency of acute cellular rejection which has also been associated with an increased severity of recurrence of HCV.

OKT3 administration has been associated with shorter time to the development of and greater severity of recurrence of hepatitis C. The NIDDK Liver Transplant Database found that steroid resistant rejection treated with antilymphocyte preparations was associated with a greater than fivefold increased risk of mortality in HCV infected recipients. These data strongly suggest that the use of antilymphocyte preparations in HCV infected recipients can lead to an increased severity of HCV recurrence associated with diminished patient and graft survival.

There are few data concerning the impact of newer immunosuppressive agents, such as sirolimus and interleukin-2 receptor antibodies on post-transplant HCV infection. The only multicenter, multinational, randomized controlled trial of sirolimus, demonstrated a *higher* incidence of rejection among HCV infected recipients randomized to sirolimus ($p = 0.055$). A multicenter, multinational, randomized placebo-controlled trial which found the use of interleukin-2 receptor antibodies to be neutral in terms of rejection rates and clinical outcomes.

Cytomegalovirus infection has also been associated with increased severity of HCV recurrence. It is not known whether the routine administration of prophylaxis for CMV infection will improve outcomes.

10.4.1.1 Treatment of HCV infection following liver transplantation. As yet, there have been no well-controlled, large clinical trials to determine the optimal management approach to treating recurrent HCV infection following liver transplantation. Patients with higher pre-LT HCV RNA titers experience mortality and graft loss rates ~30% greater than recipients with lower pre-LT HCV RNA titers. Unfortunately, antiviral therapy with interferon alpha (either as monotherapy or in combination with ribavirin) is poorly tolerated in the minority of Child's class B HCV-infected patients who meet treatment initiation criteria.

There are no large, randomized, controlled trials of antiviral therapy among transplant recipients. Those studies that have been carried out suggest that the overall efficacy of interferon and ribavirin is broadly comparable to that seen in the non-transplant setting. End of treatment virological response rates of 25–50% following combination therapy have been reported. Reversal of fibrosing cholestatic post-transplant hepatitis C infection, although reported, appears to be unusual. The high prevalences of anemia, thrombocytopenia, leucopenia, and renal insufficiency limit the tolerability, and thus efficacy of antiviral therapy in HCV-infected recipients. Based on the cumulative published experience to date, dose reduction/cessation of ribavirin alone can be expected in ~50% of recipients during ribavirin therapy. Early initiation of erythropoietin has been reported in small studies to facilitate increased tolerability of ribavirin.

Pegylated interferon alfa-2a monotherapy achieved end-of-treatment HCV RNA negativity in ~30% of patients following 48 weeks of treatment. There are no published reports of the efficacy of pegylated interferon alfa-2b and ribavirin combination therapy for treatment recurrence of HCV. Given the superior efficacy of pegylated interferon when compared to standard interferon in the non-transplant setting, future protocols for liver transplant recipients are likely, however, to incorporate combination therapy with pegylated interferon and ribavirin. The optimal timing and dosing for such therapy is not known.

Of the handful of studies describing the outcome of treating HCV with IFN in liver transplant recipients, two have suggested that IFN treatment may be associated with an increased risk of rejection. In contrast, none of the larger, more recent studies of combination therapy with interferon and ribavirin have reported an increased risk of frequency or severity of rejection. Hepatitis B immunoglobulin has moved hepatitis B infected patients from the ranks of the untransplantable to ideal candidates for liver transplantation. A randomized controlled study of hepatitis C immunoglobulin in the prevention of post-transplant HCV infection ($n = 26$) found no benefit in terms of post-transplant clinical reinfection rate or HCV RNA levels. Further anti-HCV immunoglobulin preparations are currently in various stages of development.

10.4.2 Hepatitis B

The identification of hepatitis B immunoglobulin (HBIg) as effective immunoprophylaxis has minimized the risk of recurrent hepatitis B while improving patient and graft survival [13]. Pre-transplant active viral replication, however, is associated with an increased risk of allograft infection. Clinical manifestations are similar to those associated with recurrent chronic hepatitis C. Diagnosis is made by demonstrating HBV DNA in serum or hepatitis B surface and core antigen in liver tissue. Oral agents including lamivudine have been used to date for the purpose of suppressing viral activity prior to transplant to minimize the risk of recurrence. However, concerns exist regarding long-term therapy and the potential impact of emerging YMDD mutants in 30% of patients after 1 year. Current studies are examining the use of lamivudine and adefovir in selected patients as monotherapy for preventing allograft recurrence [14].

10.4.3 Autoimmune liver diseases

Autoimmune liver diseases including PBC, PSC, and autoimmune hepatitis are known to recur after liver transplantation [15]. Previously considered a controversial topic, the recurrence of PBC following liver transplantation has now been demonstrated to be as high as 15% at 3 years and 30% at 10 years with prospective follow-up. Serum AMA status is independent of recurrence risk. Immunosuppression reduction or tapering of corticosteroids and tacrolimus-based regimens have been suggested as potential risk factors for recurrent PBC. No information is available regarding the efficacy of UDCA therapy in halting disease progression from early stage recurrent PBC.

An increasing body of evidence suggests that PSC is a recurrent disease after liver transplantation in select patients. Among 120 PSC patients undergoing liver transplantation at the Mayo Clinic, 24 (20%) individuals developed evidence for recurrent PSC using strict criteria. Cholangiography was diagnostic for recurrent PSC in 92% of cases while 46% of liver biopsies were compatible with recurrence. The identification of sustained elevations in serum alkaline phosphatase levels ($>2\times$ ULN) at least 2 years after liver transplantation may be associated with an increased risk for disease recurrence.

Recurrent autoimmune hepatitis occurs in 20–30% of patients with the original hepatic disease within 5 years of liver transplantation. Diagnostic criteria used in the non-transplant setting are also used for establishing clinical disease. Risk factors include reduced immunosuppression, corticosteroid withdrawal, and human leukocyte antigen (HLA) DR3 and DR4 allelles. Most patients are asymptomatic with liver biochemical profiles resembling acute cellular rejection. Liver biopsy is required for diagnostic confirmation. *De novo* autoimmune hepatitis has also been observed among patients transplanted for idiopathic fulminant hepatic failure or other autoimmune liver disease such as PBC and PSC. Therapy with corticosteroids and/or azathioprine is usually effective in preventing progressive injury and fibrosis.

10.4.4 Infectious hepatitis/PTLD

Other recurrent diseases include non-alcoholic steatohepatitis (especially among obese recipients or those with cryptogenic cirrhosis), alcoholic liver disease, and hepatocellular carcinoma.

Infections which may occur following liver transplantation include CMV, Epstein–Barr virus (EBV), herpes simplex virus (HSV), and rarely fungal infections. EBV infection is most commonly associated with the development of post-transplant lymphoproliferative disorder (PTLD) [16]. Common sites of involvement include the liver and gastrointestinal tract. Active infection with EBV can be detected by polymerase chain reaction (PCR) methods. Liver biopsy is confirmatory. Treatment with antiviral therapy (acyclovir) is generally ineffective. Reduction or withdrawal of immunosuppression may allow for resolution of PTLD in mild cases. Traditional chemotherapy, monoclonal antibody therapy, radiation therapy, and/or operative resection are other options.

11 CONTRACEPTION AND PREGNANCY

Amenorrhea occurs in up to 50% of women with end-stage liver disease. Restoration of fertility in women of reproductive age has been well described following liver transplantation. Pregnancy can potentially affect graft function, immunosuppressive

Table 3. Pregnancy categories for common medications used in liver transplant recipients.

Category	Medication
Category B (no evidence of risk to humans)	Prednisone
Category C (risks cannot be excluded)	Cyclosporine
	Tacrolimus
	Mycophenolate mofetil
	Sirolimus
	Ganciclovir
	Lamuvidine
	Interferon
Category D (evidence of teratogenic risk)	Azathioprine
Category X (absolute contraindication)	Ribavirn

efficacy, and potential toxicities incurred by the fetus remain important [17] (Table 3).

Pathophysiology: Hypothalamic/pituitary axis dysfunction, portosystemic shunting and increased estrogen production, and poor nutritional status contribute to pre-transplant menstrual abnormalities. Testicular feminization in men results in erectile dysfunction as well as sterility. Complete reversal of these processes has been associated with liver transplantation in the majority of individuals reported.

Clinical features: Anecdotal case reports describe the occurrence of successful pregnancies among liver transplant recipients. Subsequently, a national registry which catalogues outcomes of pregnancy among all organ recipients including liver transplantation has been developed. Overall, the majority of maternal and fetal outcomes have been favorable among liver recipients. Calcineurin-based inhibitors, MMF, and prednisone have not been associated with an increased risk of fetal complications. Azathioprine is the only immunosuppressive agent given a pregnancy class D warning given its teratogenicity at human doses. Worsening hypertension and pre-eclampsia, the most common maternal complications, occur in patients with pre-existing hypertension and renal dysfunction from immunosuppressive therapy. Despite most pregnancies being premature in nature, there has not been an increased rate of fetal malformations compared to general populations. No significant increase in graft rejection has been observed although individual reports of graft loss are known. The risk for infection with CMV, which is known to cause congenital malformations and liver disease in the fetus, is greatest within the first 3–6 months after transplantation.

Management: The rapid return of menstrual cycles can be associated with unintended pregnancy within 1–2 months after liver transplant. Counseling with regards to pregnancy risk for both men and women is strongly recommended. A delay between 1 and 2 years following transplantation is advised given the likelihood of developing a stable immunosuppression regimen and low risk for developing CMV infection. Contraception with barrier methods is preferred immediately after transplantation with hormonal treatments a possibility once satisfactory allograft function is established. Elimination of specific agents including azathioprine should be initiated with compensatory changes if necessary. Pregnancy after organ transplantation is considered high risk and requires involvement with an obstetrician trained in maternal–fetal medicine.

12 HEALTH MAINTENANCE STRATEGIES

Regularly scheduled follow-up visits afford the promise of implementing preventive health maintenance strategies. In addition to updating immunization status and cancer surveillance, the importance of screening for unique issues includes depression and substance abuse recidivism.

12.1 Immunizations

The delivery of pneumoccocal, hepatitis A and B, influenza, and tetanus toxoid vaccines are considered mandatory among patients with end-stage liver disease. The recognition of inadequate antibody response among these patients warrants a reassessment of need for repeat vaccination following liver transplantation [18]. Annual influenza vaccination and periodic pneumococcal and tetanus toxoid administration are followed based on guidelines for all adults. Uncommon immunizations such as inactivated polio vaccine, cholera, rabies, and anthrax can be safely used in liver transplant recipients if clinically indicated. Live or attenuated vaccines are contraindicated. The indication for Varicella-Zoster immunization among previously unexposed recipients is not well substantiated to date.

12.2 Cancer screening

An increased frequency of skin cancer, non-Hodgkin's lymphoma, Kaposi's sarcoma, and carcinoma of the genitourinary system are associated with chronic immunosuppression. Individuals with requiring monoclonal antibody therapy (OKT3) for steroid-resistant rejection may be at increased risk for PTLD. Discontinuation of azathioprine is recommended for individuals diagnosed with skin cancer.

Colorectal cancer screening is required among all transplant recipients beyond the age of 50 years. Colonoscopy is the preferred screening method. The presence of adenomatous polyps requires follow-up examinations every 3–5 years. Negative examinations warrant surveillance every 5 years based on increased risks from immunosuppressive therapy. A history of chronic ulcerative colitis or Crohn's colitis independent of coexisting PSC warrants annual surveillance colonoscopy with random mucosal biopsies to exclude dysplasia.

Gender-specific strategies remain important following liver transplantation. Screening for prostatic carcinoma with yearly digital rectal examination and PSA after the age of 40 years is recommended. Annual mammography to exclude breast carcinoma among average risk individuals is recommended after age 40 as well. High-risk patients (independent of chronic immunosuppression effects) should be offered surveillance at earlier ages. Annual pelvic and Papanicolau smear examinations should also be performed, even among women with a prior history of hysterectomy.

12.3 Depression

Major depression is common following liver transplantation, occurring in 5–10% of liver transplant recipients. Risk factors include pre-transplant depression, ability to gain employment, and marital status. Clinical manifestations are similar to those seen in the in non-transplant setting, including alterations in appetite, sleep hygiene, and attenuated energy level. Re-evaluation of psychological, social, and financial status are important recurring components of the post-transplant evaluation. Referral for formal psychiatric evaluation should be considered in recipients exhibiting signs of major depression. Antidepressants, such as serotonin selective re-uptake inhibitors (SSRI), have been anecdotally successful in the treatment of post-transplant depression, although adverse effect profiles of the SSRI's are poorly established in this patient population.

12.4 Substance abuse

Many transplant programs require abstinence from alcohol use for a period of 6 months or greater before considering liver transplantation. Emerging data, however, suggests that duration of abstinence or prior treatment for alcoholism do not accurately predict the risk for post-transplant recidivism. Evidence for relapse of alcoholism usually emerges beyond the first post-operative year and often remains undetected in patients who are otherwise medically compliant. The reported prevalence rates of post-transplant alcohol consumption range from 20 to 30%, with pathologic drinking occurring in 10–50% of patients who consume alcohol following liver transplantation. In addition to formal chemical dependency evaluation, a concerted effort to reinitiate treatment for refractory alcoholism is mandatory in patients with post-transplant alcohol consumption [19]. While reductions in patient and graft survival have not been associated with a pre-transplant diagnosis of alcoholism, the long-term medical and psychosocial consequences of recurrence of alcoholism are likely to be significant. A similar approach should be considered among patients returning to other forms of chemical dependency.

REFERENCES

[1] Carral, M.S., Lilly, L.B. and Levy, G.B. (2000) Immunosuppression in liver transplantation. *Semin. Liver Dis.* **20**, 523–531.

[2] The US Multicenter FK506 Liver Study Group (1994) A comparison of tacrolimus FK506 and cyclosporine

for immunosuppression in liver transplantation. *N. Engl. J. Med.* **331**, 1110–1115.

[3] Gonwa, T.A., Mai, M.L., Melton, L.B. *et al.* (2001) End stage renal disease (ESRD) following orthotopic liver transplantation (OLTx) utilizing calcineurin based immunotherapy: risk of development and treatment. *Transplantation* **72**, 1934–1939.

[4] Textor, S.C., Taler, S.J., Canzanello, V.J. *et al.* (2000) Posttransplantation hypertension related to calcineurin inhibitors. *Liver Transpl.* **6**, 521–530.

[5] Navassa, M., Bustamante, J., Marroni, C. *et al.* (1996) Diabetes mellitus after liver transplantation: prevalence and predictive factors. *J. Hepatol.* **25**, 64–71.

[6] Imagawa, D., Dawson, S., Holt, C. *et al.* (1996) Hyperlipidemia after liver transplantation: natural history and treatment with the hydroxymethylglutaryl-coenzyme A reductase inhibitor pravastatin. *Transplantation* **62**, 934–942.

[7] Hay, J.E. (1995) Bone disease after liver transplantation. *Liver Transpl. Surg.* **1**, S55–S63.

[8] Everhart, J., Lombardero, M., Lake, J. *et al.* (1998) Weight change and obesity after liver transplantation: incidence and risk factors. *Liver Transpl. Surg.* **4**, 285–296.

[9] Wiesner, R.H., Demetris, A.J., Belle, S.H. *et al.* (1998) Acute hepatic allograft rejection: incidence, risk factors, and impact on outcome. *Hepatology* **28**, 638–645.

[10] Wiesner, R.H., Batts, K.P. and Krom, R.A.F. (1999) Evolving concepts in the diagnosis, pathogenesis, and treatment of chronic hepatic allograft rejection. *Liver Transpl. Surg.* **5**, 388–400.

[11] Tung, B.Y. and Kimmey, M.B. (1999) Biliary complications of orthotopic liver transplantation. *Dig. Dis.* **17**, 133–144.

[12] Charlton, M., Seaberg, E., Wiesner, R. *et al.* (1998) Predictors of patient and graft survival following liver transplantation for hepatitis C. *Hepatology* **28**, 823–830.

[13] Shouval, D. and Samuel, D. (2000) Hepatitis B immune globulin to prevent infection following liver transplantation. A concise review. *Hepatology* **32**, 1189–1195.

[14] Perillo, R., Rakela, J., Dienstag, J. *et al.* (1999) Multicenter study of lamivudine therapy for hepatitis B after liver transplantation. *Hepatology* **29**, 1581–1586.

[15] Faust, T.W. (2000) Recurrent primary biliary cirrhosis, primary sclerosing cholangitis, and autoimmune hepatitis after transplantation. *Semin. Liver Dis.* **20**, 481–495.

[16] Paya, C.V., Fung, J.J., Nalesnik, M.A. *et al.* (1999) Epstein–Barr virus induced posttransplant lymphoproliferative disorder. *Transplantation* **68**, 1517–1525.

[17] Armenti, V.T., Wilson, G.A., Radomski, J.S. *et al.* (1999) Report from the national transplantation pregnancy registry (NTPR). Outcomes of pregnancy after liver transplantation. *Clin. Transpl.*, 101–112.

[18] Zeldin, G.A., Maygers, J., Klein, A. and Thuluvath, P.J. (2001) Vaccination, screening for malignancy, and health maintenance of the liver xtransplant recipient. *J. Clin. Gastroenterol.* **32**, 148–150.

[19] Coffman, K.L., Hoffman, A., Sher, L. *et al.* (1997) Treatment of the postoperative alcoholic liver transplant recipient with other addictions. *Liver Transpl. Surg.* **3**, 322–327.

Hepatology: A Practical Approach
B. Al Knawy, M.L. Shiffman, R.H. Wiesner (editors)

Color Plates

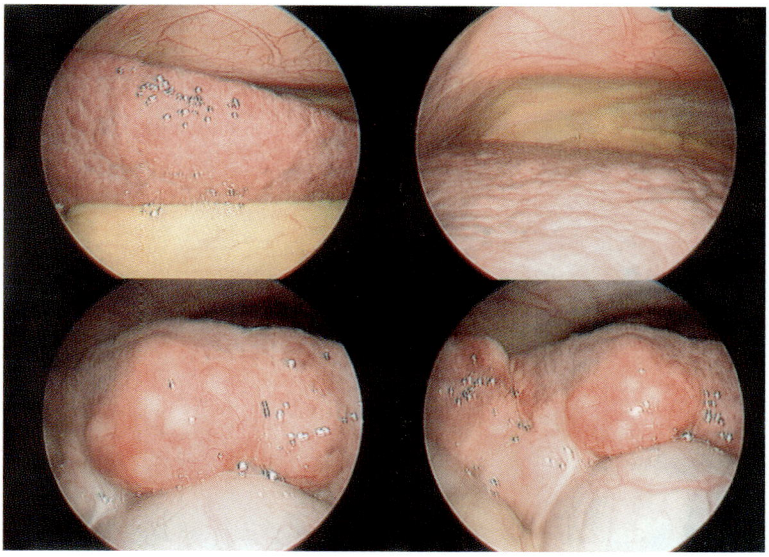

Plate I. Cirrhotic appearing liver with a relatively hypervascular and nodular lesion anterior to the gallbladder which was a biopsy-proven HCC. (See Figure 1 on Page 36.)

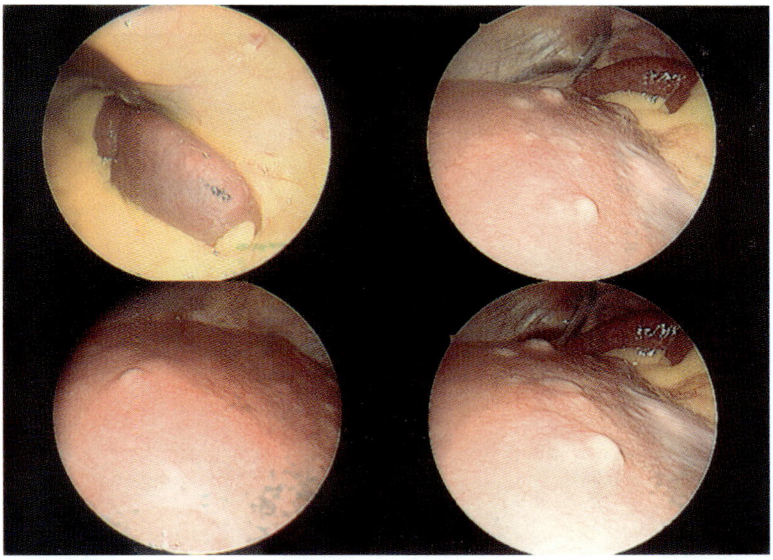

Plate II. Laparoscopy demonstrating raised, partly whitish areas, on the surface of the liver which, on biopsy, proved to be metastatic liver disease. (See Figure 2 on Page 38.)

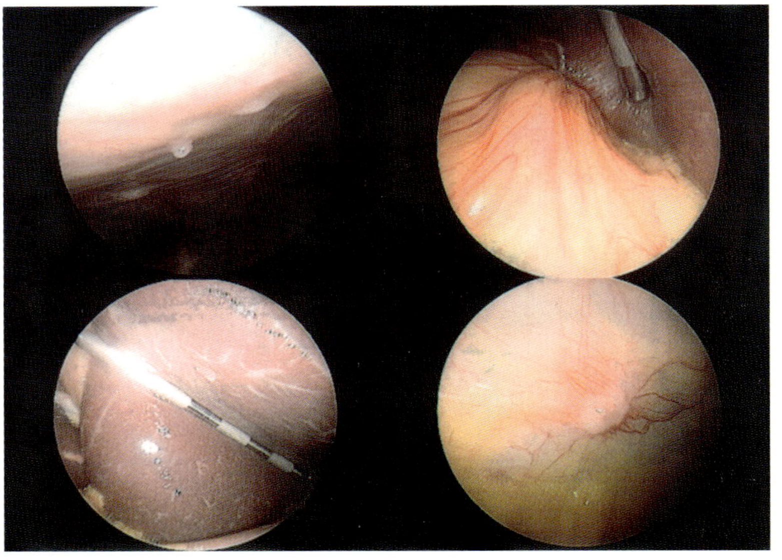

Plate III. Tiny white implants on the peritoneal surface consistent with peritoneal metastasis. (See Figure 3 on Page 38.)

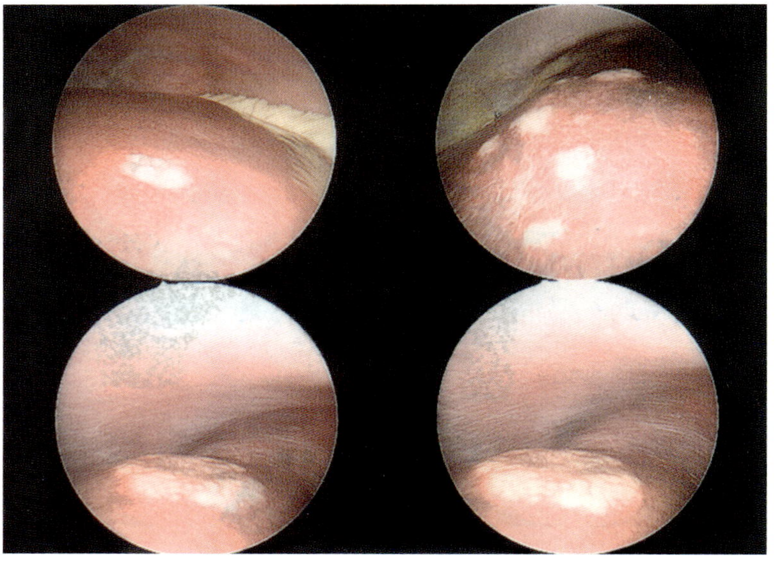

Plate IV. Large white, circumscribed areas over the liver which were due to a lymphoma on biopsy. (See Figure 4 on Page 39.)

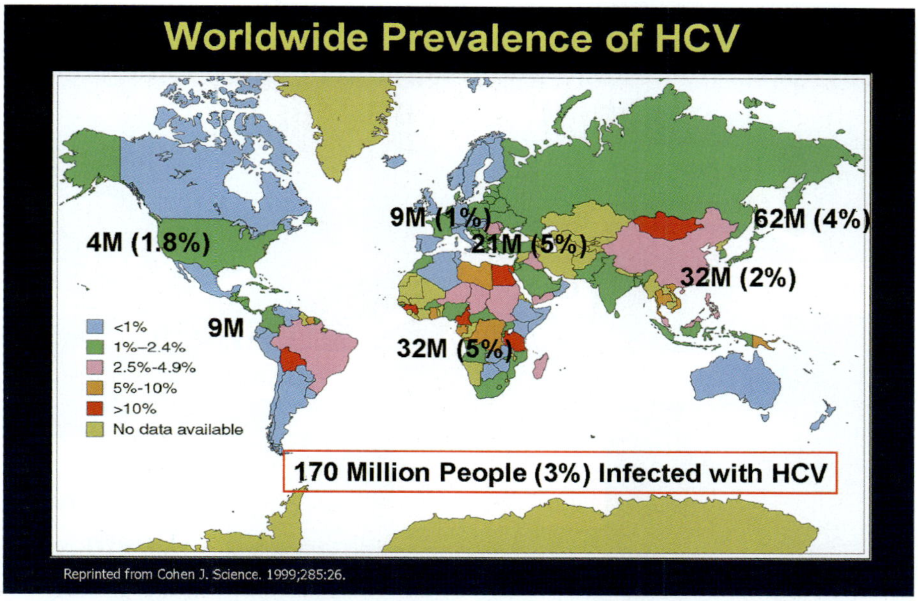

Plate V. Worldwide prevalence of HCV. (See Figure 1 on Page 88.)

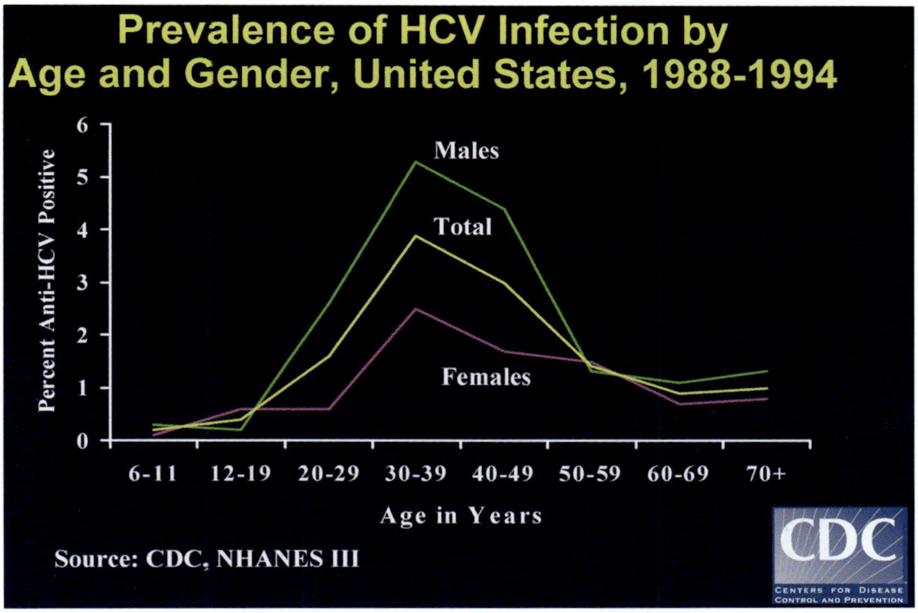

Plate VI. Age adjusted prevalence of hepatitis C infection in the United States. (See Figure 2 on Page 89.)

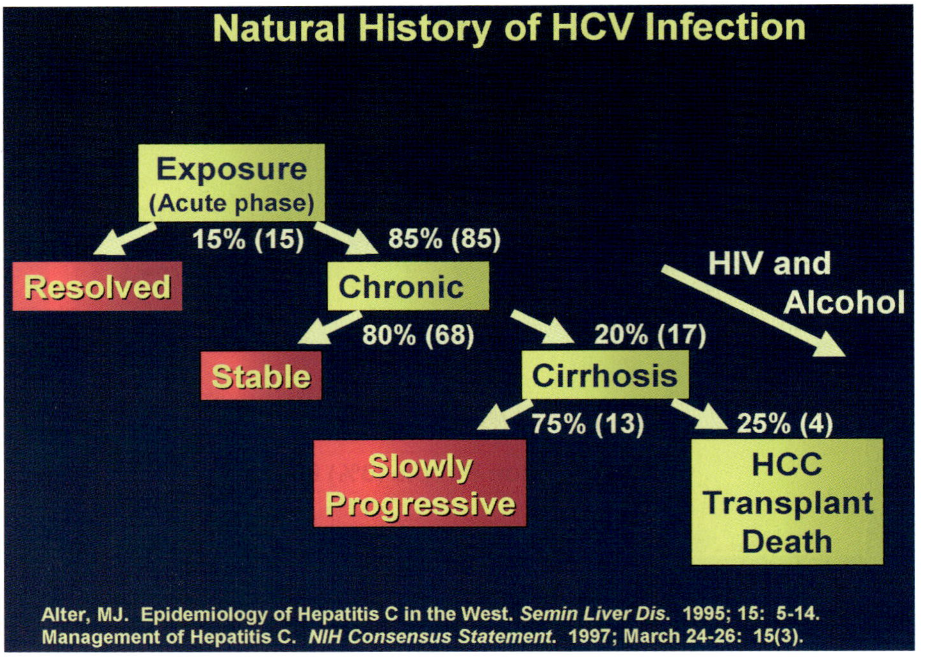

Plate VII. Natural history of chronic hepatitis C. (See Figure 3 on Page 90.)

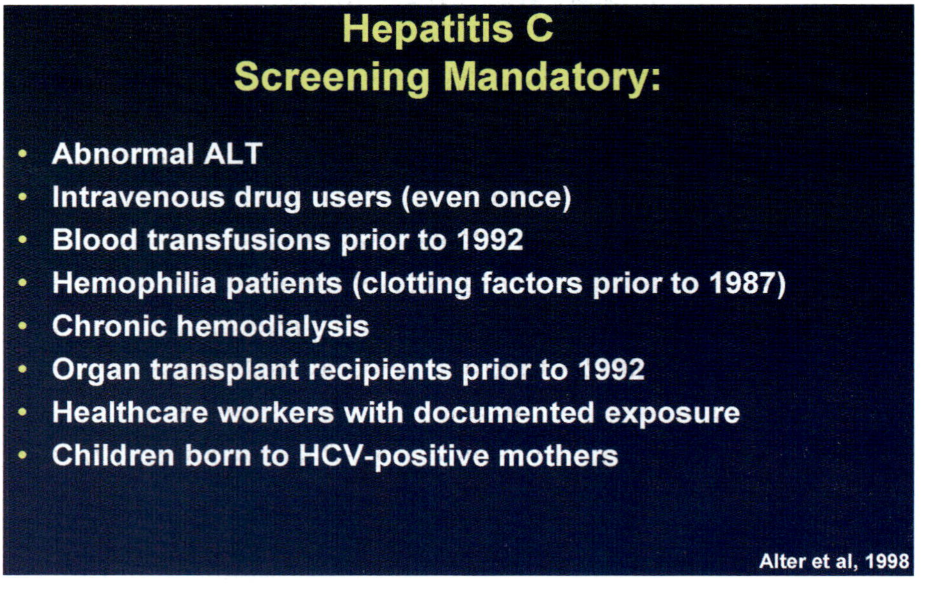

Plate VIII. Risk factors for HCV acquisition. (See Figure 4 on Page 91.)

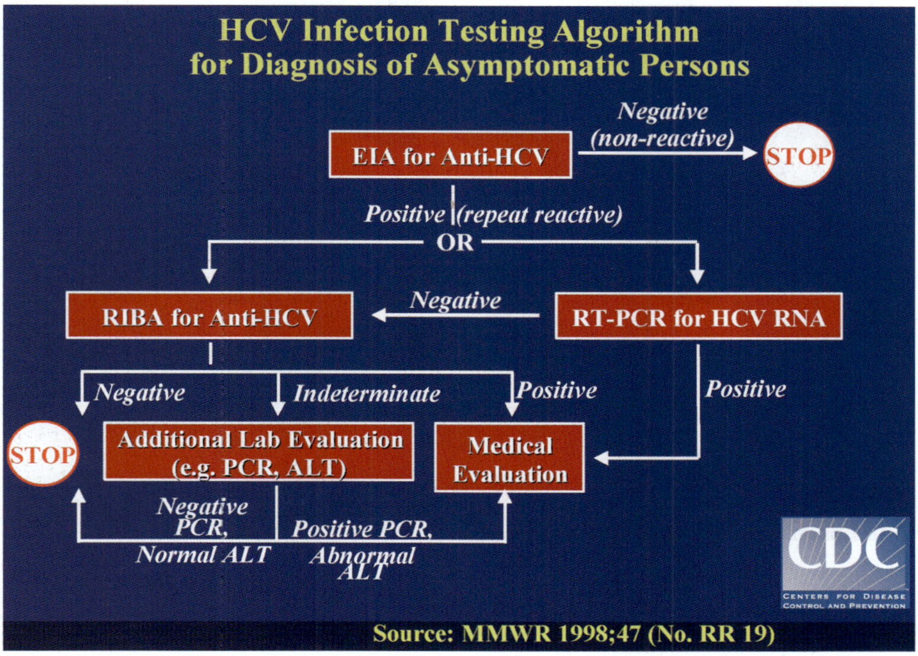

Plate IX. CDC recommendations for HCV serologic testing. (See Figure 5 on Page 92.)

HCV RNA Assays
Performance Characteristics

Assay	Type	Lower Limit Detection	Dynamic Range
Amplicor HCV v2.0	Qual	50 IU/ml	N/A
Versant HCV RNA	Qual	10 IU/ml	N/A
Monitor HCV v2.0	Quant	600 IU/ml	600-500,000
Versant v3.0	Quant	615 IU/ml	615-7,700,000
SuperQuant	Quant	30 IU/ml	30-1,470,000

Adapted from Pawlotsky, 2002

Plate X. HCV RNA assays. (See Figure 6 on Page 94.)

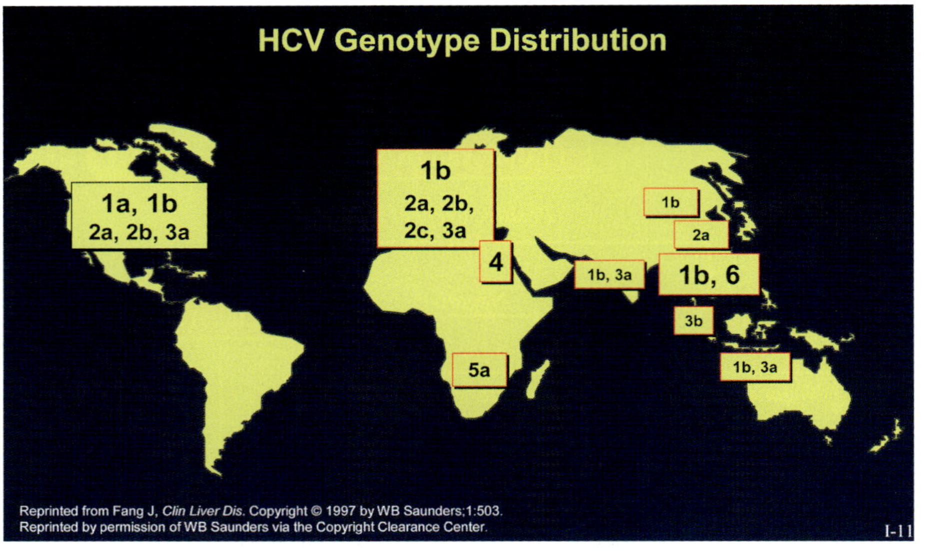

Plate XI. Geographic distribution of HCV genotypes. (See Figure 7 on Page 94.)

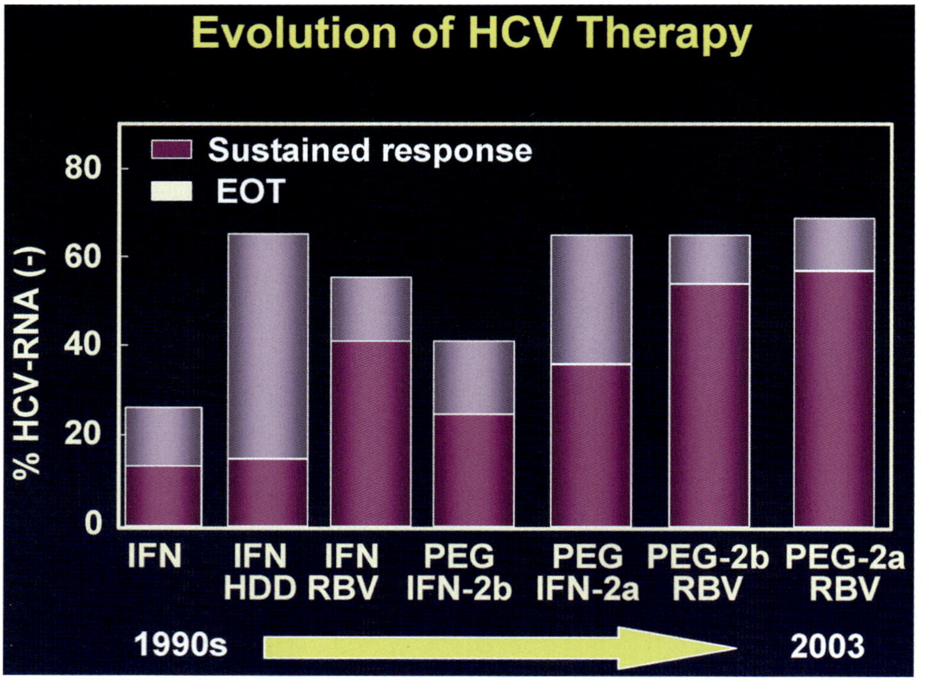

Plate XII. Improvement in antiviral therapy for chronic hepatitis C over the last decade (EOT = End of treatment response). (See Figure 8 on Page 96.)

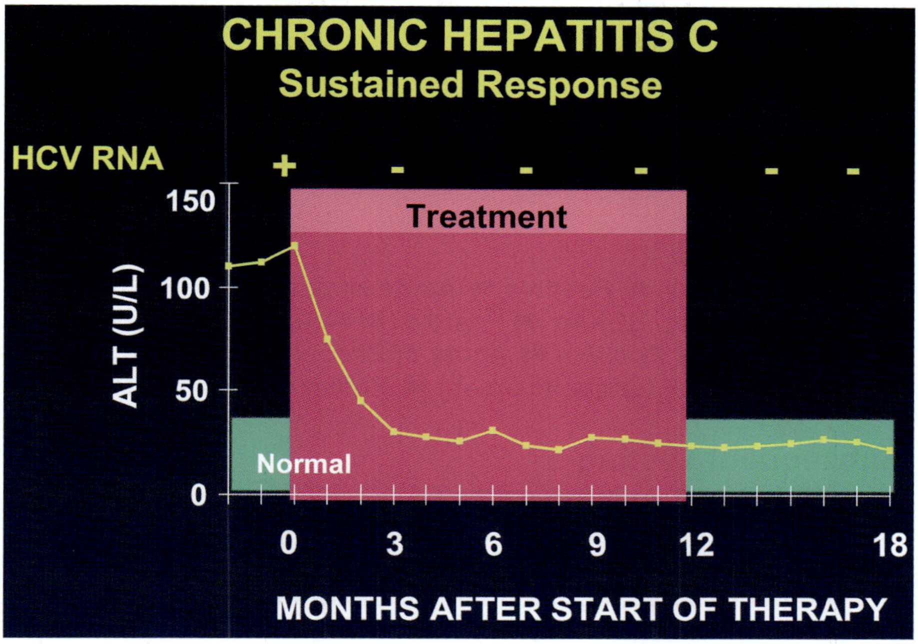

Plate XIII. Schematic of sustained virological response (SVR). (See Figure 9 on Page 97.)

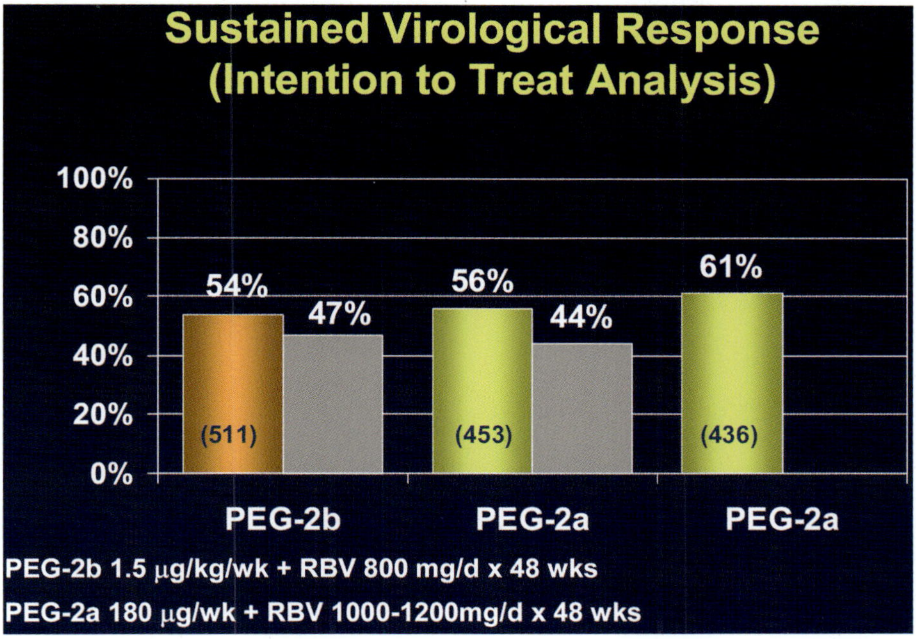

Plate XIV. Sustained virological response using peginterferon alfa-2a or peginterferon alfa-2b in combination with ribavirin (Refs. [20,21,27]). (See Figure 10 on Page 97.)

Clinical and Biochemical Diagnosis of Acute Hepatitis

↓

Medical History

- Alcoholic intake
- Hepatotoxic drugs
- Toxic exposure

↓

Initial Work-Up

- IgM anti-HAV ➡ Positive ➡ Acute Hepatitis A
- IgM anti-HBc, HBsAg ➡ Positive ➡ Acute Hepatitis B
- Anti-HCV ➡ Positive ➡ Acute or Chronic Hepatitis C
- IgM anti-HEV (endemic areas) ➡ Positive ➡ Acute Hepatitis E

↓

Subsequent Testing

- HCV RNA ➡ Acute Hepatitis C
- IgM anti-HEV (travel to endemic areas) ➡ Acute Hepatitis E
- IgM anti-HDV (positive HBsAg) ➡ Acute Hepatitis D
- Autoantibodies, γ-globulin ➡ Autoimmune Hepatitis
- Ceruloplasmin, urinary copper ➡ Wilson's Disease

↓

Investigation of Other Viral Infections

Plate XV. Diagnostic algorithm for acute hepatitis. (See Figure 1 on Page 125.)

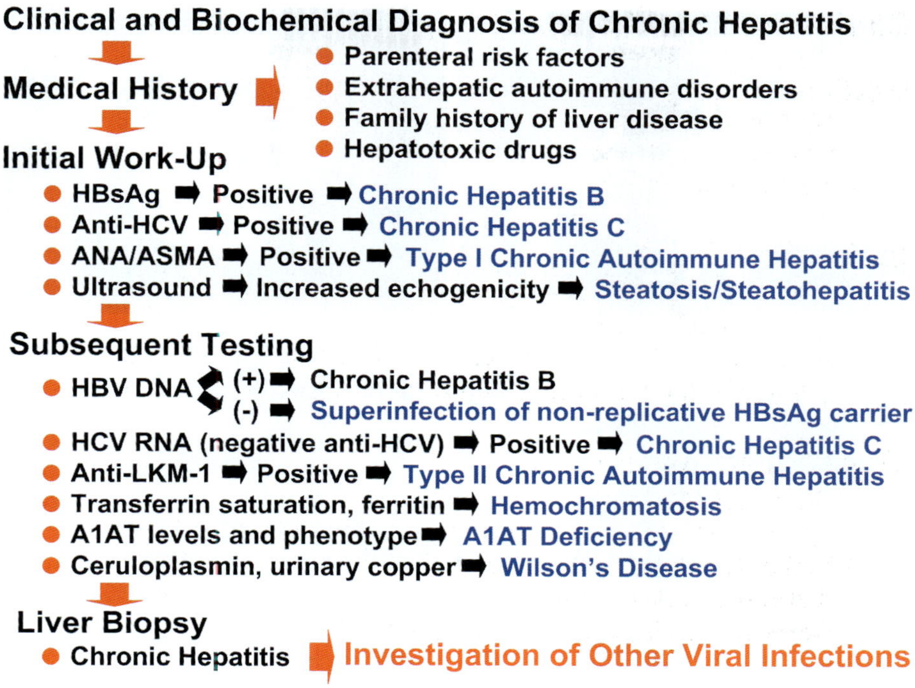

Plate XVI. Diagnostic algorithm for chronic hepatitis. (See Figure 2 on Page 126.)

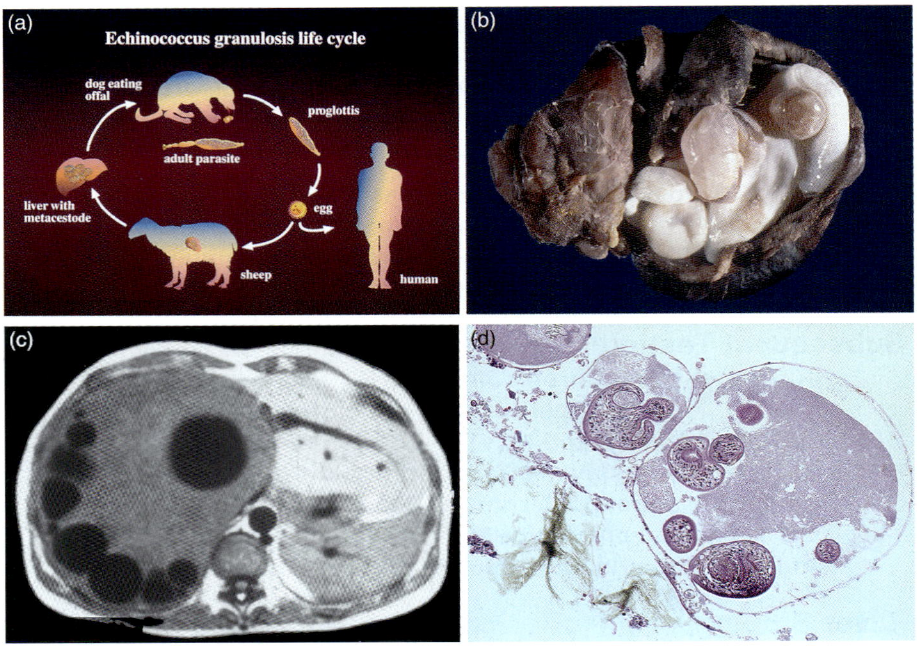

Plate XVII. (a) Life cycle of *Echinococcus granulosus*. The parasite completes the life cycle between dog, the definitive host and sheep, the intermediate host. Human beings become incidental intermediate hosts and do not complete the life cycle of the parasite. (*Source:* Khuroo, M.S. (2002) Hydatid disease: current status and recent advances. *Ann. Saudi Med.* **22**, 56–64) (b) Resected hydatid cyst liver with peripheral coating (pericyst), ivory white laminated membranes, and glistening rounded daughter cysts. (c) Hydatid cyst liver. An axial T_1-weighted MR image shows a large rounded lesion occupying the whole right lobe of the liver. The lesion reveals multiple rounded low signal lesions (daughter cysts). The remainder of the contents reveal high signal (matrix). (d) Histology of the hydatid cyst. Multiple protoscolices (both eviginated and invaginated) are seen attached to the endocyst. (See Figure 2 on Page 163.)

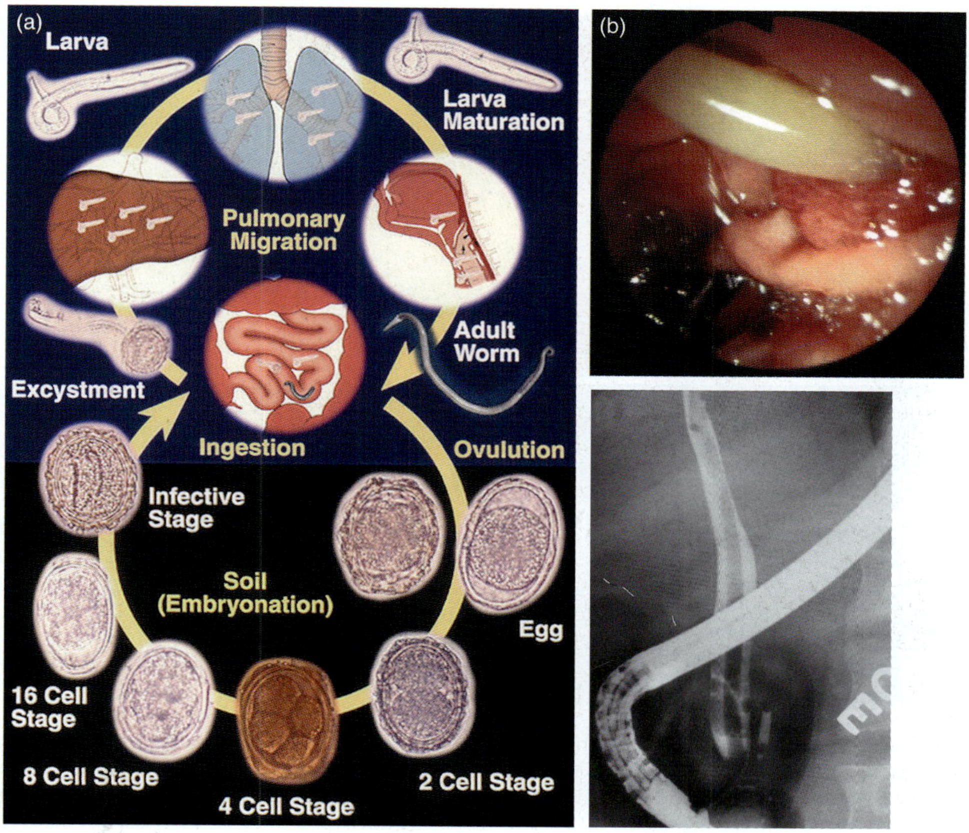

Plate XVIII. (a) Life cycle of *Ascaris lumbricoides*. (*Source*: Khuroo, M.S. (1996) Ascariasis. *Gastroenterol. Clin. N. Am.* **25**, 553–577.) (b) Endoscopic retrograde cholangiogram of a 30-year-old woman who presented with recurrent episodes of biliary colic of 7 days duration. Top panel. Duodenoscopic view of the papilla showing an Ascaride in the ampullary orifice with its tail in the duodenal lumen. Bottom panel. Cholangiogram. A long linear smooth filling defect in the common bile duct and across the papilla representing the portion of the Ascaride that had entered the bile duct. (*Source*: Khuroo *et al.* (1993) *Gastrointest. Endosc.* **39**, 680–685, Fig. 1, p. 682.) (See Figure 3 on Page 167.)

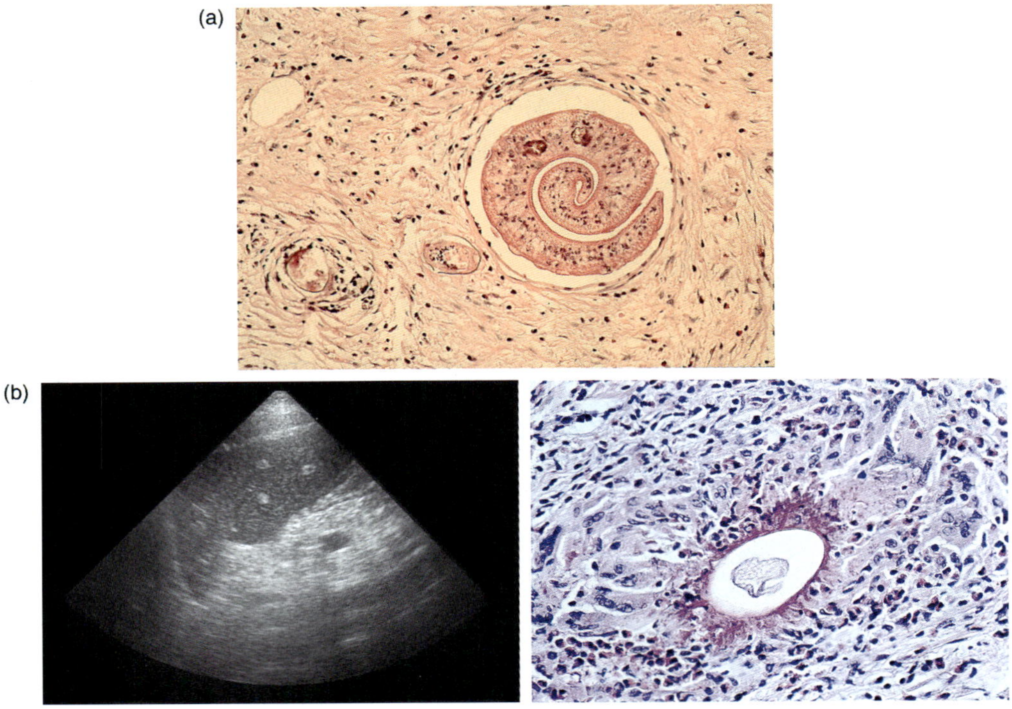

Plate XIX. (a) Microscopic examination of a mesenteric mass in a 40-year-old male who had laparotomy for intestinal obstruction. A mesenteric mass with adhesions to the bowel loops was seen at surgery. Histology of the mass shows an adult worm of *Schistosoma mansoni* curved up in the mesenteric vein. Two eggs, oval in shape and with lateral spines (*Schistosoma mansoni* eggs) are placed nearby. (b) A 30-year-old male who presented with variceal bleed secondary to hepatic schistosomiasis. Left panel: A transverse sonogram through hilum of the liver shows an echogenic mass surrounding the portal vein. Right panel: Liver biopsy shows an *S. mansoni* egg with a lateral spine. Eosinophilic fibrinoid material is surrounding the egg, the Hoeppli–Splendore reaction. (See Figure 4 on Page 169.)

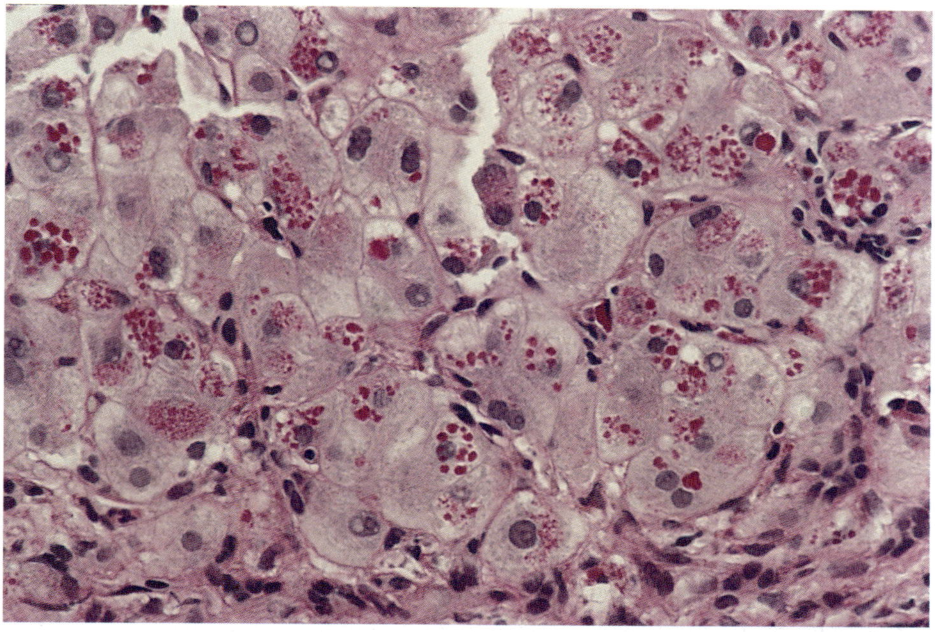

Plate XX. DPAS stain showing PAS-positive, diastase-resistant globules within the cytoplasm of numerous hepatocytes. Mild hepatocyte ballooning and a mild degree of lymphocytic interface hepatitis are also noted. (Photomicrograph courtesy of Terry Gramlich, MD, AmeriPath Inc., Oakwood Village, OH, USA.) (See Figure 1 on Page 206.)

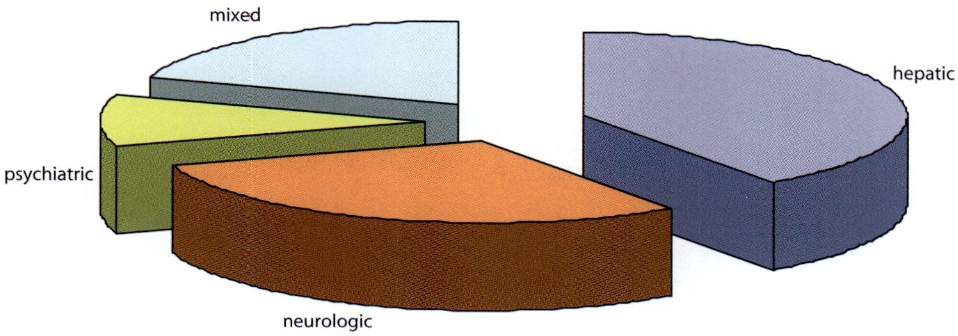

Plate XXI. Wilson's disease clinical presentation. (See Figure 1 on Page 225.)

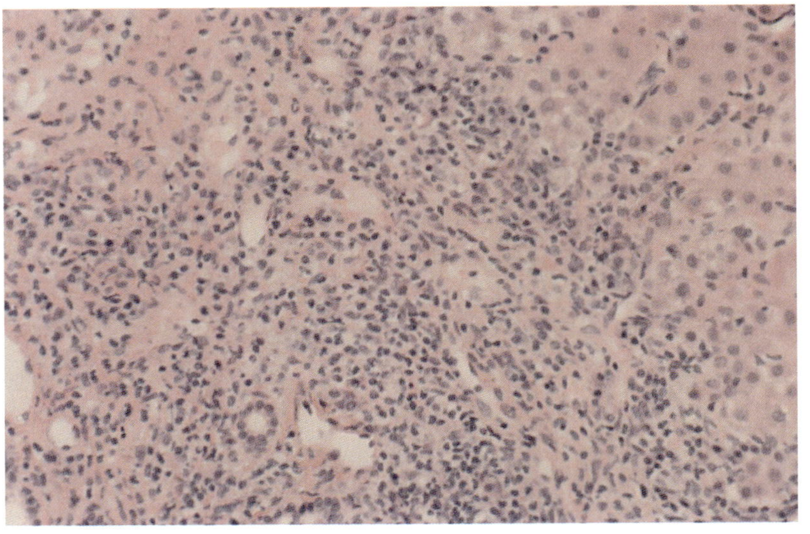

Plate XXII. *Interface hepatitis*. The limiting plate of the portal tract is disrupted by an inflammatory infiltrate in association with hepatocyte damage. Hematoxylin and eosin; original magnification, ×200. (See Figure 1 on Page 234.)

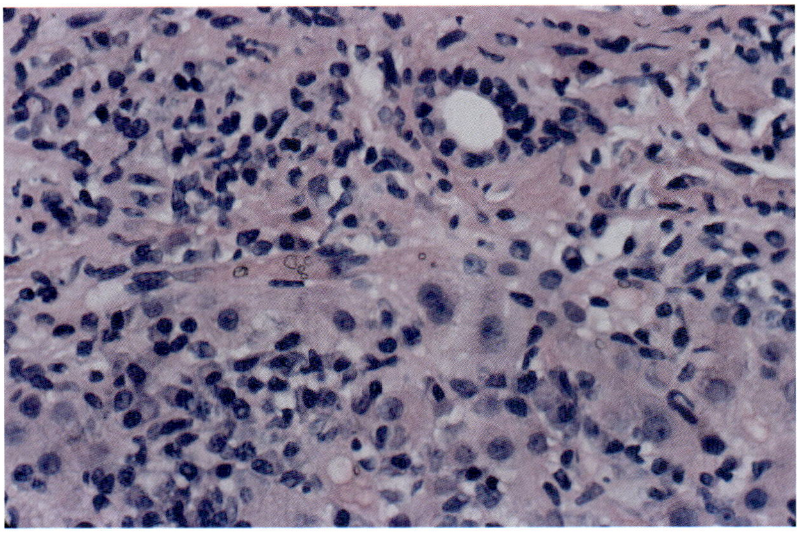

Plate XXIII. *Plasma cell infiltration*. Plasma cells, which are characterized by a perinuclear cytoplasmic halo, are present within the inflammatory infiltrate of the portal tract. Hematoxylin and eosin; original magnification, ×400. (See Figure 2 on Page 235.)

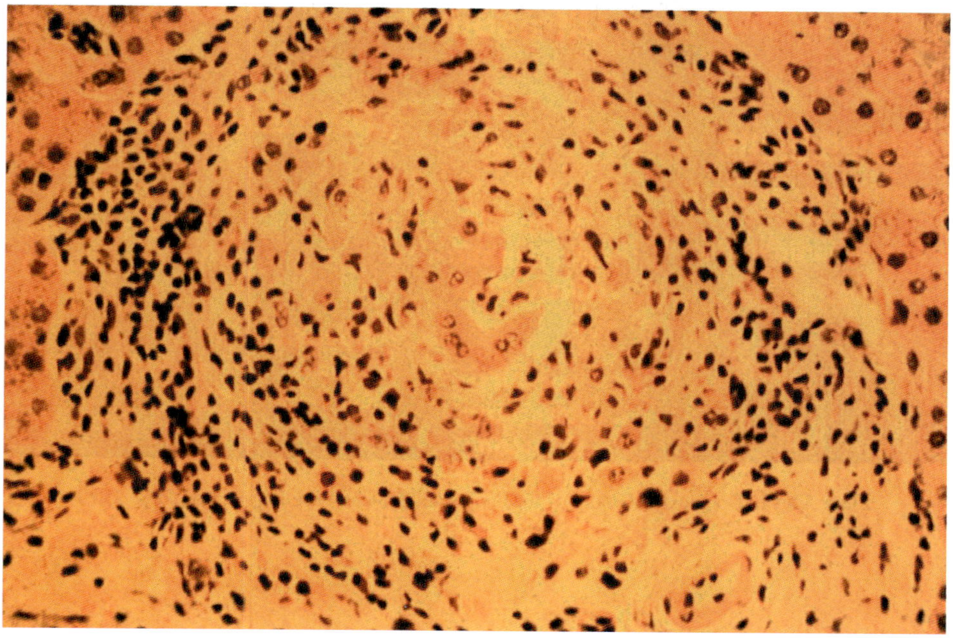

Plate XXIV. Typical bile duct lesion in PBC. (See Figure 1 on Page 250.)

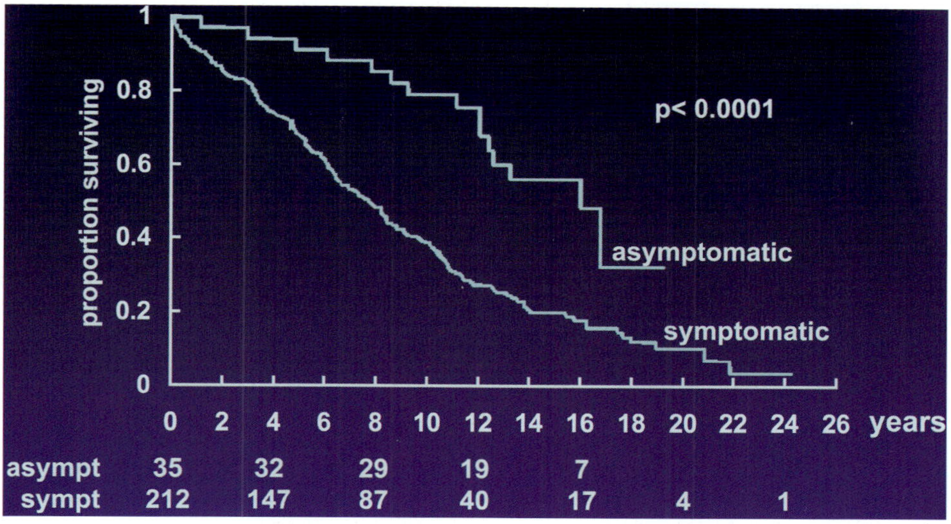

Plate XXV. PBC: long-term survival. (See Figure 2 on Page 252.)

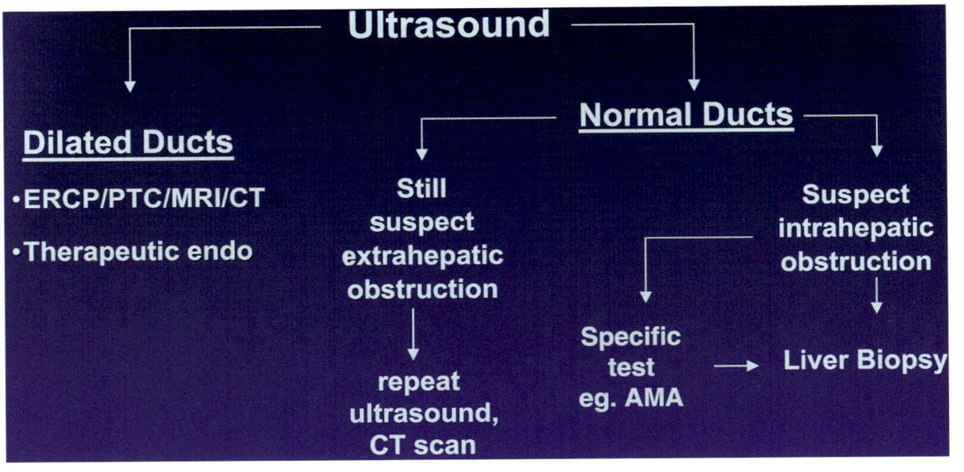

Plate XXVI. Diagnostic workup of the cholestatic patient. (See Figure 3 on Page 253.)

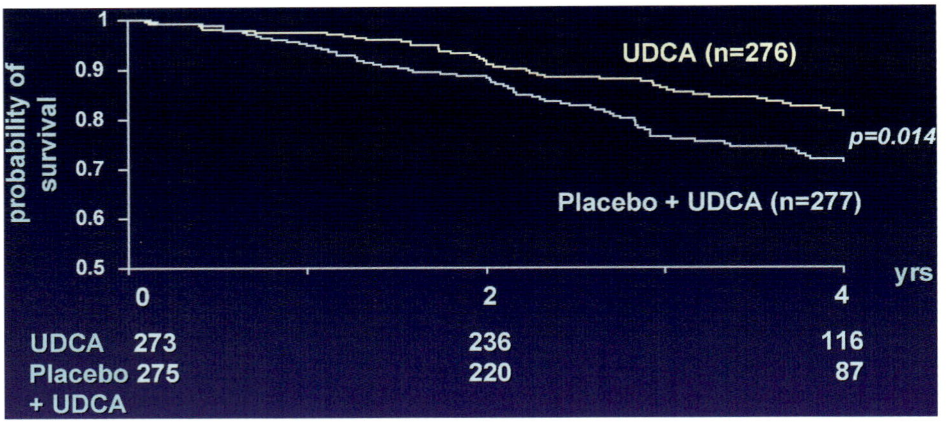

Plate XXVII. Combined analysis of RCT of UDCA in PBC. Probability of survival free of transplantation. (See Figure 4 on Page 256.)

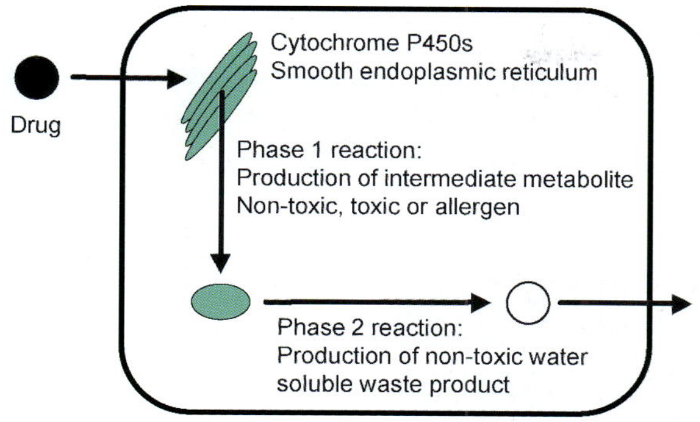

Plate XXVIII. The two step mechanism by which drugs and other compounds are metabolized by the liver. The native compound is first broken down by a cytochrome P450 enzyme located on the smooth endoplasmic reticulum. This intermediate metabolite can be non-toxic, toxic or act as an allergen and precipitate an immunologic reaction. The second step is the detoxification of this intermediate to a water-soluble non-toxic waste product. This is typically accomplished in the cytoplasm by conjugation with glucuronate, sulfate, glycine, a methyl group or water. (See Figure 1 on Page 305.)

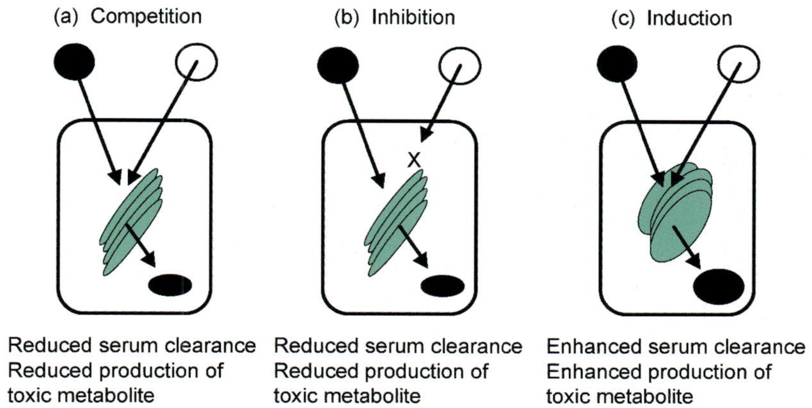

Plate XXIX. Mechanisms by which the metabolism of a drug is altered by other compounds which interact with cytochrome P450. (a) Competition for the CYP enzyme reduces the metabolism of each drug, (c) inhibition of the CYP slows the metabolism of drugs metabolized by this particular CYP enzyme and (c) induction of the CYP enhances the metabolism of the drug and leads to more rapid production of toxic metabolite. (See Figure 2 on Page 308.)

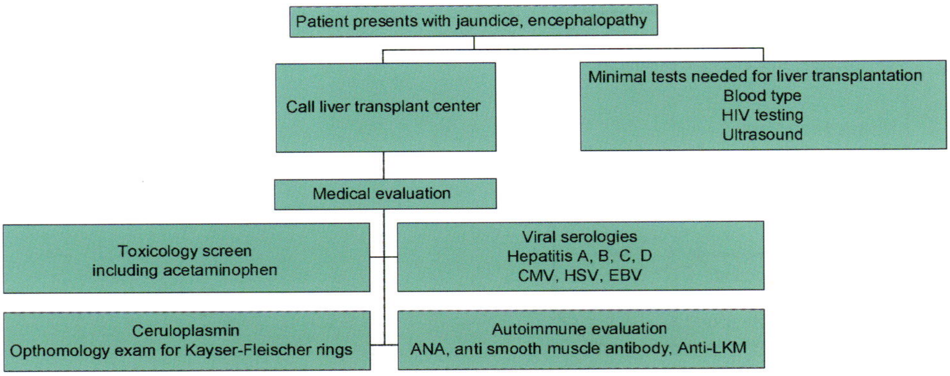

Plate XXX. Flowsheet for evaluation of FHF. (See Figure 1 on Page 321.)

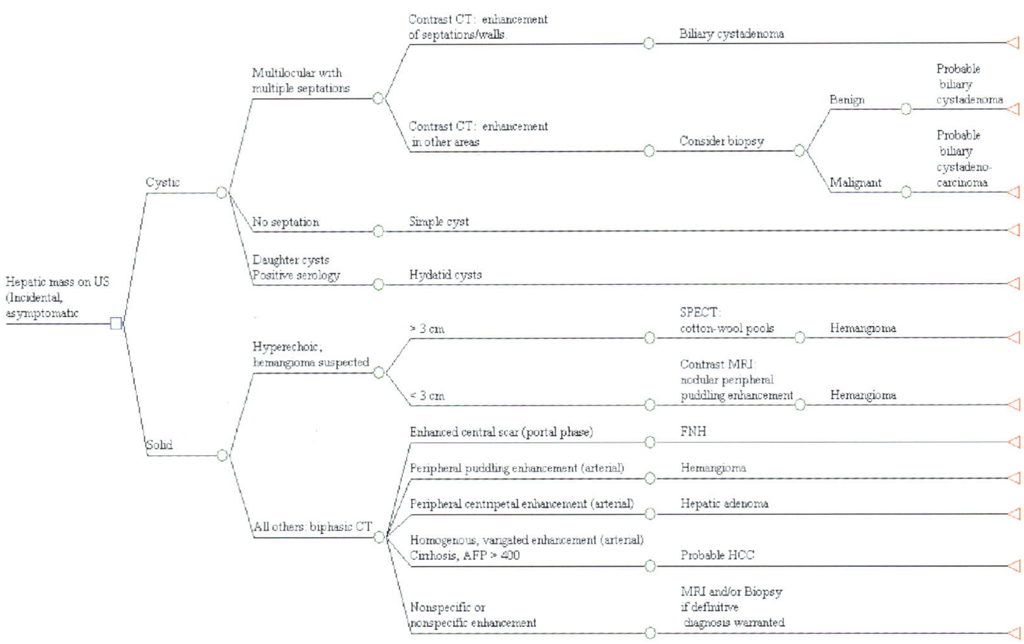

Plate XXXI. Evaluation for asymptomatic liver masses. (See Figure 1 on Page 341.)

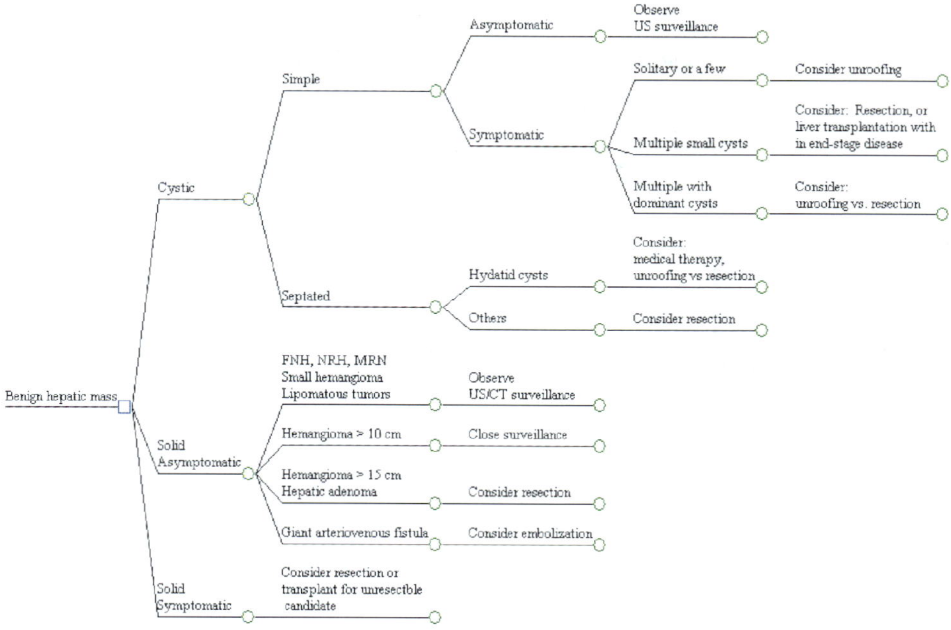

Plate XXXII. Follow-up and management of benign liver masses. (See Figure 2 on Page 341.)

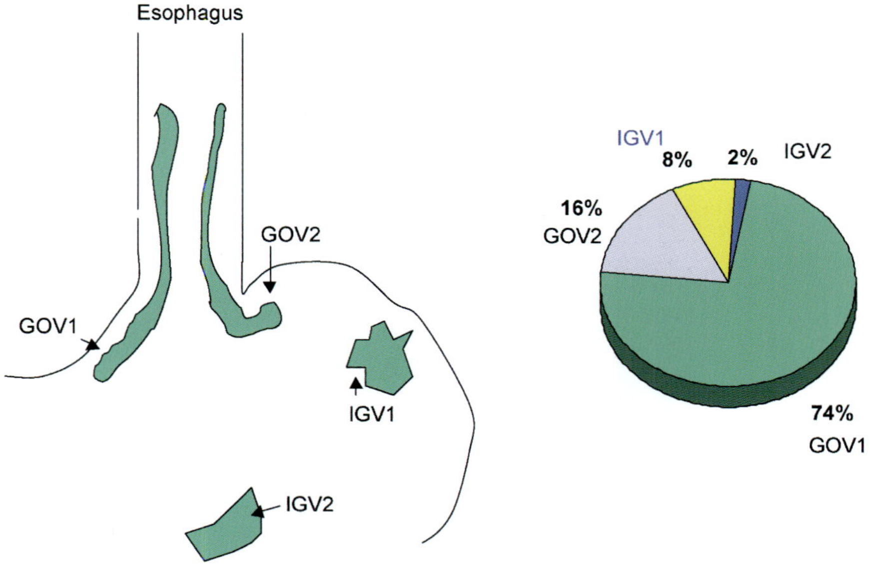

Plate XXXIII. Types and prevalence of gastric varices. Gastro-oesophageal varices (GOV) are varices in continuity with esophageal varices along the lesser curve (Type 1) or greater curve (Type 2). Isolated gastric varices (IGV) are present in the fundus (Type 1) or elsewhere in the stomach (Type 2). Based on the descriptions of Sarin *et al*. (1992) *Hepatology* **16**, 1342. (See Figure 2 on Page 363.)

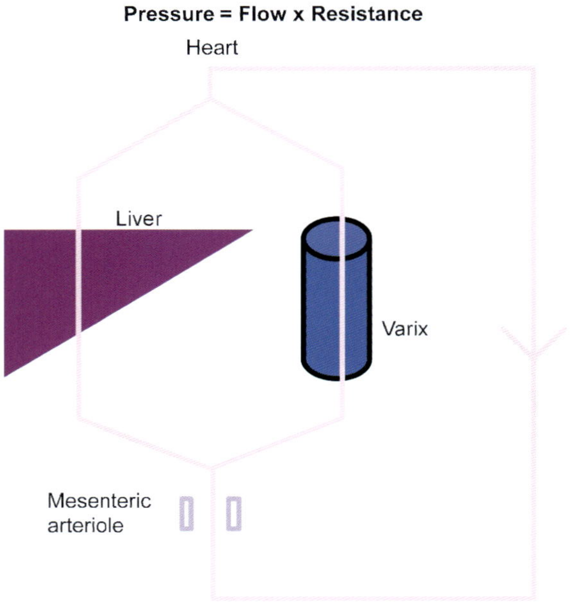

Plate XXXIV. A cartoon showing the functional anatomy of the splanchnic circulation and variceal circulation. Published with permission from Sanyal *et al*. *Clin. Liver Dis.* (See Figure 3 on Page 364.)

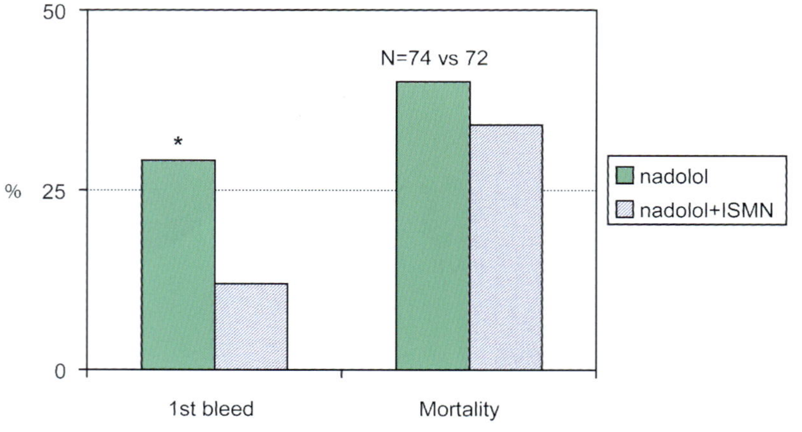

Plate XXXV. Nadolol vs Nadolol + Isosorbide mononitrate (ISMN) for primary prophylaxis of variceal hemorrhage. Combination therapy was associated with a significantly superior bleeding rate, i.e., less bleeding although the mortality data were comparable. Data from Ref. [11]. (See Figure 6 on Page 368.)

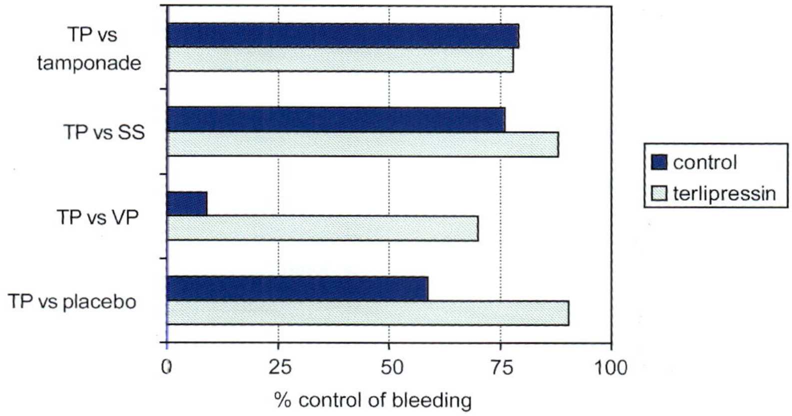

Plate XXXVI. Comparison of terlipressin (TP) vs placebo, vasopressin (VP), somatostatin (SS) or tamponade in the management of acute variceal hemorrhage. (See Figure 7 on Page 371.)

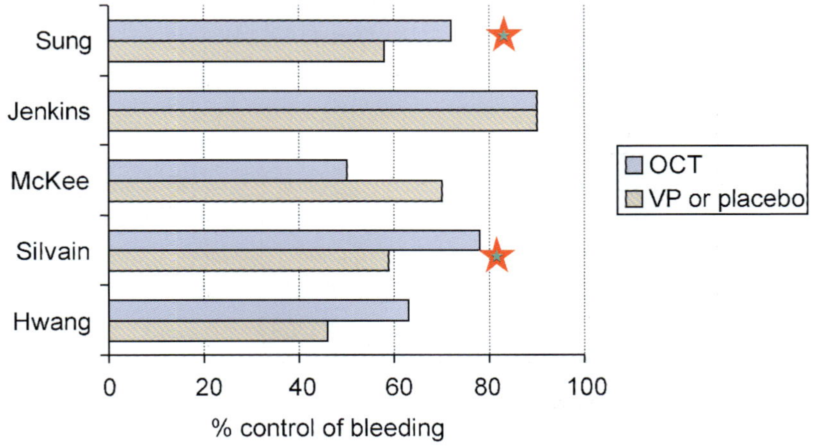

Plate XXXVII. Clinical trials demonstrating the relative efficacy of octreotide vs either vasopressin or placebo in the control of variceal hemorrhage. (See Figure 8 on Page 372.)

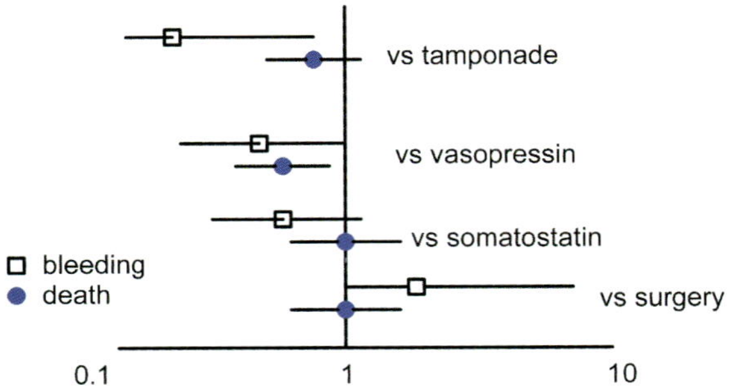

Plate XXXVIII. The relative efficacy of endoscopic sclerotherapy vs other modalities of treatment for the management of acute variceal hemorrhage. Sclerotherapy was superior to tamponade, vasopressin for prevention of bleeding. Although it appeared superior to somatostatin, this did not reach significance. Surgery was more effective than sclerotherapy for the control of bleeding but was not associated with an improvement in survival. Based on data from Ref. [22]. (See Figure 9 on Page 372.)

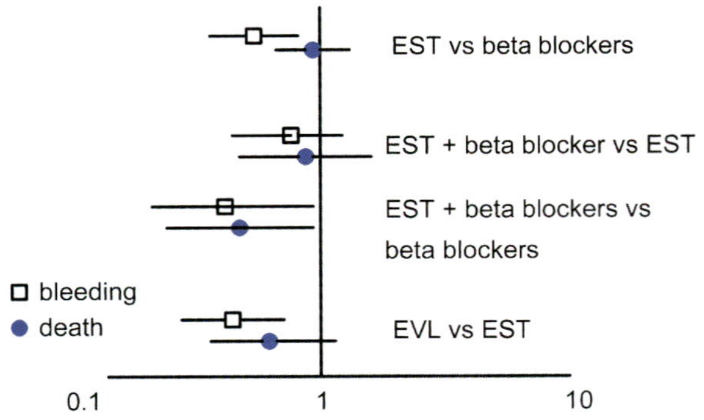

Plate XXXIX. The relative efficacy of endoscopic therapies for the prevention of recurrent variceal hemorrhage. Endoscopic sclerotherapy (EST) was associated with improved rebleeding rates compared to β-blockers but the survival data were unchanged. Endoscopic band ligation (EVL) was superior to EST for prevention of rebleeding. There was also a trend towards improved survival. Based on data from Ref. [22]. (See Figure 11 on Page 375.)

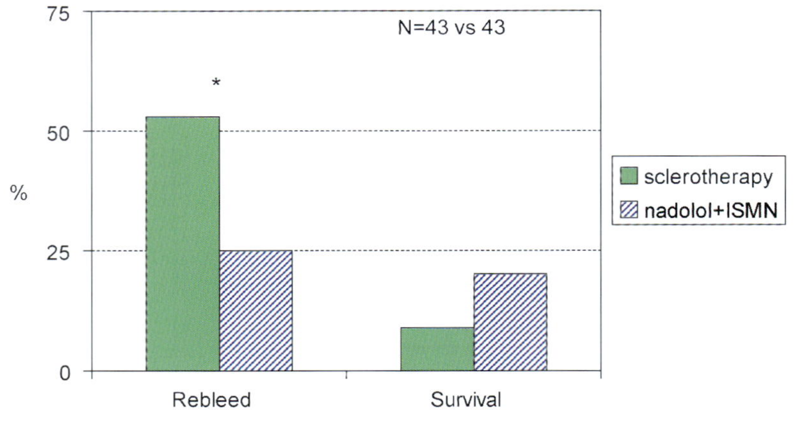

Plate XL. The effects of sclerotherapy vs nadolol and isosorbide mononitrate (ISMN) on prevention of recurrent variceal hemorrhage. Combination therapy was associated with a lower rebleed rate although the survival data were not significantly different. Based on data from Villanueva *et al.* (1996) *N. Engl. J. Med.* **334**, 1624–1629. (See Figure 12 on Page 375.)

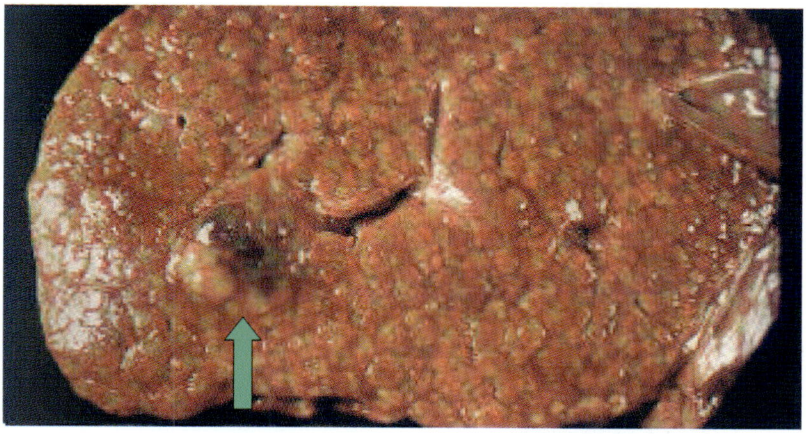

Plate XLI. Nodular HCC in a liver with cirrhosis (most common form of HCC in the most common setting). (See Figure 1 on Page 410.)

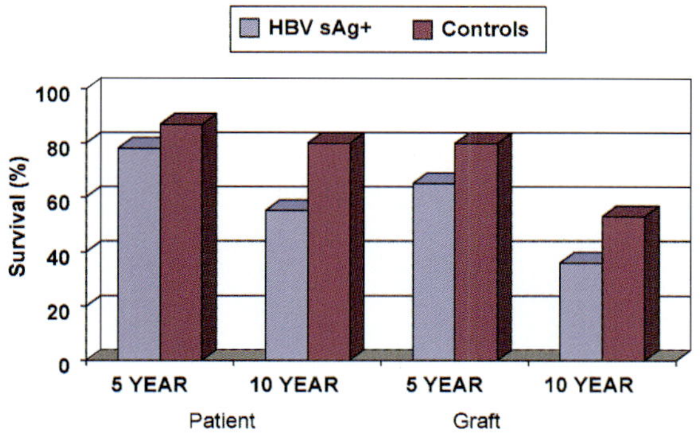

Plate XLII. Five- and 10-year patient and graft survival (%) in hepatitis B virus patients following renal transplantation (adapted from Ref. [7]). (See Figure 1 on Page 449.)

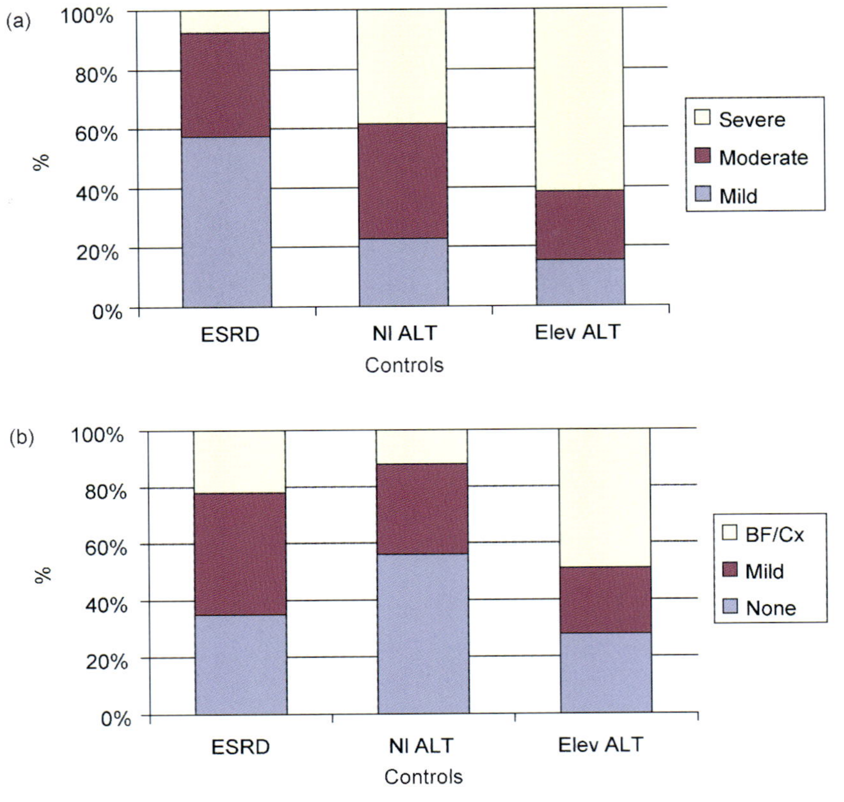

Plate XLIII. (a) Inflammation on liver biopsy in hepatitis C patients with end stage renal disease awaiting renal transplantation [9]. (b) Fibrosis on liver biopsy in hepatitis C patients with end stage renal disease awaiting renal transplantation [9]. ESRD, end stage renal disease; Nl ALT, normal ALT controls; Elev ALT, elevated ALT controls; BF/Cx, bridging fibrosis/cirrhosis; 0, no fibrosis; 1, portal fibrosis. (See Figure 2 on Page 451.)

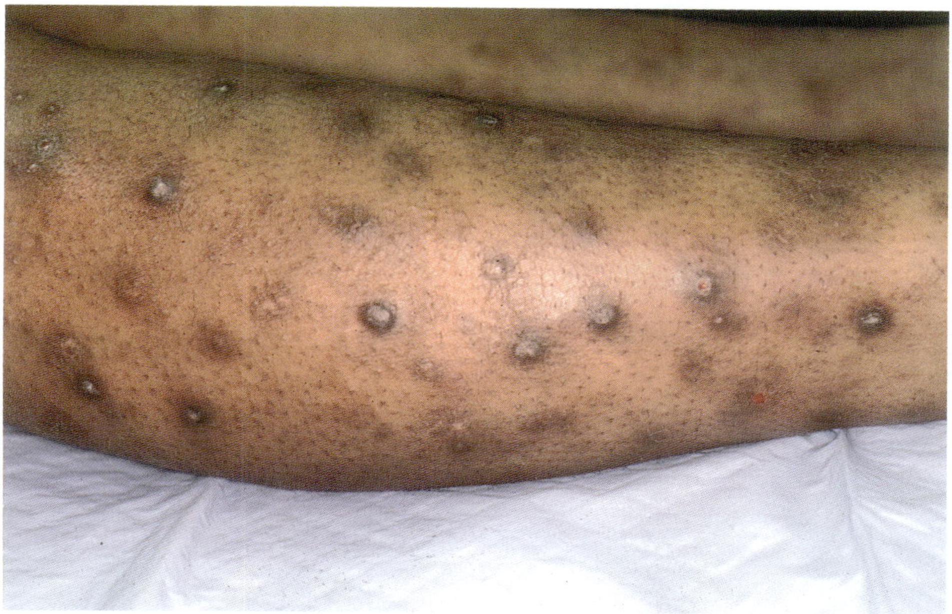

Plate XLIV. This patient presented with generalized pruritus which was subsequently shown to be related to HCV infection. Present here are the classic hyperkeratotic lesions of prurigo nodularis. (See Figure 1 on Page 458.)

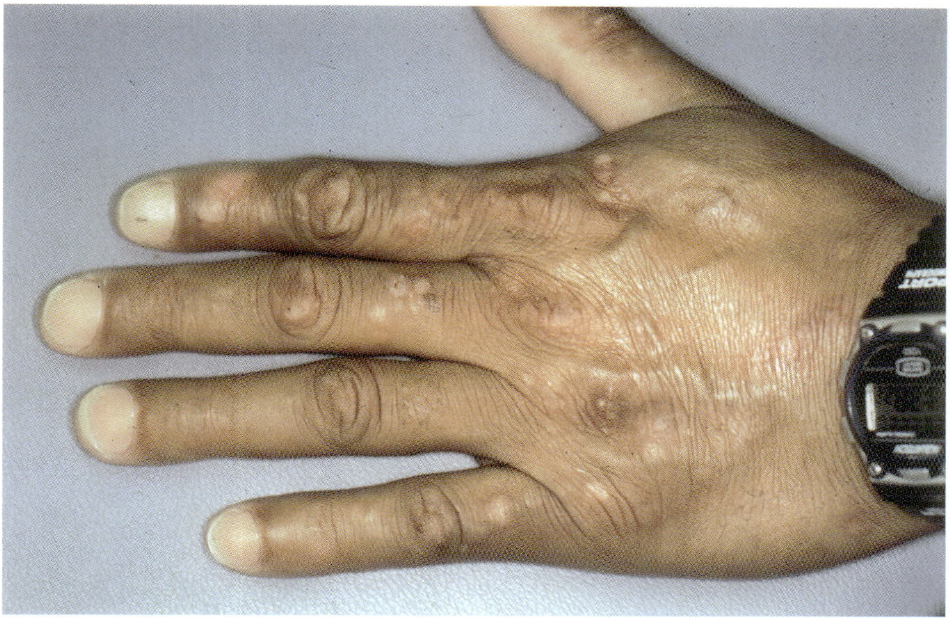

Plate XLV. This hand demonstrates two cutaneous changes associated with liver disease. The nails have the classic white, or Terry's nails. The erosions are evidence of the underlying porphyria cutanea tarda. (See Figure 2 on Page 459.)

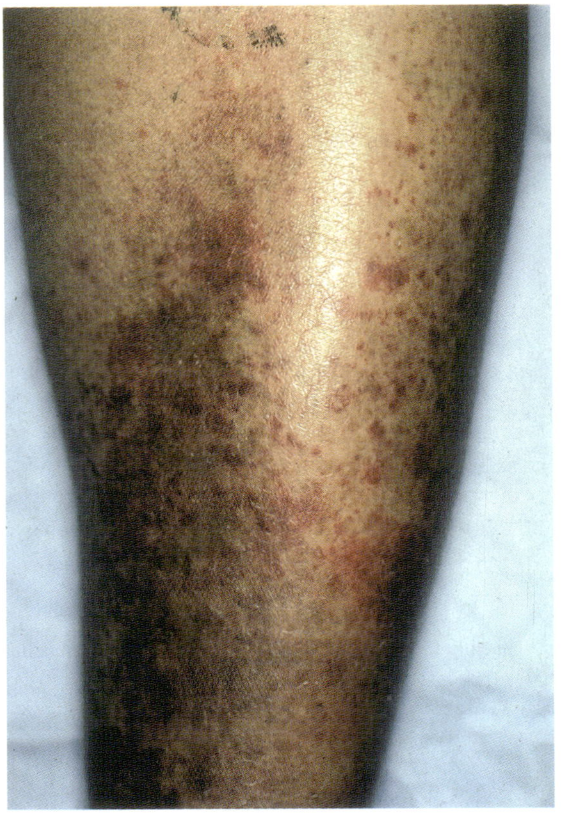

Plate XLVI. The leg of this patient demonstrates the classic palpable purpura of small vessel vasculitis from HCV-induced mixed cryoglobulinemia. (See Figure 3 on Page 462.)

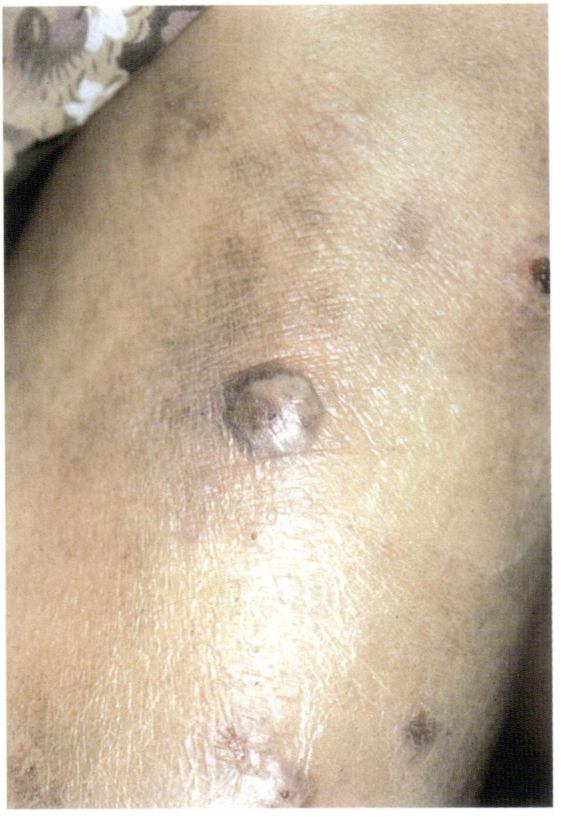

Plate XLVII. This patient presented with episodes of hepatic decompensation associated with skin lesions. Seen here are Sweet's syndrome-like lesions of the vesiculopustular eruption of hepatobiliary disease. (See Figure 4 on Page 463.)

(a)

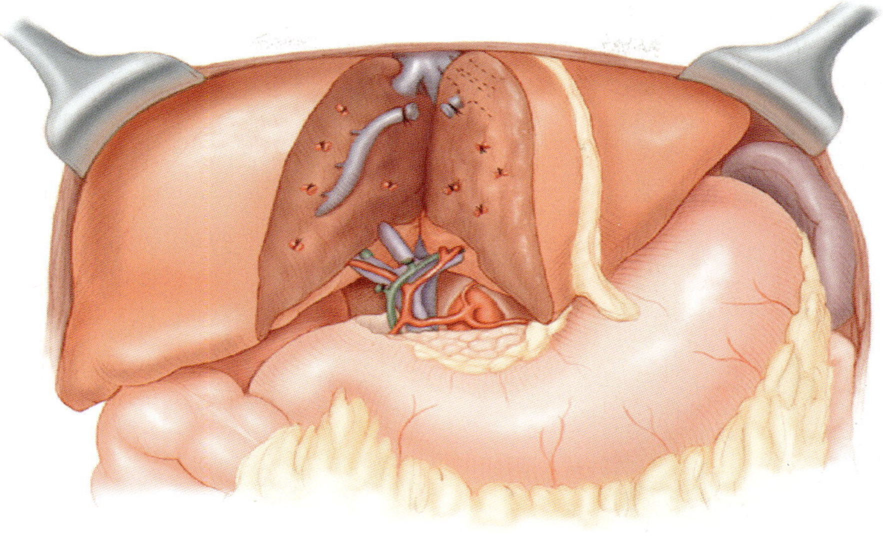

(b)

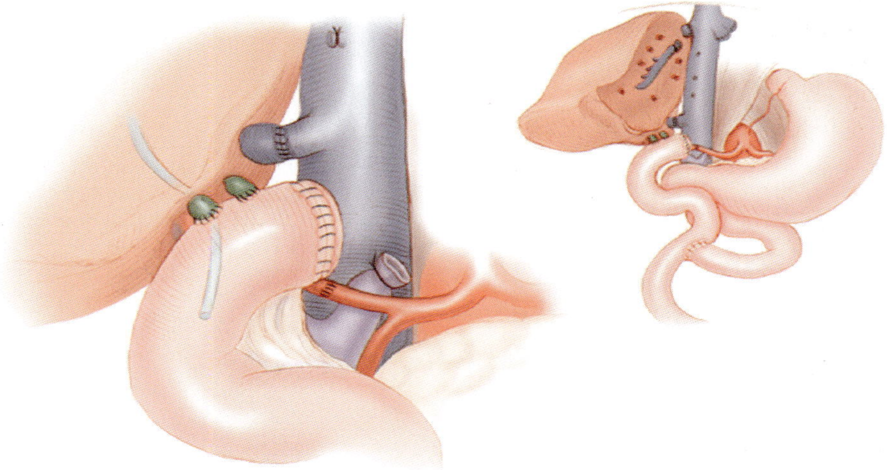

Plate XLVIII. (a) Donor hepatectomy. (b) Implantation of donor right hepatic lobe. (See Figure 3 on Page 535.)

Index

AASLD *see* The American Association for the Study of Liver Disease
AAT *see* alpha 1-antitrypsin
abdomen 6, 8, 37–39, 164
ablative non-surgical therapies 417–418
abscesses 156, 157, 158–161, 167
absorption, PEM 427
acalculous cystitis 166
acetaminophen 306, 308–309, 312–313, 318, 324–325, 502
N-acetylcysteine 312, 324–325
N-acetyl-*p*-benzoquinoneimine (NAPQI) 306, 308–309, 312, 318, 324
acquired immune deficiency syndrome (AIDS) 78, 102, 139–153, 412
acute cellular rejection 536–537
acute cholangitis 166–167
acute fatty liver of pregnancy (AFLP) 292–293
acute liver disease
    alcoholic steatohepatitis 194, 196–198
    common causes 15
    diagnosis 123–127
    HAV infection 57–65
    HBV infection 69, 73, 78
    HCV infection 88–89
    HDV infection 101, 103, 106
    sporadic viral hepatitis 118
    Wilson's disease 225
acute pancreatitis 167
acute renal failure (ARF) 443–445
acute tubular necrosis 444–445
acute variceal hemorrhage 369–373
ADAR *see* double-stranded RNA adenosine deaminase
adefovir dipivoxil 77–78, 143–144
adenoma 332–335, 340
AFLP *see* acute fatty liver of pregnancy
AFP *see* alpha-fetoprotein
AIC *see* autoimmune cholangitis
AIDS *see* acquired immune deficiency syndrome
AIH *see* autoimmune hepatitis
albumin 13
alcohol-induced liver disease 191–198, 300–301, 308–309
    asymptomatic patients 5
    cirrhosis after transplantation 520
    HCV–HIV coinfected patients 150
    hepatocellular carcinoma risk 411–412, 413
    nutritional therapy 435
    toxicity 434–435
algorithms
    abnormal liver test patients 17, 18
    acute hepatitis diagnosis 125
    arthropathy with chronic liver disease diagnosis 473
    chronic hepatitis diagnosis 126
    HBV therapies 80
    hepatocellular carcinoma surveillance/therapies 414, 417
    hepatopulmonary syndrome diagnosis 405
    imaging 29–31
    liver disease in AIDS patients 141, 142
    variceal hemorrhage management 373, 374, 377–378
alkaline phosphatase 12, 18
allograft rejection 536–537, 552
alpha 1-antitrypsin (AAT) deficiency 201–207
alpha-blockers 366, 507
alpha-fetoprotein (AFP) 413–414
Alzheimer type II astrocytosis 381
AMA *see* serum antimitochondrial antibody
amebic liver abscess 159–161
The American Association for the Study of Liver Disease (AASLD) 518
amino acid requirements 434
aminoglycoside antibiotics 508
aminotransferases 12, 15, 18, 123, 124, 126
ammonia 14, 382, 385, 386
amyloidosis 495–496
analgesics 306, 308–310, 312–313, 318, 324–325, 445, 502–505
anatomy 273–274, 362–363, 401, 535
aneurysms 276
anorexia 5
antibiotics 228, 243–244, 386, 508–509

antibodies 63, 119, 237, 481–483
see also immune...
antidepressants 512
anti-HCV antibody test 92–93
antihypertensives 506–508
anti-seizure medications 309
antiviral therapy 412
arachidonic acid 390–391
ARF *see* acute renal failure
arterial hypertension 548–549
arterial vasodilation theory 391
arteriovenous fistula 339
arthropathies 472–473, 474, 475
ascariasis 165–168
ascites 36–37, 347, 349–352
Aspergillus spp. 145, 146
asymptomatic patients 3–10, 341
augmentation therapy 206, 207
autoantibodies 243–244
autoantigens 238
autoimmune cholangitis (AIC) 235, 241, 243, 245
autoimmune hepatitis (AIH) 233–247, 296
autoimmune hepatitis and hepatitis C virus (AIH + HCV) 235, 241, 243, 245
autoimmune hepatitis and primary biliary cirrhosis (AIH + PBC) 235, 241, 243, 245, 254
autoimmune hepatitis and primary sclerosing cholangitis (AIH + PSC) 235, 241, 243, 245
autoimmune hypothyroidism 483–485
autoimmune liver disease 556
azathioprine 244–245, 246, 546

bacterial infection 147, 156–159, 319, 324, 525
band ligation 368–369
bariatric surgery 186
behavior modification 185
Behcet's disease 282
benign tumors 28–29, 331–343
benzimidazoles 164–165
Bernheim, Bertram 33
beta-blockers 366–367, 368
biliary tract problems
colic 166, 167
cystadenoma 342
excretion 223–230
post-transplant complications 539–540
stricture formation 553
bilirubin 13–14, 18
bioartificial liver 326–327
biochemical tests *see* serologic tests
biopsy 195–196, 197, 415
bleeding 13, 319, 361–378, 538–539
blood tests *see* serologic tests
blood transfusions 132, 135–136, 218
blood urea nitrogen (BUN) 443–444
bone disease 255, 550–551
branched chain amino acids 386
brucellosis 158
Budd–Chiari syndrome 278–282, 297, 304

C282Y *see* hereditary hemochromatosis
cadaveric transplantation 533
calcium pyrophosphate crystal-induced inflammatory arthritis (CPPD) 472–473
cancer *see* malignant tumors
Candida infection 145–146, 173
cardiac failure 276–278, 492–493
cardiovascular system 8–9, 276–278, 320, 323, 492–494, 523–524
Caroli's disease 342
cavernous hemangioma 25–26, 337–338
cccDNA *see* covalently closed circular DNA
CD4 T helper cells 236–237
CDC *see* Centers for Disease Control
CECT *see* contrast-enhanced computed tomography
celiac disease 488–489
cellular rejection, acute 536–537
Centers for Disease Control (CDC) 92
central nervous system 316, 319, 321–323
cerebral edema 322–323
chemoembolization 418
children 129, 176–177, 179, 181, 239
Child–Turcotte–Pugh (CTP) classification 527–528
cholangiopathy 147, 166–167, 262–263, 270
see also primary sclerosing cholangitis
cholelithiasis 498

cholestatic diseases 16, 60, 62, 291–292, 301–303
cholestyramine 254–255
chronic cholelithiasis 262
chronic liver disease
 associated renal disease 471
 common causes of hepatitis 15
 diabetes as complication 498–499
 drug-induced liver injury risk 301
 fulminant hepatic failure 317, 318
 HBV infection 69, 70, 73, 74–78, 79, 80
 HCV infection 89–90, 95
 HDV infection 103, 106
 hepatitis diagnosis 124–127
 hereditary hemochromatosis 219
 immune-mediated manifestations 465–489
 laparoscopic diagnosis 34–35
 malnutrition 423–440
 musculoskeletal diseases 471–476
 pregnancy 295–296
 Wilson's disease 225
chronic obstructive pulmonary disease (COPD) 204
chronic renal disease 449–452
circoviruses 125, 127, 134–136
cirrhosis
 see also primary biliary cirrhosis
 alcohol-induced 194, 520
 ascites 347–359
 glucose homeostasis 499
 hepatocellular carcinoma incidence 410
 hepatorenal syndrome 390, 392
 imaging 22–23
 laparoscopic diagnosis 34–35, 36
 nonalcoholic fatty liver disease 178, 180
 nutritional therapy 435
 protein loss and energy 427–428
'clay pipestem' lesions 170
clinical aspects
 alcohol-induced liver disease 194
 alpha 1-antitrypsin deficiency 203–204
 amebic liver abscess 160
 autoimmune hepatitis and overlap syndromes 239–241
 benign hepatic tumors 334
 drug-induced liver disease 301–304
 fulminant hepatic failure 319–320
 HDV infection 103–104
 hereditary hemochromatosis 213–214
 HEV infection 117–119
 nonalcoholic fatty liver disease 177, 180–181
 primary biliary cirrhosis 251–252
 primary sclerosing cholangitis 261–262
 Wilson's disease 224–226
clonorchiasis 171
CMV *see* cytomegalovirus
coagulopathy 13, 319
co-infection 74, 101, 103, 108, 139–153
collagen vascular disease 496–497
color changes in skin 456
colorectal carcinoma 264
complications
 chronic liver disease 498–499
 laparoscopy 42–43
 LDLT-specific 541–542
 post-transplantation 534–541
 primary sclerosing cholangitis 262
computed tomography (CT) 21–31
concomitant disease 443–452
conformational diseases 201–207
congenital simple cysts 339
congestive cardiac failure 492–493
congestive hepatopathy 276–278
constrictive pericarditis 494
contraception 332, 556–557
contrast-enhanced computed tomography (CECT) 159, 160
COPD *see* chronic obstructive pulmonary disease
copper 223–230
corticosteroids 546
counseling for HCV infection 95–96
covalently closed circular DNA (cccDNA) 71–72
COX-2 *see* cyclooxygenase-2
CPPD *see* calcium pyrophosphate crystal-induced inflammatory arthritis
Crohn's disease 487–488
cryoglobulinemia 447–448, 461, 462, 469–471
cryoglobulinemia-associated MPGN 477, 479

cryptogenic cirrhosis 178, 180
CT *see* computed tomography
CTP *see* Child–Turcotte–Pugh classification
cutaneous manifestations of liver disease 455–463, 483
cyclo-oxygenase-2 (COX-2) inhibitors 503
cyclosporine 546
cysts 26–27, 339
 see also hydatid disease
cytochrome P450 enzyme system 192–193, 238, 305, 306–309
cytomegalovirus (CMV) 129–130, 145, 540
cytotoxicity 236–237

demographics
 alcohol-induced liver disease 192
 autoimmune hepatitis and overlap syndromes 236
 fulminant hepatic failure 317
 hepatitis A 58–59
 liver transplants 532–533
 nonalcoholic fatty liver disease 179
 primary biliary cirrhosis 250
 primary sclerosing cholangitis 260
 protein and energy metabolism 425
depression after liver transplant 558
dermatological manifestations 455–463, 483
diabetes mellitus
 drug-induced liver disease 310, 498
 hepatocellular carcinoma risk 412
 liver involvement 497–499
post-liver transplantation 549–550
 type II, NAFLD 185
diagnosis
 see also imaging; liver biopsy; serologic tests
 alcohol-induced liver disease 194–196
 algorithms 17, 18, 29–31, 125, 126, 405, 473
 alpha 1-antitrypsin deficiency 204–205
 asymptomatic patients 3–10
 autoimmune hepatitis 233–234, 237, 241–244
 fulminant hepatic failure 320–321
 HCV infection 90–91, 92–95
 HDV infection 104–107
 hepatic vascular disorders 275, 276, 277–278, 280, 284, 285
 hepatitis types 123–127
 hepatopulmonary syndrome 402–404
 hepatorenal syndrome 393
 hereditary hemochromatosis 214–216
 HEV infection 119
 laparoscopic 33–43
 malnutrition 430–431
 nonalcoholic fatty liver disease 182–183
 primary biliary cirrhosis 252–254
 primary sclerosing cholangitis 264–265
 Wilson's disease 226–228
dialysis 395–396, 449, 450, 451
diet 184, 323–324, 423–440
 see also obesity
dilutional hyponatremia 356
discriminant function formula 194–195
diuretics 353, 505–506
DNA 69, 70, 71–72, 129, 132, 135–136, 142–144
DNA viruses *see* cytomegalovirus; Epstein–Barr virus; hepatitis B virus; Sendai virus; transfusion transmitted virus; varicella-zoster virus
double-stranded RNA adenosine deaminase (ADAR) 102
drug treatments *see* pharmacotherapy
dysplastic nodules *see* macrogenerative nodules

EBV *see* Epstein–Barr virus
echinococcosis 40, 161–165, 339, 341
eclampsia 293, 295
edema, cerebral 322–323
emphysema 204
encephalopathy *see* hepatic encephalopathy
endocrine diseases 525
endocrine glands 483–485
endoscopic treatment 267, 368–369, 371–372
 see also laparoscopic diagnosis
end-stage liver disease 347–359
energy expenditure 428–429
energy requirements 432
Entamoeba histolytica 159–160
enteric transmission 111–112, 114
epidemiology
 HAV infection 58–59
 HBV infection 68
 HCV infection 87–88

- hepatocellular carcinoma 409–411
- HEV 112–116

episodic hepatic encephalopathy 383
Epstein–Barr virus (EBV) infection 127–129
esophageal cancer 37
ethanol *see* alcohol
exercise 184–185
exocrine glands 485–487
extrahepatic manifestations 74, 90–91
extremities examinations 7–8
eyes 7, 226

face examinations 7
family screening
- *see also* genetics
- autoimmune hepatitis 245–246
- HDV 107–108
- hereditary hemochromatosis 218–220
- history-taking 5
- nonalcoholic fatty liver disease 180, 186
- Wilson's disease 230

fascioliasis 171
fatigue 5–6, 251, 254
fatty liver *see* steatosis
ferritin 216, 217
FHF *see* fulminant hepatic failure
fibrosis 302, 304
fingernails 457–458, 459
flaviviruses 125, 131–133
FNH *see* focal nodular hyperplasia
focal nodular hyperplasia (FNH) 26, 27, 335–336, 340
forward theory of ascites formation 349–350
fulminant hepatic failure (FHF) 118, 315–328, 435–436, 521
fungal liver disease 145–147

gallstones 262
gamma-aminobutyric acid–benzodiazepine receptor complex 382
gamma-glutamyltransferase 12
gas exchange abnormalities 400–402
gas insufflation 41
gastro-esophageal varices (GOV) 361–378
gastrointestinal diseases 193, 487–489, 525–526
GB virus (GBV) 131
gender 192
genetics
- *see also* family screening
- alpha 1-antitrypsin deficiency 201–207
- autoimmune hepatitis 238
- hereditary hemochromatosis 212–213, 218–220
- nonalcoholic fatty liver disease 180, 182

genotypes 93–94, 102, 112
geographical distribution 94, 114, 115
glomerular abnormalities 446–448
glomerulonephritis 476–481
glucose homeostasis 499
glycogen deposition 497
GOV *see* gastro-esophageal varices
graft dysfunction 552–556
granulomatous liver disease 147, 302, 303, 494–499

HAART *see* highly active anti-retroviral therapy
HAV *see* hepatitis A virus
HBV *see* hepatitis B virus
HCC *see* hepatocellular carcinoma
HCV *see* hepatitis C virus
HDV *see* hepatitis D virus
HE *see* hepatic encephalopathy
health food supplements 310–311
health maintenance (post-transplant) 557–558
heart *see* cardiac failure; cardiovascular system
HELLP (hemolysis, elevated liver enzymes, low platelet counts) 293
hemangioma 337–338, 340
hematology *see* serologic tests
hemochromatosis 456, 458
hemodialysis 395–396, 449, 450, 451
hemodynamics 348
hemorrhage 13, 319, 361–378, 538–539
hepatic...
- adenoma 332–335
- artery 274–276, 537–538
- cysts 26–27
- hematoma 294
- hydrothorax 357–358

infarction 275, 294
see also ischemic hepatitis
masses 296
stenosis 150
vascular disorders 273–287, 304
vein thrombosis 278–282, 297, 304
Wilson's disease 224–225
hepatic encephalopathy (HE) 316, 319, 321–322, 328, 381–386, 433–434
hepatic iron concentration (HIC) 215
hepatic iron index (HII) 215
hepatic venous pressure gradient (HVPG) 364–365
hepatitis A virus (HAV) infection 57–65
acute liver failure 60–61, 62–63
AIDS patients with liver disease 140
dermatological manifestations 460–461
fulminant hepatic failure 317
prevention 63–65
relapsing 60, 62
typical 59–60, 62
vaccines 63–65
hepatitis B virus (HBV) infection 67–81
see also hepatitis D virus infection
AIDS patients with liver disease 142–144
arthropathy 475, 476
chronic renal disease patients 449–450
dermatological manifestations 461
epidemiology 68
fulminant hepatic failure 317–318
glomerular abnormalities 446–447
glomerulonephritis 480–481
hepatitis delta virus coinfection 78
hepatocellular carcinoma 409, 410, 411, 412
HIV coinfection 78
host and viral determinants 70–71
late allograft dysfunction 555–556
natural history 69–71
pathophysiology 71–72
polyarteritis nodosa 467–469
serologic testing 72–74
transplantation 520
treatments 74–78
hepatitis C virus (HCV) infection 87–98
AIDS patients with liver disease 144–145
arthropathy 475, 476
autoimmune hepatitis overlap syndrome 235, 241, 243, 245
autoimmune hypothyroidism 484
chronic renal disease patients 450–452
counseling 95–96
dermatological manifestations 461–462
diagnosis 90–91, 92–95
glomerular abnormalities 447
HCV genotypes 93–94
hepatocellular carcinoma 409, 410, 411
hereditary hemochromatosis 219
late allograft dysfunction 553–555
liver biopsy 95
mixed cryoglobulinemia 469–471
natural history 88–90
nonalcoholic fatty liver disease 179
risk factors 91–92
Sjogren's syndrome 485
therapy 96–98
transplantation 519–520
hepatitis D virus (HDV) infection 74, 78, 101–108, 124
hepatitis E virus (HEV) infection 111–120, 124, 296, 318
hepatitis G virus (HGV) infection 127, 131–133
hepatobiliary and pancreatic ascariasis (HPA) 165–168
hepatobiliary tuberculosis 172, 174
hepatocellular adenoma 26
hepatocellular carcinoma (HCC) 23–24, 35–36, 67, 71, 187, 409–418
hepatocellular disorders 14–15
hepatocyte transplantation 327
hepatopulmonary syndrome (HPS) 399–407
hepatorenal syndrome (HRS) 389–397
hepatotoxicity 148–150, 299–313
herbs 310–311
hereditary hemochromatosis (HH) 211–220, 522
herpes simplex virus (HSV) 130–131, 145, 296–297
herpetic viruses *see* cytomegalovirus; Epstein–Barr virus; varicella-zoster virus
HEV *see* hepatitis E virus

HFE gene 211, 212
HH *see* hereditary hemochromatosis
HHC-associated arthritis 472–473
HIC *see* hepatic iron concentration
highly active anti-retroviral therapy (HAART) 139, 144
HII *see* hepatic iron index
histology 50–52, 116–117, 340
Histoplasma capsulatum 146
history of laparoscopy 33–34
HIV *see* human immunodeficiency virus
Hodgkin's lymphoma 39
hormonal changes in skin 457
HPA *see* hepatobiliary and pancreatic ascariasis
HPS *see* hepatopulmonary syndrome
HRS *see* hepatorenal syndrome
HSV *see* herpes simplex virus
human immunodeficiency virus (HIV) 78, 102, 139–153, 412
HVPG *see* hepatic venous pressure gradient
hydatid disease 40, 161–165, 339, 341
hypercholesterolemia 510
hyperemesis gravidarum 291
hyperlipidemia 185–186, 550
hypertrigliceridemia 510
hypnotics 505
hypoglycemic agents 511–512
hypolipidemic agents 509–511
hypophosphatemia 542
hypothyroidism 483–485
hypoxemia 400–402
hypoxic hepatitis *see* ischemic hepatitis

IBD *see* irritable bowel disease
idiosyncratic hepatotoxicity 306–307
IG *see* immune globulin
IGV *see* isolated gastric varices
imaging 21–31
    adenoma 340
    alcohol-induced liver disease 195
    autoimmune hepatitis and overlap syndromes 241–242
    focal nodular hyperplasia 335, 340
    fulminant hepatic failure 320
    hemangiomas 338, 340
    hepatic encephalopathy 385
    hepatitis A 62
    hepatocellular carcinoma 414–415
    hepatopulmonary syndrome 399, 400, 403–404, 405
    nonalcoholic fatty liver disease 183
    primary non-function of transplant 534
    primary sclerosing cholangitis 265
    Wilson's disease 228
immune globulin (IG) 63, 119, 481–483
immune-mediated manifestations of liver disease 465–489
immunizations 557–558
immunosuppression 256–257, 541, 546–547
inclusion body hepatocellular disease *see* alpha 1-antitrypsin deficiency
infections 147, 155–174, 319, 324, 525
    see also individual infections
infectious mononucleosis *see* Epstein–Barr virus infection
inflammatory bowel disease (IBD) 487–488
inflammatory pseudotumor 339
INH *see* isoniazid
inhalation augmentation therapy 206
insulin resistance 177, 179
insulin resistance syndrome *see* Syndrome X
interface hepatitis 233, 234, 240
interferon α (IFN-α) 74–75, 107, 143
interferons 96–98, 107
intra-abdominal malignancies 37–39
intravenous augmentation therapy 206, 207
iron 211–220
irritable bowel disease (IBD) 263–264
ischemic hepatitis 274–275, 493–494
isolated gastric varices (IGV) 363, 365
isoniazid (INH) 309

jaundice 17, 456

Kaposi's sarcoma 147–148
Kelling, Georg 33
kiss disease *see* Epstein–Barr virus infection

lab tests
    see also serologic tests
    urine 227
lactate dehydrogenase 12–13

lactulose 508
lamivudine 75–77, 107, 143
laparoscopic diagnosis 33–43
late hepatic allograft dysfunction 552–556
latent HDV infection 104
LDLT *see* live donor liver transplantation
leishmaniasis 146
leptin 180
life cycles of parasites 160, 162, 163, 166, 167, 169–172
light microscopy 49–50
lipid lowering drugs 309
lipodystrophy 151
lipomatous tumors 338–339
listing criteria for transplantation 527–528
live donor liver transplantation (LDLT) 532–534, 541–542
liver biopsy
    alpha 1-antitrypsin deficiency 205, 206
    autoimmune hepatitis and overlap syndromes 242–243
    HCV infection 95
    hepatic vascular disorders 280–281, 284
    hereditary hemochromatosis 215–216
    histopathology 50–52
    indications 47–48
    light microscopy 49–50
    pathologists' perspective 45–52
    primary sclerosing cholangitis 265
    role in evaluation 17
    special procedures 50
    tissue processing 48–49
    Wilson's disease 227–228
liver dialysis (bioartificial liver) 326–327
liver failure *see* fulminant hepatic failure
liver flukes 171–172
liver function tests *see* serologic tests
liver injury 11–13
liver metastases 24–25
liver transplantation *see* transplantation
long-term management, transplant recipients 545–558

macrogenerative nodules (MRN) 27–28, 337
magnetic resonance imaging (MRI) 21–31
malabsorption 427
malaria 173
malignant tumors
    drug-induced 304
    hepatocellular carcinoma 23–24, 35–36, 67, 71, 187, 409–418
    HIV-related liver neoplasms 147–148
    immunosuppression-related 558
    laparoscopic diagnosis 37–39
    ovarian 39
    pregnancy 297
    transplantation for hepatic malignancy 521–522
    types in liver 333
malnutrition 423–440
manganese 382–383
Mayo Risk Score calculation 257
MC *see* mixed cryoglobulinemia
medication *see* pharmacotherapy
melanosis 456
MELD *see* Model for End-Stage Liver Disease
membranous glomerulonephritis (MGN) 476–481
membranous obstruction of the vena cava (MOVC) 282–283
mesangial proliferative glomerulonephritis (MPGN) 476–481
metabolic diseases 150, 427, 522, 550–551
metabolite clearance measures 13–14
metastases 24–25, 333
metformin 185
metronidazole 508–509
MGN *see* membranous glomerulonephritis
mini-laparoscopes 42
mixed cryoglobulinemia (MC) 447–448, 461, 462, 469–471
mixed Wilson's disease 225–226
Model for End-Stage Liver Disease (MELD) scale 406
MOVC *see* membranous obstruction of the vena cava
MPGN *see* mesangial proliferative glomerulonephritis
MRI *see* magnetic resonance imaging
MRN *see* macrogenerative nodules
multiorgan infection 172–174
multiple focal hyperplasia syndrome 336
musculoskeletal diseases 471–476
mycophenolate mofetil 546

NA *see* nuclear antigens
NAFLD *see* nonalcoholic fatty liver disease

NAPQI (*N*-acetyl-*p*-benzoquinoneimine) 306, 308–309, 312, 318, 324
NASH *see* nonalcoholic steatohepatitis
NAT *see* nucleic acid testing
nausea and vomiting 5
neonates 203, 205
neoplasms *see* tumors
nephrotoxicity 445–446
nervous system 9, 225, 316, 319, 321–323, 445–446
neuropsychiatric Wilson's disease 225
newborns *see* neonates
nitrates 367–368
NNRTIs *see* non-nucleoside reverse transcriptase inhibitors
nodular regenerative hyperplasia (NRH) 336–337
nonalcoholic fatty liver disease (NAFLD) 175–187
nonalcoholic steatohepatitis (NASH)
  demographics 179
  family history 180
  hereditary hemochromatosis 219
  hypolipidemic agents 509–510
  pathophysiology 179–180
  prevalence 178
  risk factors for progression 182
  steatosis distinction 177
  transplantation 187
non-Hodgkin lymphoma 147–148
non-nucleoside reverse transcriptase inhibitors (NNRTIs) 148–150
non-selective beta-blockers 366–367
non-steroidal anti-inflammatory drugs (NSAIDs) 310, 445, 502–504
  see also acetaminophen
non-viral liver infections 155–174
NRH *see* nodular regenerative hyperplasia
NSAIDs *see* non-steroidal anti-inflammatory drugs
nuclear antigens (NA) 128
nuclear medicine studies *see* positron emission tomography
nucleic acid testing (NAT) 93
nutrition 184, 323–324, 423–440

obesity 176, 178–179, 185, 426, 439–440, 551–552
OLT (orthotopic liver transplantation) *see* transplantation
open reading frames (ORF) 112, 113
ophthalmic symptoms 226
opioids 504–505
opisthorchiasis 171–172
oral contraceptives 332
oral diabetic agents 310
ORF *see* open reading frame
ornithine–aspartate 386
orthotopic liver transplantation *see* transplantation
osteoporosis 255
outpatient liver biopsy 46
ovarian cancer 39
overfill theory of ascites formation 349
overlap syndromes 233–247, 254
oxidative stress 179–180
oxygen therapy 404

PAN *see* polyarteritis nodosa
pancreatic cancer 37
pancreatitis 167, 264
paracentesis 352, 353
paracetamol *see* acetaminophen
parasites 146–147, 161–172
pathology 195–196, 197, 227–228
pathophysiology
  alcohol-induced liver disease 192–193
  alpha 1-antitrypsin deficiency 202–203
  autoimmune hepatitis and overlap syndromes 236–239
  drug-induced liver disease 304–311
  fulminant hepatic failure 317–319
  HDV infection 102–103
  hepatitis A 59
  hepatitis B virus infection 71–72
  hepatorenal syndrome 400–402
  hereditary hemochromatosis 213
  malnutrition 426–429
  nonalcoholic fatty liver disease 179–180
  portal hypertension 363–364
  pregnancy associated liver disorders 291–292
  primary biliary cirrhosis 250–251
  primary sclerosing cholangitis 260–261
  Wilson's disease 223–224
patient preparation for laparoscopy 40–41
patient selection for transplantation 523–528

PBC *see* primary biliary cirrhosis
PCP *see Pneumocystis carinii*
PCR *see* polymerase chain reaction
PCT *see* porphyria cutanea tarda
peginterferons (PEG-IFN) 96–98, 145
peliosis hepatis 284–285, 342
PEM *see* protein energy malnutrition
penicillamine 228
pentoxifylline 197
perioperative period 531–542
PET *see* positron emission tomography
PG *see* pyoderma gangrenosum
pharmacotherapy
  acute variceal hemorrhage 370–371
  alcohol-induced liver disease 197–198
  hepatorenal syndrome 394–395
  hepatotoxicity in AIDS patients 148–150
  immunosuppression 256–257, 541, 546–547
  interactions 306, 307–308
  nonalcoholic fatty liver disease 185–186
  NSAIDs 310, 445, 502–504
    acetaminophen 306, 308–309, 312–313, 318, 324–325
  renal dysfunction 445–446
  resistance 77
  use/misuse 4, 299–313, 501–512
  variceal hemorrhage 366–369
phlebotomy 216–218
physical examinations 6–9, 430
PI*ZZ phenotype *see* alpha 1-antitrypsin deficiency
Pneumocystis carinii (PCP) 146
PNF *see* primary non-function
polyarteritis nodosa (PAN) 467–469, 475
polycystic kidney disease 448
polymerase chain reaction (PCR) 74, 132
porphyria cutanea tarda (PCT) 219–220, 455, 459–460
portal hypertension 295–296, 361, 363–364
portal vein thrombosis (PVT) 285–287
portal venous circulation 285–287
positron emission tomography (PET) 22, 25
post-operative bleeding 538–539
post-transplant complications 534–541
prednisone 244–245, 246
pre-eclamptic liver disease 293–295
pregnancy 270, 289–297, 556–557
  HEV infection 113, 114, 116, 118, 119
prerenal azotemia 444
prevalence
  alcohol-induced liver disease 191–192
  autoimmune hepatitis and overlap syndromes 236
  fulminant hepatic failure 316–317
  HAV infection 58
  HCV infection 88
  HDV infection 101–102
  hereditary hemochromatosis 212
  HEV infection 112–114
  nonalcoholic fatty liver disease 178–179
  primary sclerosing cholangitis 260
  Wilson's disease 223
prevention
  HAV infection 63–65
  HBV infection 79–80
  HDV infection 107–108
  hepatocellular carcinoma 413–414
  hepatorenal syndrome 396
  HEV infection 119–120
  nonalcoholic fatty liver disease 186
  primary biliary cirrhosis 255–256
  recurrent variceal hemorrhage 373–378
  variceal hemorrhage 365–369
primary biliary cirrhosis (PBC) 249–257
  alcohol-related 520–521
  autoimmune hepatitis overlap syndrome 235, 241, 243, 245
  autoimmune hypothyroidism 484–485
  celiac disease 488–489
  dermatological manifestations 460
  pregnancy 296
  rheumatoid-type arthritis 474
primary hepatic cancers 333
primary hyperoxaluria 522
primary non-function (PNF) 534–536
primary sclerosing cholangitis (PSC) 235, 241, 243, 245, 259–270, 521

prioritization for transplantation 527–528
propranolol 366, 507
protein 427–428, 431–432, 433–434
protein energy malnutrition (PEM) 424, 425, 439
prothrombin time (PTT) 13, 319
pruritus 6, 251, 254–255, 261, 457
PSC *see* primary sclerosing cholangitis
pseudogout 472–473
PTT *see* prothrombin time
pulmonary system 8–9, 204, 399–407, 524
PVT *see* portal vein thrombosis
pyoderma gangrenosum (PG) 463
pyogenic liver abscess 156, 157, 158–159, 167

RAAS *see* renin–angiotensin–aldosterone system
recombinant immunoblot assay (RIBA) 93
recurrent hepatic disease 553–556
recurrent variceal hemorrhage 373–378
regenerative nodules 27–28
rejection 536–537, 552
relapsing hepatitis A 60, 62
renal dysfunction
  ascites-related 348–349
  chronic liver disease 443–452, 471
  drug-induced 445–446
  fulminant hepatic failure 319–320, 324
  hepatorenal syndrome 390–391
  immune-mediated 476–483
  liver disease with ESRD 449–452
  liver transplant recipients 524–525, 547–548
  transplantation patient selection 524–525
  Wilson's disease 226
renal transplantation 451–452
renin-angiotensin-aldosterone system (RAAS) 390
replication of viruses 72
respiratory quotient 429, 433
respiratory system 8–9, 399–407, 524
reverse transcriptase polymerase chain reaction (RT-PCR) 105–106
reverse Trendelenburg 42
rheumatoid-type arthritis 474
RIBA *see* recombinant immunoblot assay
ribavirin 96–98
risk factors 91–92, 181–182, 300–301, 411–413
RNA 57, 93–94, 102, 111, 112
RNA viruses *see* hepatitis A virus; hepatitis C virus; hepatitis D virus; human immunodeficiency virus
RT-PCR *see* reverse transcriptase polymerase chain reaction
rupture of liver 294

salt 356, 434
sarcoidosis 494–495
SBP *see* spontaneous bacterial peritonitis
schistosomiasis 168–171
scleroderma 483
sclerotherapy 375
screening *see* family screening
sedatives 505
selective serotonin reuptake inhibitors (SSRIs) 512
Sendai virus (SENV) infections 132, 135–136
serine protease inhibitors 201–207
serologic tests 11–19
  acute hepatitis 125
  alcohol-induced liver disease 194–195
  ascites 351
  autoimmune hepatitis/overlap syndromes 239–240, 241
  blood urea nitrogen 443–444
  cystic hydatid disease 164
  fulminant hepatic failure 320
  HAV 61–62
  HBV 72–74
  HCV 92–93
  HDV 105, 106
  nonalcoholic fatty liver disease 182
  primary sclerosing cholangitis 264–265
  Wilson's disease 226
seroprevalence 116
serotypes 130–131
serum albumin 352
serum antimitochondrial antibody (AMA) 249–254, 257
shifting dullness sign 351
shock liver *see* ischemic hepatitis
sicca syndrome 485, 486
simple hepatic cysts 339
sirolimus 546–547
Sjogren's syndrome 485–487

skin 6–7, 455–463, 483
sodium levels 352, 356, 434
somatostatin 371
spider angiomas 455
splanchnic hemodynamics 348, 391, 394–395
spontaneous bacterial peritonitis (SBP) 356–357
SSRIs *see* selective serotonin reuptake inhibitors
staging 35, 37–39, 415
starvation 433
statins 309
steatosis
    alcohol-induced liver disease 194, 195, 196
    drug-induced liver disease 302, 303–304
    imaging 28
    NAFLD pathophysiology 179
    nonalcoholic steatohepatitis distinction 177
strongyloidosis 173
subclinical hepatotoxicity 311
substance abuse 558
super-infection 101, 103, 104, 106, 108, 118
surgery
    see also transplantation
    alcohol-induced liver disease 198
    esophageal hemorrhage 377
    hepatic vein thrombosis 281–282
    hepatis D virus infection 107
    hepatocellular carcinoma 416
    nonalcoholic fatty liver disease 186
    nutritional therapy 436
    portal decompression for variceal hemorrhage 368–369
    primary sclerosing cholangitis 267–268
    variceal hemorrhage 373
    Wilson's disease 230
sustained virological response (SVR) 97
Sweet's syndrome 463
Syndrome X 177, 178, 180
synthetic function (hepatic) 13
systemic disease 147, 274–275, 302, 303, 310, 491–499

tacrolimus 546
technetium-99-labeled macroaggregated albumin 403
tetrathiomolybdate 229
thiazolidinediones 185
thrombosis 278–282, 285–287, 297, 304, 537–538
timing of transplantation 528–529
TIPS (transjugular intrahepatic portosystemic shunt) 373, 375–378, 395
tissue processing 48–49
toxicity
    cell-mediated 236–237
    drugs 299–313, 318, 445–446, 498
    HAART 148–150
transferrin saturation 216, 217
transfusions 132, 135–136, 218
transfusion transmitted virus (TTV) 132
transjugular approach 46
transjugular intrahepatic portosystemic shunt (TIPS) 373, 375–378, 395
transmission modes 68, 114, 116, 132–133
transplantation 517–529
    AIDS patients 151
    autoimmune hepatitis 246
    cadaveric 533
    fulminant hepatic failure 321, 326, 327
    hepatitis D virus 107
    hepatocellular carcinoma 416–417
    hepatopulmonary syndrome 405, 406
    hepatorenal syndrome 396
    long-term management of recipients 545–558
    nonalcoholic fatty liver disease 186, 187
    nutritional therapy 436–437
    patient with ascites 353–354
    post-operative bleeding 538–539
    primary biliary cirrhosis 257
    primary sclerosing cholangitis 267–268
    recipient issues 531–542
    renal 451–452
trientine 228–229
trocar needles 38, 46
TTV *see* transfusion transmitted virus
tuberculosis 172, 173, 174
tumors
    see also malignant tumors
    benign 331–343
    cysts 26–27, 339

drug-induced 304
markers 263
type II diabetes (NIDDM) 185
typical hepatitis A 59–60, 62

UC *see* ulcerative colitis
UDCA *see* ursodeoxycholic acid
ulcerative colitis (UC) 263–264, 487–488
ultrasonography 183
United States (US) 176
urine 227
ursodeoxycholic acid (UDCA) 256, 257, 264, 265–266

vaccines 63–65, 120
variceal hemorrhage 361–378
varicella-zoster virus (VZV) 145
vascular disorders 273–287, 304, 318–319, 456–457, 552–553
vasoconstriction 390–391, 394–395
vasopressin 370–371
VCA *see* viral capsid antigens
veno-occlusive disease (VOD) 283–284, 302, 304
Veress needle 40–42, 43
viral capsid antigens (VCA) 128
viral hepatitis-associated arthropathy 475–476
virus particles 112, 113
vitamin requirements 432–433
VOD *see* veno-occlusive disease
VZV *see* varicella-zoster virus

waiting lists for transplants 518
water supplies 111–112, 114
weight loss/gain 6, 184
see also nutrition; obesity
West Haven Criteria for Grading Hepatic Encephalopathy 384
Wilson's disease 223–230, 296, 462, 522

zinc acetate 229–230